Handbook of
Psychopharmacology

Volume 5

Synaptic Modulators

Handbook of

Psychopharmacology

SECTION I: BASIC NEUROPHARMACOLOGY

Volume 1 Biochemical Principles and Techniques in Neuropharmacology
Volume 2 Principles of Receptor Research
Volume 3 Biochemistry of Biogenic Amines
Volume 4 Amino Acid Neurotransmitters
Volume 5 Synaptic Modulators
Volume 6 Biogenic Amine Receptors

in preparation

SECTION II: BEHAVIORAL PHARMACOLOGY IN ANIMALS

SECTION III: HUMAN PSYCHOPHARMACOLOGY

Volume 5

Synaptic Modulators

Edited by

Leslie L. Iversen
Department of Pharmacology
University of Cambridge

Susan D. Iversen
Department of Psychology
University of Cambridge

and

Solomon H. Snyder
Departments of Pharmacology and Psychiatry
The Johns Hopkins University
School of Medicine

PLENUM PRESS • NEW YORK AND LONDON

Library of Congress Cataloging in Publication Data

Main entry under title:

Handbook of psychopharmacology.

Includes bibliographies and indexes.
CONTENTS: v. 1. Biochemical principles and techniques in neuropharmacology. — v. 2. Principles of receptor research. — v. 3. Biochemistry of biogenic amines. — v. 4. Amino acid neurotransmitters. — v. 5. Synaptic modulators. — v. 6. Biogenic amine receptors.
1. Psychopharmacology. I. Iversen, Leslie Lars. II. Iversen, Susan D., 1940- III. Snyder, Solomon H., 1938- [DNLM: 1. Psychopharmacology. QV77 H236]
RC483.H36 615'.78 75-6851
ISBN 0-306-38925-8 (v. 5)

A Division of Plenum Publishing Corporation
227 West 17th Street, New York, N.Y. 10011

United Kingdom edition published by Plenum Press, London
A Division of Plenum Publishing Company, Ltd.
Davis House (4th Floor), 8 Scrubs Lane, Harlesden, London, NW10 6SE, England

Printed in the United States of America

CONTRIBUTORS TO VOLUME 5

G. BURNSTOCK, *Department of Anatomy and Embryology, University College London, London, England*

JOHN DALY, *Laboratory of Chemistry, National Institute of Arthritis, Metabolism and Digestive Diseases, National Institutes of Health, Bethesda, Maryland*

GAVRIL W. PASTERNAK, *Department of Experimental Therapeutics, The Johns Hopkins University School of Medicine, Baltimore, Maryland*

CANDACE B. PERT, *Department of Psychiatry and Behavioral Sciences, The Johns Hopkins University School of Medicine, Baltimore, Maryland*

J. H. QUASTEL, *Division of Neurological Sciences, Department of Psychiatry, University of British Columbia, Vancouver, Canada*

CATHERINE RIVIER, *The Salk Institute, Neuroendocrinology Laboratory, La Jolla, California*

SOLOMON H. SNYDER, *Department of Pharmacology, The Johns Hopkins University School of Medicine, Baltimore, Maryland*

WYLIE VALE, *The Salk Institute, Neuroendocrinology Laboratory, La Jolla, California*

RICHARD E. ZIGMOND, *M.R.C. Neurochemical Pharmacology Unit, Medical School, Cambridge, England*

CONTENTS

CHAPTER 1
Effects of Drugs on Energy Metabolism of the Brain and on Cerebral Transport
J. H. QUASTEL

1. Introduction 1
2. Drugs and Brain Cell Energetics 2
3. Neurotropic Drugs Affecting Electron and Energy Transfer 4
   3.1. Barbiturates 4
   3.2. Uncouplers of Brain Respiration 10
   3.3. Fluoroacetate 11
   3.4. Methionine Sulfoximine 12
   3.5. Chlorinated Hydrocarbon Insecticides 14
   3.6. 2-Deoxyglucose 14
   3.7. γ-Hydroxybutyrate 15
   3.8. Aminooxyacetate 15
   3.9. Haloperidol 16
4. Drugs and Brain Cell Permeabilities 17
   4.1. Tetrodotoxin 17
   4.2. Local Anesthetics: Cocaine, Procaine, Lidocaine, etc. 19
   4.3. Ouabain 21
   4.4. Protoveratrine 23
5. Drugs Affecting Cerebral Biogenic Amine Levels 24
   5.1. Reserpine 25
   5.2. Phenothiazines 26
   5.3. Imipramine 28
   5.4. Amphetamines 28
   5.5. Monoamine Oxidase Inhibitors 30

5.6. Lysergic Acid Diethylamide (LSD) 31
5.7. Amino Acid Decarboxylase Inhibitors 31
6. Ethanol 32
7. References 33

Chapter 2

Role of Cyclic Nucleotides in the Nervous System

John Daly

1. Introduction 47
2. Enzymatic Formation, Degradation, and Action of Cyclic Nucleotides 48
2.1. Adenylate Cyclases 48
2.2. Guanylate Cyclases 52
2.3. Phosphodiesterases 52
2.4. Protein Kinases 55
2.5. Phosphoprotein Phosphates 56
3. Accumulation of Cyclic Nucleotides 57
3.1. Cyclic AMP in Brain Slices 57
3.2. Cyclic GMP in Brain Slices 87
3.3. Cyclic AMP in Ganglia 88
3.4. Cyclic AMP in Cells of Neuronal or Glial Origin 91
4. Functional Roles of Cyclic Nucleotides 94
4.1. Effects on Enzymatic Processes 95
4.2. Cell Morphology, Differentiation, and Growth 97
4.3. Membrane Phenomena 98
4.4. Centrally Active Drugs and Levels of Cyclic Nucleotides in Brain 103
4.5. Behavioral Effects 106
5. Conclusion 107
6. References 107

Chapter 3

Purinergic Transmission

G. Burnstock

1. Introduction 131
2. Distribution of Purinergic Nerves 133
2.1. Gastrointestinal Tract 134
2.2. Lung and Trachea 136

2.3. Vascular System 137
2.4. Urinogenital System 140
2.5. Eye 141
2.6. CNS 141
3. Fine Structure and Histochemistry of Purinergic Nerves .. 143
3.1. Fine Structure of Purinergic Nerves 143
3.2. Histochemical Approaches to Localization of Purinergic Nerves 146
4. Electrophysiology of Purinergic Transmission 147
4.1. Inhibitory Junction Potentials 147
4.2. Postsynaptic Action of Transmitter 151
4.3. Interaction of Purinergic with Cholinergic and Adrenergic Responses in Single Cells 151
5. Physiological Roles of Purinergic Nerves 152
5.1. Reflex Relaxation of the Esophagogastric Junction ... 153
5.2. "Receptive Relaxation" of the Stomach 154
5.3. "Descending Inhibition" of Peristalsis 154
5.4. Reflex Relaxation of the Internal Anal Sphincter 154
5.5. Vomiting and Nausea 156
5.6. Bronchodilatation, Asphyxia, Asthma 157
5.7. Coughing 157
5.8. Inflammation of the Skin 157
5.9. Activities in the CNS 158
6. Evidence that ATP is the Purinergic Nerve Transmitter ... 158
6.1. Formation and Storage of ATP 159
6.2. Release of ATP 159
6.3. Direct Actions of Purine Nucleotides and Nucleosides on Smooth Muscle 162
6.4. Inactivation of ATP 162
6.5. Antagonism and Potentiation of Responses to Nerve Stimulation and ATP 163
7. Pharmacology of Adenyl Compounds and Purinergic Transmission 164
7.1. Inhibitory and Excitatory Action of Adenyl Compounds 165
7.2. Drugs That Antagonize the Action of Adenyl Compounds 168
7.3. Drugs That Potentiate the Action of Adenyl Compounds 170
8. Speculations on the Evolution and Development of Purinergic Nerves 171
9. Summary 175
10. References 177

Chapter 4

Hypothalamic Hypophysiotropic Hormones

Wylie Vale and Catherine Rivier

1. Introduction 195
2. Hypophysiotropic Hormone Action 196
   2.1. Characteristics 196
   2.2. Mechanisms of Hypophysiotropic Action of Peripheral Hormones 200
3. Thyrotropin Releasing Factor (TRF) 201
   3.1. Effect of TRF on Secretion of Other Pituitary Hormones 202
   3.2. Psychotropic Actions of TRF 203
   3.3. TRF Binding Studies 204
   3.4. TRF Structure–Function Relationship Studies 205
4. Luteinizing Hormone Releasing Factor (LRF) 209
   4.1. LRF Structure–Function Studies 210
   4.2. LRF Binding Studies 213
   4.3. Behavioral Effects of LRF 214
5. Corticotropin Releasing Factor (CRF) 214
6. Prolactin Release Inhibiting Factor (PIF) 215
7. Growth Hormone Releasing Factor (GRF) 218
8. Somatostatin-Somatotropin Release Inhibiting Factor (SRIF) 218
9. References 228

Chapter 5

Binding, Metabolism, and Action of Steroid Hormones in the Central Nervous System

Richard E. Zigmond

1. Introduction 239
2. Estrogens 241
   2.1. Determination of the Estradiol Concentration in Dissected Brain Regions 241
   2.2. Determination of the Cellular Localization of [^{3}H]Estradiol by Autoradiography 245
   2.3. Subcellular Distribution of Estradiol 252
   2.4. Developmental Changes in the Estradiol Binding System 262
   2.5. Changes in Estradiol Binding During the Estrus Cycle 266

2.6. Behavioral and Physiological Effects of Estrogen Agonists and Antagonists 267
2.7. Sites of Estrogen Action 271
2.8. Temporal Aspects of Estrogen Action 272
3. Androgens 273
3.1. Regional and Cellular Distribution of Radioactivity After an Injection of [^{3}H]Testosterone in the Castrated Male Rat 273
3.2. Testosterone Metabolism in Peripheral Tissues: The Idea of Testosterone as a "Prehormone" 274
3.3. Metabolism of Testosterone in the Brain 278
3.4. Saturability and Stereoselectivity of Androgen Retention 280
3.5. Androgen-Binding Macromolecules 280
3.6. Androgen Retention in Birds 281
3.7. Comparison of Sites of Androgen Binding and Androgen Action in the Adult 284
3.8. Androgen Binding and Action During Development 286
3.9. Chemical Specificity of Androgen Action: Is There More Than One Type of Androgen Receptor in the Brain? 288
3.10. Role of Aromatization in Androgen Action 289
4. Glucocorticoids 292
4.1. Anatomical Distribution of Corticosterone Binding Sites in the Rat 292
4.2. Saturability and Stereoselectivity of Corticosterone Retention 294
4.3. Subcellular Distribution of Corticosterone 296
4.4. Corticosterone-Binding Macromolecules in the Nucleus and Cytoplasm *in Vivo* 297
4.5. Corticosterone Binding *in Vitro* 300
4.6. Experiments on Other Glucocorticoids and Other Species 301
4.7. Metabolism of Glucocorticoids in the Brain 303
4.8. Measurements of Endogenous Glucocorticoids in the Nervous System 303
4.9. Correlations Between Corticosterone Binding and Corticosterone Action 304
5. Progestins 305
5.1. Regional Differences in the Retention of Progesterone 305
5.2. Progesterone Metabolism *in Vivo* and *in Vitro* 306
5.3. Saturability of Progesterone Retention 307

5.4. Subcellular and Cellular Localization of Progesterone 307
5.5. Role of Progesterone in Female Mating Behavior 308
5.6. Anatomical and Chemical Specificity of Progesterone Action in the Brain.................................. 309
6. Conclusion.. 311
7. References.. 312

CHAPTER 6
Opiate Receptor Mechanisms
SOLOMON H. SNYDER, GAVRIL W. PASTERNAK, and CANDACE B. PERT

1. Introduction 329
2. Biochemical Identification of Opiate–Receptor Binding... 334
3. Localization of the Opiate Receptor to Synaptic Membranes 338
4. Regional Distribution of Opiate–Receptor Binding 340
5. Effect of Destruction of Norepinephrine, Serotonin, Acetylcholine, and Dopamine Tracts on Opiate–Receptor Binding............................ 345
6. Phylogenetic Distribution of the Opiate Receptor......... 348
7. Effect of Sodium on Opiate–Receptor Binding 352
8. Toward a Theory of Addiction......................... 355
9. References.. 357

Addendum to Chapter 2................................ 361

Index 375

1

EFFECT OF DRUGS ON ENERGY METABOLISM OF THE BRAIN AND ON CEREBRAL TRANSPORT

J. H. Quastel

1. INTRODUCTION

Aspects of this subject, whose scope is now so extensive that it cannot be treated adequately within the limits of this chapter, have been reviewed extensively in recent years, e.g., Shore (1971), Mullins (1971), Dettbarn (1971), Gabay (1971), Schildkraut and Gershon (1971), Clouet (1971), Sulser and Sanders-Bush (1971), Matthyse (1973), Quastel (1967, 1970), Løvtrup (1967), Glick (1972), McGeer and McGeer (1973). Accordingly, this chapter will deal with some of the main *in vivo* and *in vitro* effects on brain cell energetics and transport processes of a number of drugs that have awakened interest either because of their therapeutic value, or because of their public interest as drugs of abuse, or because of their value as tools for research.

J. H. Quastel • Division of Neurological Sciences, Department of Psychiatry, University of British Columbia, Vancouver, Canada

2. DRUGS AND BRAIN CELL ENERGETICS

Drugs that affect brain cell energetics may be divided into several categories: (1) Those that directly block electron transfer processes or respiratory systems, leading to a fall in ATP concentration or altered NADH–NAD ratios. Such drugs may act by suppressing the rate of oxidation of NADH and include a variety of anesthetics (e.g., barbiturates), aldehydes, and steroids, or they may be potent cell poisons such as cyanide and azide that block the activity of the cytochrome system. (2) Those that inhibit the activity of the citric acid cycle, which is the major respiratory pathway in the brain, by effects on the constituent enzymes in that pathway, e.g., malonate, fluoroacetate. (3) Those that uncouple phosphorylation from oxidation so that the cell ATP concentration may fall even if the rate of oxygen consumption does not fall. Among such uncoupling drugs are the thiobarbiturates, ethyl ether, and chlorpromazine. (4) Those that compete with glucose for hexokinase, e.g., 2-deoxyglucose. Their immediate effect is to reduce the effective concentration of glucose in the brain cell or to divert ATP from its normal operations. (5) Those that react with the α-keto acids (α-ketoglutarate, oxaloacetate, or pyruvate) produced during the process of glucose breakdown and whose normal metabolism is essential for operation of the citric acid cycle. Among such drugs are aminooxyacetate and hydrazides. These drugs, however, may react primarily with an aldehyde cofactor, such as pyridoxal, that is essential for various aspects of amino acid metabolism in the brain.

When considering the effects of these and other drugs on cerebral metabolic and transport processes, it is essential to bear in mind that it is rare to find a drug that is quite specific in its behavior. Most drugs have multiple effects, optimal activities being manifest at different concentrations. In attempting, therefore, to correlate *in vivo* with *in vitro* findings, it is important to have some knowledge of the effective concentration of the drug at the site in the nervous system at which it operates optimally. Moreover, it has to be borne in mind that both the quantitative and qualitative aspects of the activity of a drug may vary according to the site of the nervous system affected. For example, cyanide or carbon monoxide poisoning, which greatly affects cell respiratory systems, has selective effects resulting in more consistent degeneration of neurons in the globus pallidus than in various other parts of the nervous system. Nitrous oxide poisoning brings about greater changes in the brain cortex and basal ganglia than in the brain stem and cerebellum in human beings (Himwich, 1951). The lenticular nucleus is especially vulnerable to agents that produce the effects of anoxia. The high rate of respiratory metabolism of the striatum (caudate nucleus) makes this tissue very susceptible to anoxic deprivation of energy (Himwich, 1951). Moreover, the brain cells of different animal species do not all have the same sensitivities to drugs; for example, respiration of human brain cortex is more sensitive to phenobarbitone (luminal) than that of rat brain cortex (Elliott and Sutherland, 1952).

The consequences of interference with brain cell energetics, leading to falls in ATP concentration, are such as to affect the kinetics of many ATP-dependent brain cell processes. These include phospholipid and phosphoprotein formation, important for the establishment of cell membranes; glutamine and acetylcholine formation; phosphorylations involved in the course of glycolytic breakdown, in the operation of the sodium pump, in the establishment of ionic gradients, or in the transport into the brain cell, against a concentration gradient, of exogenous amino acids, amines, creatine, choline, thiamine, ascorbic acid, etc. However, these various processes are not all affected to the same degree by changes in ATP concentration. Much depends on the location in the cell of the change in cell energetics and on what type of cell (e.g., glia or neuron) is primarily involved. For example, it has been concluded (Clarke *et al.*, 1970) that the effect of the convulsant fluoroacetate, a citric acid cycle inhibitor, is located for the most part, at low concentrations, in a compartment of the brain in which glutamine biosynthesis plays a major role. Yet fluoroacetate at such concentrations brings about *in vitro* little or no fall in the total brain concentration of ATP. It would seem that localized changes in ATP level may be masked by the undisturbed ATP levels present in the unaffected cells.

Another consideration that may be of importance in correlating *in vitro* with *in vivo* effects of drugs is the fact that isolated brain (in the form of slices) needs stimulation, either by application of electrical impulses or by changed cation concentrations in the bathing medium (e.g., increased K^+ or decreased Ca^{2+}) (McIlwain, 1953; Ghosh and Quastel, 1954), to produce a rate of respiration approximating that found *in vivo*. This stimulation does not occur in brain homogenates or minces. The enhanced respiration is due to an increased rate of turnover of the citric acid cycle in brain cell mitochondria, for it is highly sensitive to malonate (Takagaki *et al.*, 1958; Quastel, 1962). This is brought about by an increased concentration of ADP formed as a result of cation movements at the cell membrane. This controls the rate of oxidation of NADH and therefore the cell concentration of NAD. This, in turn, partly controls the speed of the citric acid cycle. The stimulation of brain cell membrane ATPase which is both Na^+ and K^+ dependent by increased intracellular Na^+ (brought about, for example, by electrical stimulation, the absence of Ca^{2+} from the bathing medium, or a drug such as protoveratrine) or by increased extracellular K^+ is probably the major reason for the increased brain cell concentration of ADP that is responsible for the stimulation of brain respiration *in vitro*. The stimulated brain tissue respiration has sensitivities to a variety of neurotropic drugs that approach those seen in the living animal—presumably because it is largely ADP controlled.

The ADP-stimulated respiration of mitochondria is highly sensitive to the inhibitory action of barbiturates (e.g., liver mitochondria, Aldridge and Parker, 1960; Aldridge, 1962; Chance and Hollunger, 1963).

Another consideration to be borne in mind in assessing the effects of neurotropic drugs *in vitro* is that brain tissue stimulation may cause marked falls in the concentrations of organic phosphates such as phosphocreatine (McIlwain and Gore, 1951; Heald, 1954). A fall in the concentration of this substance reduces its "buffering" ability so that a fall in brain cell ATP may occur more readily in the stimulated brain preparation than in the unstimulated. Thus a drug might have a greater suppressing effect on ATP-dependent reactions of the stimulated cell than on those of the unstimulated cell.

3. NEUROTROPIC DRUGS AFFECTING ELECTRON AND ENERGY TRANSFER

3.1. Barbiturates

3.1.1. Effects in Vivo

Glucose enters the brain apparently by a saturable carrier-mediated mechanism (Crone, 1965) with a K_m of 7.2 mM and a maximum influx rate, in the rat, of 1.13 μmol/min/g (Bachelard *et al.*, 1973). The mean net cerebral uptake of glucose in the rat calculated from arteriovenous differences at normal concentrations of glucose in the blood plasma is 0.28 μmol/min/g, which is near to the normal utilization rate of glucose in the brain of 0.3–0.35 μmol/min/g (McIlwain and Bachelard, 1971).

Barbiturate anesthesia brings about diminished utilization of glucose in the brain, both in human subjects (Himwich *et al.*, 1947; Wechsler *et al.*, 1951) and in laboratory animals (Lowry and Passoneau, 1962; Lowry *et al.*, 1964). The animal experiments indicated that there is an increase in cerebral concentration of high-energy phosphate compounds. Goldberg *et al.* (1966) suggested that, in barbiturate anesthesia, the cause of the diminished rate of glucose breakdown is inhibition at a stage prior to the formation of pyruvate. Strang and Bachelard (1973) found that intraperitoneal injection of phenobarbitone (250 mg/kg) into rats causes increased brain concentrations of glucose (100%), glucose-6-phosphate (10%), and ATP (12%) and decreased concentrations of lactate (33%) and ADP (15%). Moreover, shortly after systemic injection of radioactive glucose the rates of increase in the brain of the specific activities of glucose, lactate, glutamate, and glycogen are all halved by phenobarbitone. These results do not provide evidence for a direct effect on glucose transport into the brain (Mayman *et al.*, 1964); its accumulation may arise partly from a decrease in its rate of consumption. Even if there were an effect on glucose transport, this could not account for all the changes observed. It has been suggested (Lowry and Passoneau, 1964; Gatfield *et al.*, 1966) that there may be an effect of barbiturates *in vivo* at the stage of phosphofructokinase, an enzyme known to be inhibited by ATP with deinhibition by ADP.

The rate of oxygen consumption of the human brain diminishes by 30% in light anesthesia and by 45% in deep thiopental (pentothal) anesthesia (Wechsler *et al.*, 1951) and the specific radioactivities of brain glutamate and α-ketoglutarate fall by 45% after administration of pentobarbitone and labeled glucose (Bachelard and Lindsay, 1966).

Phenobarbitone administration to mice (300 mg/kg, intraperitoneally), reduces the uptake of radioactivity from radioactive choline into the brain by half (Diamond, 1971), and a similar reduction in acetylcholine (ACh) synthesis takes place, in mouse brain, after pentobarbital (Schuberth *et al.*, 1969). These results may be due to suppression of choline transport into the brain by effects at the brain cell membrane (Bunker and Vandam, 1965) or by depression of cerebral metabolism. Bachelard *et al.* (1966) have shown that pentobarbitone anesthesia results in the inhibition of incorporation of glucose-carbon into amino acids in the brain.

While these and similar results of the effects of barbiturate anesthesia on brain metabolism indicate a combination of effects due to (1) general depression of brain respiratory metabolism and (2) specific effects on membrane transport processes, further information on the mode of action of barbiturates *in vivo* is gained from consideration of their effects on neuronal excitation.

3.1.2. *Barbiturates and Neuronal Excitation*

Important properties of neuronal membranes are their low permeability to various ions, giving rise to high electrical resistance, and their ability to undergo specific permeability changes. Excitation of the neuron, leading to the generation of action potentials, is brought about by a series of transient changes in membrane permeability triggered by depolarization. Sequential changes in permeability to Na^+ and K^+ are of crucial importance in the development of the excitatory state. A widely held belief is that anesthetics act primarily at or near synaptic junctions (Larrabee and Posternak, 1952), some apparently acting postsynaptically. Barbiturates, at low doses, act presynaptically (Richens, 1969). Many anesthetic agents modify neurotransmission in the CNS by altering the sensitivity of neurons to various transmitter substances (e.g., Crawford, 1970; Johnson *et al.*, 1969; Bloom *et al.*, 1965) and depression by anesthetics of Ach-induced excitation occurs with neurons in the cortex (Krnjević and Phillis, 1963) and caudate nucleus (Bloom *et al.*, 1965). Neurons in the brain stem are sensitive to systemic injections of barbiturates (Rosina and Sotgiu, 1967) and to microiontophoretically applied pentobarbitone (Bradley and Wolstencroft, 1965). A characteristic effect of pentobarbitone is a depression of the spontaneous neuronal firing rate. This may be due to depression of the release of ACh (Paton and Speden, 1965; Weakly, 1969). Bradley and Dray (1973) have found that administration of pentobarbitone to rats (50 mg/kg) specifically antagonizes the excitation of neurons by exogenously applied ACh and suggest that postsynaptic antagonism of endogenously released ACh may be a contributing factor in the mode of action of pentobarbitone.

Pentobarbitone (0.3 mM) causes almost complete block of the spontaneous generation of action potentials in isolated guinea pig cerebellum (Okamoto and Quastel, 1973).

Since 2:4-dinitrophenol, as well as a moderate degree of anoxia, also selectively and reversibly blocks spontaneous firing and discharges evoked by Ach (Godfraind *et al.*, 1971), it has been suggested that general anesthetics may depress neuronal excitability by an action similar to that of 2:4-dinitrophenol or anoxia, i.e., by suppression of mitochondrial metabolism (Krnjević, 1972). Brief administration of anesthetics, including pentobarbitone, causes a temporary selective depression of the spontaneous firing and Ach-evoked response of deep pericruciate neurons of cats but relatively little change of glutamate-evoked firing, effects similar to those produced by local application of 2:4-dinitrophenol (Catchlove *et al.*, 1972). The barbiturates may act in this manner by release of Ca^{2+} from its binding sites, on suppression of mitochondrial metabolism, leading to a changed membrane permeability to K^+. According to Krnjević (1972), the anesthetic-induced increase of K^+ permeability may be effective in suppressing the cholinergic activity required for the maintenance of processes needed for the conscious state.

Such facts as these lead to the conclusion that barbiturates may reduce neuronal excitability either by suppression of mitochondrial metabolism leading to changed neuronal permeability to K^+ or by a direct action on the neuronal membrane that may be independent of metabolism or by a combination of both processes. These activities may vary according to the concentration of the anesthetic and its location in the CNS.

The depression of neuronal excitation by barbiturates leads presumably not only to the suppression of the normal functional activity of the affected cells but also to a depression of the activities of those parts of the nervous system normally controlled by the excitatory activities of the affected cells. In this way, it is possible to visualize the suppression of brain respiration *in vivo*, in barbiturate anesthesia, as due to the depression of excitatory activities of key neurons by the anesthetic rather than due to an anesthetic-induced depression of respiration throughout the nervous system. As stimulation *in vitro* of brain respiration is known to be due largely to an increased rate of glucose oxidation via the citric acid cycle, it seems reasonable to infer that the normal rate of respiration in the brain of the conscious animal is due to brain cells undergoing the constant stimulation inherent in the conscious state. This view is supported by the fact that the rate of respiration of brain *in vivo* is approximately equal to that of stimulated brain *in vitro* and that the rate of respiration of the brain of a comatose animal, or of one under deep anesthesia, is approximately that of unstimulated brain *in vitro* (for references, see Quastel, 1962, 1965). If the depressed respiration of the brain of the anesthetized animal is indeed due to the suppression of neuronal excitability, it would be expected that there will result diminished oxidative glucose utilization and diminished turnover of ATP with possibly increased levels of ATP in parts of the nervous system. Such *in vivo* effects would be a consequence of depressed cerebral activity. They would not necessarily be the same as those taking place *in vitro*, as, for example, when slices of brain cortex or other brain preparations are exposed to the anesthetics.

3.1.3. Barbiturates and Cerebral Energy Metabolism in Vitro

It was shown over 40 years ago (Quastel and Wheatley, 1932) that barbiturates and other anesthetics depress oxidative metabolism of isolated brain tissue and that there is a parallelism between the potencies of anesthetics of the same chemical type and their abilities to suppress brain respiration *in vitro*. This conclusion has been confirmed by many subsequent workers. Studies of cation-stimulated or electrically stimulated brain cortex slices or of brain mitochondria preparations have shown that anesthetics, at low pharmacologically active concentrations, bring about marked inhibitions of a number of respiratory processes (McIlwain, 1953; Ghosh and Quastel, 1954).

The barbiturate Amytal (amylobarbitone), in common with a variety of other barbiturates and anesthetics, suppresses the rate of oxidation of NADH by the cytochrome system (Ernster *et al.*, 1955; Jalling *et al.*, 1955; Estabrook and Mackler, 1957; Michaelis and Hashimoto, 1962; Chance and Hollunger, 1963). This result is in accordance with the results and conclusions of Michaelis and Quastel (1941) that the effect of certain anesthetics on brain respiration is inhibition of a process playing an intermediate role between cytochrome oxidase and a flavoprotein concerned with the oxidation of NADH. The stimulated respiration of isolated brain, which may be regarded as mainly an ADP-controlled respiration, is highly sensitive to barbiturates and other general anesthetics. Apparently the un-ionized form of the barbiturate is required for its inhibitory effect (Silberman *et al.*, 1972). The concentrations of barbiturates that inhibit mitochondrial respiration are approximately those that bring about anesthesia (Aldridge, 1962; Chance and Hollunger, 1963).

Only oxidation of substances that enable stimulation to take place, e.g., glucose or pyruvate, is affected appreciably by these neurotropic drugs at pharmacologically active concentrations. The drugs act in this way because they are able to suppress ADP-controlled NADH oxidation, and this well-known fact has made Amytal, for example, a very useful tool for the study of certain aspects of cell respiration in which NADH is involved. As it is now well known that the biological oxidation of NADH in the cell is accompanied, and indeed controlled, by the phosphorylation of ADP to ATP, it follows that the anesthetic is also inhibitory to oxidative phosphorylation. With liver mitochondria, the oxygen uptake may be depressed by barbiturates by more than 50% with an equivalent depression of the amount of phosphate esterified (Eiler and McEwen, 1949; Aldridge and Parker, 1960; Aldridge, 1962). However, thiobarbiturates such as pentothal act also as uncoupling agents, depressing the P:O ratio. This may be correlated with their activation of ATPase, in contrast to that of the oxybarbiturates which have little effect on this enzyme (Maxwell and Nickel, 1954; Andrejew and Rosenberg, 1956; Aldridge and Parker, 1960; Chance and Hollunger, 1963). Amytal suppresses the activity of ouabain-sensitive ATPase only at high concentrations, 50% inhibition occurring at 4 mM (Schwartz and Laseter, 1964).

The interference by barbiturates, and other general anesthetics, with ATP synthesis in the brain is shown by their suppression of ACh synthesis (Mann *et al.*, 1938; McLennan and Elliott, 1951; Johnson and Quastel, 1953) and by their inhibitory effects (e.g., by 1 mM pentobarbitone) on ^{32}P incorporation (from phosphate) into phosphoproteins or organic phosphorus compounds in cat brain slices respiring in presence of glucose (Findlay *et al.*, 1954) or by their suppression of ATP-dependent glutamine biosynthesis in incubated rat brain cortex slices (e.g., by 0.5 mM Amytal) (Kini and Quastel, 1959). Whether such effects as these may take place in the brain during barbiturate anesthesia is not known with certainty, as the concentrations of the anesthetic in localized parts of the brain are not known with certainty. However, Amytal (0.25 mM) at a concentration approximately that present in the blood of rats under Amytal anesthesia (Reading and Wallwork, 1969) brings about complete suppression of electrically or K^+-stimulated respiration of incubated rat brain cortex slices (Chan and Quastel, 1970). Pentothal (0.2 mM) suppresses electrically stimulated respiration and even at 0.1 mM shows a significant inhibition (Chan and Quastel, 1970); at somewhat higher concentrations it suppresses K^+-stimulated brain respiration. The barbiturates at the low concentrations that are effective *in vitro* (McIlwain, 1953; Ghosh and Quastel, 1954) have no significant inhibitory effects on the membrane-bound, ouabain-sensitive ATPase that is involved in the active transport of Na^+ and K^+ across the brain cell membranes (Chan and Quastel, 1970). This fact makes it unlikely that the barbiturate exerts its effect *in vitro* primarily by affecting permeability to Na^+ or K^+.

This is made clear by recent investigations on the effects of barbiturates and other neurotropic drugs on Na^+ influx into incubated rat brain cortex *in vitro*. Amytal (0.25 mM) or pentothal (0.5 mM), either of which blocks rat brain cortex respiration stimulated electrically or by the addition of protoveratrine (5 μM), does not diminish the influx of Na^+ that occurs under these conditions (Chan and Quastel, 1970; Shankaran and Quastel, 1972): Hillman *et al.* (1963) found that phenobarbitone (0.3 mM) has no effect on the content of Na^+ of incubated guinea pig brain cortex slices after application of electrical impulses for 10 min.

However, when there is a lack of Ca^{2+} in the incubation medium together with an augmented rate of respiration, e.g., by addition of protoveratrine or high K^+, barbiturates (Amytal 0.25 mM, pentothal 0.5 mM) bring about a diminished rate of entry of Na^+ into the incubated brain cells and an increased cell concentration of K^+ (Shankaran and Quastel, 1972). These results become understandable when they are considered in relation to the known effects of Amytal on the release of Ca^{2+} from cell mitochondria (Chappell and Crofts, 1965). Mitochondria from a variety of tissues are able to accumulate Ca^{2+} either by a respiration-dependent process or by a process requiring the presence of ATP (Lehninger *et al.*, 1963; Chappell *et al.*, 1963; Brierley *et al.*, 1963). This accumulation of Ca^{2+} by mitochondria is prevented by respiratory inhibitors, including Amytal, and by a variety of uncoupling agents (Chappell and Crofts, 1965). The suppression of mitochondrial metabolism, particularly when stimulated by ADP, by barbiturates at anesthetic concentrations is presumably sufficient to release Ca^{2+} from its bound sites in the mitochondria, and the increase of cytoplasmic Ca^{2+} causes alterations in the membrane changes in permeability to Na^+ and K^+ brought about by Ca^{2+} deficiency in the incubation medium. Such a conclusion is compatible with the view (Godfraind *et al.*, 1971; Krnjević, 1972) that anesthetic barbiturates may act by causing a rise in cytoplasmic Ca^{2+}, by suppression of mitochondrial metabolism, resulting in a changed membrane permeability to K^+.

Amytal (0.25 or 0.5 mM) or pentothal (0.25 or 0.5 mM), while having no significant effects on ACh synthesis in unstimulated brain except at high concentrations (1 mM), diminishes or abolishes the evoked release of ACh due to high K^+ or lack of Ca^{2+} in the incubation medium (Grewaal and Quastel, 1973). This fact may be correlated with the findings of Weakly (1969) that pentothal or pentobarbitone decreases the amount of transmitter released by afferent impulses or with the facts concerning the block of release of transmitter from nerve terminals by anesthetics (Thesleff and Quastel, 1965; Quastel *et al.*, 1972). The action of the barbiturate in diminishing evoked-release of ACh *in vitro* may be due to the changed permeabilities of Na^+ and K^+ brought about by release of Ca^{2+} from the mitochondria. This suggestion receives support from the fact that either pentothal or Amytal reverses the fall in ACh content of the incubated brain tissue occurring in a Ca^{2+}-free incubated medium.

It is therefore evident that a correlation between *in vivo* and *in vitro* effects of barbiturates is possible when they are considered from the standpoint of modified neuronal excitability brought about by changed cation fluxes due to depressed mitochondrial metabolism. That the barbiturates may perhaps directly affect the brain cell membrane is also evident from metabolic studies that show that Amytal, at relatively high concentrations (1 mM), causes an increased rate of anaerobic glycolysis. Such an effect may be due to changed permeabilities of the membrane to Na^+ and K^+ that may occur at these high concentrations. At anesthetic concentrations (e.g., 0.25 mM), Amytal shows but little effect on cerebral anaerobic glycolysis and then only in Ca^{2+}-free incubation media (Shankar and Quastel, 1972).

The suggestion has been made recently that the CNS-depressing effects of barbiturates (apparently in their ionized forms) may be connected with an increase in brain biogenic aldehydes, because NADP-linked aldehyde reductase of brain is inhibited by barbiturates (Erwin *et al.*, 1971), e.g., by phenobarbitone, pentobarbitone, and Amytal, that have K_i values ranging from 0.05 mM to 0.4 mM. This view would of course receive support if it could be shown that biogenic aldehydes accumulate in the brain exposed to barbiturates.

Compounds that affect, directly or indirectly, the energetics of brain cells, by interference with oxidative phosphorylation or by inhibitory effects on stimulated brain cell metabolism, include a wide variety of neurotropic substances such as alcohols, aldehydes, and steroids. Examples of these substances are chlorobutanol (chloretone), effective *in vitro* at 2 mM, tribromethanol (0.1 mM), acetaldehyde (1 mM), the steroid anesthetic Viadril (3-20-diketopregnone-21-ol) (0.2 mM) (Quastel, 1958), and nitrous oxide (Hosein *et al.*, 1955).

These substances, of diverse molecular structure, have in common surface active properties (e.g., see Seeman, 1972) that imply an affinity for certain types of membrane constituents or enzyme structures. Permeability or enzymatic changes presumably ensue whose precise nature will depend on both the specific chemical structures of the membrane or enzyme constituents and those of the related effective neurotropic drugs.

3.2. Uncouplers of Brain Respiration

Among drugs that uncouple mitochondrial respiration from phosphorylation are ethyl ether, which is active at concentrations that are present in the brain during surgical anesthesia (Hulme and Krantz, 1955), thiobarbiturates at anesthetic concentrations (Chance and Hollunger, 1963; Aldridge and Parker, 1960), chlorpromazine (Dawkins *et al.*, 1959), and acetylsalicylate (5 mM; Gonda and Quastel, 1963).

3.3. Fluoroacetate

3.3.1. Effects in Vivo

Fluoroacetate, a well-known convulsant drug, causes violent seizures accompanied by alterations of the concentration of cerebral constituents such as increased alanine and decreased glutamate, decreased aspartate and increased ammonia (Dawson, 1953; Benitez *et al.*, 1954; Stone *et al.*, 1960; Tews and Stone, 1965). Brain glutamine, however, does not increase. In rats, treatment with fluoroacetate results in a sedated phase, in which brain citrate and ammonia increase in concentration, followed by a convulsive stage in which the brain concentrations of lactate, citrate, glucose, and ammonia are high (Stewart *et al.*, 1969). Probably the increased ammonia is all of cerebral origin as the blood ammonia levels are lower than those in the brain.

These *in vivo* effects may be correlated with the following effects of fluoroacetate *in vitro.*

3.3.2. Effects in Vitro

It is well known that fluoroacetate inhibits the operation of the citric acid cycle by its conversion to fluorocitrate, which blocks the activity of aconitic hydratase (Peters, 1957) and so causes accumulation of citrate. However, fluoroacetate at low pharmacologically active concentrations does not affect the respiration of rat brain cortex slices but suppresses (at 1 mM or less) the formation of glutamine from glucose and the cerebral utilization of NH_4^+ (Lahiri and Quastel, 1963). It does not suppress the activity of glutamine synthetase. This phenomenon is difficult to explain on the basis of decreased ATP concentration in brain slices as the diminution amounts only to 30% in presence of 2 mM fluoroacetate (Abadom and Scholefield, 1962). As there is little or no fall in the rate of brain slice respiration, the effect of fluoroacetate is unlikely to be due to a suppression of mitochondrial metabolism in all the brain cells. Berl and Clarke (1969) (see also Clarke *et al.*, 1970) point out, however, that these effects would be understandable if there is compartmentation in the brain of such a nature that glutamine biosynthesis takes place largely in one compartment and if the fluoroacetate suppression of the citric acid cycle and resultant fall in ATP are largely restricted to that compartment. From this view, fluoroacetate would have a profound effect on glutamine biosynthesis without necessarily diminishing glutamate formation from glucose. This view also implies the existence of two locations of the citric acid cycle in brain cells, and may partly explain the facts that fluoroacetate blocks in brain slices the oxidation of [1-^{14}C]acetate but not that of [6-^{14}C]glucose (Gonda and Quastel, 1966) and has but little effect on the normal glucose-dependent respiration of brain cortex *in vitro.* This concept was supported and advanced by the finding (Benjamin and Quastel, 1972) that the protoveratrine stimulation of brain cortex slice respiration, which is confined to neurons because it is completely blocked by tetrodotoxin, is suppressed by malonate but not by fluoroacetate. This fact, among others, has led to the conclusion that the fluoroacetate suppression of the citric acid cycle must be confined to the glia, which appears to be the location of much of cerebral glutamine biosynthesis, and not the neurons which constitute the major site of the energy cycle in brain and where the stimulated citric acid cycle is blocked by malonate at low concentrations. The major effect of fluoroacetate (3 mM) is to bring about a diminution in the tissue content of glutamine with an increase in that of glutamate.

These effects may be correlated with those *in vivo*, where in spite of the large increase in brain ammonia due to fluoroacetate administration there is no rise in brain glutamine (rat, dog). Nadler *et al.* (1972), studying the effects of fluoroacetate administration followed by intracerebrally administered labeled aspartate, found a decrease in the formation of labeled glutamine and glutamate and considered these and other effects to be due to selective inhibition of the citric acid cycle at the site of glutamine biosynthesis.

Fluoroacetate, it may be noted, blocks cerebral active transport of acetate (Gonda and Quastel, 1966).

3.4. Methionine Sulfoximine

3.4.1. Effects in Vivo

The neurotoxic affects of methionine sulfoximine have been often described, e.g., by Proler and Kellaway (1962) and Tews and Stone (1964). Administration of methionine sulfoximine to mice in doses greater than 100 mg/kg results in intermittent convulsions within a few hours after the injection, death occurring in the convulsive period. During this period, the brain ammonia concentration rises markedly and brain glutamine concentration falls (Warren and Schenker, 1964). In dogs, intraperitoneal administration of methionine sulfoximine at 10 mg/kg causes severe generalized seizures after 16–18 h, accompanied by a large increase in the content of brain ammonia and a marked fall in that of brain glutamine. The brain glutamate concentration also falls, although not so markedly (Tews and Stone, 1965). The increase of brain ammonia is of cerebral origin as the blood concentration of ammonia remains normal. Long before the seizures due to methionine sulfoximine begin, there is a marked rise in cerebral ammonia concentration (Folbergrova *et al.*, 1969). The cerebral glutamine concentration falls at the onset of the seizures (Peters and Tower, 1959; Kolousek and Jiracek, 1959; Folbergrova, 1963, 1964). Increased cerebral concentrations of alanine and lactate and a decrease of that of aspartate are considered secondary to the elevated brain ammonia concentration.

According to Folbergrova *et al.* (1969), the cerebral concentrations of phosphocreatine and ATP in mice after severe convulsions due to methionine sulfoximine (300 mg/kg intraperitoneally) remain unchanged and there is a marked increase in cerebral glucose concentration. The content of cerebral glycogen also increases, and this seems not to be related to the seizures, as it increases before the onset of seizures. Moreover, methionine administration, which prevents the seizures, does not prevent the glycogen accumulation. There is a positive correlation between the increases of concentrations of glucose and glycogen. It has been pointed out that glycogen accumulation takes place in glial cells after certain types of brain injury (Shimizu and Hamuro, 1958).

3.4.2. *Effects in Vitro*

Methionine sulfoximine, an analogue of glutamine, inhibits cerebral glutamine synthetase competitively with respect to glutamate, some inhibition being seen at 0.01 mM. It gives about 50% inhibition at 1 mM with low glutamate concentrations (Sellinger and Weiler, 1963). It seems evident that the drug binds at the active site of the enzyme and undergoes phosphorylation there (Lamar and Sellinger, 1965; Sellinger, 1967; Ronzio and Meister, 1967, 1968).

Doubtless the rise in cerebral ammonia concentration is partly responsible for the neurological effects of methionine sulfoximine administration. One of the effects of NH_4^+ *in vitro* is to cause release of ACh from the bound form in the brain (Grewaal and Quastel, 1973; Braganca *et al.*, 1953), and this effect may perhaps be correlated with the results reported by Tower (1960) on the diminished ability of incubated brain cortex slices from methionine sulfoximine–treated cats to form bound ACh.

Warren and Schenker (1964) have shown that methionine sulfoximine administration reduces the toxicity of NH_4^+. At a dose of ammonium chloride lethal for 50% of untreated mice, no deaths were observed in any of the methionine sulfoximine–treated animals at the various time intervals studied; nevertheless, the cerebral ammonia levels were very high. The rise in brain glutamine concentration following the injection of ammonium chloride was lower in the methionine sulfoximine–treated animals than in the untreated controls. It is possible, as suggested by Warren and Schenker (1964), that the diminished toxicity of injected NH_4^+ caused by methionine sulfoximine administration is due to diminished activity of glutamine synthetase. As the major site of this enzyme appears to be in the glia, it seems to the writer that high NH_4^+ may cause a localized (glial) fall in ATP with loss of ability of glia to absorb K^+ and other substances released from neurons during excitation (Okamoto and Quastel, 1970; Benjamin and Quastel, 1972), with resultant increased neuronal activity. Suppression of glial glutamine synthetase activity by methionine sulfoximine should prevent this localized fall of ATP and hence diminish the loss of buffering capacity of the glia for K^+, and other neuroactive molecules such as glutamate, released during neuronal excitation. A localized fall of glial ATP may not be apparent in measurements of total brain tissue ATP.

3.5. Chlorinated Hydrocarbon Insecticides

Other substances, of importance as insecticides, that have potent neurological effects in rats and birds and are also associated with increased cerebral ammonia levels are a group of chlorinated hydrocarbons. Hathway *et al.* (1965) have reported an association of neurotoxicity of two structurally related insecticides, telodrin and dieldrin, with abnormally high concentrations of cerebral ammonia in rats. Hathway and Mallinson (1964) point out that telodrin administration, which in rats causes convulsions and coma, leads to increased cerebral glutamine and diminished cerebral glutamate concentrations together with an increased concentration of cerebral ammonia during seizures. They conclude that telodrin causes liberation of ammonia in the brain that occurs before the onset of convulsions and throughout their course. Cerebral pyruvate accumulates, as is known to occur in the brains of dogs treated with ammonia (Clark and Eiseman, 1958). St. Omer (1971) finds that high concentrations of brain ammonia occur in rats and cockerels poisoned acutely with lindane, dieldrin, heptachlor, and DDT. The intensities of convulsions and other neurological symptoms coincide, and correlate, with the increases of concentrations of brain ammonia. Elevated levels of brain glutamine occur in the cockerels after administration of all four insecticides but in rats only after lindane and dieldrin. It seems that cockerels are more resistant than rats to ammonia toxicity, perhaps by a greater ability to convert ammonia to glutamine. The mode of action of these substances in the brain is unknown, but the facts are consistent with the view that they interfere with brain cell energetics, involving oxidative breakdown of glucose, leading to ammonia liberation.

3.6. 2-Deoxyglucose

A substance whose effects after administration to an animal are related to the central nervous system and include convulsions and coma (Lazlo *et al.*, 1960) is the glucose analogue 2-deoxyglucose. The effects are in some measure due to diminished cerebral glucose utilization by competition with glucose or to ATP depletion. Tower (1958) has shown that incubation of cerebral cortex slices with 2-deoxyglucose results in marked depletion of phosphocreatine and adenosine polyphosphates with concomitant formation of 2-deoxyglucose-6-phosphate. It had already been shown by Harpur and Quastel (1949) that D-glucosamine, a related glucose analogue, is phosphorylated by brain hexokinase and is able to suppress ACh formation in brain preparations by competition for ATP.

2-Deoxyglucose competes with glucose for carrier-mediated transport into mammalian brain (Bidder, 1968; Bachelard, 1971) and is converted to 2-deoxyglucosephosphate, which is not further metabolized (Bachelard *et al.*, 1971). Meldrum and Horton (1973) have shown that intravenous administration of 2-deoxyglucose in the rhesus monkey affects the level of consciousness, impairs cerebral electrical activity, and diminishes the cerebral metabolic rate, provided that the molar blood ratio of 2-deoxyglucose to glucose exceeds 2:1. Horton *et al.* (1973) have shown, moreover, that after 2-deoxyglucose administration to mice at doses producing behavioral effects there is a derangement of cerebral glucose metabolism separate from the inhibition of glucose influx. They consider that this derangement is partly due to competition between 2-deoxyglucose and glucose for carrier-mediated transport and for hexokinase and partly due to inhibition by 2-deoxyglucose-6-phosphate of hexosephosphate isomerase. Such changes in cerebral glucose metabolism are considered to be responsible for the behavioral changes.

3.7. γ-Hydroxybutyrate

Another substance having distinct neurological effects whose activity seems to be concerned with brain cell energetics is γ-hydroxybutyrate, which has caused considerable interest because of the similarities between the hypnotic state it induces and the natural sleeping state (Drakontides *et al.*, 1962; Laborit, 1964). Although it is closely related chemically to GABA, it causes no change in the level of endogenous GABA in the brain (Giarman and Schmidt, 1963; Mitoma and Neubauer, 1968) and apparently no change in the overall oxygen consumption of the brain *in vitro*. Taberner *et al.* (1972) find that it increases the $1\text{-}^{14}C/6\text{-}^{14}C$ ratio in expired CO_2 in mice (given labeled glucose) by 300% and that the same effect occurs with slices of cerebral cortex from γ-hydroxybutyrate-treated rats but not with brain homogenates or with slices of kidney or diaphragm. They suggest that the drug increases the activity of the pentose phosphate pathway in brain by an increase in the activity of glucose-6-phosphate dehydrogenase, although the activity of this enzyme is not altered *in vitro* by high concentrations of γ-hydroxybutyrate. The reason for the apparent association between the increase in cerebral oxidation of glucose by the pentose pathway and the hypnotic state is still unknown.

3.8. Aminooxyacetate

The neurotropic drug aminooxyacetate, whose inhibitory effects on various aspects of brain metabolism are becoming increasingly interesting in relation to its neurological behavior, causes in the dog at doses of

5–20 mg/kg a profound depression from which recovery may occur after several hours (Tews and Stone, 1965). Such effects have been described in detail (Wallach, 1961; Roa *et al.*, 1964), convulsive activity with large doses also being observed (Wood and Peesker, 1973). Outstanding neurochemical effects *in vivo* are the increases in cerebral concentrations of γ-aminobutyrate (GABA) and ammonia and glutamine (Wallach, 1961; Tews and Stone, 1965). The aspartate level is diminished. It is possible that some of these changes are brought about by the increase in blood ammonia that follows aminooxyacetate administration (Tews and Stone, 1965), as similar changes in cerebral concentrations of glutamine and aspartate occur after administration of ammonium chloride (Berl *et al.*, 1962).

Major effects of aminooxyacetate are its inhibition of pyridoxal-dependent pathways of amino acid metabolism, presumably by its combination with pyridoxal. It inhibits glutamate transamination (Hopper and Segal, 1964), GABA transaminase (Wallach, 1961), and glutamate decarboxylase (Baxter and Roberts, 1961). When incubated rat brain cortex slices are exposed to aminooxyacetate, there ensues a diminished rate of conversion of glucose to GABA (Haber, 1965), presumably because of the block of glutamate decarboxylase activity. There occurs also depressed cerebral metabolism of GABA itself owing to the suppression of GABA transaminase. The rate of oxygen consumption of rat brain cortex slices respiring in a glucose saline medium is markedly diminished by aminooxyacetate (Haber, 1965), which evidently affects brain cell energetics by interference with glucose metabolism. The site of the "energy cycle" (Berl *et al.*, 1970), presumably the neurons (Benjamin and Quastel, 1972), is affected by aminooxyacetate, and perhaps this is partly the reason why aminooxyacetate gives rise to increased cerebral ammonia concentrations. The cerebral glutamate decarboxylase activity of aminooxyacetate-treated rats is apparently unaffected by the drug, although the activity of GABA transaminase falls considerably (Collins, 1973); this may account for the increased levels of GABA in the treated animals. Wood and Peesker (1973), however, find that cerebral glutamate decarboxylase is inhibited *in vivo*. Neal and Starr (1973) point out that aminooxyacetate increases the accumulation of labeled GABA in isolated retina by suppressing the metabolism of this amino acid. Accumulation of GABA also occurs with amphibian spinal cord after an exposure to the drug (Davidoff *et al.*, 1973) for presumably a similar reason.

3.9. Haloperidol

Haloperidol, a member of the butyrophenone neuroleptics, although differing in chemical structure from the phenothiazine drugs, has a similar activity to that of the piperazine phenothiazines. It has a marked tendency to produce extrapyramidal side-effects (Laborit and Sanseigne, 1970).

It is a potent inhibitor of glutamate dehydrogenase (Shemisa and Fahien, 1971) and inhibits GABA uptake (Iversen and Johnston, 1971). Collins (1973) finds that haloperidol reduces rat brain glutamate concentrations *in vivo* and that the rate of disappearance of labeled GABA is increased whereas that of labeled glutamate is decreased after intracisternal administration of the labeled substances. The drug has no effect on glutamate decarboxylase and GABA transaminase activities or on brain levels of GABA. Collins suggests that the behavioral effects of haloperidol are partly due to its effects on glutamate and GABA metabolism.

4. DRUGS AND BRAIN CELL PERMEABILITIES

4.1. Tetrodotoxin

Tetrodotoxin (TTX), a potent neurotoxin found in the Japanese puffer fish and elsewhere, is well known to abolish at low concentrations (e.g., 0.3 μM) the generation of action potentials in a variety of excitable tissues, including frog myelinated nerve fibers and squid giant axons, and the associated Na^+ in such tissues (Kao, 1966; Narahashi *et al.*, 1964; Nakamura *et al.*, 1965). It is considered to be a specific blocker of sodium conductance with no effect on potassium conductance. It does have, however, suppressing effects on action potentials produced in media containing salts of divalent cations only (Ca^{2+}, Sr^{2+}, Ba^{2+}, Watanabe *et al.*, 1967; Tasaki and Singer, 1966). Whereas it has no effect on the rate of respiration of rat brain cortex slices incubated in a physiological glucose medium, TTX blocks the stimulation of respiration that occurs on application of electrical impulses or in the presence of protoveratrine or in the absence of Ca^{2+} from the incubation medium (Chan and Quastel, 1967, 1970; Okamoto and Quastel, 1970). McIlwain (1967) also found that TTX inhibits the respiratory response due to electrical stimulation of incubated guinea pig cortex slices and that the K^+ content of such stimulated slices is enhanced by TTX. The fluxes of Na^+ and K^+ during such stimulation are suppressed by TTX (Swanson, 1968). The increased influx of Na^+ that occurs not only with electric pulses but also in the presence of protoveratrine is completely blocked by TTX at low concentrations (Chan and Quastel, 1970; Okamoto and Quastel, 1970). It was concluded that TTX causes its metabolic inhibitions in the brain under certain conditions by suppression of the influx of Na^+ that occurs under these conditions. TTX also diminishes the increases of uptake of Na^+ and water that may occur in rat brain cortex slices incubated in a variety of ways, e.g., the absence of glucose from the incubation medium or the presence of ouabain (Okamoto and Quastel, 1970; Hammerstad and Cutler, 1972) or the onset of anoxia (Shankar and

Quastel, 1972). It was concluded that under such circumstances action potentials are generated *in vitro*. This has been confirmed by investigations on isolated guinea pig cerebellar slices (Okamoto and Quastel, 1973) which showed that the various incubation conditions causing TTX-sensitive uptakes of water and Na^+ lead to enhanced frequencies of spontaneous action potentials *in vitro*. As it is known that glia are not electrically excitable cells and do not generate action potentials (Kuffler and Nicholls, 1966; Kuffler, 1967), it is evident that the effect of TTX in diminishing influx of Na^+ into incubated brain tissue is confined to the neurons. The suppression of increased water uptake, which is apparently mainly confined to glia (Zadunaisky *et al.*, 1965; Tower, 1967), by TTX is considered to be due to the diminution of neuronal efflux of K^+ that occurs during the generation of action potentials and that is largely taken up, together with Cl^-, by the glia, causing increased water uptake. Such water uptake takes place to maintain isoosmoticity of the glial cells if a Donnan equilibrium is to be maintained when the K^+ concentration is increased and the Na^+ concentration is decreased in the extracellular space after an action potential. Thus the glial cells have a buffering action, as far as extracellular K^+ concentration is concerned, during the generation of action potentials. This conclusion (Okamoto and Quastel, 1970) is in agreement with that of Kuffler (1967), Kuffler and Nicholls (1966), and Trachtenberg and Pollen (1970) that glial cells are selectively permeable to K^+ and as a consequence of the release of K^+ by neighboring neurons and its transient accumulation in the intracellular clefts the membrane of the glial cell becomes depolarized. As the K^+ disappears by uptake and diffusion, the glial potential returns to normal (Kuffler, 1967).

Not only are the neuronal fluxes of Na^+ and K^+ affected by the generation of action potentials but so are the fluxes of a variety of amino acids. Glutamate, GABA, aspartate, and glycine are released from rat brain cortex slices on incubation with protoveratrine (especially in a Ca^{2+}-free medium) or with ouabain, or in the absence of glucose. These releases are partially or wholly suppressed by TTX (Benjamin and Quastel, 1972). TTX, however, does not affect the release of glutamine nor does protoveratrine accelerate it. It was concluded that glutamate released from neurons during neuronal excitation is partly taken up by the glia and converted there to glutamine. This is returned to the neurons where it is hydrolyzed and converted into glutamate and GABA (Benjamin and Quastel, 1972, 1974). The movement of glutamate from neuron to glia resembles that apparently occurring with the movement of K^+ under the same conditions.

TTX also abolishes the stimulating effect of protoveratrine on Ach release from incubated rat brain slices, and it has suppressing effects (partial or complete) on the action of high K^+, sodium L-glutamate, or lack of Ca^{2+} on ACh synthesis and release (Grewaal and Quastel, 1973). Thus release of ACh from brain cells can be the result of conditions leading to the generation of action potentials or to the activation of the Na^+ current system, at the neuronal membrane, known to be suppressed by TTX. Stimulation of nerve fibers causes release of ACh (Dettbarn, 1967).

Saxitoxin, a marine neurotoxin whose pharmacological effects resemble those of TTX, is even more potent than TTX in suppressing the fluxes of Na^+ and K^+ due to electrical stimulation. The influx of Ca^{2+} into brain slices is increased by electrical stimulation, but whereas TTX blocks this increase, saxitoxin potentiates it (Bull and Trevor, 1972). Baker *et al.* (1970) have shown that in squid giant axons there is a TTX-sensitive entry of Ca^{2+} which precedes the entry of Na^+ during excitation. Ramsey and McIlwain (1970) have reported a TTX-sensitive uptake of Ca^{2+} in unstimulated guinea pig brain slices and in slices exposed to glutamate. Inhibition of Ca^{2+} influx is apparently not essential for the inhibition of Na^+ influx according to the results obtained with saxitoxin, and it would seem that at least one site of Ca^{2+} entry into the brain cells is independent of Na^+ entry.

TTX does not inhibit L-glutamate uptake into incubated rat brain slices at concentrations that inhibit the Na^+ influx caused by L-glutamate and other excitant amino acids (Balcar and Johnston, 1972). Perhaps this may be explained partly by the fact that much exogenous L-glutamate is taken up by the glia, although some must be absorbed by neurons (Okamoto and Quastel, 1972; Kuhar and Snyder, 1970). TTX also affects the inward movement of Na^+ into incubated chicken retina induced by exogenous glutamate, as judged by changes in retinal transparency (Van Harreveld and Fifková, 1972).

4.2. Local Anesthetics: Cocaine, Procaine, Lidocaine, etc.

A variety of reviews concerned with the mode of action of local anesthetics have appeared in recent years (e.g., Ariens, 1964; Watson, 1960; Ritchie and Greengard, 1966; Dettbarn, 1971; Seeman, 1972).

Both TTX and the local anesthetic lidocaine are known to block the sodium conductance associated with membrane depolarization in the axon and as a result suppress propagation of an action potential along the axon (Narahashi *et al.*, 1964; Shanes *et al.*, 1959). Lidocaine is far less potent than TTX in this respect and less specific in its activities. The inhibitory effects of local anesthetics are influenced by the presence of Na^+ and Ca^{2+} (Davis and Dettbarn, 1962; Shanes, 1958), and their main action takes place at the membrane. As the initial step in the excitation cycle in the neuron seems to be the removal of Ca^{2+} from receptor sites (Hodgkin, 1966), much work has been carried out on the relations between local anesthetics and Ca^{2+} for membrane components. Thus local anesthetics compete with Ca^{2+} for binding sites containing phosphatidylserine and they inhibit Ca^{2+} uptake in proportion to their local anesthetic potency (Dettbarn, 1971); moreover, the binding of labeled local anesthetics to phosphatidylserine is antagonized by Ca^{2+}. Competition between Ca^{2+} and local anesthetics for specific sites in the membrane is evidently of importance in the control of Na^+ and K^+ permeabilities of the membrane. The relative effectiveness of cocaine and tropine derivatives in displacing Ca^{2+} from phosphatidylserine parallels their relative effectiveness in inhibiting axonal sodium and potassium conductances (Goldman and Blaustein, 1966). Tetracaine, for example, is a more potent local anesthetic than procaine in displacing Ca^{2+} from phospholipid *in vitro* (Feinstein, 1964).

Local anesthetics (cocaine, 0.2 mM; lidocaine, 0.5 mM; and procaine, 1 mM) abolish the stimulation of brain cortex respiration *in vitro* brought about by the application of electrical impulses or the depression of acetate oxidation brought about by the same means, while having no effect on the unstimulated brain metabolism (Chan and Quastel, 1970; see also Hammerstad and Cutler, 1972). This is caused by the suppression of the inward flow of Na^+ that occurs with such stimulation. In this manner, the local anesthetics resemble TTX and differ from the barbiturates that have no such effects under similar incubation conditions. However, cocaine at high concentration (0.2 mM) brings about an increased influx of Na^+ into unstimulated incubated rat brain cortex, which may be due to some suppression of brain respiration (Ryman and Walsh, 1954). At relatively high concentrations, the local anesthetics exercise inhibitory effects on rat brain cortex respiration stimulated by high K^+ in the incubation medium (Geddes and Quastel, 1956), differing from TTX in this respect, but resembling the barbiturates. The local anesthetics, also in contrast to TTX, decrease potassium conductance in the axon membrane (Goldman and Blaustein, 1966).

The local anesthetics (cocaine, lidocaine) suppress the influx of Na^+ into rat brain cortex slices incubated aerobically in the presence of protoveratrine or of ouabain, or in the absence of glucose, but not, under the experimental conditions used, in the presence of L- or D-glutamate. They resemble TTX in this respect and differ from the barbiturates (Amytal, pentothal) used at the anesthetic concentrations that completely block potassium or electrically stimulated brain respiration (Shankaran and Quastel, 1972).

There appear to be several systems by which Na^+ can accumulate in brain cells *in vitro*. One is blocked by TTX and local anesthetics and is presumably identical to the sodium current system associated with the generation of action potentials and this is not affected by barbiturates at anesthetic concentrations. Another is manifest under conditions of Ca^{2+} deficiency, in the extracellular medium, and agumented respiratory metabolism and this is inhibited by barbiturates at anesthetic concentrations. This is presumably due, as already mentioned, to the rise in cytoplasmic Ca^{2+} caused by suppression of mitochondrial respiration, affecting membrane permeability to Na^+ and K^+.

Local anesthetics resemble TTX in another respect, that of abolishing the generation of action potentials, with resultant influx of Na^+ and efflux of K^+, at the onset of anoxia (Shankar and Quastel, 1972). They differ, however, from TTX in competitively suppressing ACh uptake into the rat brain cortex slices incubated in the presence of paraoxon to suppress the activity of cholinesterase (Liang and Quastel, 1969).

Cocaine blocks neuronal uptake of norepinephrine in brain (Dengler *et al.*, 1961; Schildkraut *et al.*, 1967) and in peripheral sympathetic nerves (Hertting *et al.*, 1961). It also inhibits uptake of 5-hydroxytryptamine (5-HT) in brain slices and synaptosomes (Blackburn *et al.*, 1967; Ross and Renyi, 1967; Segawa and Kuruma, 1968). It seems to affect norepinephrine metabolism in a manner resembling that of amphetamine.

4.3. Ouabain

Intracranial administration of ouabain leads to selective swelling of astrocytes (Venturini and Palladini, 1973), an effect shown to be associated with the suppression of membrane ATPase *in vivo* with resultant changes in brain cell contents of Na^+ and K^+. Intraventricular administration of ouabain leads to seizures in rats with accompanying increased CSF concentrations of K^+ (Donaldson *et al.*, 1972) and an increase in hippocampal 5-HT concentration and diminished norepinephrine concentration in the midbrain region (Izumi *et al.*, 1973).

As the cardiac glycosides are able to inhibit cationic fluxes without necessarily depressing respiration or glycolysis (Schatzmann, 1953; Kunz and Sulser, 1957; Maizels *et al.*, 1958; Yoshida *et al.*, 1961), it is evident that their effects are not due to energetic changes. Ouabain brings about a multiplicity of changes in *in vitro* brain metabolism and transport processes, among which are the following (Gonda and Quastel, 1962): suppression of K^+-stimulated brain respiration, suppression of influx of L-glutamate or of creatine from the extracellular medium, and increased efflux of amino acids from the brain into the incubation medium (see also Cremer, 1967). These effects are explained by the block of the sodium pump due to suppression of the activity of membrane-bound Na^+/K^+-ATPase (Dunham and Glynn, 1961; Skou, 1957, 1960; Post *et al.*, 1960). Ouabain also suppresses glutamine biosynthesis and acetate metabolism in the brain *in vitro* (Gonda and Quastel, 1966) and the active transport of ascorbic acid into the brain (Sharma *et al.*, 1963). It causes reduction of the uptake of GABA by retina (Goodchild and Neal, 1973), of the uptake of glycine by brain cortex slices (Nakazawa and Quastel, 1968), and of synaptosomal uptake of norepinephrine and 5-HT (Tissari *et al.*, 1969; Tissari and Bogdanski, 1971). It causes release of amino acids (e.g., glutamate, aspartate, glycine, taurine), partly suppressed on addition of TTX, from incubated rat brain slices (Benjamin and Quastel, 1972), loss of norepinephrine from rat midbrain slices (Yessaian *et al.*, 1971), release of ACh from synaptosomes (Haga, 1971), and stimulation of ACh release from incubated brain cortex slices (Grewaal and Quastel, 1973).

Ouabain inhibits uptake of K^+ and extrusion of Na^+ by brain slices, even after electrical stimulation (Swanson, 1968), and it has become evident that its block of the sodium pump is associated with its suppression of the Na^+/K^+-ATPase activity of the brain cell (Bonting *et al.*, 1962). The enzyme is probably located in the cell membranes of cell bodies and axons (Cummins and Hyden, 1962), a rise in its activity taking place in rat brain during development from birth. This is partly due to the proliferation of dendrites during maturation and partly due to the multiplication of nerve endings which are rich in the enzyme activity (Abdel-Latif and Abood, 1964). There is a possible relationship between ATPase activity and electrical activity (EEG) of the brain (Abdel-Latif *et al.*, 1967; Bignami *et al.*, 1966).

The site of action of ouabain is on the outer aspect of the cell membrane, for intracellular microinjection of the drug into squid giant axons fails to inhibit Na^+ efflux, although it is most effective when applied externally (Caldwell and Keynes, 1959).

Ouabain may act as pacemaker for part of brain respiration (Whittam and Blond, 1964) by controlling the fluxes of Na^+ and K^+ into the brain cell, but its effect is most evident when brain respiration has been stimulated by high external K^+ or by some conditions leading to increased inward flow of Na^+, e.g., electrical stimulation (Nakazawa and Quastel, 1968).

Ouabain brings about not only a large influx of Na^+ into incubated brain slices but also an increased water uptake (Yoshida *et al.*, 1961; Bourke and Tower, 1966). Both these processes have a TTX-sensitive component (Okamoto and Quastel, 1970), indicating that ouabain can cause an increased inward flow of Na^+ in the TTX-sensitive channel and may therefore lead to the generation of action potentials. This has been confirmed by observations on guinea pig cerebellar slices, where ouabain (0.1 mM) causes a marked increase in the frequency of spontaneous action potentials (Okamoto and Quastel, 1973). Ouabain can also cause an increased influx of Ca^{2+} with guinea pig cerebral cortex slices (Fujisawa *et al.*, 1965).

The coupling of the sodium pump with the transport of amino acids against a concentration gradient (Gonda and Quastel, 1962; Hammerstad and Cutler, 1972) accounts for the marked effect of ouabain on the release of amino acids concentration in brain cells and in the suppression of their active uptake. Many amino acids, including L- and D-glutamate, GABA, glycine, serine, alanine, proline, tyrosine, and 5-hydroxytryptophan (see Quastel, 1970, for references) are transported against a gradient, and such accumulation is Na^+ dependent (Takagaki *et al.*, 1959; Abadom and Scholefield, 1962; Lahiri and Lajtha, 1964; Nakazawa and Quastel, 1968) and sensitive to the action of ouabain.

Studies such as these point to the conclusion that amino acid influx into the brain is dependent not only on the brain cell level of ATP but also on the activity of the membrane-bound sodium–potassium-sensitive ATPase. The exit rates of amino acids (e.g., α-aminoisobutyrate, D-glutamate, and L-lysine) are largely determined by the intracellular concentrations of the amino acid (Levi *et al.*, 1965). Many metabolic inhibitors increase the efflux (Cherayil *et al.*, 1967) partly by blocking the influx. Incubations leading to the generation of action potentials (e.g., the presence of protoveratrine) lead to increased efflux of amino acids, and this is potentiated by the presence of ouabain, which blocks reuptake (Benjamin and Quastel, 1972). These effects are suppressed by TTX. Ouabain apparently may cause some release of sodium-dependent binding of amino acids, this being most marked with GABA (Shiu and Elliott, 1973). The actual level of an amino acid in the brain at any time is obviously determined by its relative rates of influx and efflux.

It has been suggested (Berl *et al.*, 1970) that the major site of action of ouabain is the compartment in which glutamine is largely synthesized, accounting for the potent effect of the drug on glutamine formation (Gonda and Quastel, 1962). The drug, however, must have various sites of action (Berl and Clarke, 1969; Rose, 1965), one of which must be the neuron to account for its partial sensitivity to TTX (Benjamin and Quastel, 1972).

4.4. Protoveratrine

Wollenberger (1955) found that very low concentrations of protoveratrine and closely related substances cause large increases in the respiratory and aerobic glycolytic rates of incubated guinea pig brain cortex slices, the same changes being found *in vivo* in animals treated with protoveratrine. He pointed out that there seemed to be a striking parallel between the effects of protoveratrine and those of electrical impulses on brain metabolism. The protoveratrine stimulation of respiration like that of electrical impulses is blocked by barbiturates and by malonate (Quastel, 1959). It is well known that veratrine alkaloids bring about marked changes in ion permeability and bioelectric phenomena (Shanes, 1958) and it has been suggested that protoveratrine and Ca^{2+} compete for membrane receptor sites (e.g., Gershfeld and Shanes, 1959). Protoveratrine changes the amino acid contents of incubated rat brain cortex slices in a manner similar to that of increased K^+, and it has been concluded that it may act by an interaction with or an antagonism to Ca^{2+} located in the brain cell membrane. Its effects are antagonized by the presence of cocaine (Kini and Quastel, 1960). Protoveratrine (10 μM) increases the influx of Na^+ and of water into incubated brain slices, as well as their respiration, and these increases are abolished by the presence of TTX (Okamoto and Quastel, 1970) or of the local anesthetics cocaine and lidocaine (Shankaran and Quastel, 1972). It causes considerable release (especially in a Ca^{2+}-deficient incubation medium) of a number of amino acids, particularly glutamate, GABA, aspartate, and glycine, and this effect is suppressed by TTX (Benjamin and Quastel, 1972). The amino acids especially affected are those considered to have transmitter properties in the CNS. Electrical stimulation of guinea pig brain slices also causes increased release of amino acids into the incubation medium (Jones and McIlwain, 1971). Since the effects of protoveratrine are presumably confined to the electrically excitable cells of the nervous system, i.e., the neurons, because they are completely blocked by TTX, it is likely that the amino acids glutamate, GABA, aspartate, and glycine released by the action of protoveratrine emanate from the neurons. Gottesfeld and Elliott (1971) have noted that rat brain cortex slices loaded with GABA, by previous incubation in its presence, lose this amino acid at a rate accelerated by protoveratrine, whose effect is blocked by TTX. A notable effect of protoveratrine is to increase, on incubation, the brain slice concentration of glutamine (Benjamin and Quastel, 1972). This may be explained by the release of glutamate from neurons, leading to an increased concentration of glutamate in the intracellular space with consequent increased uptake of glutamate by the glia and therefore an increased amount of conversion in the glia of glutamate into glutamine. Protoveratrine causes profound effects on ACh synthesis and release in incubated rat brain cortex slices. It causes a greatly increased release of ACh without concomitant increase in synthesis and entirely blocks the increased synthesis and release of ACh due to high K^+ (Grewaal and Quastel, 1973). It was suggested that the neuronal synaptic vesicles, whose integrity is presumably essential for high rates of synthesis of ACh, are substantially depleted by the large depolarization effected by protoveratrine. The drug brings about a marked acceleration of the frequency of spontaneous action potentials in guinea pig cerebellar slices, the effect being completely blocked by TTX (Okamoto and Quastel, 1973).

5. DRUGS AFFECTING CEREBRAL BIOGENIC AMINE LEVELS

Many drugs alter the concentrations of biogenic amines, including the catechol- and indolealkylamines, in the CNS and have marked effects on animal and human behavior. They have been widely used as tools to ascertain the role of biogenic amines in the pharmacological action of psychotropic or neurotropic substances. They may be grouped in at least the following three categories: (1) compounds that affect the binding and transport of amines, e.g., reserpine, phenothiazines and tricyclic antidepressants, amphetamines, and possibly alcohol; (2) inhibitors of monoamine oxidase, e.g., iproniazid; and (3) inhibitors of amino acid decarboxylase, e.g., α-methyldopa. Various reviews of the subject have appeared, e.g., Carlsson

(1966), Kopin (1966), Quastel (1965, 1967), Pletscher (1968), Sulser and Sanders-Bush (1971).

5.1. Reserpine

The well-known tranquilizing action of reserpine seems to be associated with its ability to diminish the content in the cell of amines that are known to have pharmacological activities in the nervous system, e.g., 5-HT in the brain or catecholamines in hypothalamus or in adrenergic neurons (Pletscher *et al.*, 1956; Holzbauer and Vogt, 1956). Reserpine releases 5-HT and norepinephrine from depots in the brain, perhaps by an inhibition of the uptake of these substances due to its affinity for the transport carrier involved. A single reserpine dose can deplete catecholamine and 5-HT reserves in the brain and peripheral organs for a period of days or weeks. The conclusion that the sedative action of the reserpine group of drugs is due to lowered brain levels of certain amines seems to be supported by the fact that drugs that raise these levels (e.g., monoamine oxidase inhibitors) may act as antidepressants. Reserpine-induced rigidity in rats is antagonized by monoamine oxidase inhibition and reduced by pretreatment with α-methyl-*m*-tyrosine and α-methyldopa. These results are consistent with the view that reserpine produces rigidity by depressing an inhibitory motor system in which the transmitter is an amine (Morrison and Webster, 1973). Dopamine can antagonize the effect of reserpine, but it is likely that reserpine acts by a variety of mechanisms (Laborit and Sanseigne, 1970). The antihypertensive effect of reserpine is probably related to the decrease of catecholamines in tissues and peripheral organs, and this hypotensive response is not related to the drug's central action. Reserpine acts not at the outer cell membrane but within the nerve terminal on the synaptic vesicles where amines are stored (Carlsson, 1966; Kopin, 1966). It interferes with their ability to retain norepinephrine. This substance is released from the vesicles and is deaminated by monoamine oxidase inside the nerve terminal (Sulser *et al.*, 1969). It leaves the neuron as the deaminated inactive product, and, therefore, after reserpine treatment there is no norepinephrine available to act on postsynaptic receptors. Sedation ensues (Snyder, 1970). A large dose of reserpine administered rapidly to animals leads to initial excitation prior to the sedation, and this is attributed to the release of unmetabolized norepinephrine that crosses the synaptic membrane and acts on receptor sites. A similar excitatory effect is seen when there has been pretreatment with a monoamine oxidase inhibitor. However, Brodie *et al.* (1960*a*) consider that the sedative action of reserpine is more associated with a change in brain 5-HT than with that of norepinephrine.

Reserpine and related drugs do not directly inhibit enzymes involved in the synthesis of catecholamines and 5-HT (Glowinski *et al.*, 1966*b*;

Rutledge and Weiner, 1967). They seem to inhibit the uptake of dopamine at the site where dopamine-β-hydroxylase is located, and therefore they inhibit, indirectly, the synthesis of norepinephrine from dopamine (Rutledge and Weiner, 1967). Functional recovery after reserpine is associated with reuptake and storage of exogenous amines (Iversen *et al.*, 1965; Brodie *et al.*, 1966; Lundberg and Stitzel, 1968). There may exist at the neuronal membrane a Na^+-dependent reserpine-sensitive amine carrier mechanism (Sugrue and Shore, 1970), but there seems to be normally very little interference by reserpine with neuronal amine transport. Reserpine may affect cerebral tissues so that they are less capable of storing added amines (Brodie *et al.*, 1960*b*). Thus incubated tissues taken from the pituitary, pineal, cerebral cortex, and hypothalamus of reserpinized cats are less able to absorb norepinephrine than those from normal animals (Weil-Malherbe *et al.*, 1961). Binding *in vivo* of reserpine occurs in brain subcellular components, particularly the microsomal fractions (Manara *et al.*, 1972).

Reserpine administration also affects the concentration of amino acids in those neuronal structures of the cat supplied with noradrenergic terminals (Gasserian, spinal and sympathetic ganglia, and spinal cord). The drug reduces the levels of glutamate, alanine, and glycine in dorsal root ganglia, that of glutamate in the sympathetic ganglia, and those of glutamate and aspartate in the spinal cord (Santini and Berl, 1972). It is possible that these effects are linked with those of reserpine on neuronal amino acid metabolism in specific brain compartments (Berl and Frigyesi, 1969).

5.2. Phenothiazines

Neurochemical aspects of the mode of action of the phenothiazines have been reviewed by Gabay (1971).

Chlorpromazine (CPZ) has a wide range of pharmacological properties and a variety of clinical applications. It is a depressant affecting many parts of the CNS and has its principal effects on the hypothalamus and limbic and reticular systems. The phenothiazine psychotropic drugs now number several hundred, the chief component being the phenothiazine nucleus.

CPZ at low concentrations reduces enhanced neuronal respiration due to electrical (McIlwain and Greengard, 1957) or cationic (Lindan *et al.*, 1957) stimulation, the former being the more sensitive process, indicating an effect on cation permeability at the brain cell membrane. The drug affects mitochondrial metabolism perhaps by its action at the membrane (Løvtrup, 1967). It also uncouples phosphorylation associated with the oxidation of NADH by the cytochrome system and of ferrocytochrome *c* (see Gabay, 1971, for references). It is capable of suppressing, in the brain, oxidative synthesis of ATP. It differs from the barbiturates in bringing about progressive inhibition of neuronal respiratory processes and in its high binding powers with various tissue proteins. It affects various enzymes, the effects differing according to the concentration of the drug and the nature of the enzyme. For example, Gey *et al.* (1965) have found that the level of hexosephosphates in rat brain is diminished from the normal level at the time of maximum depression following the injection of CPZ. They suggest that the drug, in common with some other depressants, acts by suppressing glucose phosphorylation. Again, glutamate dehydrogenase activity is suppressed by CPZ at quite low concentrations (e.g., 25 μM), and it is thought that this may be related to the pharmacological action of the drug (Shemisa and Fahien, 1971).

It seems unlikely, however, that the many effects of CPZ on brain respiratory and phosphorylation systems are directly related to the action of phenothiazines as antipsychotic agents, the concentrations required for significant effects being on the whole much higher than those required for effects on behavior. It seems more likely that their activities at low concentrations are associated with alterations in membrane permeability to cations and perhaps especially to biogenic amines. Giarman and Schanberg (1962) found that the drug frees 5-HT from its bound condition and increases its amount in the brain. The increased monoamine concentrations resulting from administration of monoamine oxidase inhibitors are diminished by CPZ. This drug, as well as several other phenothiazines, causes release of particle-bound epinephrine in adrenal gland preparations. Altered cell membrane permeability may explain why CPZ diminishes the uptake of circulatory norepinephrine in heart and adrenal medulla (Axelrod *et al.*, 1961). In fact, there is much information pointing to changes in permeability brought about by CPZ (Bulle, 1957; Bauer and Leonhardt, 1956; Christensen *et al.*, 1958). CPZ suppresses the activity of neurons in the reticular system excited by norepinephrine and potentiates the inhibitory effects of norepinephrine on other responsive cells, possibly by inhibiting reuptake (Schanberg *et al.*, 1967). A number of centrally active drugs, including the phenothiazines, inhibit catecholamine uptake into synaptosomes prepared from various areas of rat brain (Horn *et al.*, 1971). Many of the drugs have markedly different affinities for the dopamine neurons of the corpus striatum as compared with those for the norepinephrine neurons in other brain regions.

According to Matthyse (1973), enhancement of dopamine turnover is a characteristic of the antipsychotic group of the phenothiazines, but it is not clear whether the effects of these drugs on dopamine metabolism are related to their effects on the mental state or only to their extrapyramidal side effects. The enhancement of turnover is considered to be a consequence of blockade of dopamine receptor sites (see Horn, Chap. 6, Vol. 2; York, Chap. 2, Vol. 6).

5.3. Imipramine

The isosteric replacement of sulfur in the phenothiazine nucleus with an ethylene bridge yields a major antidepressant drug, imipramine. It is a potent inhibitor of the reuptake process at the cell membrane of norepinephrine (Carlsson, 1966; Kopin, 1966) that is released at the synapse both in peripheral sympathetic nerves and in the brain (Glowinski and Axelrod, 1964). (For a review of the role of biogenic amines in mediating the action of antidepressant drugs, see Schildkraut and Gershon, 1971.) It would seem that the antidepressant action of the tricyclic agents is due to enhancement of central adrenergic transmission by block of reuptake of centrally released norepinephrine (Carlsson and Waldeck, 1965), but a change in its metabolism may also be involved (see Iversen, Chap. 7, Vol. 3; Horn, Chap. 6, Vol. 2).

Studies of the effects of tricyclic antidepressants on the metabolism of biogenic amines suggest (Schildkraut and Gershon, 1971) that these drugs may inhibit the deamination of norepinephrine by mitochondrial amine oxidase. This effect need not necessarily be due to direct inhibition of the enzyme, but, perhaps, by an effect at the membrane these drugs may prevent the amine from reacting with the enzyme (Schildkraut *et al.*, 1964). Imipramine will reverse reserpine sedation if it is administered before the reserpine; its effect is to suppress the inactivation of released norepinephrine (Snyder, 1970). Carlsson *et al.* (1968) consider that another process that may be involved is the selective inhibition of reuptake of 5-HT by the appropriate neurons.

5.4. Amphetamines

Recent data indicate that many of the central actions of amphetamine, including locomotor stimulation and sterotyped behavior, are mediated through brain catecholamines (Stein and Wise, 1969; Stein, 1964; Glowinski *et al.*, 1966*a*; Carr and Moore, 1969). Its effects are potentiated by desmethylimipramine (Sulser *et al.*, 1966), which brings about an increase in the brain concentration of *d*-amphetamine owing to an inhibition of the *p*-hydroxylation of this drug. However, there is a possiblity that the enhancement of the action of amphetamine by the tricyclic antidepressant may be due partly to block of reuptake of catecholamines released by amphetamine at adrenergic receptor sites (Sulser and Sanders-Bush, 1971).

Amphetamine treatment of animals causes a lowering of brain norepinephrine but not of brain 5-HT. It seems that the excitatory effect of the drug may be explained by the fact that released norepinephrine is metabolized primarily by *O*-methylation, partly outside the presynaptic neuron. Large decreases in the effects of amphetamine are observed if the norepinephrine levels in the brain are depleted by α-methyl-*p*-tyrosine, an inhibitor of norepinephrine biosynthesis (Weissman *et al.*, 1966). This action of amphetamine is restored by giving dihydroxyphenylalanine (Randrup and Munkvad, 1966; Weissman *et al.*, 1966). The excitatory effects of amphetamine are potentiated by monoamine oxidase inhibitors that presumably act by suppressing the oxidation of the released norepinephrine (Stein and Wise, 1971). The exact nature of the releasing action of amphetamine on norepinephrine is not known. There is reason to believe that the drug does not simply displace norepinephrine from storage sites but that it potentiates its release both by its ability to inhibit monoamine oxidase and by its ability to prevent reuptake of the released transmitter (Stein and Wise, 1971). Glowinski *et al.* (1966*a*) consider that the suppression of monoamine oxidase activity *in vivo* is a cause of the effect of amphetamine on the amine breakdown, but the results of Rutledge (1970) indicate that this may be largely due to an inhibition of neuronal uptake of norepinephrine.

Amphetamine or methamphetamine alters the levels of various biogenic amines in the brain (Smith, 1965; Sanan and Vogt, 1962; Moore and Lariviere, 1963), but the magnitude and type of change may vary with the dose of the drug and the time after administration (Cook and Schanberg, 1968).

d-Amphetamine is more potent than *l*-amphetamine in inhibiting catecholamine uptake by norepinephrine neurons, but they are about equally active in inhibiting catecholamine uptake by the dopamine neurons of the corpus striatum (Taylor and Snyder, 1970). Results of these *in vivo* studies agree with those of earlier *in vitro* studies on the inhibition of uptake of catecholamines by the two isomers into synaptosomes from striatal and nonstriatal brain areas (Coyle and Snyder, 1969; see also Baldessarini, Chap. 2, Vol. 3; Iversen, Chap. 7, Vol. 3).

Low doses of α-methyl-*p*-tyrosine block much of the activity of amphetamine but not of *p*-chloramphetamine except at very high doses. It is known that the chlorinated amphetamines cause a marked long-lasting and selective depletion of cerebral 5-HT (see Sulser and Sanders-Bush, 1971, for references). The accumulation of 5-HT in brain is reduced when animals, after receiving a monoamine oxidase inhibitor, are treated with *p*-methoxyamphetamine or *p*-chlormethamphetamine (Meek and Fuxé, 1971). The drugs appear to release neuronally accumulated 5-HT into the extraneuronal space, either by direct displacement of 5-HT from binding sites or by an action on the nerve cell membrane, perhaps by processes similar to those exercised by amphetamine in the release of norepinephrine and dopamine (Carlsson *et al.*, 1966).

Amphetamine stimulates ACh release from the cerebral cortex (Hemsworth and Neal, 1968), possibly through its catecholamine releasing properties from adrenergic nerve endings. This stimulation *in vivo* is inhibited by the pretreatment of the animals (cats) with α-methyl-*p*-tyrosine

(Nistri *et al.*, 1972). The results support the view that amphetamine increases ACh output at the cerebral cortex by the release of catecholamines from adrenergic nerve endings and these, in turn, stimulate cholinergic pathways.

5.5. Monoamine Oxidase Inhibitors

Many amine analogues, e.g., amphetamines, ephedrine, and iproniazid, are competitive inhibitors of monoamine oxidase (MAO) (see Mussachio, Chap. 1, Vol. 3; Greene and Grahame-Smith, Chap. 4, Vol. 3), and in fact the first example of competitive inhibition of MAO by a psychoactive amine analogue, amphetamine, was described (Mann and Quastel, 1940) in the same year that sulfanilamide was shown to exert its bactericidal action by competition with its analogue *p*-aminobenzoate. It is now believed that MAO plays an important role in controlling the amounts of norepinephrine, 5-HT, and dopamine stored in the brain (Horita, 1970). Its inhibition leads to increases in the concentrations of the bound and free forms of the amine. This is due to suppression of amine breakdown while its synthesis proceeds unaffected.

A potent inhibitor of the enzyme is iproniazid (Zeller *et al.*, 1955), which, in contrast to amphetamine, is highly active in this respect *in vivo*. The drug affects 5-HT and tyramine oxidations similarly, so that its administration leads to a marked increase of endogenous 5-HT. This is increased still further by giving a dose of tryptophan or 5-hydroxytryptophan, which produces abnormalities of electrical potential and mental disturbances (Udenfriend *et al.*, 1957; Shore and Brodie, 1957). Increase of brain 5-HT by iproniazid parallels the potentiation of central effects.

The harmala alkaloids (harmaline and harmine) are potent reversible MAO inhibitors. They are active at 0.1 μM and 10 times more active *in vitro* than the powerful hydrazine derivatives (Freter *et al.*, 1958). Brain levels of catecholamines are increased after administration of such MAO inhibitors (Shore *et al.*, 1957). α-Ethyltryptamine is a stronger inhibitor than amphetamine of MAO (Greig *et al.*, 1961) and brings about marked increases in brain concentrations of 5-HT and epinephrine.

The excitation that occurs in various animal species after administration of MAO inhibitors is associated with increased cerebral levels of norepinephrine (Spector *et al.*, 1963) and normetanephrine (Pletscher, 1968). On giving MAO inhibitors to cats there is an increase in concentration of 5-HT in the effluent from perfused cerebral ventricles (Goodrich, 1969).

The excitation caused by MAO inhibitors has been variously attributed to increased levels of norepinephrine, dopamine, or 5-HT. The inhibitors antagonize the depressant activity of reserpine (Chessin *et al.*, 1957; Spector *et al.*, 1963; Graeff *et al.*, 1965).

It is of interest to compare briefly the effects of various psychotropic drugs that influence catecholamine metabolism and transport at the brain cell membrane (Snyder, 1970). The MAO inhibitors cause an accumulation of norepinephrine in the nerve terminal with possibly a leakage into the synaptic cleft. Reserpine releases norepinephrine within the nerve terminal and, with inactivation by MAO, sedation occurs after the amine has been lost from the brain. Amphetamine releases brain norepinephrine into the synaptic cleft and blocks its reuptake. The released amine then affects postsynaptic receptors. Imipramine drugs inhibit norepinephrine reuptake into nerve terminals and potentiate the activities of synaptically released catecholamines.

5.6. Lysergic Acid Diethylamide (LSD)

LSD elicits effects similar to those brought about by drugs that increase 5-HT levels in the CNS (Page and Carlsson, 1970). It has been thought to owe its potent hallucinogenic effects, perhaps by its possession of an indole nucleus, to interference with the physiological action of 5-HT in the brain (Gaddum, 1954); see, however, Bebbington and Brimblecombe (1969). The various changes brought about by LSD are similar to those following administration of tryptamine, suggesting an action of LSD at tryptamine receptor sites (Martin and Sloan, 1970). The drug increases the 5-HT content of rats brain within 10 min of its administration, but it does not affect synthesis of 5-HT from 5-hydroxytryptophan either *in vivo* or *in vitro*. After inhibition of synthesis of 5-HT (by α-propyldopacetamide), LSD decreases the rate of amine depletion in serotoninergic neurons (Page and Carlsson, 1970). It would seem that serotonin receptor stimulation may be responsible for some of the behavioral effects of LSD.

5.7. Amino Acid Decarboxylase Inhibitors

Various aspects of the inhibition of α-amino acid decarboxylation have been reviewed by Clark (1963).

The formation of GABA by glutamate decarboxylation, which has an important role as an inhibitory transmitter in the CNS, is affected by amino acid decarboxylase inhibitors, which therefore may greatly affect the cerebral concentrations of this transmitter. Interference with amino acid decarboxylation *in vitro* can be brought about by amino acid analogues such as α-methyltryptophan or α-methylhistidine. 2-Hydroxy- and 2:5-dihydroxytryptophan are inhibitors of 5-hydroxytryptophan decarboxylase (Freter *et al.*, 1958).

In vivo inhibition of dihydroxyphenylalanine decarboxylation can be brought about by administration of α-methyldopa, which is clinically used as an antihypertensive agent that can occasionally precipitate psychotic depression. The relevant decarboxylase is competitively inhibited by α-methyldopa, which brings about a rapid fall in the concentrations of cerebral dopamine and norepinephrine. There is also a fall in cerebral 5-HT. The drug inhibits dopamine formation when exogenous dihydroxyphenylalanine and certain other amino acids are administered (Sourkes and D'Iorio, 1963). Pletscher *et al.* (1964) consider that the decrease of norepinephrine in various tissues by α-methyldopa is related more to a displacement or release mechanism rather than wholly to an inhibition of the relevant decarboxylase. α-Methyldopa is also decarboxylated to form α-methyldopamine, and this can be converted to α-methylnorepinephrine, which may be stored in the norepinephrine synaptic vesicles. It may be liberated, on nerve stimulation, as a "false transmitter." If depression is related to a deficiency of norepinephrine at synapses in the brain (Schildkraut, 1965), the production of an inactive false transmitter by α-methyldopa might explain why this drug can cause depression (Snyder, 1970). The amine-depleting action of α-methyldopa is matched by that of the related substance β-methyl-*m*-tyrosine, which can cause a rapid depletion of both cerebral dopamine and norepinephrine (Sourkes, 1962).

6. ETHANOL

Various aspects of the mode of action of ethanol in the CNS have been reviewed by Wallgren (1966, 1971) and will be touched on only briefly in this chapter.

The depressant action of ethanol in the body is shown by the diminished oxygen consumption and glucose utilization in the human brain in heavy alcohol intoxication, with blood alcohol levels of about 0.3% or more, while the cerebral blood flow increases (Fazekas *et al.*, 1955). *In vivo* observations of cerebral metabolites after alcohol administration (Wallgren, 1971) are consistent with the conclusion that the depression caused by alcohol leads to diminished activities of cerebral glycolytic processes, and those of the citric acid cycle, similar to what is observed with general depressants and described earlier in this chapter.

Ethanol and higher alcohols have little or no suppressing effects at anesthetic concentrations on mitochondrial respiration (Wolpert *et al.*, 1956; Beer and Quastel, 1958). They act presumably at the cell membrane, affecting cation transport, for they are able to suppress the stimulation of brain cortex respiration *in vitro* by K^+ (Beer and Quastel, 1958; Majchrowicz, 1965) or by electrical pulses (Wallgren and Kulonen, 1960). Electrically stimulated brain cortex respiration is more sensitive than K^+-stimulated respiration to ethanol. Depression of electrically stimulated brain respiration occurs at concentrations of alcohols compatible with reversibility *in vivo* (Lindbohm and Wallgren, 1962). It appears that the effect of ethanol at relatively small concentrations is linked with the changes of cation permeabilities associated with neuronal excitation. The alcohols do not uncouple oxidative phosphorylation (Truitt *et al.*, 1956) but can affect cerebral microsomal ATPase (Järnefelt, 1961), the action being competitive with K^+ and not with Na^+ (Israël *et al.*, 1965). Ethanol seems to act directly on excitation in squid giant axons (Moore, 1966), particularly sodium conductance. It seems likely that the pharmacological effects of ethanol are largely connected with cation permeability changes at the neuronal membrane.

7. REFERENCES

Abadom, P. N., and Scholefield, P. G., 1962, Amino acid transport in brain cortex slices, *Canad. J. Biochem. Physiol.* **40:**1575–1618.

Abdel-Latif, A. A., and Abood, L. G., 1964, Biochemical studies on mitochondria and other cytoplasmic fractions of developing rat brain, *J. Neurochem.* **11:**9–15.

Abdel-Latif, A. A., Brody, J., and Ramahi, H., 1967, Studies on Na-K-ATPase of nerve endings and appearance of electrical activity in developing rat brain, *J. Neurochem.* **14:**1133–1141.

Aldridge, W. N., 1962, in: *Ciba Foundation Symposium on Enzymes and Drug Action* (J. L. Mongar and A. V. S. de Reuck, eds.), p. 155, Churchill, London.

Aldridge, W. N., and Parker, V. H., 1960, Barbiturates and oxidative phosphorylation, *Biochem. J.* **76:**47–56.

Andrejew, A., and Rosenberg, A. J., 1956, Action de chlorpromazine, 2:4dinitrophenol, penthiobarbital et soneryl sur l'activité de ATP-ase, *C. R. Soc. Biol. Paris* **150:**681–683.

Ariens, E. J. (ed.), 1964, *Molecular Pharmacology*, Academic Press, New York.

Axelrod, J., Whitby, L. G., and Hertting, G., 1961, Effect of psychotropic drugs on the uptake of ^{3}H-norepinephrine by tissues, *Science* **133:**383–384.

Bachelard, H. S., and Lindsay, J. R., 1966, Effects of neurotropic drugs on glucose metabolism in rat brain *in vivo, Biochem. Pharmacol.* **15:**1053–1058.

Bachelard, H. S., Gaitonde, M. K., and Vrba, R., 1966, Effects of psychotropic drugs on the utilization of glucose carbon atoms in the brain, heart and liver of the rat, *Biochem. Pharmacol.* **15:**1039–1043.

Bachelard, H. S., 1971, Specificity and kinetic property of monosaccharide uptake into guinea pig cerebral cortex *in vitro, J. Neurochem.* **18:**213–222.

Bachelard, H. S., Clark, A. G., and Thompson, M. F., 1971, Cerebral cortex hexokinases, *Biochem. J.* **123:**707–715.

Bachelard, H. S., Daniel, P. M., Love, E. R., and Pratt, O. E., 1973, Transport of glucose into the brain of rat *in vivo, Proc. Roy. Soc. Lond. Ser. B* **183:**71–82.

Baker, P. F., Hodgkin, A. L., and Ridgeway, E. B., 1970, Two phases of Ca^{++} entry during the action potentials in giant axons of *Loligo, J. Physiol.* **208:**80P.

Balcar, V. J., and Johnston, G. A. R., 1972, Glutamate uptake by brain slices and its relation to the depolarization of neurons by acidic amino acids, *J. Neurobiol.* **3:**295–301.

Bauer, K. F., and Leonhardt, H., 1956, A contribution to the pathological physiology of the blood brain barrier, *J. Comp. Neurol.* **106:**363–370.

BAXTER, C. F., and ROBERTS, E., 1961, Elevation of GABA in brain: Selective inhibition of GABA-α-ketoglutaric acid transaminase, *J. Biol. Chem.* **236:**3287–3294.

BEBBINGTON, A., and BRIMBLECOMBE, R. W., 1969, Actions of some psychotomimetics on the CNS, *Brit. Med. Bull.* **25:**293–298.

BEER, C. T., and QUASTEL, J. H., 1958, Effects of aliphatic alcohols on the respiration of rat brain cortex slices and rat brain mitochondria, *Canad. J. Biochem. Physiol.* **36:**543–556.

BENITEZ, D., PSCHEIDT, G. R., and STONE, W. E., 1954, Formation of ammonium ions in the cerebrum in fluoroacetate poisoning, *Am. J. Physiol.* **176:**488–492.

BENJAMIN, A. M., and QUASTEL, J. H., 1972, Locations of amino acids in brain slices from the rat: Tetrodotoxin-sensitive release of amino acids, *Biochem. J.* **128:**631–646.

BENJAMIN, A. M., and QUASTEL, J. H., 1974, Fate of L-glutamate in the brain, *J. Neurochem.* **23:**457–464.

BERL, S., and CLARK, D. D., 1969, Compartmentation of amino acid metabolism, in: *Handbook of Neurochemistry*, Vol. 2 (A. Lajtha, ed.), pp. 447–472, Plenum Press, New York.

BERL, S., and FRIGYESI, T. L., 1969, Effect of reserpine on the turnover of glutamate, glutamine, aspartate and GABA, labelled with (1-^{14}C)-acetate, in caudate nucleus, thalamus, sensorimotor cortex (cat), *Brain Res.* **14:**683–695.

BERL, S., TAKAGAKI, G., CLARKE, D. D., and WAELSCH, H., 1962, Metabolic components *in vivo*: Ammonia and glutamic acid metabolism in brain and liver, *J. Biol. Chem.* **237:**2562–2569.

BERL, S., CLARKE, D. D., and NICKLAS, W. J., 1970, Compartmentation of citric acid cycle metabolism in brain. Effects of aminooxyacetate, ouabain and Ca^{++}, *J. Neurochem.* **17:**999–1007.

BIDDER, T. G., 1968, Hexose translocation across the blood–brain interface, *J. Neurochem.* **15:**867–874.

BIGNAMI, A., PALLADINI, G., and VENTURINI, G., 1966, Na-K-ATPase in the developing chick brain, *Brain Res.* **3:**207–209.

BLACKBURN, K. J., FRENCH, P. C., and MERRILLS, R. J., 1967, 5-Hydroxytryptamine uptake in rat brain *in vitro, Life Sci.* **6:**1653–1663.

BLOOM, F. A., COSTA, E., and SALMOIRAGHI, G. C., 1965, Anesthesia and the responsiveness of individual neurons of the caudate nucleus of the cat to Ach, norepinephrine and dopamine, *J. Pharmacol. Exp. Ther.* **150:**244–252.

BONTING, S. L., CARRAVAGGIO, L. L., and HAWKINS, N. M., 1962, Studies on Na-K-ATPase: Correlation with cation transport sensitive to cardiac glycosides, *Arch. Biochem. Biophys.* **98:**413–419.

BOURKE, R. S., and TOWER, D. B., 1966, Fluid compartmentation and electrolytes of cat cerebral cortex *in vitro, J. Neurochem.* **13:**1071–1099.

BRADLEY, P. B., and DRAY, A., 1973, Modification of the responses of brain stem neurones to transmitter substances by anesthetic agents, *Brit. J. Pharmacol.* **48:**212–224.

BRADLEY, P. B., and WOLSTENCROFT, J. H., 1965, Actions of drugs on single neurones in the brain stem, *Brit. Med. Bull.* **21:**15–18.

BRAGANCA, B. M., FAULKNER, P., and QUASTEL, J. H., 1953, Effects of inhibitors of glutamine synthesis on the inhibition of Ach synthesis in brain slices by ammonium ions, *Biochim. Biophys. Acta* **10:**83–88.

BRIERLEY, G. P., MURER, E., BACHMANN, E., and GREEN, D. E., 1963, Studies on ion transport: Accumulation of phosphate and magnesium ions by heart mitochondria, *J. Biol. Chem.* **238:**3482–3489.

BRODIE, B. B., FINGER, K. F., ORLANS, F. B., QUINN, G. P., and SULSER, F., 1960*a*, Evidence that tranquilising action of reserpine is associated with changes in brain serotonin and not in brain norepinephrine, *J. Pharmacol. Exp. Ther.* **129:**250–256.

BRODIE, B. B., DENGLER, H. J., TITUS, E., and WILSON, C. W. M., 1960*b*, Inhibition of the uptake of catecholamines in brain tissue by reserpine, *J. Physiol.* **154:**37P.

BRODIE, B. B., COMER, M. S., COSTA, E., and DLABAC, A., 1966, Role of brain serotonin in the mechanism of the central action of reserpine, *J. Pharmacol. Exp. Ther.* **152:**340–349.

Bull, R. J., and Trevor, A. J., 1972, Saxitoxin, tetrodotoxin and the metabolism and cation fluxes in isolated cerebral tissues, *J. Neurochem.* **19:**999–1009.

Bulle, P. H., 1957, Effects of reserpine and chlorpromazine in prevention of cerebral edema and reversible cell damage, *Proc. Soc. Exp. Biol. Med.* **94:**553–556.

Bunker, J. P., and Vandam, L. D., 1965, Effects of anesthesia on metabolism and cellular functions, *Pharm. Rev.* **17:**183–263.

Caldwell, P. C., and Keynes, R. D., 1959, Effect of ouabain on the efflux of Na^+ from a squid giant axons, *J. Physiol.* **148:**8P.

Carlsson, A., 1966, Pharmacological depletion of catecholamine stores, *Pharmacol. Rev.* **18:**541–549.

Carlsson, A., and Waldeck, B., 1965, Mechanisms of amine transport in the cell membranes of adrenergic nerves, *Acta Pharmacol.* **22:**293–300.

Carlsson, A., Fuxé, K., Hamberger, B., and Lindqvist, M., 1966, Biochemical and histochemical studies on the effects of imipramine-like drugs and of amphetamine on central and peripheral catecholamine neurons, *Acta Physiol. Scand.* **67:**481–497.

Carlsson, A., Fuxé, K., and Unterstedt, U., 1968, Effect of imipramine on central 5-HT neurons, *J. Pharm. Pharmacol.* **20:**150–151.

Carr, L. A., and Moore, K. E., 1969, Norepinephrine release from brain by *d*-amphetamine *in vivo, Science* **164:**322–323.

Catchlove, R. F. H., Krnjević, K., and Maretic, H., 1972, Similarity between effects of general anesthetics and dinitrophenol on cortical neurons, *Canad. J. Physiol. Pharmacol.* **50:**1111–1114.

Chan, S. L., and Quastel, J. H., 1967, Tetrodotoxin effects on brain metabolism *in vitro, Science* **156:**1752–1753.

Chan, S. L., and Quastel, J. H., 1970, Effects of neurotropic drugs on sodium influx into rat brain cortex *in vitro, Biochem. Pharmacol.* **19:**1071–1085.

Chance, B., and Hollunger, G., 1963, Inhibition of electron and energy transfer in mitochondria, *J. Biol. Chem.* **278:**418–431.

Chappell, J. B., and Crofts, A. R., 1965, Calcium ion accumulation and volume changes of isolated liver mitochondria, *Biochem. J.* **95:**378–386.

Chappell, J. B., Cohn, M., and Greville, G. D., 1963, in: *Energy-Linked Functions of Mitochondria* (B. Chance, ed.), p. 319, Academic Press, New York.

Cherayil, A., Kandera, J., and Lajtha, A., 1967, Cerebral amino acid transport. Effect of inhibitors on exit, *J. Neurochem.* **14:**105–115.

Chessin, M., Kramer, E. R., and Scott, C. T., 1957, Modification of the pharmacology of reserpine and serotonin by iproniazid, *J. Pharmacol. Exp. Ther.* **119:**453–460.

Christensen, J., Feng, Y. S. L., Polley, E., and Wase, A. W., 1958, Influence of chlorpromazine on transport of ions into cerebral tissue, *Fed. Proc.* **17:**358.

Clark, G. M., and Eiseman, B., 1958, Studies in ammonia metabolism: Biochemical changes in brain tissue of dogs during ammonia induced coma, *New Engl. J. Med.* **259:**178–180.

Clark, W. G., 1963, Inhibition of amino acid decarboxylases, in: *Metabolic Inhibitors,* Vol. 1 (R. M. Hochster and J. H. Quastel, eds.), pp. 315–381, Academic Press, New York.

Clarke, D. D., Nicklas, W. J., and Berl, S., 1970, Tricarboxylic acid cycle metabolism in brain: Effects of fluoroacetate and fluorocitrate, *Biochem. J.* **120:**345–351.

Clouet, D. H., 1971, Alteration of brain metabolism by narcotic analgesic drugs, in: *Handbook of Neurochemistry,* Vol. 6 (A. Lajtha, ed.), pp. 479–499, Plenum Press, New York.

Collins, G. G. S., 1973, Effects of aminooxyacetate, thiosemicarbazide and haloperidol on the metabolism of glutamate and GABA in rat brain, *Biochem. Pharmacol.* **22:**101–111.

Cook, J., and Schanberg, S., 1968, Effect of methamphetamine on norepinephrine metabolism in brain, *Pharmacologist* **10:**195.

Coyle, J. T., and Snyder, S. H., 1969, Catecholamine uptake by synaptosomes and in homogenates of rat tissue: Stereospecificity in different areas, *J. Pharmacol. Exp. Ther.* **170:**221–231.

CRAWFORD, J. M., 1970, Anesthetic agents and the chemical sensitivity of cortical neurons, *Neuropharmacology* **9:**31–46.

CREMER, J. E., 1967, Studies on brain cortex slices: Influence of inhibitors on retention of K^+ and amino acids with glucose or pyruvate as substrate, *Biochem. J.* **104:**223–228.

CRONE, C., 1965, Facilitated transfer of glucose from blood into brain tissue, *J. Physiol.* **181:**103–113.

CUMMINS, J., and HYDEN, H., 1962, ATP levels and ATPase in neurons, glia and neuronal membranes of the vestibular nucleus, *Biochim. Biophys. Acta* **60:**271–275.

DAVIDOFF, R. A., GRAYSON, V., and ADAIR, R., 1973, GABA-transaminase inhibitors and presynaptic inhibition in the amphibian spinal cord, *Am. J. Physiol.* **224:**1230–1234.

DAVIS, F. A., and DETTBARN, W. D., 1962, Depolarizing action of Ca^{++} depletion in frog nerve and its inhibition by compounds acting on the Ach system, *Biochim. Biophys. Acta* **63:**349–357.

DAWKINS, M. J. R., JUDAH, J. D., and REES, K. R., 1959, Mechanism of action of chlorpromazine, *Biochem. J.* **73:**16–23.

DAWSON, R. M. C., 1953, Cerebral amino acids in fluoroacetate-poisoned, anesthetised and hypoglycaemic rats, *Biochim. Biophys. Acta* **11:**548–552.

DENGLER, H. G., SPIEGEL, H. E., and TITUS, E. O., 1961, Effect of drugs on the uptake of isotopic norepinephrine by cat tissues, *Nature* **191:**816–817.

DETTBARN, W. D., 1967, The Ach system in peripheral nerve, *Ann. N.Y. Acad. Sci.* **144:** Art. 2, p. 483.

DETTBARN, W. D., 1971, Local anesthetics, in: *Handbook of Neurochemistry*, Vol. 6 (A. Lajtha, ed.), pp. 423–440, Plenum Press, New York.

DIAMOND, I., 1971, Choline metabolism in brain, *Arch. Neurol.* **24:**333–339.

DONALDSON, J., MINICH, J., and BARBEAU, A., 1972, Ouabain induced seizures in rats, *Canad. J. Biochem.* **50:**888–896.

DRAKONTIDES, A. B., SCHNEIDER, J. A., and FUNDERBARK, W. H., 1962, Some effects of sodium γ-hydroxybutyrate on the CNS, *J. Pharmacol. Exp. Ther.* **135:**275–284.

DUNHAM, E. T., and GLYNN, I. M., 1961, ATP-ase activity and the active movements of alkali metal ions, *J. Physiol.* **156:**274–293.

EILER, J. P., and MCEWEN, W. K., 1949, Effect of pentobarbital on aerobic phosphorylation in brain homogenates, *Arch. Biochem.* **20:**163–165.

ELLIOTT, H. W., and SUTHERLAND, V. C., 1952, The oxygen uptake of human cerebral cortex and the effects of some inhibitors, *J. Cell. Comp. Physiol.* **40:**221–241.

ERNSTER, L., LOW, H., and LINDBERG, O., 1955, The action of Amytal on the oxidation of NADH in rat liver mitochondria, *Acta Chem. Scand.* **9:**200–201.

ERWIN, V. G., TABAKOFF, B., and BRONAUGH, R. L., 1971, Inhibition of a NADPH-linked aldehyde reductase from bovine brain by barbiturates, *Mol. Pharmacol.* **7:**169–176.

ESTABROOK, R. S., and MACKLER, B., 1957, Enzymatic and spectrophotometric studies of a reduced NADoxidase preparation from heart muscle, *J. Biol. Chem.* **229:**1091–1103.

FAZEKAS, J. F., ALBERT, S. N., and ALMAN, R. W., 1955, Influence of chlorpromazine and alcohol on cerebral neurodynamics and metabolism, *Am. J. Med. Sci.* **230:**128–132.

FEINSTEIN, M. B., 1964, Reaction of local anesthetics with phospholipids: A possible chemical basis for anesthesia, *J. Gen. Physiol.* **48:**357–374.

FINDLAY, M., SKICKLAND, K. P., and ROSSITER, R. J., 1954, Incorporation of radioactive phosphate into non-nucleotide protein-bound phosphorus fractions of respiring cat brain slices, *Canad. J. Biochem. Physiol.* **32:**504–514.

FOLBERGROVA, J., 1963, Effect of methionine sulfoximine on the protein metabolism of brain cortex slices, *J. Neurochem.* **10:**775–782.

FOLBERGROVA, J., 1964, Free glutamine levels in the rat brain *in vivo* after methionine sulfoximine administration, *Physiol. Bohemoslav.* **13:**21–27.

FOLBERGROVA, J., PASSONEAU, J. V., LOWRY, O. H., and SCHULTZ, D. W., 1969, Glycogen, ammonia, and related metabolites in the brain during seizures evoked by methionine sulfoximine, *J. Neurochem.* **16:**191–203.

FRETER, K., WEISSBACH, H., REDFIELD, B., UDENFRIEND, S., and WITKOP, B., 1958, Analogs of 5-hydroxy-tryptamine, and -tryptophan, as inhibitors of the biosynthesis and breakdown of serotonin, *J. Am. Chem. Soc.* **80:**983–987.

FUJISAWA, H., KAJIKAWA, K., OHI, Y., HOSHIMOTO, Y., and YOSHIDA, H., 1965, Movement of radioactive Ca^{++} in brain slices and influence of protoveratrine, ouabain, KCl and cocaine, *Jap. J. Pharmacol.* **15:**327–334.

GABAY, S., 1971, Phenothiazines; Neurochemical aspects of their mode of action, in: *Handbook of Neurochemistry* (A. Lajtha, ed.) **6:**325–348, Plenum Press, New York.

GADDUM, J. H., 1954, in: Hypertension; Humoral and Neurogenic Factors, *Ciba Foundation Symposium,* p. 75, Churchill, London.

GATFIELD, P. D., LOWRY, O. H., SCHULTZ, D. W., and PASSONEAU, J. V., 1966, Regional energy reserves in mouse brain and changes with ischemia and anesthesia, *J. Neurochem,* **13:**185–195.

GEDDES, H., and QUASTEL, J. H., 1956, Effects of local anesthetics on respiration of rat brain cortex *in vitro, Anesthesiology* **17:**666–671.

GERSHFELD, N. L. and SHANES, A. M., 1959, Antagonism of veratrine by Ca^{++} in monolayers of stearic acid, *Science* **129:**1427–1428.

GEY, K. F., RUTIHAUSER, M., and PLETSCHER, A., 1965, Suppression of glycolysis in rat brain *in vivo* by chlorpromazine, reserpine and phenobarbital, *Biochem. Pharmacol.* **14:**507–514.

GHOSH, J. J., and QUASTEL, J. H., 1954, Narcotics and brain respiration, *Nature,* Lond. **174:**28–31.

GIARMAN, N. J., and SCHANBERG, S. M., 1962, Drug induced alterations of subcellular distribution of 5HT in rat brain, *Biochem. Pharmacol.* **9:**93–96.

GIARMAN, N. J., and SCHMIDT, K. F., 1963, Some neurochemical aspects of the depressant action of γ-butyrolactone in the CNS, *Brit. J. Pharmacol. Chemother.* **20:**563–568.

GLICK, N., 1972, Inhibition of transport reactions, in: *Metabolic Inhibitors,* Vol. 3 (R. M. Hochster, M. Kates, and J. H. Quastel, eds.), pp. 1–45, Academic Press, New York.

GLOWINSKI, J., and AXELROD, J., 1964, Inhibition of uptake of ^{3}H-norepinephrine in the intact rat brain by imipramine and related compounds, *Nature* **204:**1318–1319.

GLOWINSKI, J., AXELROD, J., and IVERSEN, L. L., 1966*a*, Regional studies of catecholamines in rat brain: Effects of drugs on the disposition and metabolism of ^{3}H-norepinephrine and ^{3}H-dopamine, *J. Pharmacol. Exp. Ther.* **153:**30–41.

GLOWINSKI, J., IVERSEN, L. L., and AXELROD, J., 1966*b*, Storage and synthesis of norepinephrine in the reserpine treated rat brain, *J. Pharmacol. Exp. Ther.* **151:**385–399.

GODFRAIND, J. M., KAWAMURA, H., KRNJEVIĆ, K., and PUMAIN, R., 1971, Actions of dinitrophenol and some other metabolic inhibitors or cortical neurones, *J. Physiol.* **215:**199–222.

GOLDBERG, N. D., PASSONEAU, J. V., and LOWRY, O. H., 1966, Effects of changes in brain metabolism on the levels of citric acid cycle intermediates, *J. Biol. Chem.* **241:**3997–4003.

GOLDMAN, D. E., and BLAUSTEIN, M. P., 1966, Ions, drugs and the axon membrane, *Ann. N.Y. Acad. Sci.* **137:** Art. 2, 967–981.

GONDA, O., and QUASTEL, J. H., 1962, Effects of ouabain on cerebral metabolism and transport mechanisms *in vitro, Biochem. J.* **84:**394–406.

GONDA, O., and QUASTEL, J. H., 1963, Effects of acetylsalicylate and 2:4-dinitrophenol on metabolism and transport in rat brain cortex *in vitro, Canad. J. Biochem. Physiol.* **41:**435–454.

GONDA, O., and QUASTEL, J. H., 1966, Transport and metabolism of acetate in rat brain cortex *in vitro, Biochem. J.* **100:**83–94.

GOODCHILD, M., and NEAL, M. J., 1973, Uptake of ^{3}H-GABA by the retina, *Brit. J. Pharmacol.* **47:**529–542.

GOODRICH, C. A., 1969, Effect of monoamine oxidase inhibitors on 5-hydroxy-tryptamine output from perfused cerebral ventricles of anesthetised cat, *Brit. J. Pharmacol.* **37:**87–93.

GOTTESFELD, Z., and ELLIOTT, K. A. C., 1971, Factors that affect binding and uptake of GABA by brain tissue, *J. Neurochem.* **18:**683–690.

GRAEFF, F. G., LEME, J. G., and ROCHE E SILVA, M., 1965, Role played by catechol and indoleamines in the central actions of reserpine after monoamineoxidase inhibition, *Int. J. Neuropharmacol.* **4:**17–26.

GREIG, M. E., SEAY, P. H., and FREYBURGER, W. A., 1961, The pharmacology of etryptamine, *J. Neuropsychiat.* **2:**131–135 (Suppl. 1).

GREWAAL, D. S., and QUASTEL, J. H., 1973, Control of synthesis and release of radioactive Ach in brain slices from the rat, *Biochem. J.* **132:**1–14.

HABER, B., 1965, Effects of hydroxylamine and aminooxyacetate on the cerebral *in vitro* utilisation of glucose, fructose, glutamate and GABA, *Canad. J. Biochem.* **43:**865–876.

HAGA, T., 1971, Synthesis and release of ^{14}C-Ach in synaptosomes, *J. Neurochem.* **18:**781–798.

HAMMERSTAD, J. P., and CUTLER, R. W. P., 1972, Na^+ movements and the spontaneous and electrically stimulated release of GABA and glutamate from rat cortical slices, *Brain Res.* **47:**401–413.

HARPUR, R. P., and QUASTEL, J. H., 1949, Relations between Ach synthesis and metabolism of carbohydrates and *d*-glucosamine in the CNS, *Nature* **164:**779–784.

HATHWAY, D. E., and MALLINSON, A., 1964, Chemical studies in relation to convulsive conditions, *Biochem. J.* **90:**51–60.

HATHWAY, D. E., MALLINSON, A., and AKINTONWA, D. A., 1965, Effects of dieldrin, picrotoxin and telodrin on the metabolism of ammonia in brain, *Biochem. J.* **94:**676–686.

HEALD, P. J., 1954, Rapid changes in creatine phosphate level in cerebral cortex slices, *Biochem. J.* **57:**673–679.

HEMSWORTH, B. A., and NEAL, M. J., 1968, Effect of central stimulant drugs on the release of Ach from the cerebral cortex, *Brit. J. Pharm. Chemother.* **32:**543–550.

HERTTING, G., AXELROD, J., and WHITBY, L. G., 1961, Effects of drugs on the uptake and metabolism of ^{3}H-norepinephrine, *J. Pharmacol. Exp. Ther.* **134:**146–153.

HILLMAN, H. H., CAMPBELL, W. J., and MCILWAIN, H., 1963, Membrane potentials in isolated and electrically stimulated mammalian cerebral cortex, *J. Neurochem.* **10:**325–339.

HIMWICH, H., 1951, *Brain Metabolism and Cerebral Disorders*, pp. 298–301, Williams and Wilkins, Baltimore.

HIMWICH, W. A., HOMBURGER, E., MARESCA, R., and HIMWICH, H. E., 1947, Brain metabolism in man: unanesthetized and in pentothal narcosis, *Am. J. Psychiat.* **103:**689–696.

HODGKIN, A. L., 1966, *The Nature of the Nerve Impulse*, p. 108, University Press, Liverpool.

HOLZBAUER, M., and VOGT, M., 1956, Depression by reserpine of the noradrenaline concentration in the hypothalamus of the cat, *J. Neurochem.* **1:**8–11.

HOPPER, S., and SEGAL, H. L., 1964, Comparative properties of glutamic-alanine transaminases from several sources, *Arch. Biochem. Biophys.* **105:**501–505.

HORITA, A., 1970, Pharmacology of monoamine oxidase inhibitor antidepressants, in: *Principles of Psychopharmacology* (W. G. Clarke and J. del Giudice, eds.), pp. 279–287, Academic Press, New York.

HORN, A. S., COYLE, J. T., and SNYDER, S. H., 1971, Catecholamine uptake by synaptosomes from rat brain, *Mol. Pharmacol.* **7:**66–80.

HORTON, R. W., MELDRUM, B. S., and BACHELARD, H. S., 1973, Enzymic and cerebral metabolic effects of 2-deoxyglucose, *J. Neurochem.* **21:**507–520.

HOSEIN, E. A., STACHIEWICZ, E., BOURNE, W., and DENSTEDT, O. F., 1955, The influence of nitrous oxide on the metabolic activity of brain tissue, *Anesthesiology* **16:**708–715.

HULME, N. A., and KRANTZ, J. C., 1955, Effect of ethylether on oxidative phosphorylation in the brain, *Anesthesiology* **16:**627–631.

ISRAËL, Y., KALANT, H., and LAUFER, I., 1965, Effects of ethanol on microsomal ATPase, *Biochem. Pharmacol.* **14:**1803–1814.

IVERSEN, L. L., and JOHNSTON, G. A. R., 1971, GABA uptake in rat CNS: Comparison of uptake in slices and homogenates and effects of some inhibitors, *J. Neurochem.* **18:**1939–1950.

IVERSEN, L. L., GLOWINSKI, J., and AXELROD, J., 1965, Uptake and storage of ^{3}H-norepinephrine in the reserpine treated rat heart, *J. Pharmacol. Exp. Ther.* **150:**173–183.

IZUMI, K., DONALDSON, J., MINNICH, J., and BARBEAU, A., 1973, Ouabain-induced seizures in rats: Relationship to brain monoamines, *Canad. J. Biochem.* **51:**198–203.

JALLING, O., LINDBERG, O., and ERNSTER, L., 1955, On the effect of substituted barbiturates on mitochondrial respiration, *Acta Chem. Scand.* **9:**198–199.

JÄRNEFELT, J., 1961, Inhibition of brain microsomal ATPase by depolarizing agents, *Biochim. Biophys. Acta* **48:**111–116.

JOHNSON, E. S., ROBERTS, M. H. T., and STRAUGHAN, D. W., 1969, Responses of cortical neurons to monoamines under differing anesthetic conditions, *J. Physiol.* **203:**261–280.

JOHNSON, W. J., and QUASTEL, J. H., 1953, A comparison of the effects of narcotics and of 2:4-dinitrophenol on sulfanilamide acetylation, *J. Biol. Chem.* **205:**163–171.

JONES, D. A., and MCILWAIN, H., 1971, Amino acid production and translocation in incubated and superfused tissues from the brain, *J. Neurobiol.* **2:**311–326.

KAO, C. Y., 1966, Tetrodotoxin, saxitoxin and their significance in the study of excitation phenomena, *Pharmacol. Rev.* **18:**997–1049.

KINI, M. M., and QUASTEL, J. H., 1959, Carbohydrate-amino acid interrelations in brain cortex *in vitro, Nature* **184:**252–256.

KINI, M. M., and QUASTEL, J. H., 1960, Effects of veratrine and cocaine on cerebral carbohydrate–amino acid interrelations, *Science* **131:**412–414.

KOLOUSEK, J., and JIRACEK, U., 1959, Stickstoff Metabolismus des Gehirns und der Leber bei Ratten nach einer Applikation von Methionine sulfoximine, *J. Neurochem.* **4:**178–181.

KOPIN, J., 1966, Biochemical aspects of release of norepinephrine and other amines from synpathetic nerve endings, *Pharmacol. Rev.* **18:**513–523.

KRNJEVIĆ, K., 1972, Excitable membranes and anesthetics, in: *Cellular Biology and Toxicity of Anesthetics*, (B. R. Fink, ed.), pp. 3–9, Williams and Wilkins, Baltimore.

KRNJEVIĆ, K., and PHILLIS, J. W., 1963, Ach sensitive cells in the cerebral cortex, *J. Physiol.* **166:**296–327.

KUFFLER, S. W., 1967, Neuroglial cells: Physiological properties and a K^+-mediated effect of neuronal activity on the glial membrane potential, *Proc. Roy. Soc. Lond. Ser. B* **168:** 1–21.

KUFFLER, S. W., and NICHOLLS, J. G., 1966, The physiology of neuroglial cells, *Ergeb. Physiol.* **57:**1–90.

KUHAR, M. J., and SNYDER, S. H., 1970, The subcellular distribution of free ^{3}H-glutamic acid in rat cerebral cortex slices, *J. Pharmacol. Exp. Ther.* **171:**141–152.

KUNZ, H. A., and SULSER, F., 1957, Uber die Hemming des activen Kationen transport durch Herz glykoside, *Experientia* **13:**365–367.

LABORIT, H. M., 1964, Sodium 4-hydroxybutyrate, *Int. J. Neuropharmacol.* **3:**433–457.

LABORIT, H. M., and SANSEIGNE, A., 1970, Pharmacology of antipsychotic drugs, in: *Principles of Psychopharmacology* (W. G. Clark and J. del Giudice, eds.), pp. 259–267.

LAHIRI, S., and LAJTHA, A., 1964, Cerebral amino acid transport *in vitro*: Some requirements and properties of uptake, *J. Neurochem.* **11:**77–86.

LAHIRI, S., and QUASTEL, J. H., 1963, Fluoroacetate and the metabolism of ammonia in brain, *Biochem. J.* **89:**157–163.

LAMAR, C., and SELLINGER, O. Z., 1965, Inhibition *in vivo* of cerebral glutamine synthetase and glutamine transferase by methionine sulfoximine, *Biochem. Pharmacol.* **14:**489–506.

LARRABEE, M. G., and POSTERNAK, J. M., 1952, Selective action of anesthetics on synapses and axons in mammalian sympathetic ganglia, *J. Neurophysiol.* **15:**91–99.

LAZLO, J., HUMPHREYS, S. R., and GOLDIN, A., 1960, Effects of glucose analogs (2-deoxyglucose) on experimental tumors, *J. Natl. Cancer Inst.* **24:**267–281.

LEHNINGER, A. L., ROSSI, C. S., and GREENAWALT, J. W., 1963, Respiration dependent accumulation of inorganic phosphate and Ca^{++}, *Biochem. Biophys. Res. Commun.* **10:**444–448.

LEVI, G., CHERAYIL, A., and LAJTHA, A., 1965, Cerebral amino acid transport. Heterogeneity of exit, *J. Neurochem.* **12:**757–770.

LIANG, C. C., and QUASTEL, J. H., 1969, Effects of drugs on the uptake of Ach in rat brain cortex slices, *Biochem. Pharmacol.* **18:**1187–1194.

LINDAN, O., QUASTEL, J. H., and SVED, S., 1957, Biochemical studies on chlorpromazine, *Canad. J. Biochem.* **35:**1135–1144.

LINDBOHM, R., and WALLGREN, H., 1962, Changes in respiration of rat brain cortex slices induced by some aliphatic alcohols, *Acta Pharmacol. Toxicol.* **19:**53–58.

LØVTRUP, S., 1967, On the correlation between psychic action, chemical effects, and physical properties of chlorpromazine and imipramine, in: *Molecular Basis of Some Aspects of Mental Activity*, Vol. 2 (O. Walaas, ed.), pp. 39–73, Academic Press, New York.

LOWRY, O. H., and PASSONEAU, J. V., 1962, Application of quantitative histochemistry to the pharmacology of the nervous system, *Biochem. Pharmacol.* **9:**173–180.

LOWRY, O. H., and PASSONEAU, J. V., 1964, The relationships between substrates and enzymes of glycolysis in brain, *J. Biol Chem.* **239:**31–42.

LOWRY, O. H., PASSONEAU, J. V., HASSELBERGER, F. X., and SCHULTZ, D. W., 1964, Effect of ischemia on known substrates and cofactors of the glycolytic pathway in brain, *J. Biol. Chem.* **239:**18–30.

LUNDBERG, P., and STITZEL, R. E., 1968, Studies on the relationship between adrenergic nerve function and granular uptake mechanisms, *Brit. J. Pharmacol.* **33:**98–104.

MAIZELS, M., REMINGTON, M., and TRUSCOE, R., 1958, Effects of certain physical factors and of cardiac glycosides on Na^+ transfer by mouse ascites tumor cells, *J. Physiol.* **140:**61–79.

MAJCHROWICZ, E., 1965, Effects of aliphatic alcohols and aldehydes on the metabolism of K^+ stimulated rat brain cortex slices, *Canad. J. Biochem.* **43:**1041–1051.

MANARA, L., CARMINATI, P., and MENNINI, T., 1972, *In vivo* persistent binding of ^{3}H-reserpine to rat brain subcellular components, *Eur. J. Pharmacol.* **20:**109–113.

MANN, P. J. G., and QUASTEL, J. H., 1940, Benzedrine and brain metabolism, *Biochem. J.* **34:**414–431.

MANN, P. J. G., TENNENBAUM, M., and QUASTEL, J. H., 1938, On the mechanism of Ach formation in brain *in vitro*, *Biochem. J.* **32:**243–261.

MARTIN, W. R., and SLOAN, J. W., 1970, Effects of infused tryptamine in man, *Psychopharmacologia* **18:**231–237.

MATTHYSE, S., 1973, Antipsychotic drug actions, *Fed. Proc.* **32:**200–205.

MAXWELL, R. G., and NICKEL, V. S., 1954, Chelating agents, barbiturates and stimulation of rat brain ATPase, *Proc. Soc. Exp. Biol. Med.* **86:**846–848.

MAYMAN, C. I., GATSFIELD, P. D., and BRECKENBRIDGE, B. MC. L., 1964, The glucose content of brain in anesthesia, *J. Neurochem.* **11:**483–487.

MCGEER, E. G., and MCGEER, P., 1973, Amino acid hydroxylase inhibitors, in: *Metabolic Inhibitors*, Vol. 4 (R. M. Hochster, M. Kates, and J. H. Quastel, eds.), pp. 45–105, Academic Press, New York.

MCILWAIN, H., 1953, Effects of depressants on the metabolism of stimulated cerebral tissues, *Biochem. J.* **53:**403–412.

MCILWAIN, H., 1967, Tetrodotoxin and the cation content, excitability and metabolism of isolated mammalian cerebral tissues, *Biochem. Pharmacol.* **16:**1389–1396.

MCILWAIN, H., and BACHELARD, H. S., 1971, *Biochemistry and the CNS*, 4th ed., Churchill, London.

MCILWAIN, H., and GORE, M. B. R., 1951, Actions of electrical stimulation and of 2:4-dinitrophenol on the phosphates in sections of mammalian brain *in vitro*, *Biochem. J.* **50:**24–28.

MCILWAIN, H., and GREENGARD, O., 1957, Excitants and depressants of the CNS in isolated electrically stimulated cerebral tissues, *J. Neurochem.* **1:**348–357.

MCLENNAN, H., and ELLIOTT, K. A. L., 1951, Effects of convulsant and narcotic drugs on Ach synthesis, *J. Pharmacol. Exp. Ther.* **103:**35–43.

MEEK, J. L., and FUXE, K., 1971, Serotonin accumulation after monoamine oxidation inhibition: Effects of some antidepressants and hallucinogens, *Biochem. Pharmacol.* **20:**693–706.

MELDRUM, B. S., and HORTON, R. W., 1973, Cerebral functional effects of 2-deoxy-D-glucose and 3-O-methylglucose in Rhesus monkeys, *Electroenceph. Clin. Neurophysiol.* **35:**59–66.

MICHAELIS, M., and HASHIMOTO, S., 1962, Action of chloretone on reduced cozymase oxidation by cytochrome *c*, *Nature* **194:**680–681.

MICHAELIS, M., and QUASTEL, J. H., 1941, Site of action of narcotics in respiratory processes, *Biochem. J.* **35:**518–533.

MITOMA, C., and NEUBAUER, S. E., 1968, γ-Hydroxybutyric acid and sleep, *Experientia* **24:**12–13.

MOORE, J. W., 1966, Effects of ethanol on ionic conductances in the squid axon membrane, *Psychosom. Med.* **28:**450–457.

MOORE, K. E., and LARIVIERE, E. W., 1963, Effects of *d*-amphetamine and restraint on the content of norepinephrine and dopamine in rat brain, *Biochem. Pharmacol.* **12:**1283–1288.

MORRISON, A. B., and WEBSTER, R. H., 1973, Reserpine rigidity and adrenergic neurons, *Neuropharmacology* **12:**725–733.

MULLINS, L. J., 1971, Anesthetics, in: *Handbook of Neurochemistry*, Vol. 6 (A. Lajtha, ed.), pp. 395–423, Plenum Press, New York.

NADLER, J. V., HORWITCH, P., and COOPER, J. R., 1972, Effects of sodium fluoroacetate on the metabolism of *N*-acetylaspartate and aspartate in mouse brain, *J. Neurochem.* **19:**2107–2118.

NAKAMURA, Y., NAKAJIMA, S., and GRUNDFEST, H., 1965, Action of tetrodotoxin on electrogenic components of squid giant axons, *J. Gen. Physiol.* **48:**985–996.

NAKAZAWA, S., and QUASTEL, J. H., 1968, Effects of inorganic salts and of ouabain on some metabolic responses of rat brain cortex slices to cationic and electrical stimulation, *Canad. J. Biochem.* **46:**355–362.

NARAHASHI, T., MOORE, J. W., and SCOTT, W. R., 1964, Tetrodotoxin blockage of sodium conductance increase in lobster giant axons, *J. Gen. Physiol.* **47:**965–974.

NEAL, M. J., and STARR, M. S., 1973, Effect of inhibitors of GABA transaminase on the accumulation of GABA by the retina, *Brit. J. Pharmacol.* **47:**543–555.

NISTRI, A., BARTIOLINI, A., DEFENU, G., and PEPEU, G., 1972, Investigations into the release of Ach from cerebral cortex of the cat: Effects of amphetamine, of scopolamine and of septal lesions, *Neuropharmacology* **11:**665–674.

OKAMOTO, K., and QUASTEL, J. H., 1970, Tetrodotoxin sensitive uptake of ions and water by slices of rat brain *in vitro*, *Biochem. J.* **120:**37–47.

OKAMOTO, K., and QUASTEL, J. H., 1972, Uptake and release of glutamate in cerebral cortex from the rat, *Biochem. J.* **128:**1117–1124.

OKAMOTO, K., and QUASTEL, J. H., 1973, Spontaneous action potentials in isolated guinea pig cerebellar slices: Effects of amino acids and conditions affecting sodium and water uptake, *Proc. Roy. Soc. Lond. Ser. B* **184:**83–90.

PAGE, I. H., and CARLSSON, A., 1970, Serotonin, in: *Handbook of Neurochemistry*, Vol. 4 (A. Lajtha, ed.), pp. 251–262, Plenum Press, New York.

PATON, W. D. M., and SPEDEN, R. N., 1965, Uptake of anesthetics and their actions on the CNS, *Brit. Med. Bull.* **21:**44–48.

PETERS, E. L., and TOWER, D. B., 1959, Glutamic acid and glutamine metabolism in cerebral cortex after seizures induced by methionine sulfoximine, *J. Neurochem.* **5:**80–90.

PETERS, R. A., 1957, Mechanism of toxity of *Dichapetalum cymosum*, *Advan. Enzymol.* **18:**113–159.

PLETSCHER, A., 1968, in: *Psychopharmacology: A Review of Progress 1957–1967* (D. H. Efron, ed.), pp. 649–654, Government Printing Office, Washington, D.C.

PLETSCHER, A., SHORE, P. A., and BRODIE, B. B., 1956, Serotonin as a mediator of reserpine action in brain, *J. Pharmacol. Exp. Ther.* **116:**84–89.

PLETSCHER, H., BURKARD, W. P., and GEY, K. F., 1964, Effect of monoamine releasers and decarboxylase inhibitors on endogenous 5-hydroxyindole derivatives in brain, *Biochem. Pharmacol.* **13:**385–390.

POST, R. L., MERRITT, C. R., KINSOLVING, C. R., and ALBRIGHT, C. D., 1960, Membrane ATPase as a participant in the active transport of Na^+ and K^+ in the human erythrocyte, *J. Biol. Chem.* **235:**1796–1802.

PROLER, M., and KELLAWAY, P., 1962, The methionine sulfoximine syndrome in the cat, *Epilepsia 4th Ser.* **3:**117–130.

QUASTEL, D. M. J., HACKETT, J. T., and OKAMOTO, K., 1972, Presynaptic action of central depressant drugs, *Canad. J. Physiol. Pharmacol.* **50:**279–284.

QUASTEL, J. H., 1958, Enzymatic basis of drug action, in: *Proc. Internat. Symp. Enz. Chem. Tokyo, 1957,* pp. 510–521, Maruzen, Tokyo.

QUASTEL, J. H., 1959, Enzymatic mechanisms of the brain: Effects of some neurotropic agents, in: *Biochemistry of the Central Nervous System,* Vol. 3 (F. Brucke, ed.), pp. 90–114, Proc. Fourth Int. Cong. Biochem., Vienna, Pergamon Press, London.

QUASTEL, J. H., 1962, Effects of electrolytes on brain metabolism, in: *Neurochemistry,* 2nd ed. (K. A. C. Elliott, I. H. Page, and J. H. Quastel, eds.), pp. 226–237, Thomas, Springfield, Ill.

QUASTEL, J. H., 1965, Effects of drugs on the metabolism of the brain *in vitro, Brit. Med. Bull.* **21:**49–56.

QUASTEL, J. H., 1967, Effects of neurotropic drugs on brain metabolism *in vitro,* in: *Molecular Basis of Some Aspects of Mental Activity,* Vol. 2 (O. Walaas, ed.), pp. 19–37, Academic Press, New York.

QUASTEL, J. H., 1970, Transport processes at the brain cell membrane, in: *Neurosciences Research,* Vol. 3 (S. Ehrenpreis and O. C. Solnitzky, eds.), pp. 1–41, Academic Press, New York.

QUASTEL, J. H., and WHEATLEY, A. H. M., 1932, Narcosis and oxidations of the brain, *Proc. Roy. Soc. Lond. Ser. B* **112:**60–79.

RAMSEY, R. L., and MCILWAIN, H., 1970, Calcium content and exchange in neocortical tissues during the cation movements induced by glutamates, *J. Neurochem.* **17:**781–787.

RANDRUP, A., and MUNKVAD, J., 1966, Role of catecholamines in the amphetamine excitatory response, *Nature* **211:**540.

READING, H. W., and WALLWORK, J., 1969, Oxidation of succinate and pyruvate in rat brain and its effect on barbiturate anesthesia, *Biochem. Pharmacol.* **18:**2211–2214.

RICHENS, A., 1969, Microelectrode studies in the frog isolated spinal cord during depression by general anesthetic agents, *Brit. J. Pharmacol.* **36:**312–319.

RITCHIE, J. M., and GREENGARD, P., 1966, On the mode of action of local anesthetics, *Ann. Rev. Pharmacol.* **6:**405–430.

ROA, P. D., TEWS, J. K., and STONE, W. E., 1964, A neurochemical study of thiosemicarbazide seizures and their inhibition by aminooxyacetate, *Biochem. Pharmacol.* **13:**477–487.

RONZIO, R. A., and MEISTER, A., 1967, Attachment of methionine sulfoximine to the active site of glutamine synthetase, *Fed. Proc.* **26:**389.

RONZIO, R. A., and MEISTER, A., 1968, Phosphorylation of methionine sulfoximine by glutamine synthetase, *Proc. Natl. Acad. Sci.* **59:**164–170.

ROSE, S. P. R., 1965, Effects of ouabain, glutamate and cations on phosphate incorporation in brain slices, *Biochem. Pharmacol.* **14:**589–601.

ROSINA, A., and SOTGIU, M. L., 1967, Effects of intravertebral injection of a barbiturate on unit-activity in the lower brain stem, *Brain Res.* **6:**510–522.

ROSS, S. B., and RENYI, A. L., 1967, Accumulation of ^{3}H-5-hydroxytryptamine in brain slices, *Life Sci.* **6:**1407–1415.

RUTLEDGE, C. O., 1970, The mechanisms by which amphetamine inhibits oxidative deamination of norepinephrine in the brain, *J. Pharmacol. Exp. Ther.* **171:**188–195.

RUTLEDGE, C. O., and WEINER, H., 1967, Effect of reserpine on the synthesis of norepinephrine in the isolated rabbit heart, *J. Pharmacol. Exp. Ther.* **157:**290–302.

RYMAN, B. E., and WALSH, E. O'F., 1954, Site of inhibitory action of cocaine on cellular respiration, *Biochem. J.* **58:**111–115.

SANAN, S., and VOGT, M., 1962, Effects of drugs on the noradrenaline content of brain and peripheral tissue, *Brit. J. Pharmacol.* **18:**109–127.

SANTINI, M., and BERL, S., 1972, Effects of reserpine and monoamine oxidase inhibitors on the levels of amino acids in sensory ganglia, sympathetic ganglia and spinal cord, *Brain.Res.* **47:**167–176.

SCHANBERG, N. J., and SCHANBERG, S. M., 1962, Drug induced alterations of the sub-cellular distribution of serotonin in rat brain, *Biochem. Pharmacol.* **9:**93–96.

SCHANBERG, S. M., SCHILDKRAUT, J. J., and KOPIN, I. J., 1967, Effect of psychoactive drugs on ^{3}H-norepinephrine metabolism in brain, *Biochem. Pharmacol.* **16:**393–399.

SCHATZMANN, H. J., 1953, Herzglykoside als Hemmstoffe fur den aktiven K^+ und Na^+ transport durch die erythrocyten Membran, *Helv. Physiol. Acta* **11:**346–354.

SCHILDKRAUT, J. J., 1965, The catecholamine hypothesis of affective disorders: A review of supporting evidence, *Am. J. Psychiat.* **122:**509–522.

SCHILDKRAUT, J. J., and GERSHON, S. S., 1971, Antidepressants and related drugs, in: *Handbook of Neurochemistry*, Vol. 6 (A. Lajtha, ed.) pp. 357–386, Plenum Press, New York.

SCHILDKRAUT, J. J., KLERMAN, G. L., HAMMOND, R., and FRIEND, D. G., 1964, Excretion of 3-methoxy-4-hydroxymandelic acid in depressed patients treated with antidepressant drugs, *J. Psychiat. Res.* **2:**257–266.

SCHILDKRAUT, J. J., SCHANBERG, S. M., BREESE, G. R., and KOPIN, I. J., 1967, Norepinephrine metabolism and drugs used in the affective disorders, *Am. J. Psychiat.* **124:**600–608.

SCHUBERTH, J., SPARF, B., and SUNDWALL, A., 1969, A technique for the study of Ach turnover in mouse brain *in vivo, J. Neurochem.* **16:**695–700.

SCHWARTZ, A., and LASETER, A. H., 1964, A Na^+- and K^+-stimulated ATP-ase from cardiac tissue: Effects of ouabain and other agents that modify enzyme activity, *Biochem. Pharmacol.* **13:**337–348.

SEEMAN, P., 1972, The membrane actions of anesthetics and tranquilisers, *Pharmacol. Rev.* **24:**583–655.

SEGAWA, T., and KURUMA, I., 1968, Influence of drugs on uptake of 5-HT by nerve ending particles of rabbit brain stem, *J. Pharm. Pharmacol.* **20:**320–322.

SELLINGER, O. Z., 1967, Inactivation of glutamine synthetase by methionine sulfoximine, *Biochim. Biophys. Acta* **132:**514–516.

SELLINGER, O. Z., and WEILER, P., 1963, Nature of inhibition *in vitro* of cerebral glutamine synthetase by methionine sulfoximine, *Biochem. Pharmacol.* **12:**989–1000.

SHANES, A. M., 1958, Electrochemical aspects of physiological and pharmacological action in excitable cells, *Pharmacol. Rev.* **10:**59–103.

SHANES, A. M., TREYGANG, W. H., GRUNDFEST, H., and AMATNIK, E., 1959, Anesthetic and calcium action in the voltage-clamped squid axon, *J. Gen. Physiol.* **42:**793–802.

SHANKAR, R., and QUASTEL, J. H., 1972, Effects of tetrodotoxin and anesthetics on brain metabolism and transport during anoxia, *Biochem. J.* **126:**851–867.

SHANKARAN, R., and QUASTEL, J. H., 1972, Effects of anesthetics on sodium uptake into rat brain cortex *in vitro, Biochem. Pharmacol.* **21:**1763–1773.

SHARMA, S. K., JOHNSTONE, R. N., and QUASTEL, J. H., 1963, Active transport of ascorbic acid in adrenal cortex and brain cortex *in vitro, Canad. J. Biochem. Physiol.* **41:**597–604.

SHEMISA, D. A., and FAHIEN, L. A., 1971, Modifications of glutamate dehydrogenase by various drugs which affect behaviour, *Mol. Pharmacol.* **7:**8–25.

SHIMIZU, N., and HAMURO, Y., 1958, Deposition of glycogen and changes in some enzymes in brain wounds, *Nature* **181:**781–782.

SHIU, P. C., and ELLIOTT, K. A. C., 1973, Binding and uptake of amino acids by brain tissue, *Canad. J. Biochem.* **51:**121–128.

SHORE, P. A., 1971, Reserpine: A survey of its pharmacology, in: *Handbook of Neurochemistry*, Vol. 6 (A. Lajtha, ed.), pp. 349–356, Plenum Press, New York.

SHORE, P. A., and BRODIE, B. B., 1957, LSD-like effects elicited by reserpine in rabbits pretreated with iproniazid, *Proc. Soc. Exp. Biol.* **94:**433–435.

SHORE, P. A., MEAD, J. A. R., KUNTZMAN, R. G., SPECTOR, S. and BRODIE, B. B., 1957, On the physiological significance of monoamine oxidase in brain, *Science* **126:**1063–1064.

SILBERMAN, A., YU, C.-T., and LAM, K.-W., 1972, Alleviation of barbiturate inhibition on the oxidative activity of mitochondrial particles by alkali, *Res. Commun. Chem. Pathol. Pharmacol.* **4:**115–119.

SKOU, J. C., 1957, Influence of some cations on an ATPase from peripheral nerves, *Biochim. Biophys. Acta* **23:**394–401.

SKOU, J. C., 1960, Further investigations on a Mg^{++} + Na^{+}-activated ATPase possibly related to the active linked transport of Na^{+} and K^{+} across the nerve membrane, *Biochim. Biophys. Acta* **42:**6–23.

SMITH, C. B., 1965, Effects of *d*-amphetamine on brain amine content and locomotor activity of mice, *J. Pharmacol. Exp. Ther.* **147:**96–102.

SNYDER, S. H., 1970, Catecholamines, brain function and how psychotropic drugs act, in: *Principles of Psychopharmacology* (W. G. Clark and J. del Giudice, eds.), pp. 115–125, Academic Press, New York.

SOURKES, T. L., 1962, *Biochemistry of Mental Disease*, p. 358, Harper and Row, New York.

SOURKES, T. L., and D'IORIO, A., 1963, Inhibition of catecholamine metabolism, in: *Metabolic Inhibitors*, Vol. 2 (R. M. Hochster and J. H. Quastel, eds.), pp.79–98, Academic Press, New York.

SPECTOR, S., HIRSCH, C. W., and BRODIE, B. B., 1963, Association of behavioural effects of pargyline with increase in brain norepinephrine, *Int. J. Neuropharmacol.* **2:**81–93.

STEIN, L., 1964, Self-stimulation of the brain and the central stimulant action of amphetamine, *Fed. Proc.* **23:**836–849.

STEIN, L., and WISE, C. D., 1969, Release of norepinephrine from hypothalamus and amygdala, *J. Comp. Physiol. Psychol.* **67:**189–198.

STEIN, L., and WISE, C. D., 1971, Behavioural pharmacology of central stimulants, in: *Principles of Psychopharmacology* (W. G. Clark and J. del Giudice, eds.), pp. 313–325, Academic Press, New York.

STEWART, G. G., ABBS, E. T., and ROBERTS, D. J., 1969, Biochemical effects of fluoroacetate admininstration in rat brain, heart and blood, *Biochem. Pharmacol.* **19:**1861–1866.

ST. OMER, V., 1971, Investigations into mechanisms responsible for seizures induced by chlorinated hydrocarbon insecticides, *J. Neurochem.* **18:**365–374.

STONE, W. E., TEWS, J. K., and MITCHELL, E. N., 1960, Chemical concomitants of convulsive activity in the cerebrum, *Neurology* **10:**241–248.

STRANG, R. H. C., and BACHELARD, H. S., 1973, Rates of cerebral glucose utilization in rats anesthetized with phenobarbitone, *J. Neurochem.* **20:**987–996.

SUGRUE, M. F., and SHORE, P. A., 1970, Further evidence for a Na^{+} dependent, optically specific, reserpine-sensitive amine carrier mechanism in the adrenergic neuron, *Pharmacologist* **12:**214.

SULSER, F., and SANDERS-BUSH, E., 1971, Effect of drugs on amines in the CNS, *Ann. Rev. Pharmacol.* **11:**209–230.

SULSER, F., OWENS, M. L., and DINGELL, J. V., 1966, Mechanism of amphetamine potentiation by desipramine, *Life Sci.* **5:**2005–2010.

SULSER, F., OWENS, M. L., STRADA, S. J., and DINGELL, J. V., 1969, Modification by desipramine of the availability of norepinephrine released by reserpine in rat hypothalamus *in vivo*, *J. Pharmacol. Exp. Ther.* **168:**272–282.

SWANSON, P. D., 1968, Effects of tetrodotoxin and ouabain on electrically stimulated cerebral cortex slices, *Biochem. Pharmacol.* **17:**129–141.

TABERNER, P. B., RICK, J. T., and KERKUT, G. A., 1972, The action of γ-hydroxybutyrate on cerebral glucose metabolism, *J. Neurochem.* **19:**245–254.

TAKAGAKI, G., HIRANO, S., and TSUKADA, Y., 1958, Effects of some inhibitors on the metabolism of guinea pig brain slices, *J. Biochem. Tokyo* **45:**41–48.

TAKAGAKI, G., HIRANO, S., and NAGATA, Y., 1959, Some observations on the effect of D-glutamate on glucose metabolism, and accumulation of K^{+}, in brain cortex slices, *J. Neurochem.* **4:**124–134.

TASAKI, I., and SINGER, I., 1966, Membrane macromolecules and nerve excitability: A physico-chemical interpretation of excitation in squid giant axons, *Ann. N.Y. Acad. Sci.* **137:**792–806.

TAYLOR, T., and SNYDER, S. H., 1970, Amphetamine: Differentiation by *d*- and *l*-isomers of behaviour involving brain norepinephrine or dopamine, *Science* **168:**1487–1489.

TEWS, J. K., and STONE, W. E., 1964, Effects of methionine sulfoximine on levels of free amino acids and related substances in the brain, *Biochem. Pharmacol.* **13:**543–545.

TEWS, J. K., and STONE, W. E., 1965, Free amino acids and related compounds in brain and other tissues: Effects of convulsant drugs, in: *Progress in Brain Research*, Vol. 16: *Horizons in Neuropsychopharmacology* (W. A. Himwich and J. P. Schadé, eds.), pp. 135–163, Elsevier, New York.

THESLEFF, S., and QUASTEL, D. M. J., 1965, Neuromuscular pharmacology, *Ann. Rev. Pharnacol.* **5:**263–284.

TISSARI, A. H., and BOGDANSKI, D. F., 1971, Biogenic amine transport: Comparison of effects of ouabain and K^+ deficiency in transport of 5-HT and norepinephrine by synaptosomes, *Pharmacology* **5:**225–234.

TISSARI, A. H., SCHÖNHÖFER, P. S., BOGDANSKI, D. F., and BRODIE, B. B., 1969, Mechanism of biogenic amine transport: Relation between Na^+ and mechanism of ouabain blockade of accumulation of 5-HT and norepinephrine by synaptosomes, *Mol. Pharmacol.* **5:**593–604.

TOWER, D. B., 1958, Effects of 2-deoxy-D-glucose on metabolism of slices of cerebral cortex incubated *in vitro*, *J. Neurochem.* **3:**185–205.

TOWER, D. B., 1960, *Neurochemistry of Epilepsy* (I. N. Kugelmass, ed.), pp. 174–175, Thomas, Springfield, Ill.

TOWER, D. B., 1967, *Brain Edema* (I. Klatzo and F. Seitelberger, eds.), pp. 313, 318, Springer, New York.

TRACHTENBERG, M. C., and POLLEN, D. A., 1970, Neuroglia: Biophysical properties and physiological function, *Science* **167:**1248–1252.

TRUITT, E. B., BELL, F. K., and KRANTZ, J. G., 1956, Effects of alcohols and acetaldehyde on oxidative phosphorylation in brain, *Quart, J. Stud. Alcohol* **17:**594–600.

UDENFRIEND, S., WEISSBACH, H., and BOGDANSKI, D. F., 1957, Increase of tissue serotonin following administration of its precursor, 5-hydroxy-tryptophan, *J. Biol. Chem.* **224:**803–810.

VAN HARREVELD, A., and FIFKOVÁ, E., 1972, Effects of metabolic inhibitors on the release of glutamate from the retina, *J. Neurochem.* **19:**1439–1450.

VENTURINI, G., and PALLADINI, G., 1973, ATPase activity, Na and K content in guinea pig cortex after ouabain treatment *in vivo*, *J. Neurochem.* **20:**237–239.

WALLACH, D. P., 1961, Studies on the GABA pathway, *Biochem. Pharmacol.* **5:**232–331.

WALLGREN, H., 1960, Effects of alcohol on biochemical processes in the CNS, *Psychosom. Med.* **28:**431–442.

WALLGREN, H., 1971, Alcohol, in: *Handbook of Neurochemistry*, Vol. 6 (A. Lajtha, ed.), pp. 509–523, Plenum Press, New York.

WALLGREN, H., and KULONEN, E., 1960, Effects of ethanol on respiration of rat brain cortex slices, *Biochem. J.* **75:**150–158.

WARREN, K. S., and SCHENKER, S., 1964, Effect of an inhibitor of glutamine synthesis (methionine sulfoximine) on ammonia toxicity and metabolism, *J. Lab. Clin. Med.* **64:**442–449.

WATANABE, A., TASAKI, I., SINGER, I., and LERMAN, L., 1967, Effects of tetrodotoxin on excitability of squid giant axons in sodium free media, *Science* **155:**95–97.

WATSON, P. G., 1960, The mode of action of local anesthetics, *J. Pharm. Pharmacol.* **12:**257–292.

WEAKLY, J. N., 1969, Effects of barbiturates on "quantal" synaptic transmission in spinal motor neurons, *J. Physiol.* **204:**63–77.

WECHSLER, R. L., DRIPPS, R. D., and KETY, S. S., 1951, Blood flow and oxygen consumption of the human brain during anesthesia produced by thiopental, *Anesthesiology* **12:**308–314.

WEIL-MALHERBE, H., WHITBY, L. G., and AXELROD, J., 1961, Uptake of circulating ^{3}H-norepinephrine by the pituitary gland and various areas of the brain, *J. Neurochem.* **8:**55–64.

WEISSMAN, A., KOE, B. K., and TENEN, S. S., 1966, Antiamphetamine effects following inhibition of tyrosine hydroxylase, *J. Pharmacol. Exp. Ther.* **151:**339–352.

WHITTAM, R., and BLOND, D. M., 1964, Respiratory control by an ATPase involved in active transport in brain cortex, *Biochem. J.* **92:**147–158.

WOLLENBERGER, A., 1955, Action of protoveratrine on metabolism of cerebral cortex, *Biochem. J.* **61:**68–80.

WOLPERT, H., TRUITT, E. B., BELL, F. K., and KRANTZ, J. C., 1956, Anesthesia: Effect of certain narcotics on oxidative phosphorylation, *J. Pharmacol. Exp. Ther.* **117:**358–361.

WOOD, J. D., and PEESKER, S. J., 1973, Role of GABA metabolism in the convulsant and anticonvulsant actions of aminooxyacetate, *J. Neurochem.* **20:**379–387.

YESSAIAN, N. H., ARMENIAN, A. R., KAZAROVA, E. K., and BUNIATIAN, H. C., 1971, On the involvement of inorganic ions in the effect of GABA on brain 5-HT and norepinephrine, *J. Neurochem.* **18:**307–321.

YOSHIDA, H., NUKADA, T., and FUJISAWA, H., 1961, Effects of ouabain on ion transport and metabolic turnover of phospholipids of brain slices, *Biochim. Biophys. Acta* **48:**614–615.

ZADUNAISKY, J. A., WALD, F., and DE ROBERTIS, E., 1965, Osmotic behaviour and glial changes in isolated frog brains, *Prog. Brain Res.* **15:**196–218.

ZELLER, E. A., BARSKY, J., and BERMAN, E. R., 1955, Amine oxidases: Inhibition of monoamine oxidase by isonicotinyl-isopropylhydrazine, *J. Biol. Chem.* **214:**267–274.

2

ROLE OF CYCLIC NUCLEOTIDES IN THE NERVOUS SYSTEM

John Daly

1. INTRODUCTION

The complexity of the central nervous system makes investigation and elucidation of the factors involved in the establishment, regulation, and integration of neuronal function a formidable task. However, on the molecular level a variety of evidence indicates that the nucleotides cyclic AMP and cyclic GMP are involved in regulatory roles associated with neuronal function. Cyclic AMP regulates prime functions in many other tissues: gluconogenesis in liver, lipolysis in fat, secretion in endocrine glands. Definitive roles for cyclic GMP have as yet not been established (*cf.* Goldberg *et al.*, 1973). These cyclic nucleotides are formed from intracellular ATP and GTP, respectively, by the action of cyclase enzymes. The cyclic nucleotides are degraded by phosphodiesterases to their respective 5′-phosphates. The diverse biological effects of cyclic nucleotides appear to be manifested through activation of protein kinases which specifically phosphorylate enzymes and other functional proteins and thus alter their properties. The specificity and nature of the effects of cyclic nucleotides presumably depend, therefore, not only on the intracellular site of generation of the cyclic nucleotide but also on the substrate specificity of the activated kinases and

John Daly ● Laboratory of Chemistry, National Institute of Arthritis, Metabolism, and Digestive Diseases, National Institutes of Health, Bethesda, Maryland

the accessibility of endogenous protein substrates. Termination of the physiological effects initiated by the cyclic nucleotides presumably occurs via the action of phosphoprotein phosphatases which hydrolyze the phosphorylated proteins. In certain instances, levels of cyclic AMP and cyclic GMP appear to be interrelated; increases in one nucleotide are accompanied by decreases in the other, suggesting a functional interrelationship.

The mechanisms involved in the formation and role of cyclic nucleotides in nervous tissue have been investigated on many levels: (1) with cell-free preparations, (2) with incubated brain slices, (3) with cells of neuronal or glial origin, (4) with functional ganglia or discrete central neurons, (5) in intact animals. With cell-free preparations, the endogenous levels of nucleotides and the levels and properties of cyclases, phosphodiesterases, and cyclic nucleotide–dependent protein kinases have been investigated. With brain slices from control animals and in animals subjected to prior drug treatment, the effects of putative neurotransmitters, other regulatory agents, electrical stimulation, and various drugs on the intracellular accumulation of cyclic AMP have been studied. Cultured cells of neuronal or glial origin have provided simpler systems for studying the effects of such agents. Regulatory roles for cyclic AMP have been investigated in functional ganglia and certain central neurons. The effect of centrally active drugs on levels of brain cyclic nucleotides and the behavioral effects of administered cyclic AMP and its derivatives have been studied in whole animals. The present chapter attempts to survey the results of such investigations with emphasis on their relevance to possible roles of cyclic nucleotides in the central nervous system.

2. ENZYMATIC FORMATION, DEGRADATION, AND ACTION OF CYCLIC NUCLEOTIDES

2.1. Adenylate Cyclases

Brain contains high levels of adenylate cyclases, plasma membrane enzymes whose activity in intact cells is regulated by receptor(s) exposed to extracellular space (for a comprehensive review on adenylate cyclases, see Perkins, 1973). Levels of adenylate cyclase vary considerably in different brain regions (Klainer *et al.*, 1962; Weiss and Costa, 1968; Williams *et al.*, 1969; Weiss, 1971), with high levels in gray matter and low in white matter. Levels of cyclic AMP also vary considerably in different brain regions (Ebadi *et al.*, 1971*a,b*; Schmidt *et al.*, 1971, 1972; Steiner *et al.*, 1972; Kodama *et al.*, 1973; Volicer and Gold, 1973; Wellmann and Schwabe, 1973) and probably reflect both the activity of cyclases and phosphodiesterases and the availability of ATP. Measurements of endogenous levels of cyclic AMP in brain are, however, complicated by rapid postdecapitation changes, the magnitude of which depends on the brain region and species (see Section 3.1). In brain homogenates, high levels of both adenylate cyclase and cyclic AMP have been detected in synaptosomal fractions (De Robertis *et al.*, 1967; Goldberg *et al.*, 1970; Krishna *et al.*, 1970; Weller *et al.*, 1972; Johnson *et al.*, 1973). Immunofluorescent assay of cyclic AMP in rat cerebellar slices revealed pronounced fluorescence in Purkinje neurons and granule cells (Bloom *et al.*, 1972*b*; Siggins *et al.*, 1973). The molecular layer, which consists predominantly of Purkinje dendrites and parallel fibres, was weakly fluorescent, while white matter was unreactive. The extent of fluorescence in Purkinje neurons increased greatly after decapitation. Adenylate cyclase and to a lesser extent phosphodiesterase activity increased proximal to a constriction of the sciatic nerve (Bray *et al.*, 1971).

Adenylate cyclase activity in brain homogenates is enhanced by magnesium or manganese ions, while calcium ions may have either stimulatory or inhibitory effects (Bradham *et al.*, 1970; McCune *et al.*, 1971; Bradham, 1972; Johnson and Sutherland, 1973; Perkins, 1973; von Hungen and Roberts, 1973*a*,*b*). A soluble heat-stable factor was reported to activate membranal adenylate cyclase in brain homogenates (Kauffman *et al.*, 1972; *cf.* Weiss and Costa, 1968). Fluoride ion stimulates adenylate cyclases in most cell-free preparations, including those from brain (Perkins and Moore, 1971; Johnson and Sutherland, 1973; Katz and Tenenhouse, 1973*a*; Perkins, 1973; Swislocki and Tierney, 1973), but has no effect on accumulations of cyclic AMP in whole cells. The activation of adenylate cyclases by fluoride in homogenates from rodent cerebral cortex was antagonized by lithium ions (Dousa and Hechter, 1970; Forn and Valdecasas, 1971). Phenothiazines inhibit fluoride-activated adenylate cyclases in brain homogenates (Uzunov and Weiss, 1971). Brain adenylate cyclases have also been reported to be inhibited by adenosine (McKenzie and Bar, 1973), alloxan (Cohen and Bitensky, 1969), and sulfhydryl reagents (Ferrendelli *et al.*, 1973*b*).

Endogeneous levels of brain cyclic AMP and both basal and fluoride-activated cyclase in homogenates increased in rats after birth until about 9–18 days of age (Schmidt *et al.*, 1970; Hommes and Beere, 1971; Weiss, 1971; Kauffman *et al.*, 1972; Schmidt and Robison, 1972; Kohrman, 1973; Perkins and Moore, 1973*b*; Singhal, 1973). The basal levels of cyclase then declined markedly, while fluoride-activated levels declined less markedly. In hamster cerebrum, adult levels of cyclase are threefold greater than in young animals (Weiss *et al.*, 1971). Levels of cyclic AMP also increase during maturation of mice, with a large increase in forebrain and small increases in cerebellum and brain stem (Steiner *et al.*, 1972).

Adenylate cyclase measured with exogenous ATP in cell-free preparations retains little of the receptor-mediated regulation of activity which is usually seen with cell-free preparations from other tissues. Thus, although significant intracellular accumulations of cyclic AMP can result from incubations of brain slices with certain biogenic amines, adenosine, or prostaglandins, the cyclases in homogenates from the same tissue usually show marginal or no enhancement of activity with the same compounds (Klainer *et al.*, 1962; Burkard and Gey, 1968; Williams *et al.*, 1969; Krishna *et al.*, 1970; Rall and Gilman, 1970; Sattin and Rall, 1970; Abdulla and McFarlane, 1972; Kodama *et al.*, 1973). Norepinephrine and dopamine have been reported to enhance cyclic AMP formation in cell-free preparations from rat cerebral cortex, but the degree of activation was small, especially in the presence of optimal concentrations of calcium ions (McCune *et al.*, 1971; von Hungen and Roberts, 1973*a,b*). The effect of norepinephrine was blocked by β-antagonists, while the effects of dopamine were antagonized by haloperidol. Another group reported that dopamine had no effect on cyclases in preparations from rat cortex, hippocampus, or cerebellum, but that norepinephrine significantly enhanced cyclase activity (Walker and Walker, 1973*b*). Cyclase activity in cell-free preparations from caudate nucleus was reported to be somewhat enhanced by both dopamine and norepinephrine. The effects of dopamine were prevented by haloperidol, the effects of norepinephrine by β-antagonists (Walker and Walker, 1973*a,b*). Katz and Tenenhouse (1973*b*) reported that epinephrine or ouabain elicited a small increase in cyclase activity in cell-free preparations from rat cerebral cortex. These effects were not observed when the cyclase was maximally activated by manganese ions or when calcium ions were absent. Both α- and β-antagonists reduced the responses to epinephrine. A fourth group reported that dopamine, apomorphine, and norepinephrine but not isoproterenol activated cyclases in preparations from rat caudate nucleus (Kebabian *et al.*, 1972). The effects of both dopamine and norepinephrine were inhibited by haloperidol, α-antagonists, and chlorpromazine. Catecholamine-mediated activations of cyclases in cell-free preparations from rat, ox, dog, and cat brain have also been reported (Klainer *et al.*, 1962; Rigberg *et al.*, 1969; Janiec *et al.*, 1970; Kohrman, 1973; Palmer, 1973*a*), but in these reports as in most other studies less than a twofold increase in cyclase activity was observed. The degree of activation of cyclases by catecholamines in rat brain preparations depended on the age of the animal (Walker and Walker, 1973*b*). Acetylcholine was reported to inhibit cyclases in rat striatal homogenates (Walker and Walker, 1973*a*). After osmotic disruption of neuronal and glial-enriched fractions from different brain regions, norepinephrine was found to elicit small increases in cyclase activity in virtually all rat neuronal and glial fractions (Palmer, 1973*a*). Dopamine elicited small increases in cyclase activity in neuronal fractions from rat cerebral cortex, midbrain, and striatum and in glial fractions from cerebellum and striatum. Histamine elicited small increases in neuronal fractions from rabbit cortex and hippocampus and in glial fraction from rabbit hippocampus. Cyclases in homogenates from bovine superior cervical ganglion were activated less than twofold by dopamine or norepinephrine (Kebabian and Greengard, 1971). No studies on the effect of GTP on hormone responses of brain adenylate cyclases have apparently been reported (*cf.* Birnbaumer, 1973, and references therein). Recently, prostaglandin has been reported to enhance adenylate cyclase activity in rat brain homogenates (Collier and Roy, 1974). This effect was antagonized by morphine. (For further reports on activation of cyclases, see *Addendum*).*

In view of the large, often complete, and certainly variable loss of receptor-mediated activation of adenylate cyclases which occurs during cellular disruption of nervous tissue, caution must be exercised in any extrapolation of *in vitro* results to the relative levels and responsiveness of the cyclases in a particular brain region. However, a method of brain homogenization in Krebs–Ringer buffer that affords vesicular preparations which retain receptor-modulated adenylate cyclases and which in other ways exhibit characteristics of intact cell systems has now been reported (Chasin *et al.*, 1974). Thus the resuspended particulate preparation from guinea pig cerebral cortex, cerebellum, and hippocampus labeled with radioactive adenine (see Section 3.1) responded to various agents with large accumulations of intravesicular radioactive cyclic AMP. Epinephrine elicited twofold, six- to twentyfold, and 1.3-fold increases in cyclic AMP levels in preparations from cortex, cerebellum, and hippocampus, respectively, while histamine caused elevations of three- to fourfold in cortical and three- to eightfold in hippocampal homogenates. Both adenosine and exogenous cyclic AMP elicited a twofold increase in radioactive cyclic AMP in hippocampal preparations. In one experiment, epinephrine elevated endogenous levels of cyclic AMP in cerebellar preparations by 32-fold while elevating radioactive cyclic AMP by seventeenfold. The effects of epinephrine in cortical preparations were antagonized by an α-antagonist, while in cerebellar preparations a β-antagonist was effective. The stimulatory effects of adenosine and cyclic AMP were antagonized by theophylline. Histamine and epinephrine had additive effects in hippocampal preparations. Fluoride did not stimulate cyclic AMP formation, nor did exogenous ATP serve as a substrate for the responsive adenylate cyclases. The responses apparently occur in vesicular entities with sedimentation properties similar to those reported for synaptosomes. Such preparations with responses similar to those found in brain slices would appear to provide a valuable research tool.

In contrast to the usual marginal activations with homogenates of nervous tissue, cultured glioma cells yield homogenates whose adenylate cyclase activity assayed with exogenous ATP was increased four- to twelvefold by catecholamines via interaction with a β-receptor (Schimmer, 1971, 1973; Jard *et al.*, 1972; Opler and Makman, 1972; Schwartz *et al.*, 1973). High concentrations of dopamine were stimulatory, while histamine, serotonin, tyramine, tryptamine, prostaglandin, and acetylcholine had no effect and adenosine and theophylline were inhibitory. Lithium and sodium ions

*The *Addendum* begins on p. 361.

were reported to significantly enhance the stimulatory effects of epinephrine (Schimmer, 1971, 1973). Fluoride stimulated the cyclase in glioma homogenates (Perkins *et al.*, 1971).

2.2. Guanylate Cyclases

The levels of guanylate cyclases and cyclic GMP are usually at least tenfold lower than the levels of adenylate cyclases and cyclic AMP in brain tissue (Goldberg *et al.*, 1969, 1970, 1973; Hardman and Sutherland, 1969; Ishikawa *et al.*, 1969; White and Aurbach, 1969; Boehme, 1970; Ferrendelli *et al.*, 1970, 1972, 1973*a*; Steiner *et al.*, 1970, 1972; Kuo *et al.*, 1972; Gorodis and Morgan, 1973). Very high levels of cyclic GMP are found in cerebellum, where in certain species (rat and mouse) its levels approach those of cyclic AMP. Cyclic GMP levels in rat cerebellum are low at birth and begin a profound increase at the eighth day after birth (Steiner *et al.*, 1972). Increases in other brain regions are less marked. The levels of GTP, the substrate for this cyclase, are much lower in brain tissue than levels of ATP (Goldberg *et al.*, 1970, 1973) and rapidly decrease after decapitation (Steiner *et al.*, 1972). Manganese and to a lesser extent magnesium ions activate guanylate cyclases, while calcium ions, ATP, and other nucleoside triphosphates can be inhibitory (White and Aurbach, 1969; Boehme, 1970; Gorodis and Morgan, 1973). Fluoride ions have no effect on basal activity, nor has activation by hormones or other factors been reported. In brain as in other tissues, the major portion of guanylate cyclase activity does not appear to be membrane bound (Gorodis and Morgan, 1973; Bensinger *et al.*, 1974). The distribution in homogenate fractions from brain is similar to that of soluble neuronal marker enzymes such as glutamate decarboxylase and tyrosine hydroxylase.

2.3. Phosphodiesterases

Levels of cyclic AMP phosphodiesterases vary considerably in different brain regions of various species (Drummond and Perrott-Yee, 1961; Weiss and Costa, 1968; Breckenridge and Johnston, 1969; Williams *et al.*, 1969; Yamamoto and Massey, 1969; Dalton *et al.*, 1974), being high, for example, in gray matter of cortex and in hypothalamus, intermediate in cerebellum, and low in spinal cord. Phosphodiesterase activity was found in both soluble and membrane fractions from brain homogenates and was associated with both soluble and membrane fractions from lysed synaptosomes (Cheung and Salganicoff, 1967; De Robertis *et al.*, 1967; Weiss and Costa, 1968; Gaballah and Popoff, 1971*a*; Thompson and Appleman, 1971*b*; Miki and Yoshida, 1972; Johnson *et al.*, 1973). A histochemical assay demonstrated that most of the phosphodiesterase activity which survived glutaraldehyde fixation in rat cortical slices was localized at postsynaptic membranes on dendritic processes (Florendo *et al.*, 1971). Theophylline inhibited this phosphodiesterase activity. In an earlier study by another group with a similar assay, glial cells were found to be stained heavily compared to neuronal cells in slices of rabbit cerebral cortex and cerebellum (Shanta *et al.*, 1966; *cf.* Breckenridge and Johnston, 1969). Phosphodiesterase activity in cerebral cortex is not decreased after lesion of the medial forebrain nerve bundle, nor does it decrease in the denervated superior cervical ganglion (Breckenridge and Johnston, 1969) or pineal gland (Weiss, 1971), all of which is consonant with a postsynaptic localization for a significant portion of this enzyme in such tissues.

The phosphodiesterase activity in brain increases during maturation of rodents (Gaballah and Popoff, 1971*a*; Weiss, 1971; Weiss *et al.*, 1971; Kauffman *et al.*, 1972; Schmidt and Robison, 1972), although in one study no change or even a decrease was reported for rats (Hommes and Beere, 1971).

A number of different phosphodiesterases are present even in the soluble fractions from homogenates of brain tissue (Brooker *et al.*, 1968; Beavo *et al.*, 1970; Cheung, 1970; Kakiuchi *et al.*, 1971, 1972; Monn and Christianson, 1971; Thompson and Appleman, 1971*a,b,c*; Campbell and Oliver, 1972; Cehovic *et al.*, 1972; Russell *et al.*, 1972; Uzunov and Weiss, 1972; Appleman *et al.*, 1973). A phosphodiesterase with a high affinity for cyclic AMP and another with a low affinity occur in most brain regions. These "two" enzymes follow different development patterns in rat (Weiss and Strada, 1972). Preliminary data on human phosphodiesterases provide no evidence for two enzymes in brain tissue (Kodama *et al.*, 1971). The proportions of the various phosphodiesterases vary in different brain regions and their activation and inhibition profiles differ markedly. Certain of these enzymes are activated by imidazole, histamine, proteolytic enzymes, protein factors in brain homogenates, or calcium ions (Cheung, 1967*b*, 1969, 1970; 1971*a,b*; Kakiuchi and Yamazaki, 1970*a,b,c*; Kakiuchi *et al.*, 1972, 1973; McNeill *et al.*, 1972; Miki and Yoshida, 1972; Uzunov and Weiss, 1972). Presumably, all of the various phosphodiesterases require magnesium ions for maximal activity. The hydrolysis of cyclic AMP by certain phosphodiesterases including "particulate" " brain phosphodiesterases has been reported to be stimulated by low concentrations of cyclic GMP (Beavo *et al.*, 1971). Inhibition of brain phosphodiesterases has been reported for a variety of compounds, including theophylline and other methylxanthines, imidazole(s), imidazopyrazines, a benzopyrimidine, papaverine, dipyridamole, chlordiazepoxide, diazepam, imipramine and other tricyclic antidepressants, chlorpromazine and other phenothiazines, 3,4-ch-alkoxybenzyl-2-imidazolidinones such as RO 20-1724, tolbutamide, apomorphine, reserpine derivatives, dihydroergotamine, l-ethyl-4-(isopropylidenehydrazine)-l*H*-pyrazolo[3,4*b*]pyridine-5-carboxylic acid ethyl ester

(SQ 20,009), ATP, cyclic GMP, adenosine, puromycin, 6-mercapturopurine, phentolamine, etc. (Cheung, 1966, 1967*a*; Honda and Imamura, 1968; Vernikos-Danellis and Harris, 1968; Abdulla and Hamadah, 1970; Goldberg *et al.*, 1970; Ramsden, 1970; Roberts and Simonsen, 1970; Sattin and Rall, 1970; Amer and Browder, 1971; Goldfine *et al.*, 1971; Iwangoff and Enz, 1971, 1972; Kodama *et al.*, 1971; Mandel, 1971; Poech and Kukovetz, 1971; Mizon *et al.*, 1971; Schmidt *et al.*, 1970; Sheppard and Wiggan, 1971; Uzunov and Weiss, 1971; Amer *et al.*, 1972; Beer *et al.*, 1972; Chasin *et al.*, 1972; McNeill *et al.*, 1972; Pichard *et al.*, 1972; Sheppard *et al.*, 1972; Weinryb *et al.*, 1972; Berndt and Schwabe, 1973; Furlanut *et al.*, 1973; Nahorski *et al.*, 1973; Dalton *et al.*, 1974). Correlations between potency as *in vitro* inhibitors of brain phosphodiesterase and efficacy in a conflict test for a number of compounds led to a proposal that antianxiety drugs may act via elevations of brain cyclic AMP (Beer *et al.*, 1972; Horovitz *et al.*, 1972). The functional significance of different phosphodiesterase enzymes even in one brain region, however, is as yet unknown. Certain of the inhibitors do possess quite different inhibitory activity toward the various isolated isozymes (Fertel *et al.*, 1973).

Different forms of phosphodiesterases have been reported in retina, a preparation that includes both photoreceptor, bipolar and ganglion cells (Pannbacker *et al.*, 1972; Farber and Lolley, 1973; Schmidt and Lolley, 1973). Certain phosphodiesterases were shown to develop in retina during maturation of DBA mice, but not in C3H mice, the latter a strain whose photoreceptors undergo degeneration.

Phosphodiesterases are present in homogenates from cultured glioma and neuroblastoma cells (Perkins *et al.*, 1971; Jard *et al.*, 1972; Schwartz *et al.*, 1973; Uzunov *et al.*, 1973). At least two forms are present in rat glioma cells, while mouse neuroblastoma cells and human glioma cells appear to have only one. In glioma cells a significant portion of the enzyme activity is particulate.

Certain phosphodiesterases of brain appear to hydrolyze both cyclic AMP and cyclic GMP and to be inhibited to similar extents with various agents, while other enzymes appear to be more or less specific for one of the cyclic nucleotides and to be differentially affected by various agents (Drummond and Perrott-Yee, 1961; Cheung, 1967*a*, 1970, 1971*a,b*; Brooker *et al.*, 1968; Beavo *et al.*, 1970, 1971; Roberts and Simonsen, 1970; Kakiuchi *et al.*, 1971, 1973; Thompson and Appleman, 1971*b,c*; Williams *et al.*, 1971; Campbell and Oliver, 1972; Appleman *et al.*, 1973; Goldberg *et al.*, 1973; Dalton *et al.*, 1974). The efficacy of a variety of other cyclic nucleotides including 8-benzylthio and butyryl derivatives of cyclic AMP as substrates and/or inhibitors of brain phosphodiesterases has been reported (Drummond and Powell, 1970; Muneyama *et al.*, 1971; Cehovic, 1972; Meyer *et al.*, 1972; Harris *et al.*, 1973; Jastorff and Bar, 1973; Miller *et al.*, 1973*a*; Simon *et al.*, 1973).

The presence of such a variety of phosphodiesterases in brain homogenates with differing affinities for cyclic nucleotides and influenced *in situ* to varying degrees by calcium ions, protein activators, ATP, etc., makes any extrapolation of results on phosphodiesterase activity in homogenates to phosphodiesterase-controlled degradation of cyclic nucleotides in morphological compartments of the intact functioning brain extremely difficult.

2.4. Protein Kinases

In homogenates of brain tissue, protein kinases are present which are activated by cyclic AMP and which catalyze the phosphorylation of serine residues in a variety of protein substrates including glycogen synthetase, histones, ribosomes, synaptosomes, synaptic vesicles, and microtubules (Goldberg and O'Toole, 1969; Kuo and Greengard, 1969*a,b*, 1970*a,b*; Miyamoto *et al.*, 1969*a,b*; Goldberg *et al.*, 1970; Gaballah and Popoff, 1971*b*; Johnson *et al.*, 1971; Maeno *et al.*, 1971; Murray and Froscio, 1971; Schmidt and Robison, 1972; Inoue *et al.*, 1973; Schmidt and Sokoloff, 1973; Weller and Rodnight, 1973). Other protein kinases are present which are not activated by cyclic AMP (Walinder, 1972). The cyclic AMP–activated protein kinases require magnesium or manganese ions and are inhibited by calcium ions, ADP, and adenosine (see above references) and by a protein factor isolated from muscle (Walsh *et al.*, 1971). Cyclic GMP activates these kinases, but only at high concentrations. A factor from brain was reported to inhibit cyclic AMP–dependent kinases and to activate cyclic GMP–dependent kinases (Kuo and Greengard, 1973). The activation of brain protein kinases by various analogues of cyclic AMP has been extensively studied (Miyamoto *et al.*, 1969*b*; Kuo and Greengard, 1970*a*; Kuo *et al.*, 1970; Bauer *et al.*, 1971; Muneyama *et al.*, 1971; Meyer *et al.*, 1972, 1973; Jones *et al.*, 1973; Miller *et al.*, 1973*a,b*; Simon *et al.*, 1973).

Cyclic AMP–dependent protein kinases are found to be associated in brain homogenates with both soluble protein fractions and particulate fractions, including those enriched in synaptosomes. Small amounts are associated with nuclei. At least two soluble forms were detected from brain (Miyamoto *et al.*, 1971). Cyclic nucleotide–activated kinases from brain as from other tissues are dissociable into regulatory units which bind cyclic AMP and the functional catalytic units (Inoue *et al.*, 1973). The relatively inactive complex made up of regulatory and catalytic units is dissociated and thereby activated upon binding of cyclic AMP. Histones and other basic proteins may also alter the association of regulatory and catalytic units (Miyamoto *et al.*, 1971). Cyclic AMP–dependent phosphorylation of ribosomes but not of histones appears to increase in brain preparations during maturation of rats (Gaballah *et al.*, 1971; Schmidt and Robison, 1972; Schmidt and Sókoloff, 1973). Cyclic AMP–activated protein kinases have been reported in glioma cells (Perkins *et al.*, 1971; Jard *et al.*, 1972; Opler and Makman, 1972) and neuroblastoma cells (Greengard and Kuo, 1970).

A cyclic AMP–elicited increase in rates of intrinsic phosphorylation of membrane proteins by ATP occurs with synaptosomes, neurotubular fractions, and certain microsomal preparations from brain, but not with synaptic vesicles from brain or with membranes from peripheral crab nerves (Goodman *et al.*, 1970; Weller and Rodnight 1970, 1973; Johnson *et al.*, 1971; Schmidt and Robison, 1972; Schmidt and Sokoloff, 1973). Further studies on protein kinase activity in neurotubular proteins have been reported (Rappaport *et al.*, 1972; Soifer *et al.*, 1972). Certain of the above preparations contain adenylate cyclases capable of generating cyclic AMP under the conditions of assay (Weller and Rodnight, 1971). Phosphorylation of two protein components of a synaptic membrane preparation was greatly increased by cyclic AMP (Johnson *et al.*, 1973; Ueda *et al.*, 1973). The cyclic AMP–elicited increase in phosphorylation of synaptic membranes was markedly decreased in preparations from electrically shocked animals (Appel and Locher, 1973).

Cyclic GMP–activated protein kinases catalyzing the phosphorylation of histones would appear to be present in brain preparations, to require magnesium ions for activity, and to be inhibited by calcium ions (Greengard and Kuo, 1970; Hofmann and Sold, 1972). Cerebellar levels were higher than those of cortical tissue.

It should be clear that *in vitro* studies on the protein kinases of brain preparations have begun to provide insights into the possible nature of the various endogenous protein substrates whose phosphorylation cyclic nucleotides regulate in the central nervous system. In intact cells or tissue slices, such studies are complicated by high turnover rates of protein phosphate (see Section 4.1 and Kinase references in the *Addendum*).

2.5. Phosphoprotein Phosphates

The presence of phosphoprotein phosphates and their relevance to cyclic AMP–dependent mechanisms have not been studied extensively. The enzyme occurs in brain and is associated with membranes (Weller and Rodnight, 1971; Maeno and Greengard, 1972). In rat cerebral cortical homogenates, at least three phosphoprotein phosphates were present, with a major fraction of total activity associated with synaptic membranes. Magnesium and calcium ions had little effect on basal activity, while manganese ions increased enzyme activity in certain fractions. The rate of dephosphorylation of membranal preparations was not accelerated by cyclic AMP.

3. ACCUMULATION OF CYCLIC NUCLEOTIDES

The complexity of the interrelationships of the cyclases, phosphodiesterases, protein kinases, and phosphoprotein phosphatases with macromolecular factors, magnesium, manganese, and calcium ions, and levels of ATP and GTP and in addition the existence of multiple enzyme forms with differing properties even within one cell make it difficult or impossible to extrapolate results obtained with homogenates to the functional operation of cyclic nucleotide systems in intact cells. Studies on the accumulation of cyclic nucleotides in brain slices, ganglia, and cultured cells under various conditions can, however, provide pertinent information.

The extent of accumulation of cyclic AMP in intact cells will be influenced by a number of factors: (1) the basal levels of adenylate cyclases and the availability of ATP as a substrate; (2) the degree of activation of this enzyme by biogenic amines, adenosine, and other compounds; (3) the levels and properties of cyclic nucleotide phosphodiesterases; and (4) the levels of cyclic AMP–dependent protein kinases with binding sites that presumably sequester cyclic AMP. The subcellular distribution and availability of ions such as calcium and magnesium with their abilities to inhibit or activate these systems will be important in determining the extent of accumulation of cyclic AMP. Similar factors would be involved in the cyclic GMP–generating systems of intact cells. Two methods have been extensively used to study the factors regulating accumulations of cyclic AMP in such preparations. Either endogenous levels of cyclic AMP are measured or the extent of formation of radioactive cyclic AMP from intracellular radioactive adenine nucleotides labeled during a prior incubation of the preparation with radioactive adenine or adenosine is ascertained. Combination of the two methods can provide information relevant to compartmentalization of adenine nucleotides either within a cell or in different cells of a complex tissue such as that represented by a brain slice. The adenine or adenosine used in the prelabeling technique is incorporated into intracellular nucleotides by the action of adenine phosphoribosyltransferase or adenosine kinase, respectively (Shimizu and Daly, 1972*a*; Shimizu *et al.*, 1972). In the case of adenosine, a prior uptake process may be rate limiting at low concentrations (Huang and Daly, 1974*a*).

3.1. Cyclic AMP in Brain Slices

Accumulation of cyclic AMP and to a lesser extent cyclic GMP has been investigated in brain slices from different brain regions and a variety of species. The results indicate that in spite of its heterogeneity the brain slice provides a valuable tool for the study of the factors involved in the regulation of cyclic nucleotides in the central nervous system.

After sacrifice of animals, cyclic AMP levels rise rapidly in brain tissue (Breckenridge, 1964; Goldberg *et al.*, 1967, 1970; Kakiuchi and Rall, 1968*a*; Ditzion *et al.*, 1970; Steiner *et al.*, 1970, 1972; Schmidt *et al.*, 1970, 1971; Sattin, 1971; Uzunov and Weiss, 1971, 1972; Weiss and Strada, 1972). The increase is particularly large in cerebellum. Postdecapitation increases in cyclic AMP levels occur in developing rat brain at a time when a norepinephrine-sensitive cyclase cannot be detected in brain slices (Schmidt *et al.*, 1970). Adenosine-sensitive cyclases are present at this time (Perkins and Moore, 1973*b*). Prior treatment of adult rats with dopa and a monoamine oxidase inhibitor reduces postdecapitation increases in cyclic AMP (Paul *et al.*, 1970*a*). The cerebellar increase in cyclic AMP is blocked by prior treatment of rats with phenothiazines, compounds which antagonize norepinephrine effects on cyclases in cerebellar slices, or by prior treatment with lithium salts or chlorprothixene (Uzunov and Weiss, 1971, 1972). Pretreatment of adult rabbits with chlorpromazine reduces the postdecapitation increase in cyclic AMP in cerebral cortex, while pretreatment with reserpine to deplete norepinephrine or with an antihistaminic, diphenhydramine, has no effect (Kakiuchi and Rall, 1968*a*). Central depressants such as barbiturates, ethanol, papaverine, and, to a lesser degree, ether and halothane block the increase in brain cyclic AMP to varying extents in a variety of species (Kakiuchi and Rall, 1968*a*; Ditzion *et al.*, 1970; Goldberg *et al.*, 1970; Paul *et al.*, 1970*a*; Volicer and Gold, 1973). Ethanol in lower concentrations enhances the postdecapitation increases in cyclic AMP. Methylxanthines, which have been shown to have activities as central stimulants, phosphodiesterase inhibitors, and as antagonists of adenosine-sensitive cyclases in brain slices, reduce postdecapitation increases in cyclic AMP (Goldberg *et al.*, 1970; Paul *et al.*, 1970*a*; Sattin, 1971). The increases in rat cerebellar cyclic AMP levels were lower after a 12-h dark period as compared to the increases seen after 12 h of light (Weiss and Strada, 1972).

Clearly, the factors involved in postdecapitation increases in cyclic AMP levels of brain are not established. Release of norepinephrine or histamine does not appear to be of prime importance. Instead, the data suggest that intense electrical activity and anoxia following decapitation lead to an accumulation of adenosine within the tissue and that adenosine-mediated increases of cyclic AMP result. Fortunately, cyclic AMP in brain slices returns to low stable levels after incubation for 20–90 min in aerated medium. Most experiments with brain slices have been carried out after such prior incubations. Basal levels of cyclic AMP in brain slices are low, in most instances between 10 and 60 pmol/mg protein. The cyclic AMP–generating systems in slices appear to remain functional for at least 2 h.

Brain slices from rabbit, guinea pig, rat, and mouse have been extensively studied. In most investigations, chopped tissue of 200–300 μm has been used. In certain studies on electrical stimulation tangential slices of cortex have been used. Profound differences in the extent of accumulation of cyclic AMP elicited by stimulatory agents are observed in the various species and/or brain regions. Presumably, such differences in responses of brain slices to biogenic amines, adenosine, depolarization, and drugs reflect similar differences in the intact brain. However, differential losses or alterations in responses during preparation of brain slices cannot be excluded. Time courses for the accumulation of cyclic AMP in response to biogenic amines, adenosine, and depolarizing conditions have been reported for slices from different species and different brain regions. Under most conditions, maximal accumulations are reached within 3–10 min. With ouabain, nearly 15 min is required. The maximal accumulation of cyclic AMP is in most cases maintained or decreases slowly during a subsequent 10–20 min of incubation. It should be stressed that accumulations of cyclic AMP have been frequently measured and compared at a single time point between 4 and 15 min and at a single high concentration of the stimulatory agent. The biogenic amines histamine, norepinephrine, and serotonin have in most brain slice preparations an EC_{50} for accumulation of cyclic AMP between 1 and 20 μM, while adenosine has an EC_{50} of about 30 μM. The true EC_{50} values for norepinephrine and adenosine are significantly lower because of active uptake processes within the brain slice. The increases in endogenous levels of cyclic AMP in brain slices have in most instances been reflected by similar increases in accumulation of radioactive cyclic AMP derived from intracellular adenine nucleotides labeled during a prior incubation with radioactive adenine or adenosine. The following sections will discuss the effects of biogenic amines, adenosine, depolarization, and other factors on the accumulation of cyclic AMP in brain slices from various species or orders that have been extensively studied. In cat brain slices labeled with adenine, norepinephrine elicited significant increases in levels of radioactive cyclic AMP in tissue from cortex (fivefold), cerebellum (fivefold), and hypothalamus (less than threefold) and had no significant effect in slices from caudate nucleus (Forn and Krishna, 1971). Histamine elicited significant increases only in cerebellar (twofold) and hypothalamic (twofold) slices. Serotonin, dopamine, and carbachol had no significant effect. In adenine-labeled brain slices from the frog *Rana pipiens*, (nor)epinephrine, histamine, serotonin, and carbachol had no significant effect on levels of radioactive cyclic AMP (Forn and Krishna, 1971).

The effects of various agonists and antagonists on levels of cyclic AMP will be seen in the following sections to differ remarkably in different brain regions and in the same region from different strains or species of animals (Table 1). However, as will be apparent, even for the same brain region from the same species, results are often quantitatively different. Such differences would appear to be due to many factors, among which the following appear to be relevant: (1) experimental variables involving removal of brain tissue and slice preparation, length of incubation before use, amount and aeration of slices in the medium, measurement of either radioactive cyclic AMP in

TABLE 1

Effect of Various Agents on Levels of Cyclic AMP in Incubated Brain Slices[a]

Brain region	Putative neuromodulators				Depolarizing agents			
	(Nor)-epinephrine	Histamine	Adenosine	Prostaglandin	K^+ (40–60 mM)	Veratridine	Ouabain	Electrical stimulation
Rabbit								
Cerebral cortex	±	+++	+*	±	±	+++*	+++*	
Cerebellum	++(β)	++		±				
Guinea pig								
Cerebral cortex	±(α)	++	+++	±	++	+++	+++*	++
Cerebellum	++(β)	±	+++	±	±	++	+	++
Rat								
Cerebral cortex	++(α,β)	±	++	± or +	++*	++	++*	
Cerebellum	+(β)	±	+	±				
Mouse								
Cerebral cortex	++(β)	±	++		± to +++	++	++*	
Cerebellum	++	±	+++		++			

[a]Supramaximal concentrations of amines, adenosine, veratridine, and ouabain were employed. A marginal or no accumulation of cyclic AMP (zero- to twofold increase) is designated by ±, a small accumulation (two- to fourfold increase) by +, an intermediate accumulation (four- to fifteenfold increase) by ++, and a large accumulation (more than fifteenfold increase) by +++. If only accumulations of radioactive cyclic AMP in prelabeled slices have been measured, the data are marked with an asterisk. Types of receptors are designated in parentheses as α-adrenergic (α) or β-adrenergic (β). References pertinent to these data are cited in the text. Glutamate in high concentrations has now been found to stimulate cyclic AMP formation in guinea pig cortical slices (see *Addendum*, Shimizu *et al.*, 1974).

prelabeled slices or of endogenous cyclic AMP, method of determination of protein concentration, and, finally, subtle factors related to each individual investigator's experimental techniques; (2) biological variability of individual animals and of groups of animals dependent on source, history, and season; (3) inadequate experimentation, i.e., insufficient to compensate for the biological and technical variables.

3.1.1. Rabbit

In cerebral cortical slices, norepinephrine has no effect or elicits a less than threefold increase in levels of cyclic AMP, while in cerebellar slices a three- to fifteenfold increase in cyclic AMP occurs (Kakiuchi and Rall, 1968*a,b*; Shimizu *et al.*, 1969, 1970*a*; Forn and Krishna, 1971; Krishna *et al.*, 1970; Schmidt and Robison, 1971; Berti *et al.*, 1972; Kuo *et al.*, 1972). The effect of norepinephrine in cerebellar slices is completely blocked by a β-antagonist, dichloroisoproterenol, is unaffected by an α-antagonist, phenoxybenzamine, and is partially antagonized by relatively high concentrations of chlorpromazine or diphenhydramine (Kakiuchi and Rall, 1968*b*). Isoproterenol elicits an accumulation similar to that elicited by norepinephrine, providing further evidence that β-receptors are involved in norepinephrine-elicited accumulation of cyclic AMP in rabbit cerebellum. The maximal accumulations in cyclic AMP elicited by norepinephrine decline more rapidly in cerebellar than in cortical slices (Kakiuchi and Rall, 1968*a,b*). Norepinephrine has either no effect or elicited only a twofold increase in cyclic AMP levels in slices from hypothalamus, hippocampus, caudate nucleus, and brain stem (Kakiuchi and Rall, 1968*a*; Krishna *et al.*, 1970; Schmidt and Robison, 1971). With adenine-labeled slices from caudate nucleus, a much larger stimulation by norepinephrine has been reported (Shimizu *et al.*, 1969). This study was done in the presence of caffeine, a weak phosphodiesterase inhibitor. α-Methylnorepinephrine was nearly as active as norepinephrine in cerebellar slices (Shimizu *et al.*, 1970*d*). Norepinephrine elicited accumulations of cyclic AMP in slices from frontal cortex, hypothalamus, and hippocampus of newborn rabbits (Schmidt and Robison, 1971). The effect reached a maximum 9–14 days after birth and then declined to finally disappear in slices from adults. The stimulatory effects of norepinephrine were nearly constant in cerebellar slices throughout maturation to adulthood.

Histamine elicited large accumulations in both cortical (five- to thirtyfold increase) and cerebellar (three- to tenfold) slices (Kakiuchi and Rall, 1968*a,b*; Shimizu *et al.*, 1969, 1970*a,c*; Forn and Krishna, 1971, Krishna *et al.*, 1970; Berti *et al.*, 1972; Kuo *et al.*, 1972; Palmer *et al.*, 1972*a*). The maximal levels of cyclic AMP attained during histamine stimulation were maintained for an extended period of cortical slices, but not in cerebellar slices. The effects of histamine were antagonized by phenoxybenzamine, chlorpromazine, and antihistamines (Kakiuchi and Rall, 1968*a,b*; Palmer *et al.*, 1972*a*) and by lithium ions (Forn and Valdecasas, 1971). Histamine analogues and homologues such as betazole, 3-(2-aminoethyl)-1,2,4-triazole, ω-*N*-methylhistamine, and ω-*N,N*-dimethylhistamine elicited accumulations of cyclic AMP in cortical slices (Shimizu *et al.*, 1970*c*). The accumulation of cyclic AMP elicited in cortical slices by histamine increased during the first 8 days postpartum and then declined to adult levels (Palmer *et al.*, 1972*a*).

Combinations of histamine and norepinephrine had nearly additive effects on cyclic AMP levels in cortical and cerebellar slices (Kakiuchi and Rall, 1968*a,b*; Huang *et al.*, 1971). Evidence for separate histamine and norepinephrine receptors was obtained in studies on amine restimulation with cerebellar slices in the presence of theophylline (Kakiuchi and Rall, 1968*b*). Histamine did not elicit an accumulation of cyclic AMP in slices that had been previously stimulated with histamine. Similarly, norepinephrine did not elicit an accumulation in slices previously stimulated with norepinephrine. However, the slices did respond to norepinephrine after a prior stimulation with histamine and to histamine after a prior stimulation with norepinephrine.

Serotonin has either no or only a small stimulatory effect on cyclic AMP levels in cerebellar or cortical slices (Kakiuchi and Rall, 1968*a,b*; Forn and Krishna, 1971; Shimizu *et al.*, 1970*d*). β-Phenylethylamine and *N*-methyltryptamine had marginal activity in cerebellar slices (Shimizu *et al.*, 1970*c,d*). Dopamine, tyramines, octopamines, amphetamine, spermine and other polyamines, glycine, γ-aminobutyric acid, glutamate, and prostaglandin had virtually no effect on cyclic AMP levels in cortical and/or cerebellar slices (Kakiuchi and Rall, 1968*a,b*; Forn and Krishna, 1971; Shimizu *et al.*, 1970*c,d*; Berti *et al.*, 1972; Kuo *et al.*, 1972; Lee *et al.*, 1972). Indeed, certain of these agents such as acetylcholine in cerebellar slices (Kuo *et al.*, 1972) cause a slight decrease in basal levels of cyclic AMP.

Adenosine elicited a 3.5-fold increase in radioactive cyclic AMP in adenine-labeled cortical slices (Berti *et al.*, 1972). Depolarizing agents, which in slices from other rodents appear to elicit accumulations of cyclic AMP by mechanisms involving at least in part the formation and intermediacy of adenosine, elicit large accumulations of cyclic AMP in rabbit cerebral cortical slices (Rall and Sattin, 1970; Shimizu *et al.*, 1970*a,d*; Shimizu and Daly, 1972*b*). Thus veratridine, batrachotoxin, and ouabain elicited thirty-, forty-, and hundredfold increases, respectively, in cyclic AMP levels. Potassium ions (40 mM), in contrast, were only marginally effective. Combinations of veratridine with either norepinephrine or histamine had greater than additive effects.

The effects of theophylline, a relatively weak inhibitor of brain phosphodiesterase and also an antagonist of adenosine, on accumulations of cyclic AMP in brain slices were first studied in cortical and cerebellar preparations from rabbit, where in slices prepared at 4 °C it potentiated the effects of norepinephrine or histamine (Kakiuchi and Rall, 1968*a,b*). Potentiation of the effects of histamine by theophylline was confirmed in adenine-labeled cortical slices prepared in the cold (Shimizu *et al.*, 1970*b*). In later studies by Rall and Sattin (1970) using rabbit cortical slices prepared at room temperature, theophylline did not potentiate the effect of histamine. It was suggested that theophylline would potentiate amines only in slices prepared in the cold. However, others using adenine-labeled rabbit cortical slices reported no potentiation of histamine effects by theophylline regardless of the temperature at which the slices were prepared (Forn and Krishna, 1971). Theophylline has little or no effect on histamine responses in guinea pig cortical slices prepared either at room temperature or in the cold (Kakiuchi *et al.*, 1969; Rall and Sattin, 1970; Shimizu *et al.*, 1970*a*; Shimizu and Daly, 1972*b*; Schultz and Daly, 1973*b*; Huang and Daly, 1974*a*). Caffeine, which is a weaker phosphodiesterase inhibitor and a weaker adenosine antagonist than theophylline, was, however, reported to potentiate histamine responses in guinea pig cortical slices (Shimizu *et al.*, 1969). Theophylline has little or no effect on norepinephrine-elicited accumulation of cyclic AMP in guinea pig (Shimizu and Daly, 1972*b*) or rat (Forn and Krishna, 1970) cortical slices. More active phosphodiesterase inhibitors, which do not antagonize, indeed potentiate adenosine-mediated accumulations of cyclic AMP, have now proven more useful than theophylline in studies on the role of phosphodiesterase in brain slices (see below). However, theophylline is still useful in such preparations as an adenosine antagonist.

3.1.2. Guinea Pig

Norepinephrine and epinephrine elicit only a small (Kakiuchi *et al.*, 1969; Shimizu *et al.*, 1969, 1970*a*, 1973; Sattin and Rall, 1970; Chasin *et al.*, 1971, 1973; Huang *et al.*, 1971; Kodama *et al.*, 1971; Huang and Daly, 1972; Shimizu and Daly, 1972*b*; Zanella and Rall, 1973) or insignificant (Forn and Krishna, 1971; Schultz and Daly, 1973*a*; Huang and Daly, 1974*a*) accumulation of cyclic AMP in cerebral cortical slices. The response is fully manifest at birth (Schmidt *et al.*, 1970). In cerebellar slices, norepinephrine elicits an eight-to twentyfold increase in levels of cyclic AMP (Chasin *et al.*, 1971, 1973; Zanella and Rall, 1973). β-Antagonists block the stimulatory effect of the catecholamine in cerebellar slices, while α-antagonists are ineffective and antihistamines cause only a marginal inhibition. In contrast, the stimulatory effects of epinephrine in cortical slices are blocked by α-antagonists, while being only slightly antagonized by antihistamines and unaffected by β-antagonists. Thus in guinea pig cortical slices, epinephrine apparently activates adenylate cyclases by interaction with a classical α-receptor. The marginal activity of a pure β-agonist, isoproterenol (Chasin *et al.*, 1973), is compatible with this interpretation. Epinephrine elicits a small accumulation of cyclic AMP in slices from hippocampus and amygdala, but not from diencephalon and brain stem. The effects of epinephrine are blocked in both regions by α-antagonists, and partially blocked by an antihistamine. Propranolol partially antagonizes the effect of epinephrine in slices from amygdala.

Histamine elicits a three- to twentyfold increase in levels of cyclic AMP in cerebral cortical slices (Kakiuchi *et al.*, 1969; Shimizu *et al.*, 1969, 1970*a,c*, 1973; Forn and Krishna, 1971; Krishna *et al.*, 1970; Rall and Sattin, 1970; Sattin and Rall, 1970; Shimizu and Daly, 1970, 1972*b*; Chasin *et al.*, 1971, 1973; Huang *et al.*, 1971; Kodama *et al.*, 1971; Huang and Daly, 1972, 1974*b*; Schultz and Daly, 1973*a,b,c,d*; Shimizu and Okayama, 1973; Zanella and Rall, 1973; Schultz, 1974*a,b*). The effect of histamine is blocked by antihistamines, while α- and β-antagonists have marginal or no inhibitory action (Chasin *et al.*, 1971, 1973; Shimizu and Daly, 1972*b*; Schultz and Daly, 1973*b*; Zanella and Rall, 1973). In cerebellar slices, histamine has either marginal (Zanella and Rall, 1973) or no (Chasin *et al.*, 1971) effect on cyclic AMP levels. Histamine has no effect in slices from diencephalon or brain stem and only a small effect in amygdala, while eliciting a greater than eightfold increase in cyclic AMP in hippocampal slices (Chasin *et al.*, 1973). The latter effect is not blocked by α- and β-antagonists and is only partially blocked by classical H_1-antihistamines such as chlorpheniramine and pyrilamine.

Serotonin has either marginal (Shimizu *et al.*, 1970*d*; Chasin *et al.*, 1971) or no (Huang *et al.*, 1971; Huang and Daly, 1972) effect on cyclic AMP levels in cerebral cortical slices and has no effect in cerebellar slices (Chasin *et al.*, 1971). Marginal effects of serotonin have been reported with slices from hippocampus, amygdala, diencephalon, and brain stem (Chasin *et al.*, 1973). A variety of other agents including dopamine, prostaglandin, polypeptide hormones, acetylcholine, glycine, γ-aminobutyric acid, glutamate, and *N,O*-dibutyryl cyclic AMP had no significant effect on cyclic AMP levels in cerebral cortical slices (Shimizu *et al.*, 1970*c,d*; Chasin *et al.*, 1971, 1973; Zanella and Rall, 1973), nor did dopamine or acetylcholine have significant effects in slices from hippocampus, amygdala, diencephalon, and brain stem.

In contrast to results with rabbit and rat cortical slices, histamine and (nor)epinephrine have much greater than additive effects on levels of cyclic AMP in guinea pig cerebral cortical slices (Huang *et al.*, 1971, 1973; Chasin *et al.*, 1973; Schultz and Daly, 1973*a*). The synergism occurs only with the physiologically active levorotatory catecholamine. A local anaesthetic, cocaine, did not prevent the synergism, which was, however, completely blocked by α-antagonists and partially blocked by the antihistamine diphenhydramine. Thus the synergism appears to involve interaction of the catecholamine with α-receptors and histamine with H_1-receptors. Consonant with this, isoproterenol did not potentiate the accumulation of cyclic AMP elicited by histamine. The partial blockade of the effect of combinations of histamine and norepinephrine by theophylline (Huang *et al.*, 1973;

Schultz and Daly, 1973*b*; Huang and Daly, 1974*a*) suggests that adenosine is involved to some extent in this synergistic interaction. Similar synergisms between histamine and norepinephrine are seen in slices of guinea pig hippocampus (Chasin *et al.*, 1973). Slightly greater than additive effects may occur in cortical slices with combinations of histamine and serotonin (Huang *et al.*, 1971).

Adenosine elicits a fifteen- to fiftyfold increase in levels of endogenous cyclic AMP in cortical slices (Sattin and Rall, 1970; Somerville and Smith, 1972; Schultz and Daly, 1973*a,b,c,d*; Zanella and Rall, 1973; Huang and Daly, 1974*a,b*). In early studies with adenine-labeled slices, a relatively low seven- to tenfold increase in radioactive cyclic AMP levels was elicited by adenosine (Shimizu *et al.*, 1969, 1970*a,d*; Shimizu and Daly, 1970, 1972*b*; Huang *et al.*, 1971, 1972), but in later experiments from the same laboratory (Shimizu *et al.*, 1973; Schultz and Daly, 1973*a,b,c*; Huang and Daly, 1974*a,b*) and by Somerville and Smith (1972) twenty- to thirtyfold increases were consistently observed with adenine-labeled slices. The reason for the differences was not apparent. Adenosine elicits a fifty- to sixtyfold increase in cyclic AMP in cerebellar slices (Zanella and Rall, 1973).

Adenosine, in addition to stimulating formation of cyclic AMP from intracellular radioactive adenine nucleotides, is incorporated by phosphorylation into nucleotides that then serve as precursors of cyclic AMP (Sattin and Rall, 1970; Shimizu and Daly, 1970; Schultz and Daly, 1973*a*). In guinea pig cortical slices, incorporation of exogenous 0.1 mM adenosine represents less than 20% of the total accumulation of cyclic AMP after 10 min of incubation (Schultz and Daly, 1973*a*), while in mouse cortical slices it represents about 40% (Skolnick and Daly, 1974*c*). Theophylline, which competitively blocks the stimulatory effect of adenosine in cortical slices (Sattin and Rall, 1970), does not significantly inhibit the incorporation of adenosine into intracellular nucleotides that serve as precursors of cyclic AMP (Shimizu *et al.*, 1969; Sattin and Rall, 1970; Huang and Daly, 1974*a*). Furthermore, agents such as dipyridamole, papaverine, hexobendine, and 6-(*p*-nitrobenzylthio)guanosine that do effectively inhibit active uptake of adenosine into cortical slices concomitantly potentiate the accumulation of cyclic AMP elicited by low concentrations of adenosine (Huang and Daly, 1974*a*). These and other observations provide strong evidence for an extracellular adenosine receptor which serves to activate cyclic AMP–generating system(s) in brain slices. Attempts to demonstrate such an extracellular site for adenosine action using a nonpermeating quaternary analogue of the blocking agent theophylline were not successful (Schultz and Daly, 1973*b*), apparently because the quaternary analogue was no longer an effective antagonist at the extracellular adenosine receptor.

A large number of compounds structurally related to adenosine have been screened for agonist or antagonist activity in guinea pig cortical slices (Sattin and Rall, 1970; Shimizu *et al.*, 1970*d*; Huang *et al.*, 1972; Schrier and

Gilman, 1973; Huang and Daly, 1974*a*). ATP, ADP, and AMP were active in stimulating cyclic AMP formation, but their activity appeared to be dependent on a prior hydrolysis to adenosine. Almost any alteration in the ribose moiety of adenosine as in the 3′-*O*-methyl derivative, the 5′-esters other than phosphates, and 2′-deoxy, 3′-deoxy, arabinoside, xyloside, and carbocyclic analogues caused a complete loss of stimulatory activity. 5′-Deoxyadenosine, however, retained approximately one-third the agonist activity of adenosine. Most of these analogues including 5′-deoxyadenosine were adenosine antagonists, as are the xanthine derivatives, theophylline, caffeine, and 3-isobutyl-1-methylxanthine. Alterations in the purine portion of adenosine as in tubercidin, 8-azadenosine, 6-*N,N*-dimethyladenosine, 1-methyladenosine, and inosine resulted in virtual loss of both agonist and antagonist activity. Certain substituted adenosines such as the 2-chloro, 2-hydroxy, 2-amino, 6-*N*-phenyl, 6-*N*-methyl, or 8-methylamino derivatives did retain agonist activity. 8-Bromoadenosine did not exhibit agonist activity, nor did any natural nucleosides except adenosine. The effects of adenosine in cortical slices were not antagonized by α- or β-antagonists or by antihistamines (Somerville and Smith, 1972; Schultz and Daly, 1973*d*). In fact, compounds of this type which have local anesthetic activity such as phentolamine, propranolol, and pheniramine and local anesthetics such as procaine and cocaine slightly potentiated the effects of adenosine. However, in another study cocaine was reported to have no apparent effect on adenosine-elicited accumulation of radioactive cyclic AMP in adenine-labeled cortical slices (Shimizu *et al.*, 1973). Cocaine does potentiate the effects of low concentrations of biogenic amines in cortical slices (Huang *et al.*, 1971). In another rodent (rat), propranolol and phentolamine did not potentiate the effect of adenosine in cerebral cortical slices (Schultz and Daly, 1973*e*). A β-antagonist, sotalol, which has little local anesthetic activity, partially blocked the effect of adenosine in guinea pig cerebellar slices (Zanella and Rall, 1973).

In cerebral cortical slices, combinations of adenosine with norepinephrine, histamine, or serotonin have much greater than additive effects on accumulation of cyclic AMP (Sattin and Rall, 1970; Shimizu *et al.*, 1970*a*; Huang *et al.*, 1971; Schultz and Daly, 1973*a,b,c,d*; Zanella and Rall, 1973; Huang and Daly, 1974*a,b*). Combinations of adenosine and norepinephrine or histamine also have synergistic effects in cerebellar slices. Representative results are shown in Table 2. The magnitude of amine-elicited accumulations will thus be dependent on levels of endogenous adenosine within the slice. Indeed, the magnitudes of amine effects are greatly increased by the presence of compounds that would inhibit reuptake of adenosine, and this increase is antagonized by theophylline (Huang and Daly, 1974*a*). The synergistic interactions between adenosine and amines appear to be mediated in cortical slices by receptors similar to those mediating the effect of adenosine or amines alone. Thus isoproterenol, a pure β-antagonist

TABLE 2

Representative Effects of Various Agents on the Accumulation of Cyclic AMP in Guinea Pig Cerebral Cortical or Cerebellar Slices

	Cyclic AMP[a] (pmol/mg protein)		
	Cerebral cortex		Cerebellum
Agent (0.1 mM)	(A)	(B)	(C)
None	11	14	6
Histamine	80	75	8
Norepinephrine	18	13	140
Serotonin	—	14	—
Adenosine	300	220	350
Adenosine + histamine	800	900	470
Adenosine + norepinephrine	600	900	560
Adenosine + serotonin	—	600	—

[a]Data from (A) Sattin and Rall (1970), (B) Schultz and Daly (1973*a*), (C) Zanella and Rall (1973).

without effect in cortical slices, does not synergistically interact with adenosine (Schultz and Daly, 1973*d*). The synergistic effects of adenosine–(nor)epinephrine combinations are blocked by α-antagonists, partially blocked by chlorpromazine and dromoran, either partially blocked or unaffected by antihistamines, and unaffected by β-antagonists (Huang and Daly, 1972; Schultz and Daly, 1973*d*). The adenosine–histamine combination is antagonized by antihistamines, dromoran, and chlorpromazine, either partially blocked or unaffected by α-antagonists, and unaffected by a β-antagonist. The adenosine–serotonin combination is blocked by methysergide, either unaffected or partially blocked by phenoxybenzamine, and unaffected by β-antagonists, chlorpromazine, and dromoran. Synergistic effects of amine–adenosine combinations are blocked by an adenosine antagonist, theophylline (H. Duck Mah and J. W. Daly, unpublished results). At low concentrations of adenosine, the synergistic effects of amine–adenosine combinations are greatly potentiated by compounds that block uptake of adenosine (Huang and Daly, 1974*a*). Stimulatory effects of adenosine on accumulation of cyclic AMP occur at lower concentrations of the riboside when histamine is present in the incubation medium (Huang *et al.*, 1971).

Adenosine will elicit repetitive accumulations of cyclic AMP in cortical slices (Sattin and Rall, 1970; Schultz and Daly, 1973*c*). However, biogenic amines will elicit only one accumulation, after which the slices are unresponsive to amines unless adenosine is present (Schultz and Daly, 1973*c*). Thus it would appear that the presence of adenosine maintains amine-receptor mechanisms in a responsive state. An intermediate incubation with adenosine does not restore amine responsiveness to slices previously incubated with amines, although these same slices will respond normally to an adenosine–amine combination. The partial retention of amine responsiveness in amine-stimulated slices in the presence of phosphodiesterase inhibitors and the lack of effect of many phosphodiesterase inhibitors on adenosine-mediated accumulations of cyclic AMP led to the proposal that loss of amine responsiveness is due to an amine- or cyclic AMP-mediated increase in phosphodiesterase activity and that adenosine prevents or negates this increased activity of phosphodiesterase (Schultz and Daly, 1973*b,c*). Recently, however, certain phosphodiesterase inhibitors have been shown to be effective in potentiating adenosine-mediated accumulation of cyclic AMP (Schultz, 1974*a,b*).

Depolarizing agents such as batrachotoxin, veratridine, ouabain, and high concentrations (30–140 mM) of potassium ions greatly elevate cyclic AMP levels (ten- to fortyfold) in guinea pig cortical slices (Rall and Sattin, 1970; Shimizu *et al.*, 1970*a,b,d,* 1973; Shimizu and Daly, 1970, 1972*a,b*; Huang *et al.*, 1971, 1973*a*; Huang and Daly, 1972, 1974*b*; Schultz and Daly, 1973*a,b,c*; Zanella and Rall, 1973). Electrical pulsation (Kakiuchi *et al.*, 1969; Somerville and Smith, 1972; Huang *et al.*, 1973*a*; Reddington *et al.*, 1973; Zanella and Rall, 1973), elevated concentrations of cholinium and ammonium ions, or replacement of sodium ions with sucrose (Rall and Sattin, 1970; Shimizu and Daly, 1972*b*) also increase cyclic AMP levels. Depolarization is apparently requisite to the resultant accumulation of cyclic AMP since compounds with local anesthetic activity such as procaine, cocaine, chlorpromazine, dromoran, diphenhydramine, dichlorisoproterenol, and propranolol antagonize the effects of the depolarizing agents and of electrical pulsation (Kakiuchi *et al.*, 1969; Shimizu *et al.*, 1970*d*; Huang *et al.*, 1972; Shimizu and Daly, 1972*b*; Somerville and Smith, 1972; Zanella and Rall, 1973). The stimulatory effects of veratridine, batrachotoxin, electrical stimulation, and to a lesser extent ouabain are antagonized by agents such as tetrodotoxin and saxitoxin which specifically block sodium channels (Shimizu *et al.*, 1970*d*; Huang *et al.*, 1972; Shimizu and Daly, 1972*b*; Reddington *et al.*, 1973). These agents have little effect on the accumulation elicited by elevated concentrations of potassium ions or histamine. Replacement of sodium with lithium ions antagonizes the effects of batrachotoxin and ouabain, while the stimulatory effect of histamine is unchanged (Shimizu and Daly, 1972*b*). Lithium ions have been reported to antagonize the accumulation of cyclic AMP elicited by histamine in rabbit cortical slices and by norepinephrine in rat cortical and hypothalamic slices but not by norepinephrine in brain stem (Forn and Valdecasas, 1971; Palmer *et al.*, 1972*b*).

Membrane depolarization might itself activate adenylate cyclases, but it would appear more likely that depolarization-evoked formation or release of specific activators is involved. Depolarization in brain slices by batrachotoxin, veratridine, ouabain, potassium ions, or electrical pulsation reduces ATP levels and results in increased levels of adenosine within the slice and an enhanced efflux of adenosine from the slice (Pull and McIlwain, 1972*a,b*, 1973; Shimizu *et al.*, 1970*a*, 1972*a*; Heller and McIlwain, 1973; Huang *et al.*, 1973*a*; Kuroda and McIlwain, 1973; Schultz and Daly, 1973*a*; Huang and Daly, 1974*b*). If the "released" adenosine is responsible for the enhanced accumulation of cyclic AMP, its effects and hence those of depolarizing agents and electrical pulsation should be blocked by theophylline. Indeed, the effects of batrachotoxin, veratridine, and electrical pulsation in cortical slices are blocked nearly completely (more than 80%) by theophylline (Kakiuchi *et al.*, 1969; Shimizu *et al.*, 1970*b*; Shimizu and Daly, 1972*b*; Somerville and Smith, 1972; Huang *et al.*, 1973*a*; Zanella and Rall, 1973). The accumulation elicited by ouabain or potassium ions is only partially blocked (50–60%) by theophylline, indicating that with certain depolarizing agents factors other than adenosine are involved in the activation of cyclic AMP–generating systems. Adenosine deaminase in the medium reduces by 70–90% the accumulation of cyclic AMP elicited by veratridine, 100 mM potassium ions, or electrical pulsation in cortical slices, while having little effect on accumulations of cyclic AMP elicited by ouabain or a histamine–norepinephrine combination (Huang *et al.*, 1973*a*). Such results provide evidence for the release of adenosine into extracellular space as a requisite to the accumulation of cyclic AMP elicited by certain depolarizing agents.

The accumulations of cyclic AMP elicited in cortical slices by adenosine and by electrical pulsation are similar in magnitude, while the maximal accumulations elicited by veratridine, batrachotoxin, ouabain, and potassium ions are much greater, but again for all depolarizing agents of similar magnitude (Shimizu *et al.*, 1970*b*; Shimizu and Daly, 1972*b*; Somerville and Smith, 1972; Huang *et al.*, 1973*a*; Zanella and Rall, 1973). Combinations of 40 mM potassium ions with adenosine or in one case with 5′-AMP had much greater than additive effects on cyclic AMP levels in cortical slices (Rall and Sattin, 1970; Huang *et al.*, 1971; Shimizu and Daly, 1972*b*; Zanella and Rall, 1973). Combinations of submaximal stimulatory concentrations of the other depolarizing agents either with each other or with 40 mM potassium ions or with adenosine had nearly additive effects, while at supramaximal concentrations their effects were not additive (Shimizu *et al.*, 1970*b*; Shimizu and Daly, 1972*b*). Combinations of adenosine and electrical pulsation had either less than additive (Zanella and Rall, 1973) or at least additive (Somerville and Smith, 1972) effects. Availability of ATP and the differential effects of exogenous adenosine or adenosine "released" during depolarization at both receptor and catalytic sites of adenylate cyclases could be involved in some of the observed differences in extent of accumulation of cyclic AMP with the various agents. Although adenosine did not appear to inhibit adenylate cyclases in cell-free brain preparations from guinea pig (Sattin and Rall,

1970), it has been reported to inhibit cyclases in another brain preparation (McKenzie and Bar, 1973) and in preparations from other tissues (*cf.* references in Huang and Daly, 1974*a*).

Combinations of a depolarizing agent such as batrachotoxin, veratridine, ouabain, potassium and cholinium ions, or electrical pulsation with a biogenic amine such as norepinephrine, histamine, or serotonin had greater than additive effects on levels of cyclic AMP in guinea pig cortical slices (Kakiuchi *et al.*, 1969; Rall and Sattin, 1970; Shimizu *et al.*, 1970*a,d*; Huang *et al.*, 1971; Huang and Daly, 1972, 1974*b*; Shimizu and Daly, 1972*a,b*; Schultz and Daly, 1973*a,c*; Zanella and Rall, 1973).

The effects of a variety of catecholamines, phenolic amines, serotonin analogues, histamines, and various antagonists have been studied in the presence of 40 mM potassium ions (Shimizu *et al.*, 1970*a*; Huang and Daly, 1972). The results were similar to those discussed above for the amine agonists and antagonists except that the effects of the amines were much more pronounced and blocking agents with local anesthetic activity were more active as antagonists against amine–potassium ion combinations than against the amine itself. The synergism between histamine and potassium ions, unlike that between histamine and adenosine, was only partially blocked by theophylline (Rall and Sattin, 1970).

Initially, the observation that the accumulation elicited by depolarizing agents in cortical slices was antagonized in calcium-free medium was interpreted to be indicative of an excitation–secretion coupling step requiring calcium ion prior to activation of adenylate cyclase. Calcium ion dependency occurs with 40 mM and 100 mM potassium ions and with ouabain, batrachotoxin, and veratridine (Shimizu *et al.*, 1970*b*; Shimizu and Daly, 1972*b*; Zanella and Rall, 1973). However, calcium ions are not clearly required for the stimulatory effect of electrical pulsation (Zanella and Rall, 1973). High concentrations of magnesium ion, a calcium antagonist, block the increase in cyclic AMP elicited by 40 mM potassium ions and ouabain, have little effect on the increase elicited by veratridine and batrachotoxin, and potentiate the response to electrical pulsation or to histamine (Shimizu and Daly, 1972*b*; Zanella and Rall, 1973). The absence of calcium ions has little effect on the accumulation of cyclic AMP elicited by adenosine (H. Shimizu, unpublished results). Magnesium ions appear to either decrease (Shimizu and Daly, 1972*b*) or increase (Rall and Sattin, 1970) the accumulation of cyclic AMP elicited by 100 mM potassium ions. The absence of calcium ions greatly increases the "release" of adenosine from cortical slices, while partially or completely antagonizing further increases in efflux of adenosine elicited, respectively, by veratridine (H. Shimizu, unpublished results) or electrical pulsation (McIlwain, 1972; Pull and McIlwain, 1973).

Clearly, the nature of the effects of depolarizing agents on cyclic AMP levels and the involvement of adenosine formation, calcium ions, and other factors in this enhanced accumulation of cyclic AMP are not fully resolved even in guinea pig cerebral cortical slices where the phenomena have been extensively studied. Further differences appear to obtain with slices from other brain regions. In cerebellar slices, electrical pulsation elicits a six- to fourteenfold increase in cyclic AMP levels which is antagonized by the adenosine antagonist theophylline but not significantly lowered in calcium-free medium or by the presence of 14 mM magnesium ion (Zanella and Rall, 1973). In fact, under calcium-free conditions, basal levels of cyclic AMP are increased threefold. Ouabain and veratridine elicit, respectively, fourfold and eightfold increases in cyclic AMP levels. Potassium ions (40 mM) have no effect on levels of cyclic AMP in cerebellar slices and partially *antagonize* the increase in levels of cyclic AMP elicited by adenosine. In both cortical and cerebellar slices, combinations of potassium ions and amines or of adenosine and amines have greater than additive effects on cyclic AMP levels.

Prostaglandins have no effect on basal or adenosine-elicited levels of cyclic AMP in guinea pig cortical or cerebellar slices, nor does a preincubation of slices with indomethacin to inhibit synthesis of prostaglandins alter subsequent responses to norepinephrine, adenosine, or potassium ions (Zanella and Rall, 1973). Prostaglandins have no effect on cyclic AMP levels in cortical slices from a variety of mammals (Robison *et al.*, 1970*b*; Shimizu *et al.*, 1970*c,d*; Berti *et al.*, 1972). However, in two independent investigations prostaglandins E_1 and E_2 elicited accumulations of cyclic AMP in cortical slices from Sprague–Dawley rats (Berti *et al.*, 1972; Kuehl *et al.*, 1972). A lack of effect of prostaglandins in rat cerebellar slices has been cited as unpublished observations of E. C. Palmer. Recent studies (K. Dismukes and J. Daly, unpublished results) confirm and extend the reports on stimulation of cyclic AMP in rat brain slices by prostaglandins of the E series.

Certain psychotropic drugs in high concentrations have been reported to elicit accumulations of cyclic AMP in guinea pig cortical slices. These include prenylamine, phenothiazines such as chlorpromazine, and tricyclic antidepressants such as desipramine and chlorimipramine (Huang and Daly, 1972, 1974*b*). In one report, only tricyclic antidepressants appeared to increase cyclic AMP levels (Kodama *et al.*, 1971). These compounds are reported to be inhibitors of both phosphodiesterases and adenylate cyclases (see above), but their effects on levels of cyclic AMP appear due primarily to their ability to cause depletion of ATP and resultant formation and efflux of adenosine (Huang and Daly, 1974*b*). The maximal accumulation of cyclic AMP occurs only after 7–15 min and is blocked by theophylline, but not by a local anesthetic, cocaine. Attempts to demonstrate the expected synergistic interactions between "released" adenosine and biogenic amines were presumably thwarted in the case of chlorpromazine and chlorimipramine by antagonism of amine receptors by such tricyclic compounds. It was proposed that these compounds reduce ATP levels by a nonspecific interference with oxidative phosphorylation and that the resultant "release" of adenosine elicits cyclic AMP formation from remaining intracellular ATP.

Certain metabolic inhibitors such as 2,4-dinitrophenol, cyanide, and azide elicited small accumulations of cyclic AMP, while others such as 2-deoxyglucose, malonate, and oligomycin had no effect or in the case of quinones prevented accumulations of cyclic AMP. 2,4-Dinitrophenol and cyanide partially antagonized accumulations of cyclic AMP elicited by other agents (Shimizu and Daly, 1972*b*; Huang and Daly, 1974*b*). Such studies illustrate the profound difficulties associated with the study of the effects of metabolic inhibitors or depolarizing conditions in cyclic AMP–generating systems of brain slices. Thus a particular depolarizing agent may reduce ATP and lead to accumulation of adenosine in one compartment without significant effects on ATP levels in compartments associated with adenylate cyclases, while another agent may more rapidly reduce ATP levels in the adenylate cyclase compartment. The first situation could lead to a high accumulation of cyclic AMP, while the second might not affect or might reduce cyclic AMP levels. Differential effects on calcium mobilization might also be expected to occur with different agents.

Release of cyclic AMP to the medium does not appear to be a significant phenomenon with brain slices under a variety of conditions including electrical stimulation (Kakiuchi and Rall, 1968*b*; Sattin and Rall, 1970; Pull and McIlwain, 1972*a,b*). Release occurred from rabbit cortical slices under control and amine-stimulated conditions at a rate of approximately 10–20 pmol/mg protein/10 min. The presence of a high-affinity uptake system for cyclic AMP reported in rat cortical slices (Johnston and Balcar, 1973) would certainly reduce the net efflux of the cyclic nucleotide.

The enhanced release of adenosine with neuronal depolarizing agents such as veratridine suggests that adenosine formation and release are occurring primarily from neuronal compartments, but the results with depolarizing agents or metabolic inhibitors have not as yet provided any evidence as to the site of formation of cyclic AMP. Thus with respect to the role and regulation of cyclic AMP in the central nervous system *in vitro*, investigations of the various depolarizing agents have posed more questions than they have answered. Furthermore, the relevance of such artificial depolarizations to regulatory mechanisms in the intact brain has not been established. A study of the formation of cyclic AMP in the isolated piriform cortex or superior colliculus on stimulation of their respective innervating tracts might provide exciting results. Stimulation of these tracts does result in slightly enhanced release of adenosine into the medium from these isolated preparations (Heller and McIlwain, 1973).

Definitive studies on the role of phosphodiesterases in the responses of cyclic AMP–generating systems in brain slices have now begun. In earlier studies, theophylline or caffeine was often routinely added to incubation media, but the effects were variable (see above). Theophylline was subsequently found to be relatively ineffective in brain slices as a phosphodiesterase inhibitor and, in addition, to be an adenosine antagonist. Caffeine is much less active as an adenosine antagonist (Shimizu *et al.*, 1969; Sattin and

Rall, 1970; Huang *et al.*, 1972) but is also less active as a phosphodiesterase inhibitor. The phosphodiesterase inhibitors isobutylmethylxanthine, papaverine, and dibutyryl cyclic AMP significantly potentiate amine-elicited accumulations of cyclic AMP in guinea pig cerebral cortical slices (Schultz and Daly, 1973*b,c,d*). Isobutylmethylxanthine is, however, also an adenosine antagonist (Huang *et al.*, 1972; Schultz and Daly, 1973*b*). None of these inhibitors potentiates adenosine responses, nor does isobutylmethylxanthine or papaverine significantly retard the disappearance of cyclic AMP in slices previously stimulated with a combination of adenosine–histamine–norepinephrine and inhibitor. Potent phosphodiesterase inhibitors such as diazepam and RO 20-1724 have now been found to potentiate both adenosine- and amine-elicited accumulations of cyclic AMP in cortical slices (Schultz, 1974*a,b*). Other phosphodiesterase inhibitors, chlordiazepoxide and SQ 20009, were much less effective in augmenting amine-elicited accumulations and, respectively, had no effect or partially antagonized adenosine responses. Recently, low concentrations of the phosphodiesterase inhibitors papaverine, dipyridamole, and hexobendine were found to potentiate amine responses primarily by inhibition of adenosine reuptake processes, resulting in synergistic amine–adenosine interactions (Huang and Daly, 1974*a*). Such potentiations of amine responses were antagonized by theophylline. Papaverine does increase the net efflux of adenosine from perfused brain preparations (Heller and McIlwain, 1973). Diazepam, RO 20-1724, and SQ 20009 are relatively weak antagonists of adenosine uptake, while chlordiazepoxide is a potent inhibitor (H. Duck Mah and J. W. Daly, unpublished results).

3.1.3. Rat

Norepinephrine elicited a two- to twentyfold increase in cyclic AMP levels in cortical slices from Sprague-Dawley, Holtzman, Wistar, and several other strains of rats (Forn and Krishna, 1971; Krishna *et al.*, 1970; Rall and Sattin, 1970; Schmidt *et al.*, 1970; Shimizu *et al.*, 1970*a*; Forn and Valdecasas, 1971; Uzunov and Weiss, 1971, 1972; Palmer, 1972, 1973*b*; Schmidt and Robison, 1972; Weiss and Strada, 1972; French and Palmer, 1973; Huang *et al.*, 1973*b*; Kalisker *et al.*, 1973; Palmer *et al.*, 1973; Perkins and Moore, 1973*a,b*; Schultz and Daly, 1973*e*; Walker and Walker, 1973*a*; Skolnick and Daly, 1974*a*). Isoproterenol elicits an accumulation of cyclic AMP that is only about one-half the magnitude of that elicited by norepinephrine (Huang *et al.*, 1973*b*; Perkins and Moore, 1973*a,b*; Schultz and Daly, 1973*e*). Epinephrine elicits an accumulation intermediate to those evoked by isoproterenol and norepinephrine. The response to isoproterenol in cortical slices is blocked by β-antagonists and is unaffected by α-antagonists. The response to (nor)epinephrine has been reported to be only partially blocked by either α- or β-antagonists and to be completely blocked by combinations of the two types of adrenergic antagonists. A twofold increase in cyclic AMP levels elicited by norepinephrine in thick cortical slices from Wistar rats was reported to be completely blocked by propranolol and to be unaffected by phenoxybenzamine (French and Palmer, 1973). No response to norepinephrine or isoproterenol is seen in cortical slices of newborn rats (Schmidt *et al.*, 1970); Schmidt and Robison, 1972; Perkins, 1973; Perkins and Moore, 1973*b*). The responses to both amines develop in parallel between 8 and 13 days after birth and then decline to adult levels. Norepinephrine elicits significant increases in cyclic AMP levels in slices from cerebellum (two- to eightfold) (Forn and Krishna, 1971; Krishna *et al.*, 1970; Rall and Sattin, 1970; Uzunov and Weiss, 1971, 1972; Palmer *et al.*, 1973), caudate nucleus (fourfold) (Forn and Krishna, 1971), hypothalamus (two- to eightfold) (Forn and Krishna, 1971; Palmer and Burks, 1971; Palmer *et al.*, 1971, 1972*b*, 1973; Palmer, 1972, 1973*b*), hippocampus (threefold) (Palmer *et al.*, 1973), midbrain (fourfold) (Palmer *et al.*, 1973), striatum (two- to fourfold) (Palmer *et al.*, 1973; Walker and Walker, 1973*a*), combined midbrain-striatum (two- to sixfold) (Skolnick and Daly, 1974*a*), and brain stem (two- to fivefold) (Palmer and Burks, 1971; Uzunov and Weiss, 1971, 1972; Palmer, 1972; Palmer *et al.*, 1973). Basal levels of cyclic AMP in cerebellar slices were in some reports (Palmer, 1972; Palmer *et al.*, 1973) as high as 200–350 pmol/mg protein and were reduced by 50% on incubation with theophylline. Basal levels of cyclic AMP in cerebellar slices have also been reported as low as 60 pmol/mg protein (Rall and Sattin, 1970). In both reports, cerebellar levels were about 10 times greater than cortical levels. In hypothalamus isoproterenol elicited an accumulation of cyclic AMP lower than that elicited by norepinephrine (Palmer *et al.*, 1973). Epinephrine and α-methylnorepinephrine elicited accumulations of cyclic AMP in hypothalamus intermediate in magnitude to those elicited by norepinephrine and isoproterenol. Responses to norepinephrine in hypothalamus were blocked nearly completely by either α-antagonists or β-antagonists. Preliminary experiments indicated that responses to isoproterenol were also antagonized by either phentolamine or propranolol. In whole hypothalami, norepinephrine, epinephrine, and dopamine but not serotonin slightly increased levels of cyclic AMP (Gunaga and Menon, 1973). Estradiol also increased cyclic AMP levels slightly, but only after 40 min of incubation. This delayed effect was prevented by either phentolamine or propranolol.

A variety of other agents have been reported to inhibit responses to norepinephrine in slices from different brain regions. These include the serotonin antagonists LSD and BOL in hypothalamus and brain stem (Palmer and Burks, 1971), serotonin in hypothalamus and midbrain but not in cerebrum, brain stem, and cerebellum (Palmer *et al.*, 1973), chlorpromazine and other psychoactive phenothiazines in cerebrum, brain stem, cerebellum, and hypothalamus (Palmer *et al.*, 1971, 1972*b*; Uzunov and Weiss, 1971, 1972), chlorprothixene and impramine in hypothalamus and brain stem (Palmer *et al.*, 1972*b*; Uzunov and Weiss, 1972), protriptyline in cortex and hypothalamus (Palmer, 1973), amphetamines in hypothalamus

(Palmer, 1973), and lithium ions in cerebral cortex and hypothalamus but not in brain stem (Forn and Valdecasas, 1971; Palmer *et al.*, 1972*b*). The following compounds have been reported *not* to affect responses to norepinephrine: amphetamine and prostaglandin in a variety of brain regions, protriptyline and haloperidol in hypothalamus and brain stem, and cocaine in cerebral cortex, hypothalamus, and brain stem (Palmer *et al.*, 1971, 1972*b*, 1973; Palmer, 1973*b*).

Histamine has either marginal (Krishna *et al.*, 1970; Rall and Sattin, 1970; Shimizu *et al.*, 1970*a*; Berti *et al.*, 1972) or no significant (Forn and Krishna, 1971; Palmer *et al.*, 1973; Schultz and Daly, 1973*e*) effect on cyclic AMP levels in cerebral cortical slices. Histamine did elicit significant accumulations of cyclic AMP in the presence of phosphodiesterase inhibitors and these accumulations were blocked by antihistamines (Schultz and Daly, 1973*e*). Histamine had no significant effect in slices from cerebellum, hypothalamus, midbrain, or hippocampus, but did elicit a small increase in slices from caudate nucleus (Forn and Krishna, 1971; Krishna *et al.*, 1970; Palmer *et al.*, 1973). Combinations of histamine and norepinephrine had effects no greater (Schultz and Daly, 1973*e*) or only marginally greater (Huang *et al.*, 1971; Palmer *et al.*, 1973) than those elicited by norepinephrine alone.

Effects of amphetamine, serotonin, dopamine, carbachol, tyramine, and prostaglandins on accumulations of cyclic AMP were not detected in studies on slices from various brain regions (Forn and Krishna, 1971; Krishna *et al.*, 1970; Huang *et al.*, 1973*b*; Palmer *et al.*, 1973; Schultz and Daly, 1973*e*), and a variety of amines (dopamine, phenylephrine, metaraminol, octopamine, norephedrine, and *p*-hydroxynorephedrine) had no effect or lowered levels of cyclic AMP in hypothalamic slices (Palmer *et al.*, 1973). Prostaglandins E_1 and E_2 were, however, reported to elicit a four- to fivefold increase in levels of radioactive cyclic AMP in adenine-labeled cortical slices from Sprague-Dawley rats (Berti *et al.*, 1972; Kuehl *et al.*, 1972). Theophylline potentiated the effect of the prostaglandin. Dopamine has been reported to elevate levels of cyclic AMP by twofold in striatal slices (Walker and Walker, 1973*a*). Norepinephrine elicited a similar increase. Pargyline increased basal levels of cyclic AMP in slices from cerebral cortex, hypothalamus, and brain stem (Palmer, 1973*b*; Palmer *et al.*, 1973). Bufotenine, *N,N*-dialkyltryptamines, LSD, mescaline, psilocybin, and ibotenic acid were reported to elicit a twofold increase in cyclic AMP in slices of brain stem (Uzunov and Weiss, 1972). These increases were blocked by trifluoperazine.

Adenosine increases cyclic AMP levels two- to 25-fold in cortical slices (Rall and Sattin, 1970; Murray and Froscio, 1971; Berti *et al.*, 1972; Huang *et al.*, 1973*b*; Perkins and Moore, 1973*b*; Schultz and Daly, 1973*a*; Skolnick and Daly, 1974*a*), threefold in cerebellar slices (Rall and Sattin, 1970), and five- to sixfold in midbrain–striatal slices (Skolnick and Daly, 1974*a*). Responses to adenosine are absent in cortical slices from newborn rats and develop slowly between days 6 and 14 after birth (Perkins, 1973; Perkins and Moore, 1973*b*). Combinations of adenosine and norepinephrine have greater than additive effects on cyclic AMP levels in cortical, cerebellar, and midbrain–striatal slices (Rall and Sattin, 1970; Huang *et al.*, 1973*b*; Perkins and Moore, 1973*b*; Schultz and Daly, 1973*e*; Skolnick and Daly, 1973*a*). Adenosine–isoproterenol combinations have greater than additive effects in cortical slices. Responses to adenosine–norepinephrine combinations steadily increase in cortical slices during days 5–14 after birth. Responses to the combination of amine and adenosine were seen at least 5 days before norepinephrine alone elicited an accumulation of cyclic AMP. Adenosine and histamine combinations have been reported to have effects marginally (Rall and Sattin, 1970) or significantly (Huang *et al.*, 1973*b*; Schultz and Daly, 1973*e*) greater than those of adenosine alone in cortical slices. Adenosine–serotonin combinations had effects no greater than adenosine alone. The effects of amines in the presence of adenosine were antagonized by the same agents that antagonized responses to the amine alone in cortical slices (Perkins and Moore, 1973*b*; Schultz and Daly, 1973*e*). The response to norepinephrine in cortical slices can be elicited only once (Schultz and Daly, 1973*a*) but the preparation remains responsive to norepinephrine in combination with adenosine. (However see *Addendum*, Skolnick *et al.*, 1975.)

The depolarizing agents veratridine, batrachotoxin, ouabain, and potassium ions increase cyclic AMP levels by eight- to twentyfold in cortical slices (Shimizu *et al.*, 1970*a*; Huang *et al.*, 1973*b*; Skolnick and Daly, 1974*a*). Combinations of veratridine and either histamine or norepinephrine had greater than additive effects.

The effects of norepinephrine, isoproterenol, and histamine in cortical slices are potentiated by the phosphodiesterase inhibitors papaverine and isobutylmethylxanthine (Schultz and Daly, 1973*e*). Norepinephrine-elicited accumulations were not potentiated by theophylline (Forn and Krishna, 1971).

The effects of norepinephrine, isoproterenol, adenosine, an adenosine–norepinephrine combination, and veratridine on cyclic AMP levels in cortical and midbrain–striatal slices have been compared in four strains of rats (Skolnick and Daly, 1974*a*). The responses of the norepinephrine-sensitive cyclic AMP–generating systems in midbrain–striatal slices were inversely correlated in these strains with the responses of the corresponding systems in cerebral cortical slices. The magnitude of the norepinephrine responses in midbrain–striatal slices was inversely correlated with the levels of tyrosine hydroxylase in this tissue. Such correlations were not observed with the other stimulatory agents.

3.1.4. *Mouse*

Norepinephrine elicits a two- to twelvefold increase in cyclic AMP levels and histamine only a marginal increase in cerebral cortical slices from various strains of mice (Forn and Krishna, 1971; Krishna *et al.*, 1970; Rall and Sattin, 1970; Isräel *et al.*, 1972; Shimizu and Daly, 1972*a*; Schultz and Daly, 1973*e*; Skolnick and Daly, 1974*b,c*). Epinephrine elicits a response similar to that of norepinephrine, while isoproterenol elicits a significantly lower accumulation of cyclic AMP (Schultz and Daly, 1973*e*). Propranolol effectively antagonizes all three catecholamines, while phentolamine has only marginal effects.

Adenosine elicits a four- to seventeenfold increase in cyclic AMP levels in cortical slices from mice of various strains (Rall and Sattin, 1970; Schultz and Daly, 1973*e*; Skolnick and Daly, 1974*b,c*) and a thirtyfold increase in cerebellar slices from Swiss-Webster mice (Ferrendelli *et al.*, 1973*a*). Combinations of adenosine and norepinephrine have additive or greater than additive effects on cyclic AMP in cortical slices, while the effects of combinations of adenosine and either histamine or serotonin are equal to or only marginally greater than those of adenosine alone.

Veratridine elicits a four- to eighteenfold increase in cyclic AMP levels in cortical slices from two mouse strains (Shimizu and Daly, 1972*a*; Skolnick and Daly, 1974*b,c*). In cortical slices from three different mouse strains (C57Bl/6J, NIH general purpose white, and Swiss-Webster), 40–64 mM potassium ions elicited, respectively, a marginal increase (Skolnick and Daly, 1974*b*), a threefold increase (Shimizu and Daly, 1972*a*), and a sixtyfold increase (Ferrendelli *et al.*, 1973*a*) in levels of cyclic AMP. Combined effects of potassium ions and either norepinephrine or histamine appeared less than additive in cortical slices from NIH general purpose mice. In cerebellar slices from Swiss-Webster mice, 64 mM potassium ions elicited a transient thirteenfold increase in cyclic AMP levels which returned to only threefold above basal levels by 5 min. Higher concentrations of potassium ions elicited a 150-fold transient increase in cyclic AMP levels in Swiss-Webster cerebellar slices. The effects of potassium ions were blocked by theophylline.

Glutamate (3–30 mM) elicited a significant increase in cyclic AMP levels in cerebellar slices from Swiss-Webster mice (Ferrendelli *et al.*, 1974). This response was blocked by theophylline and reduced under calcium-free conditions, suggesting that a depolarization-evoked "release" of adenosine is involved. Under calcium-free conditions, levels of cyclic AMP were, however, significantly increased in mouse cerebellar slices. Glycine (1.0 mM) elicited a transient small increase and γ-aminobutyric acid (0.5 mM) a small decrease in cyclic AMP levels of cerebellar slices.

3.1.5. *Primates*

In rhesus monkey, norepinephrine and histamine had either a marginal effect (Shimizu and Daly, 1972*a*) or no effect (Forn and Krishna, 1971) on accumulations of radioactive cyclic AMP in adenine-labeled cortical slices. Norepinephrine elicited a twofold increase in levels of cyclic AMP in cerebellar slices and a fivefold increase in hypothalamic slices, but had no effect in slices from caudate nucleus (Forn and Krishna, 1971). Histamine did not have significant effects in slices from cerebellum, caudate nucleus, or hypothalamus. Serotonin, dopamine, and carbachol had no significant effects in any region. Depolarizing agents such as 40 mM potassium ions, batrachotoxin, and veratridine elicited three- to fivefold increases in cyclic AMP levels (Shimizu and Daly, 1972*a*). Ouabain elicited a tenfold increase. A combination of veratridine and histamine appeared to have greater than additive effects.

In squirrel monkey, the effects of various agents and combinations of agents on the levels of radioactive cyclic AMP in adenine-labeled slices from functional neocortical areas (polysensory, auditory, and visual) and from limbic cortex have been investigated (Skolnick *et al.*, 1973). Norepinephrine elicited a four- to fivefold increase in all regions. Histamine had no significant effects in the neocortical slices. Serotonin elicited a twofold increase in slices from polysensory cortex and had smaller effects in other regions. Adenosine elicited a ten- to thirtyfold increase in all cortical regions. Combinations of adenosine and norepinephrine had greater than additive effects, while the effects of combinations of adenosine and serotonin were not significantly greater than the effects of adenosine alone.

Two different groups, one in Italy (Fumagalli *et al.*, 1971; Berti *et al.*, 1972) and one in Japan (Shimizu *et al.*, 1971; Kodama *et al.*, 1973), have studied the formation of cyclic AMP in slices from human brain tissue. Tissue was obtained as surgical samples during operations for aneurysm, glioma, glioblastoma, meningioma, medulloblastoma, and acoustic neurinoma. Most of the results were obtained with adenine-labeled slices. In cortical slices, norepinephrine elicited either three- to fourfold increases (Fumagalli *et al.*, 1971; Berti *et al.*, 1972) or twelve- to fortyfold increases (Shimizu *et al.*, 1971; Kodama *et al.*, 1973). Norepinephrine also increased endogenous levels of cyclic AMP fifteenfold (Kodama *et al.*, 1973). Epinephrine and isoproterenol elicited greater increases in levels of radioactive cyclic AMP than did norepinephrine (Shimizu *et al.*, 1971; Kodama *et al.*, 1973). β-Antagonists prevented the response to norepinephrine, while α-antagonists were only marginally effective. Theophylline caused a slight inhibition of the response to norepinephrine. Norepinephrine elicited a two- to fivefold increase in radioactive cyclic AMP in cerebellar slices (Fumagalli *et al.*, 1971). Histamine either had no effect (Fumagalli *et al.*, 1971) or elicited a two- to sixfold increase (Shimizu *et al.*, 1971; Kodama *et al.*, 1973) in levels of radioactive cyclic AMP in cortical slices. Histamine had marginal effects in cerebellar slices, while serotonin had no effect in cortical or cerebellar slices (Fumagalli *et al.*, 1971) or elicited a marginal accumulation of radioactive cyclic AMP in cortical slices (Shimizu *et al.*, 1971; Kodama *et al.*, 1973). Adenosine elicited either a twofold (Berti *et al.*, 1972) or a five- to sixfold increase (Kodama *et al.*, 1973) in cortical slices. Veratridine elicited twenty- to fortyfold increases in cortical slices (Shimizu *et al.*, 1971; Kodama *et al.*, 1973). A combination of veratridine and norepinephrine elicited a fiftyfold increase in levels of radioactive cyclic AMP, which then represented a remarkable 70% of the total radioactive nucleotides in the slice. Prostaglandins had no effects in cortical slices (Berti *et al.*, 1972).

3.1.6. Conversion of Adenine- and Adenosine-Labeled Nucleotides to Cyclic AMP

After incubation of guinea pig cortical slices with low concentrations of radioactive adenine or adenosine, nearly all of the radioactivity was present as adenine nucleotides (Shimizu *et al.*, 1969; Shimizu and Daly, 1972*a*). The initial accumulation of adenine-labeled nucleotides in the slice showed a K_m of about 2×10^{-5} M, which is remarkably similar to that of adenine phosphoribosyltransferase from the same tissue (Shimizu and Daly, 1972*a*). A large fraction (30–40%) of the adenine-labeled nucleotides in guinea pig cortical slices can be converted subsequently to cyclic AMP under certain conditions. Unfortunately, attempts to define the morphological distribution of radioactivity in these labeled slices have not been successful. Results of autoradiographic studies on guinea pig cortical slices labeled by incubation with radioactive adenine at first suggested that a major fraction of the radioactivity in the slice was associated with synaptic structures (F. Bloom, M. Huang, and J. W. Daly, unpublished results). However, subsequent studies indicated that from 50 to 60% of the total radioactivity had been lost from the slice during fixation. Attempts to minimize these losses were not particularly successful, but did afford autoradiographs in which significant radioactivity was detected in nonsynaptic structures. Similarly, more than 50–60% of the total radioactivity in homogenates from control and electrically stimulated adenine-labeled guinea pig cortical slices was found in soluble fraction, while only much smaller percentages were found to be associated with mitochondrial and synaptosomal fractions (Kuroda and McIlwain, 1973). However, adenosine-labeled nucleotides were associated to a significantly higher extent with synaptosomal fractions than were the adenine-labeled nucleotides. This result is perhaps relevant to the observations that adenosine-labeled nucleotides are less effective than adenine-labeled nucleotides as precursors of cyclic AMP in guinea pig cortical slices (Shimizu and Daly, 1970).

Incorporation of radioactive adenine into guinea pig cortical slices was not inhibited by the copresence of a neuronal depolarizing agent, veratridine, during short incubations (H. Shimizu, unpublished results), but was reduced in rat brain slices during prolonged incubation in the presence of a similar veratrum alkaloid, protoveratrine (Glick and Quastel, 1972). High concentrations of potassium ions had no effect on incorporation of adenine during prolonged incubation. Incorporation of low concentrations of adenine was not effectively blocked by an adenine phosphoribosyltransferase inhibitor, 4-aminopyrazolo[4,5-*d*]pyrimidine (H. D. Mah and J. W. Daly, unpublished results). Prior incubations of guinea pig cortical slices with high concentrations of adenine did not reduce the subsequent incorporation of 4 μM radioactive adenine (Schultz and Daly, 1973*a*), indicating that the levels of the cosubstrate, phosphoribosyl pyrophosphate, of the transferase enzyme were not exhausted during the prior incubation. Similarly, the rate of incorporation of radioactive adenine into steady-state levels of cyclic AMP elicited by histamine, adenosine, a combination of histamine and norepinephrine, or a combination of adenosine, histamine, and norepinephrine was in all instances proportional to the steady-state levels of cyclic AMP, suggesting that even when adenine is incorporated into cyclic AMP at rates of greater than 10 pmol/mg protein/min the steps from adenine to ATP prior to the adenylate cyclase reaction are not rate limiting (Schultz and Daly, 1973*a*).

The subsequent percent conversion of adenine-labeled nucleotides to cyclic AMP elicited by veratridine was unaffected by a twofold change in the concentration (7 to 13 μM) of the radioactive adenine used to label guinea pig cortical slices (Shimizu and Daly, 1970). The percent conversion elicited by histamine was relatively independent of the duration of the adenine-labeling period (Shimizu *et al.*, 1969) except when short labeling periods of less than 10–15 min were employed (Shimizu and Okayama, 1973). After short labeling periods, the subsequent percent conversion of labeled nucleotides to cyclic AMP appeared much greater, suggestive of an initial incorporation of adenine into a small compartment of nucleotides intimately associated with adenylate cyclases, followed by equilibration with a somewhat larger compartment. However, in another study the percent conversion of radioactive adenine nucleotides formed from [^{3}H]adenine *during* stimulation with histamine either alone or in combination with norepinephrine, adenosine, or veratridine was not markedly greater than the percent conversion of the nucleotides labeled in the same guinea pig cortical slices during a prior 40 min incubation with [^{14}C]adenine (Schultz and Daly, 1973*a*). The compartments of nucleotides which serve as precursors for cyclic AMP and which are labeled during a 40 min incubation with radioactive adenine do not undergo further equilibration with other compartments as reflected in the constancy of the 35–40% conversion of labeled nucleotides elicited by a veratridine–histamine combination of various time intervals of up to 50 min after the prior labeling of the slice (Shimizu *et al.*, 1970*c*).

Incorporation of adenosine into intracellular nucleotides in guinea pig cortical slices appears dependent on both an active uptake process and on the action of adenosine kinase. Virtually all of the intracellular radioactivity was present as adenine nucleotides after incubation with low concentrations of radioactive adenosine (Shimizu *et al.*, 1972). The apparent K_m for the uptake and incorporation of radioactive adenosine was about 2×10^{-5} M in guinea pig cortical slices, a value which is similar to that of adenosine kinase from the same source. Analogues of adenosine which inhibit the kinase also inhibited incorporation of adenosine. However, other compounds that have been reported to be weak inhibitors of adenosine kinases were potent inhibitors of incorporation of low concentrations of radioactive adenosine, presumably at uptake sites (Huang and Daly, 1974*a*). The copresence of a neuronal depolarizing agent, veratridine, inhibited incorporation of adenosine (Shimizu and Daly, 1970), while another depolarizing agent, ouabain, had virtually no effect (Shimizu *et al.*, 1972). Cleavage of adenosine to adenine followed by incorporation of the adenine did not appear a significant pathway with guinea pig cortical slices (Shimizu *et al.*, 1972). The percent conversions of [^{3}H]adenine-labeled nucleotides to cyclic AMP elicited by histamine, adenosine, veratridine, or 125 mM potassium ions in guinea pig cerebral cortical slices were in each case approximately 1.8 times greater than the percent conversions of [^{14}C]adenosine-labeled nucleotides (Shimizu *et al.*, 1969; Shimizu and Daly, 1970). Such results clearly indicated a more specific incorporation of adenine into compartments of nucleotides serving as precursors of cyclic AMP, but gave no evidence for the existence of functional compartments labeled to differing extents and stimulatable by different agents. Similarly, levels of radioactive cyclic AMP in adenine-labeled slices after stimulation with biogenic amines, adenosine, veratridine, and combinations of these agents represented in each instance approximately 10% of the total endogenous cyclic AMP measured in guinea pig cortical slices in parallel experiments under the same conditions (Schultz and Daly, 1973*a*). The increase elicited by these agents in levels of radioactive cyclic AMP and in levels of endogenous cyclic AMP occurred over similar time courses and to similar extents in parallel experiments. The disappearance of radioactive and endogenous cyclic AMP after removal of the stimulatory agent(s) by washing also followed similar time courses (Schultz and Daly, 1973*b*). With histamine stimulations, both radioactive and endogenous cyclic AMP were measured simultaneously (Schultz and Daly, 1973*a*). An initial histamine-elicited accumulation of endogenous cyclic AMP was maximal in approximately 2 min and appeared responsible for a transient 50% reduction in the specific activity of cyclic AMP. The results are consonant with two compartments of adenine nucleotides responding to histamine, one of which responds with a transient accumulation of cyclic AMP from a less highly labeled compartment of nucleotides, superimposed on a more sustained accumulation of cyclic AMP from a more highly labeled compartment. Isobutylmethylxanthine potentiated the histamine-elicited accumulation of both radioactive and endogenous cyclic AMP by twofold, while papaverine potentiated the accumulation of radioactive cyclic AMP by twofold and the accumulation of endogenous cyclic AMP by only 1.5-fold (Schultz and Daly, 1973*b*). The time course for disappearance of cyclic AMP after histamine stimulation, washing, and further incubation in the presence of the phosphodiesterase inhibitor isobutylmethylxanthine was also suggestive of a two-compartment system.

During repetitive restimulations of cyclic AMP accumulations in guinea pig cortical slices by adenosine or an adenosine–histamine–norepinephrine combination, the specific activity of cyclic AMP decreased slightly, presumably due to the continued incorporation of the nonradioactive stimulant, adenosine, into the cyclic AMP (Schultz and Daly, 1973*c*). The percent conversion of radioactive adenine nucleotides to cyclic AMP with amines, adenosine, veratridine, and combinations of these agents was approximately threefold higher than the percent conversion of total adenine nucleotides to cyclic AMP under the same conditions in parallel experiments (Schultz and Daly, 1973*a*). The results suggest that the specific activities of the cyclic AMP that accumulates after stimulation with each of various agents were similar and were approximately threefold higher than the specific activity of total adenine nucleotides. Indeed, the specific activities of cyclic AMP in adenine-labeled cortical slices stimulated by histamine, adenosine, or veratridine, or by combinations of either veratridine–histamine or of adenosine–histamine–norepinephrine were found to be quite similar (Shimizu and Okayama, 1973). However, the specific activity of the cyclic AMP in these stimulated slices appeared to be about 40% higher than in control slices. The specific activity of cyclic AMP in slices incubated with histamine was approximately fivefold higher than that of ATP. In these experiments, no change in the specific activity of cyclic AMP was noted during the time course of stimulation with histamine. In experiments from another laboratory, the specific activities of cyclic AMP after stimulation of adenine-labeled guinea pig cortical slices with norepinephrine or histamine were similar, but in each case appeared lower than the specific activity of control levels of cyclic AMP (Chasin *et al.*, 1973). In guinea pig hippocampal slices, specific activities of control and histamine-stimulated levels of cyclic AMP were similar, while the specific activity in norepinephrine-stimulated slices appeared to be lower. The specific activities of cyclic AMP and ATP have also been compared in guinea pig cortical slices that have been pulse labeled with radioactive adenine for 5 min under control conditions and in slices in which steady-state levels of cyclic AMP were already elevated 1.5- or eightfold by the presence of norepinephrine or histamine, respectively (Rall and Sattin, 1970). The specific activity of cyclic AMP in control and norepinephrine-stimulated slices was 2.3–2.6 times that of ATP, while the specific activity of cyclic AMP in histamine-stimulated slices was 7 times that of ATP. Although adenosine is apparently incorporated less specifically into compartments of nucleotides serving as precursors of cyclic AMP, comparison of the specific activity of ATP–ADP to that of the cyclic AMP which accumulated in guinea pig cortical slices incubated with radioactive 0.1 mM adenosine revealed that the specific activity of cyclic AMP was about 3 times greater than that of ATP–ADP (Sattin and Rall, 1970). Thus, although some evidence for distinct functional compartments in guinea pig cortical slices labeled to differing extents with adenine or adenosine and stimulatable to various degrees with different agents has been obtained, the results from various laboratories are somewhat contradictory and have as yet provided little in the way of insights into the morphological entities with which adenine or adenosine-labeled nucleotides are associated in guinea pig cortical slices. Studies on the effects of depolarizing conditions that perhaps differentially affect neurons and glia (*cf.* Hertz, 1966; Glick and Quastel, 1972), on the levels of radioactive ATP, and on the efflux of radioactive adenosine from adenine-labeled guinea pig cortical slices have also not provided unambiguous answers. Radioactive adenosine is released under control conditions from adenine- or adenosine-labeled slices, and this efflux is increased under a variety of depolarizing conditions (Shimizu *et al.*, 1970*a*, 1972; McIlwain, 1972; Pull and McIlwain, 1972*a,b*; Heller and McIlwain, 1973; Huang *et al.*, 1973*b*; Kuroda and McIlwain, 1973; Schultz and Daly, 1973*a*; Huang and Daly, 1974*b*). Both radioactive and endogenous ATP are decreased in the slices under these conditions (Huang *et al.*, 1973*a*; Huang and Daly, 1974*b*). Interestingly, the specific activity of the adenosine released by electrical stimulation is 1.4–2.7 times greater than the specific activity of the total adenine nucleotides of the adenine-labeled slice (Kuroda and McIlwain, 1973).

Compartmentalization of labeled adenine nucleotides has not been studied extensively except in guinea pig cortical slices. With adenine-labeled slices from rat cerebral cortex, a preliminary report indicated that during incubation with norepinephrine the specific activity of cyclic AMP sharply increased during the first minutes followed by a decrease to original levels (Krishna *et al.*, 1970), suggestive of an initial utilization of more highly labeled adenine nucleotides. Another group reported that the specific activity of cyclic AMP was similar in control and isoproterenol- and norepinephrine-stimulated slices from rat cortex (Perkins, 1973; Perkins and Moore, 1973*a,b*).

The formation of cyclic AMP from endogenous nucleotides and from adenine- and adenosine-labeled nucleotide has been thoroughly studied in cortical slices from C57Bl/6J mice (Skolnick and Daly, 1974*c*). In contrast to results with guinea pig cortical slices, a comparison of the ratio of the percent conversion to cyclic AMP of [^{14}C]adenine-labeled nucleotides to that of [^{3}H]adenosine-labeled nucleotides revealed a clear dependency of the stimulatory agent; with veratridine the ratio was 1.4, with norepinephrine 2.2, with adenosine–norepinephrine 2.0, and with adenosine and adenosine–histamine 3.0. The specific activity of cyclic AMP in both adenine- and adenosine-labelled slices after incubation with norepinephrine, adenosine, adenosine–amine combinations, and veratridine was dependent on the stimulatory agent. For example, in adenosine-labeled cortical slices the specific activity of cyclic AMP was about 50% lower in the norepinephrine-stimulated preparation compared to the veratridine-stimulated preparation. The specific activity of cyclic AMP was lowest when adenosine or adenosine–norepinephrine was used as the stimulatory agent, but, at least in part, this was due to a marked incorporation of the exogenous adenosine into the accumulating cyclic AMP. Thus exogenous adenosine contributed approximately 40% of the adenine nucleotide precursor for cyclic AMP during a 9–15 min incubation of mouse cortical slices with 0.1 mM radioactive adenosine. During stimulation of adenine-labeled slices with norepinephrine, adenosine, or veratridine, there appeared to be a trend toward a gradual decrease in the specific activity of cyclic AMP.

Cyclic AMP formation was also investigated in the quaking mouse, a mutant derived from the C57Bl/6J strain (Skolnick and Daly, 1974*b*). Both in the quaking mouse and in heterozygous mice that contain one quaking gene but do not exhibit the hypomyelination and tremor characteristic of the quaking mouse, biochemical alterations in nucleotide metabolism were manifest in cortical slices. Higher rates of incorporation of adenine and adenosine into intracellular nucleotides of the slice were observed in the quaking mouse and the heterozygous mouse as compared to the parent C57Bl/6J strain. However, the increase in incorporation occurred into compartments not associated with adenylate cyclases. Thus the percent conversion of radioactive nucleotides to cyclic AMP in cortical slices from these strains containing the mutant gene was markedly lower than that seen with the parent strain after stimulation with norepinephrine, adenosine, or veratridine, but not after an adenosine–norepinephrine combination. The absolute accumulations of both radioactive and endogenous cyclic AMP were similar in slices from quaking mice, heterozygous mice, and the parent strain except with adenosine as the stimulatory agent. In the latter case, the absolute accumulations were significantly lower in slices from the quaking and heterozygous mice. The ratio of conversions of [^{14}C]adenine- and [^{3}H]adenosine-labeled nucleotides to cyclic AMP in slices from quaking and heterozygous mice were, as in the parent strain, dependent on the stimulatory agent.

3.1.7. Effects of Drug and Other Treatments of Animals on the Cyclic AMP–Generating Systems in Brain Slices

Chronic or acute treatments of animals with drugs or protocols which interfere with or augment mechanisms involving putative neurotransmitters in the central nervous system might be expected to result in compensatory changes in the responsiveness of cyclic AMP–generating systems to these same neurotransmitters. Such changes could then be investigated in brain slices. Indeed, treatment of rats with intraventricular 6-hydroxydopamine to destroy presynaptic noradrenergic nerve terminals results in a long-term potentiation of norepinephrine- and isoproterenol-elicited accumulations of cyclic AMP in slices from cerebral cortex, hypothalamus, and brain stem (Palmer, 1972; Weiss and Strada, 1972; Huang *et al.*, 1973*b*; Kalisker *et al.*, 1973). Cerebellar levels of cyclic AMP were extremely high in the reported experiments (Palmer, 1972), and norepinephrine elicited a similar small increase in cyclic AMP levels in slices from both control and 6-hydroxydopamine-treated animals. Accumulations of cyclic AMP elicited by interaction of catecholamines with either α- or β-receptors appear in both cases to be approximately doubled in cortical slices from the 6-hydroxydopamine-treated rats (Huang *et al.*, 1973*b*; Kalisker *et al.*, 1973). Lack of presynaptic uptake of norepinephrine accounts for a shift in the dose–response curve for this catecholamine. However, approximately 4 days after treatment postsynaptic changes occur which appear to be responsible for the increase in the magnitude of the maximal accumulations of cyclic AMP elicited by norepinephrine and isoproterenol. Responses to adenosine, dopamine, serotonin, veratridine, and combinations of adenosine with serotonin or histamine are not increased or are only marginally increased after 6-hydroxydopamine treatment. The maximal accumulation elicited by an adenosine–norepinephrine combination is, however, significantly increased. Intraventricular administration of dihydroxytryptamines, agents which cause selective degeneration of serotonin nerve terminals, have no significant or only marginal effects on accumulations of cyclic AMP elicited by any of the above agents. In the presence of phosphodiesterase inhibitors, the accumulations of cyclic AMP elicited by norepinephrine and isoproterenol are still significantly greater in slices from 6-hydroxydopamine-treated rats, suggesting that the increase in maximal accumulations of cyclic AMP reflects changes in formation and not degradation of cyclic AMP.

Total levels of adenylate cyclase and phosphodiesterase activity in homogenates of rat cerebral cortex are marginally decreased by the 6-hydroxydopamine treatment (Kalisker *et al.*, 1973), suggesting that measurement of total levels of these enzymes is of limited use in establishing the functional level of specific cyclic AMP-generating systems in brain. Others have, however, reported significantly higher adenylate cyclase activity in cerebral cortical homogenates from rats that had received a single intracisternal injection of norepinephrine, serotonin, or histamine (Chou *et al.*, 1971*a,b*).

Chronic treatment of mice with morphine has been reported to increase adenylate cyclase activity in cerebral homogenates, to have no effect on phosphodiesterase activity, and to reduce protein kinase activity (Chou *et al.*, 1971*a*; Clark *et al.*, 1972; Naito and Kuriyama, 1973). Chronic or acute treatment of rats with morphine did not appear to result in significant increases in the magnitude of the accumulation of cyclic AMP elicited in cortical slices by norepinephrine, adenosine, or veratridine or in hypothalamic slices by norepinephrine (M. Huang, A. K. S. Ho, and J. W. Daly, unpublished results).

Prior treatment of rats with reserpine, an agent which reduces brain levels of norepinephrine and serotonin, results in an increase in the magnitude of the accumulation of cyclic AMP elicited by norepinephrine in slices from cortex, hypothalamus, and hippocampus (Palmer *et al.*, 1973). Significant potentiation was not seen in slices from cerebellum, midbrain, or brain stem. Pretreatment of rabbits with reserpine appears to have little effect on accumulations of cyclic AMP elicited by serotonin, norepinephrine, or histamine in cerebellar slices (Kakiuchi and Rall, 1968*b*). Pretreatment of rats with a phenothiazine tranquilizer results in a marked decrease in the accumulation of cyclic AMP elicited by *N,N*-dimethyltryptamine in slices from brain stem (Uzunov and Weiss, 1972).

A greater accumulation of cyclic AMP is elicited by electrical stimulation in guinea pig cortical and cerebellar slices from animals pretreated with reserpine (Kakiuchi *et al.*, 1969; Zanella and Rall, 1973). The accumulation of cyclic AMP elicited by electrical stimulation is also significantly increased in cerebellar slices from 6-hydroxydopamine-treated guinea pigs. Responses of cerebellar slices to adenosine do not appear to be significantly greater after either pretreatment.

It is perhaps relevant that postsynaptic cyclic AMP–generating systems in pineal glands become more responsive to norepinephrine or isoproterenol after 6-hydroxydopamine or reserpine treatment, after denervation, or after exposure of animals to continuous light (Weiss and Costa, 1967; Weiss, 1969; Weiss and Strada, 1972; Deguchi and Axelrod, 1973). Maximal levels of cyclic AMP elicited by catecholamines are increased in pineal glands, but in contrast to results with brain slices from 6-hydroxydopamine-treated animals the affinity of catecholamines for the β-receptors modulating adenylate cyclase activity is also apparently greatly increased (Deguchi and Axelrod, 1973).

Pretreatment of rats with the monoamine oxidase inhibitor pargyline increases basal levels of cyclic AMP in incubated slices of cortex, hypothalamus, brain stem, hippocampus, and cerebellum, but does not apparently alter responses to norepinephrine (Palmer *et al.*, 1971, 1973). Chronic treatment of mice with ethanol increases adenylate cyclase activity in cortical homogenates and basal levels of radioactive cyclic AMP in adenine-labeled cortical slices (Isräel *et al.*, 1972; Kuriyama and Isräel, 1973). A significant accumulation of cyclic AMP in cortical slices is no longer elicited by norepinephrine after chronic alcohol treatment, while histamine still has a marginal stimulatory effect. During ethanol withdrawal, the accumulation of cyclic AMP elicited by norepinephrine is enhanced in rat cerebral cortical slices, but not in slices from hypothalamus (French and Palmer, 1973). The increase appears primarily due to α-adrenergic mechanisms. Neonatal thyroidectomy has little effect on the development of norepinephrine-sensitive cyclic AMP–generating systems in rat brain, although endogenous levels of cyclic AMP appeared somewhat lower in thyroidectomized rats (Schmidt and Robison, 1972; Singhal *et al.*, 1973). Insulin administration to hypoglycemic rats was reported to cause a slight increase in adenylate cyclase activity and a slight decrease in phosphodiesterase activity in brain homogenates (Hetenyi and Singhal, 1973). Adenylate cyclase and cyclic AMP levels were increased and phosphodiesterase levels were decreased after freezing techniques had been used to form unilateral epileptogenic foci in rat cerebral cortex (Walker *et al.*, 1973). Similar but less pronounced changes occurred in the control lateral cortex. Adrenalectomy or treatment of rats with methylxanthines or hydrocortisone had no effect on phosphodiesterase levels in cerebral cortex (Vernikos-Danellis and Harris, 1968). Neonatal infection or malnutrition resulted in an apparent increase in phosphodiesterase activity in brain and a decrease in cyclic AMP levels (Lee and Dubos, 1972).

3.2. Cyclic GMP in Brain Slices

Cyclic GMP levels in whole brain, cortex, and cerebellum do not undergo marked changes on decapitation (Goldberg *et al.*, 1970; Steiner *et al.*, 1970, 1972). Levels of this nucleotide were reported to be stable in slices after a period of incubation (Ferrendelli *et al.*, 1973*a*). Basal levels of cyclic GMP in brain slices are usually less than 1 pmol/mg protein except in cerebellar slices, where, in rat and mouse, levels as high as 10 pmol/mg protein have been observed. Significant release of cyclic GMP from slices was not detectable (Ferrendelli *et al.*, 1973*a*).

In rabbit cerebral cortical slices, acetylcholine and muscarinic agonists elicit a transient twofold increase in cyclic GMP levels (Lee *et al.*, 1972; Kuo *et al.*, 1972). Maximal levels of less than 2 pmol/mg protein are attained in about 2 min. The responses are prevented by a muscarinic blocking agent, atropine, but not by a nicotinic blocking agent, hexamethonium. In rabbit cerebellar slices, acetylcholine also elicits a two- to threefold transient increase in cyclic GMP levels. Maximal levels of less than 5 pmol/mg protein are attained in about 1 min. Histamine increases cyclic GMP levels two- to threefold in rabbit cerebral cortical slices but has no effect in cerebellar slices. Norepinephrine has no effect or reduced cyclic GMP levels in rabbit cortical slices. In cerebellar slices from Swiss-Webster mice, acetylcholine has no apparent effect on the high basal levels (4–8 pmol/mg protein) of cyclic GMP (Ferrendelli *et al.*, 1973*a*). Neither adenosine nor guanosine has any effect on cyclic GMP levels in mouse cerebellar slices.

Depolarizing agents such as veratridine, ouabain, and high concentrations of potassium ions elevate cyclic GMP levels in mouse cerebellar slices by about thirtyfold (Ferrendelli *et al.*, 1973*a*, 1974). The effects of potassium ions are significant at 30 mM and increase up to 120 mM. The effects of submaximal stimulatory concentrations of the depolarizing agents are additive. Potassium ions increase cyclic GMP levels in mouse cortical slices by tenfold. In both brain regions, accumulation of cyclic GMP is maximal in about 6 min. Atropine does not prevent the effects of depolarizing agents in cerebellar slices, nor does theophylline prevent the effects of potassium ions.

Depolarizing agents do not have any effect on cyclic GMP levels in calcium-free media and the effects of potassium ions are partially blocked by high concentrations of magnesium ions. The results suggest that a calcium-mediated excitation-coupling process is responsible for the release of a stimulatory substance, which is not adenosine or acetylcholine. This substance is then responsible for the elevation of cyclic GMP elicited by the depolarizing agents.

Amino acids which are putative excitatory and inhibitory neurotransmitters in the central nervous system elevate cyclic GMP levels in mouse cerebellar slices (Ferrendelli *et al.*, 1974). Glutamate (10 mM) causes a rapid tenfold increase in cyclic GMP levels. This increase is slightly potentiated by theophylline. Glycine (1 mM) and γ-aminobutyric acid (5 mM) elicit a slower threefold and twofold increase, respectively, in levels of cyclic GMP. In both cases, the increase is further potentiated by the presence of theophylline. Theophylline also increases basal levels of cyclic GMP in cerebellar slices. The possible role of release of these amino acids in depolarization-evoked accumulation of cyclic AMP is uncertain. Maximal stimulatory concentrations of glutamate and potassium ions are no more effective than potassium ions alone. It should be pointed out that glutamate itself is considered a depolarizing agent in brain slices. The stimulatory effects of the amino acids on cyclic GMP accumulation in all cases require calcium ions in the medium. The effects of glutamate and glycine are additive, while the effects of combinations of γ-aminobutyric acid with either glutamate or glycine are not additive. Further studies on agents that affect cyclic AMP and/or cyclic GMP levels in brain slices should provide insights as to the interrelationships or lack of interrelationships in levels of these cyclic nucleotides.

A preliminary report on determination of cyclic GMP in tissue labeled by a prior incubation with radioactive guanine has appeared (Kuo and Kuo, 1973).

3.3. Cyclic AMP in Ganglia

The effects of electrical stimulation and various amines on cyclic AMP levels have been investigated in ganglion preparations from both mammals and lower organisms. The results with the various ganglion preparations suggest that biogenic amine–elicited increases in cyclic AMP levels are probably associated with inhibitory synaptic transmission.

In rabbit superior cervical ganglia (McAfee *et al.*, 1971; Schorderet *et al.*, 1972; Kalix *et al.*, 1974) preganglionic stimulation elicits a 2.5- to fivefold increase in cyclic AMP levels. Postganglionic stimulation has no effect, nor does stimulation of the cervical vagus nerve have any effect on cyclic AMP levels in the nerve or in the nodose ganglion, a ganglion with nerve cell bodies but no synapses. The elevation of cyclic AMP elicited by preganglionic stimulation or by carbachol in the rabbit superior cervical ganglion is blocked by atropine and by spiroperidol and phentolamine, but is not significantly affected by hexamethonium or by β-antagonists. The increase in cyclic AMP is potentiated by phosphodiesterase inhibitors. The results were explained as follows: Preganglionic stimulation elicits a release of acetylcholine which in turn by interaction with muscarinic receptors on the interneurons elicits a release of dopamine. The dopamine elicits an accumulation of cyclic AMP in the adrenergic cell body by interaction with a receptor that can be blocked by α-antagonists or spiroperidol. Direct acetylcholine-mediated transmission which is blocked by hexomethonium does not appear to be involved in the formation of cyclic AMP.

Subsequent studies with adenine-labeled slices of bovine superior cervical ganglia demonstrated that both dopamine and at higher concentrations norepinephrine will elicit about a tenfold increase in radioactive cyclic AMP (Kebabian and Greengard, 1971). Dopamine elicits a similar increase in endogenous cyclic AMP. Responses to dopamine are inhibited by α-antagonists but not by β-antagonists. β-Antagonists do, however, reduce the effects of norepinephrine. In contrast, cyclic AMP levels in cultured rat superior cervical ganglion are transiently elevated eight- to twentyfold by (nor)epinephrine and isoproterenol, while even higher concentrations of dopamine or phenylephrine have only marginal effects (Cramer *et al.*, 1973*a*). The effects of norepinephrine are antagonized by both phentolamine and propranolol, with the β-antagonist much more effective. During culture of ganglia for 2 days, both basal levels of cyclic AMP and responses to isoproterenol decrease markedly. Under these conditions the adrenergic cell bodies survive and develop sprouts, while presynaptic terminals and interstitial cells degenerate (cited in Cramer *et al.*, 1973*a*), suggesting that the isoproterenol-sensitive cyclases are not uniquely located in adrenergic cell bodies. However, the threefold increase in cyclic AMP levels that is elicited in rat superior cervical ganglion *in vivo* by isoproterenol is virtually lost when the adrenergic cell bodies have been destroyed by prior treatment with 6-hydroxydopamine (Otten *et al.*, 1974). Basal levels of cyclic AMP are only slightly reduced in the ganglia from 6-hydroxydopamine-treated rats. Interestingly, more than 60 min is required in normal rats before a second injection of isoproterenol will elicit a transient accumulation of cyclic AMP in the superior cervical ganglion similar in magnitude to that of the first isoproterenol-elicited accumulation.

Histamine elicits a two- to eightfold increase in cyclic AMP levels in cultured rat superior cervical ganglia (Lindl and Cramer, 1974). Efflux of cyclic AMP into the medium is also increased. Epinephrine and histamine elicit similar increases in levels and efflux of radioactive cyclic AMP in adenine-labeled ganglia. The histamine-elicited increase in cyclic AMP levels is blocked by probenecid, while the efflux is unaffected. Epinephrine-elicited responses are unaffected by probenecid. The histamine-elicited increase in cyclic AMP levels is antagonized by both H_1- (diphenhydramine) and H_2- (burimamide) antagonists, but not by a β-antagonist. Burimamide alone elicits an increase in cyclic AMP levels.

Dopamine- and norepinephrine-sensitive adenylate cyclases would also appear to be present in ganglion cells of the retina (Brown and Makman, 1972, 1973). Thus in intact bovine retina dopamine, (nor)epinephrine, and the depolarizing agents ouabain and high concentrations of potassium ions elicit a twofold increase in cyclic AMP levels. The effects of dopamine and the depolarizing agents on cyclic AMP levels are additive. Adenosine, serotonin, and histamine have no effect. In homogenates of bovine and rat retina, the catecholamines and apomorphine activate adenylate cyclases. The activation by dopamine is blocked by α-antagonists, haloperidol, and chlorpromazine, while the effect of epinephrine is inhibited by both α- and β-antagonists. Theophylline but not nerve growth factor increases levels of cyclic AMP in chick dorsal root ganglia (Frazier *et al.*, 1973).

In the abdominal ganglion of *Aplysia* labeled during a prior incubation with radioactive adenine, electrical stimulation of nerves leads to a twofold increase of levels of radioactive cyclic AMP in the ganglion but not in the nerves (Cedar and Schwartz, 1972; Cedar *et al.*, 1972). There is, however, no increase in endogenous cyclic AMP levels. High concentrations of magnesium which prevent synaptic transmission prevent the increase in radioactive cyclic AMP, while depolarization of ganglionic neurons with ouabain or glutamate has no effect on cyclic AMP levels. Adenosine, carbachol, glutamate, norepinephrine, and histamine have no significant effects on cyclic AMP levels in the ganglion and the adenosine antagonist theophylline has no effect on the elevations of cyclic AMP elicited by electrical stimulation. Serotonin and dopamine do cause a threefold increase in levels of radioactive cyclic AMP. In other experiments, serotonin caused an eightfold and dopamine a sixfold increase in endogenous levels of cyclic AMP. The data suggest that serotonin and/or dopamine is released by electrical stimulation of the abdominal ganglia and activates postsynaptic adenylate cyclases. In cockroach thoracic ganglion, levels of cyclic AMP are increased by octopamine, dopamine, serotonin, and relatively high concentrations of norepinephrine (Nathanson and Greengard, 1973). In addition, these amines stimulate adenylate activity in homogenates. The effects of combinations of octopamine, dopamine, and serotonin are additive in homogenates, suggesting the presence of separate receptors. The effects of octopamine and dopamine are antagonized by phentolamine. Catecholamines have also been reported to activate adenylate cyclases from cockroach brain (Rojakovick and March, 1972).

3.4. Cyclic AMP in Cells of Neuronal or Glial Origin

Cells from fetal mouse brain in reaggregation cultures respond to norepinephrine or isoproterenol with a four- to sixfold increase in cyclic AMP levels (Seeds and Gilman, 1971). This response develops during culture and is manifest at 9 days but not at 15 h. Theophylline does not further potentiate the catecholamine-elicited accumulation of cyclic AMP. Thus with respect to cyclic AMP generation these cultures containing proportions of neurons and glia probably similar to those in the immature mouse brain exhibit certain properties similar to those of brain slice preparations. In surface cultures of fetal rat brain, where extensive multiplication of cells, presumably mainly glial cells, has taken place, isoproterenol elicits a remarkable sixty- to hundredfold increase in cyclic AMP levels (Gilman and Schrier, 1972; Schrier and Gilman, 1973). The response develops during culture and is maximal after about 14 days. The response to isoproterenol is blocked by a β-antagonist and is virtually unaffected by an α-antagonist. Theophylline has little effect on the response. Norepinephrine appears to elicit only a seventeenfold increase in cyclic AMP levels, but a complete dose–response curve for norepinephrine was not reported. These results contrast to responses in rat brain slices, where both α- and β-receptors appear involved in stimulated formation of cyclic AMP and where norepinephrine elicits a much greater accumulation of the cyclic nucleotide than does isoproterenol (see Section 3.1.3). Adenosine and prostaglandin elicit twelve- and thirtyfold increases, respectively, in levels of cyclic AMP in the surface cultures of rat fetal brain cells. Adenosine–catecholamine combinations do not have synergistic effects on cyclic AMP formation. Serotonin and high concentrations of potassium ions have no effect.

Cultured cells derived from various neuromas of rat, mouse, or human origin have been investigated with regard to accumulations of cyclic AMP. The results are relevant to the role of glial and neuronal cells in responses of cyclic AMP–generating systems in brain slices to different agents, although it should be stressed that tumor cell lines may show greatly altered enzyme levels or hormone responsiveness compared to that of the parent tumor cells or to that of normal cells. For example, levels of adenylate cyclase in cultured hamster astrocytes are reduced 50% after virus-induced transformation (Weiss *et al.*, 1971) and clones of glioma cells often lose responses to various agents (see Perkins, 1973).

Glioma cell lines from rat, mouse, or human respond at certain times during culture to the catecholamines (nor)epinephrine and isoproterenol with remarkable thirty- to 4000-fold increases in levels of intracellular cyclic AMP (Clark and Perkins, 1971; Gilman and Nirenberg, 1971*a*; Schultz *et al.*, 1972; Gilman and Minna, 1973; Perkins, 1973; Schwartz *et al.*, 1973; Browning *et al.*, 1974*a,b*; S. E. Pfeiffer, unpublished results). Isoproterenol is the most effective of the catecholamines, but the maximal accumulations are similar with either isoproterenol or norepinephrine. β-Antagonists block the responses to catecholamines, while α-antagonists are ineffective. A B_1-antagonist, practolol, is relatively ineffective (Gilman and Minna, 1973). The effects of isoproterenol are not antagonized by prostaglandin or carbachol. In one study with rat glioma cells the maximal responses to norepinephrine were not seen until many days after the cells had become confluent (Schwartz *et al.*, 1973), while in another study with human glioma cells the maximal responses to norepinephrine were attained before the cells had formed a confluent monolayer and declined markedly during further culture (Clark and Perkins, 1971). Lithium ions potentiated the norepinephrine-elicited accumulation of cyclic AMP in rat glioma cells (Schimmer, 1973).

Histamine has no effect in rat glioma cells (Gilman and Nirenberg, 1971*a*; Schultz *et al.*, 1972), and elicits a four- to twentyfold increase in cyclic AMP levels in certain clones of a human glioma cell line (Clark and Perkins, 1971; Perkins, 1973). Propranolol does not prevent the effect of histamine. The magnitude of the response to histamine increases only slightly after the cells have formed monolayers. Combinations of histamine and norepinephrine do not appear to have additive effects. Serotonin, carbachol, and dopamine have either no or only marginal effects on cyclic AMP levels in rat glioma cells (Gilman and Nirenberg, 1971*a*).

In human glioma cells after one stimulation with norepinephrine and washing, reintroduction of norepinephrine does not elicit another accumulation of cyclic AMP (Clark and Perkins, 1971), while introduction of histamine does elicit an accumulation of cyclic AMP. Such results are reminiscent of those seen with brain slices. However, with rat glioma cells norepinephrine can cause repetitive accumulations of cylic AMP (Schultz *et al.*, 1972). The magnitude of the accumulation of cyclic AMP markedly declines during repetitive stimulations with norepinephrine except when a phosphodiesterase inhibitor, papaverine, is present, suggesting that elevations of intracellular cyclic AMP result in an increase of an associated phosphodiesterase activity (see Section 4.1 and Browning *et al.*, 1974*a,b*).

Adenosine either alone or in combination with norepinephrine or histamine has no or only a marginal effect on cyclic AMP levels in certain glioma cells (Gilman and Nirenberg, 1971*a*; Schultz *et al.*, 1972). Adenosine does increase cyclic AMP levels in a human glioma cell line, and its effects are blocked by theophylline and potentiated by papaverine (Perkins, 1973; Clark *et al.*, 1974). Inhibition of uptake of adenosine into the cells by dipyridamole does not antagonize the adenosine-elicited accumulation of cyclic AMP, providing evidence for an extracellular site of adenosine action. Dipyridamole, unlike papaverine, does not potentiate the effects of norepinephrine. Combinations of adenosine and norepinephrine have effects no greater than those due to norepinephrine alone. Veratridine has no significant effects in glioma cells (Schultz *et al.*, 1972).

In some rat glioma cells, prostaglandin has no or marginal effects either alone or in the presence of a phosphodiesterase inhibitor (Gilman and Nirenberg, 1971*a*; Hamprecht and Schultz, 1973*b*, while in other rat glioma cells prostaglandin elicits at least a twofold accumulation of cyclic AMP which is not potentiated by theophylline (Minna and Gilman, 1973). Prostaglandin elicits an accumulation of cyclic AMP in human glioma cells which is slightly enhanced by theophylline (Perkins, 1973). The effects of prostaglandin and norepinephrine are nearly additive.

The phosphodiesterase inhibitors papaverine and isobutylmethylxanthine greatly potentiate the effects of norepinephrine in rat glioma cells and retard the disappearance of cyclic AMP in cells previously incubated with norepinephrine (Schultz *et al.*, 1972; Browning *et al.*, 1974*a,b*; Hamprecht and Schultz, 1973*b*). Theophylline has virtually no effect on the magnitude of the accumulation of cyclic AMP elicited by norepinephrine (Clark and Perkins, 1971; Schultz *et al.*, 1972). Papaverine is a potent inhibitor of oxidative metabolism in glioma cells in addition to its effects on phosphodiesterase (Browning *et al.*, 1974*a*).

Rat glioma cells incorporate radioactive adenine into intracellular nucleotides which are converted to cyclic AMP during incubations of such labeled cells with norepinephrine or isoproterenol (Schultz *et al.*, 1972). However, the percent conversion of radioactive nucleotides to cyclic AMP appeared much lower than conversions of total endogenous nucleotides to cyclic AMP. The specific activities of cyclic AMP in control and norepinephrine-stimulated human glioma cells were similar (Perkins, 1973).

In mouse neuroblastoma cells lines, prostaglandins E_1 and E_2 elicit a three- to tenfold increase in levels of cyclic AMP (Gilman and Nirenberg, 1971*b*; Gilman and Minna, 1973; Hamprecht and Schultz, 1973*a,b*; Prasad *et al.*, 1973*a,b*; Sheppard and Prasad, 1973). Adenosine elicits a twofold increase in certain cell lines (Blume *et al.*, 1973; Schultz and Hamprecht, 1973). Isoproterenol, (nor)epinephrine, histamine, serotonin, dopamine, acetylcholine, and carbachol have no significant effects either alone or in some cases in the presence of phosphodiesterase inhibitors (Gilman and Nirenberg, 1971*b*; Gilman and Minna, 1973; Hamprecht and Schultz, 1973; Schultz and Hamprecht, 1973). Cyclic AMP levels in neuroblastoma cells have been reported to be elevated by butyric acid, by 5-bromodeoxyuridine, and by the absence of serum in the culture medium (Sheppard and Prasad, 1973; Prasad *et al.*, 1973*b*). 5-Bromodeoxyuridine has little effect on cyclic AMP levels in glioma cells, but does cause a subsequent reduction in the magnitude of the accumulation of cyclic AMP elicited by norepinephrine (Schwartz *et al.*, 1973). The latter effect may be related to the increase in phosphodiesterase activity in cells cultured in the presence of the uridine derivative. Phosphodiesterase inhibitors such as papaverine, RO 20-1724, isobutylmethylxanthine, and diazepam elevate basal levels of cyclic AMP in neuroblastoma cells, and greatly potentiate the effects of prostaglandin and adenosine, while other phosphodiesterase inhibitors such as theophylline and chlordiazepoxide potentiate the effects of prostaglandin by only twofold or less (Blume *et al.*, 1973; Gilman and Minna, 1973; Hamprecht and Schultz, 1973*a,b*; Prasad, 1973*a*; Schultz and Hamprecht, 1973; Sheppard and Prasad, 1973).

The effects of adenosine in the presence of a phosphodiesterase inhibitor are competitively inhibited by theophylline (Blume *et al.*, 1973). Analogues of adenosine such as guanosine, isoguanosine, 2- and 3′-deoxyadenosines, and adenine arabinoside in combination with a phosphodiesterase inhibitor were virtually inactive under conditions where adenosine elicits a twenty- to fortyfold accumulation of cyclic AMP (Blume *et al.*, 1973; Schultz and Hamprecht, 1973). After stimulation of neuroblastoma cells with prostaglandin E_1 or adenosine and washing, readdition of the same stimulant elicited a second accumulation of cyclic AMP (Schultz and Hamprecht, 1973). Phosphodiesterase inhibitors were present in these restimulation experiments.

In adenine-labeled neuroblastoma cells, prostaglandin E_1 either alone or with a phosphodiesterase inhibitor elicited accumulations of radioactive cyclic AMP (Hamprecht and Schultz, 1973*a*). However, as was the case with glioma cells, the percent conversion of adenine-labeled nucleotides to cyclic AMP was markedly less than the conversion of total endogenous nucleotides to cyclic AMP.

All hybrid clones derived from fusion of neuroblastoma and glioma cell lines respond to prostaglandin E_1, while the norepinephrine response of the parent glioma cells is not expressed in hybrids even in the presence of a phosphodiesterase inhibitor (Hamprecht and Schultz, 1973*a*). Similar results were obtained with hybrids of glioma or neuroblastoma cells with other somatic cells (Gilman and Minna, 1973; Minna and Gilman, 1973).

4. FUNCTIONAL ROLE OF CYCLIC NUCLEOTIDES

Evidence for specific roles of cyclic nucleotides, in particular cyclic AMP, in intact cells and in whole animals has been based primarily on attempted correlations between alterations in (1) metabolic pathways, (2) cell differentiation and growth, (3) membrane function, and (4) behavioral effects and the probable alterations in intracellular levels of the cyclic nucleotide in relevant morphological compartments. Enhanced intracellular levels of cyclic AMP or a functionally "equivalent" analogue are expected as a result of the following: (1) the presence of high concentrations of extracellular cyclic AMP, *N,O*-dibutyryl cyclic AMP, *N*-butyryl cyclic AMP, 8-benzylthio cyclic

AMP, etc.; (2) the presence of a phosphodiesterase inhibitor such as theophylline, papaverine, or RO 20-1724; and/or (3) the presence of an agent that is a stimulant of cyclic AMP–generating systems in neuronal or glial cells, i.e., biogenic amines, adenosine, prostaglandin, or depolarizing agents. Antagonists of the stimulatory agents may also be employed to advantage. The difficulties in establishing such correlations are apparent. Nonspecific or non cyclic AMP–related effects of the nonphysiological concentrations of cyclic AMP analogues, phosphodiesterase inhibitors, or stimulatory agents, lack of effects of these agents on the relevant cyclic AMP–generating system, perhaps masked by pronounced effects on non-relevant compartments or systems, requirements for only a virtually undetectable increase and/or a sustained increase in cyclic AMP for a particular response, and various feedback controls on cyclic AMP formation represent only a few of the problems in attempts to establish a role for cyclic nucleotides in intact cells or organisms.

4.1. Effects on Enzymatic Processes

Attempts to demonstrate correlations of alterations of metabolic parameters such as glycogen synthetase and phosphorylase a activity, glucose oxidation, lactate production, and oxygen consumption with levels of cyclic AMP in brain tissue have been rather unsuccessful (for a discussion, see Rall and Gilman, 1970; for data on glycogen levels, see Mrsulja, 1972*a,b*). Levels of adenosine in perfusates from stimulated brain preparations do appear correlated with lactate production (Heller and McIlwain, 1973), but the extent of adenosine-mediated accumulation of cyclic AMP was not determined. Relatively low concentrations (0.1 mM) of exogenous cyclic AMP inhibit aerobic glycolysis in rabbit forebrain slices, while 1 mM cyclic AMP stimulates aerobic glycolysis and respiration (Dittmann and Herrmann, 1970). In another report, cyclic AMP was found to have no effect on glycolysis in guinea pig cortical slices (Takagaki, 1972). Intraventricular dibutyryl cyclic AMP enhances *in vivo* glycolysis in mouse brain (Leonard, 1972). Electrical stimulation, norepinephrine, serotonin, and histamine increase the turnover of protein phosphate in guinea pig cortical slices, while adenosine, another stimulant of the cyclic AMP–generating systems in slices, has no effect on the turnover of protein phosphate and blocks the increase in turnover elicited by histamine, but not that elicited by electrical pulsation (Reddington *et al.*, 1973). High concentrations of potassium ions appear to increase the rate of turnover of protein phosphate. In cultures of rat glioma cells, dibutyryl cyclic AMP, (nor)epinephrine, histamine, and papaverine were found to stimulate glycolysis (Opler and Makman, 1972; Newburgh and Rosenberg, 1972; Browning *et al.*, 1974*a,b*). The effect of norepinephrine is blocked by propranolol. Norepinephrine has no effect on glycolysis in neuroblastoma cells. Elevations of cyclic AMP in glioma cells are also accompanied by an increase in lactate dehydrogenase activity (Schwartz *et al.*, 1973, and references therein). Glutamine synthetase activity in cultured retinas is enhanced by cyclic AMP (Chader, 1971).

Exogenous dibutyryl cyclic AMP or conditions that elevate intracellular levels of cyclic AMP result in a compensatory increase in phosphodiesterase activity in glioma (Schwartz *et al.*, 1973; Uzunov *et al.*, 1973) and neuroblastoma cells (Prasad and Kumar, 1973). Cycloheximide prevents the norepinephrine-elicited increase in a specific phosphodiesterase in rat glioma cells and the dibutyryl cyclic AMP–elicited increase in phosphodiesterase in mouse neuroblastoma cells.

Cyclic AMP–dependent mechanisms have been implicated in the control of metabolic pathways involved in the synthesis and/or inactivation of putative neurotransmitters and neuroregulatory factors. These include increases in levels of acetylcholine receptors, acetylcholinesterase, choline acetyltransferase, and tyrosine hydroxylase in cultured neuroblastoma cells (Furmanski *et al.*, 1971; Prasad and Vernadakis, 1972; Siman-Tov and Sachs, 1972, 1973; Waymire *et al.*, 1972; Prasad *et al.*, 1972, 1973*a*; Prasad and Mandal, 1973; Richelson, 1973) and increases in levels of acetylcholinesterase in cultured fetal chick and rat brain cells (Werner *et al.*, 1971; Schrier and Shapiro, 1973; Shapiro, 1973) and of choline acetyltransferase in the chick brain cells. In the rat brain cells, levels of the latter enzyme were decreased. Dibutyryl cyclic AMP increases prostaglandin synthesis in neuroblastoma and glioma cells (Hamprecht *et al.*, 1973), and cyclic AMP increases prostaglandin E_1 synthesis in rat brain homogenates (Abdulla and McFarlane, 1972). The dibutyryl analogue increases levels of glutamate decarboxylase in glioma and fetal rat brain cells and acetylcholine esterase in at least one line of glioma cells (Schrier and Shapiro, 1973). Catechol-*O*-methyltransferase levels are not affected in neuroblastoma cells by dibutyryl cyclic AMP or prostaglandin (Prasad and Mandal, 1972). Levels of tyrosine hydroxylase, dopamine-β-hydroxylase, and norepinephrine in cultured rat superior cervical ganglia are elevated by dibutyryl cyclic AMP, theophylline, and potassium ions (Keen and McLean, 1972*a,b*; Makay and Iverson, 1972; Silberstein *et al.*, 1972). Dibutyryl cyclic AMP and potassium ions increase levels of tyrosine hydroxylase, dopamine-β-hydroxylase, monoamine oxidase, and dopa decarboxylase in cultured mouse superior cervical ganglion (Goodman *et al.*, 1974). A role for cyclic AMP in the transynaptic induction of tyrosine hydroxylase *in vivo* by stress or reserpine has been questioned (Goodman *et al.*, 1974; Otten *et al.*, 1973, 1974).

Dibutyryl cyclic AMP at low concentrations increases the rate of synthesis of dopamine in rat striatal preparations (Goldstein *et al.*, 1973). Intraventricular dibutyryl cyclic AMP increases the apparent rate of serotonin and dopamine synthesis in brain (Tagliamonte *et al.*, 1971*a,b,c*; Forn *et al.*, 1972). The methylxanthines enhance apparent turnover of norepinephrine *in vivo* in brain, perhaps due to an increased rate of release (Berkowitz *et al.*, 1970; Waldeck, 1971; Corrodi *et al.*, 1972). It is uncertain whether this effect is related to their activity as phosphodiesterase inhibitors. Others have reported that intraventricular epinephrine or intraperitoneal theophylline or SQ 20009 increases the turnover rate for dopamine and serotonin in brain (Burkard and Bartholini, 1973). It is perhaps relevant that cyclic AMP–dependent mechanisms appear to control the synthesis of melatonin from serotonin in pineal gland by effects on levels of serotonin *N*-acetyltransferase activity (Klein *et al.*, 1973, and references therein).

4.2. Cell Morphology, Differentiation, and Growth

Morphological differentiation in cultured cells has been found to be elicited by dibutyryl cyclic AMP, and by compounds known to cause intracellular accumulations of cyclic AMP. Neuroblastoma cells extend long neuritic processes under such conditions (Furmanski *et al.*, 1971; Prasad and Hsie, 1971; Lim and Mitsunobu, 1972; Prasad, 1972*a,b*; Prasad and Sheppard, 1972*b*; Monard *et al.*, 1973; Prasad *et al.*, 1972, 1973*a,b*; Sheppard and Prasad, 1973), while glioma cells become spindle shaped (Lim and Mitsunobu, 1972; Schwartz *et al.*, 1973). Butyrate elevates cyclic AMP in neuroblastoma cells, but does not cause differentiation (Sheppard and Prasad, 1973). Conversely, X-irradiation and the presence of factors released from glial or glioma cells elicit differentiation of neuroblastoma cells but do not measurably increase levels of cyclic AMP (Prasad and Vernadakis, 1972; Prasad *et al.*, 1973*b*; Monard *et al.*, 1973). Dibutyryl cyclic AMP and theophylline have mainly toxic effects on human glioma cells and dibutyryl cyclic AMP causes membrane proliferation in human neuroblastoma cells (MacIntyre *et al.*, 1972). Cycloheximide, an inhibitor of protein synthesis, prevents both neuritic outgrowths and long-term elevations of cyclic AMP elicited by a phosphodiesterase inhibitor in neuroblastoma cells (Lim and Mitsunobu, 1972; Sheppard and Prasad, 1973). The differentiated neuroblastoma cells no longer retain tumorigenic potency and do not react as readily with cancer cell agglutinins such as concanavalin A (Prasad, 1972*c*; Prasad and Sheppard, 1972*a*).

Cultured fetal rat brain cells undergo morphological differentiation into multipolar cells which resemble mature astrocytes when exposed to mono- or dibutyryl cyclic AMP or to a dialyzed soluble protein from brain homogenates (Lim *et al.*, 1973; Shapiro, 1973). Prostaglandin E_1 has no effect and norepinephrine was not tested. In cultured dorsal root ganglion cells from chick embryos (Hier *et al.*, 1972, 1973; Roisen *et al.*, 1972*a,b,c,d*; Frazier *et al.*, 1973; Roisen and Murphy, 1973) and in cultured dorsal root ganglion cells from rat or mouse (Haas *et al.*, 1972), dibutyryl cyclic AMP elicits a marked increase in formation and extension of neuritic processes.

Protein synthesis appears necessary with rodent ganglia since neurite elongation is blocked by cycloheximide. Cyclic AMP mechanisms do not appear to be involved in the neurite extension elicited in ganglia by nerve growth factor (Hier *et al.*, 1972, 1973; Frazier *et al.*, 1973).

A unifying theory on the mechanisms involved in cyclic AMP–elicited changes in cell morphology is that the cyclic nucleotide either enhances formation of microtubules or stabilizes microtubules. Evidence for such stabilization of microtubules systems in tissue slices by cyclic AMP has been reported (Gillespie, 1971). The observations that differentiated neuroblastoma cells no longer retract neuritic processes in the cold after exposure to dibutyryl cyclic AMP (Kirkland and Burton, 1972) and that dibutyryl cyclic AMP reverses the inhibition of neurite extension elicited by a colchicine derivative (Roisen *et al.*, 1972*c*) are also compatible with the hypothesis of a cyclic AMP–dependent enhanced formation or stabilization of microtubules. Nerve growth factor but not dibutyryl cyclic AMP stimulates synthesis of microtubule protein in cultured chick dorsal root ganglion cells (Hier *et al.*, 1972).

Studies on differentiation in the various cultured cells thus provide evidence suggestive of a role for cyclic AMP in the process of maturation and assembly of the central nervous system. These studies, however, appear less relevant to the role of cyclic AMP in the mature, fully developed brain unless such cyclic AMP–dependent mechanisms are involved in the formation of new intracellular connections. After lesion of rat sciatic nerve, dibutyryl cyclic AMP injected intramuscularly near the site of the lesion does greatly accelerate restoration of muscle innervation by this nerve (Pichichero *et al.*, 1973). The large increase in cyclic AMP observed near the site of crushing of a rat sciatic nerve (Appenzeller and Palmer, 1972) might possibly serve a function in the normal regenerative processes.

4.3. Membrane Phenomena

4.3.1. Central Neurons

A role for norepinephrine-elicited increases in cyclic AMP levels in the modulation of spontaneous electrical activity in the rat and rabbit cerebellar Purkinje cells has been firmly established by the extensive studies of Bloom, Hoffer, Siggins and coworkers (Hoffer *et al.*, 1969, 1970, 1971*a,b,c*, 1972; Siggins *et al.*, 1969, 1971*a,b,c,d,e*, 1973; Woodward *et al.*, 1971; Bloom *et al.*, 1972*a,b,c*). Rat cerebellar Purkinje cells normally exhibit (1) irregular high-frequency bursts of electrical spike activity due to excitation by climbing fibers, (2) rapid irregular single action potentials, and (3) long pauses of nonspike activity. A variety of agents slow the discharge rates in these cells when administered microiontophoretically. These include tyramine, amphetamine, histamine, serotonin, γ-aminobutyric acid, glycine, and the catecholamines (nor)epinephrine and isoproterenol (Hoffer *et al.*, 1971*c*; Siggins *et al.*, 1971*c*; Bloom *et al.*, 1972*c*). The inhibitory effects of norepinephrine on discharge rates are prevented by the β-antagonist sotalol, but not by another β-adrenergic-antagonist, *N*-isopropyl-4-nitrophenethanolamine, or by lysergic acid diethylamide. Dibutyryl cyclic AMP and cyclic AMP have inhibitory effects similar to those of norepinephrine but more rapid in onset. Both the cyclic AMP derivatives and the catecholamines increase the frequency of long pauses in spike activity (Hoffer *et al.*, 1970). Surprisingly, cyclic GMP has a similar inhibitory effect (Hoffer *et al.*, 1971*b*). ATP is excitatory. The inhibitory effects of cyclic AMP, cyclic GMP, and norepinephrine are potentiated by theophylline and its ethylenediamine salt, aminophylline, and by papaverine (Siggins *et al.*, 1969, 1971*c*; Hoffer *et al.*, 1971*b*). The methylxanthines either on parenteral or microiontophoretic application have some inhibitory effects on discharge rates. Prostaglandin E_1 has effects opposite to those of norepinephrine and cyclic AMP. Thus it increases the rate of spontaneous discharge by reducing the frequency of long pauses in spike activity. Prostaglandin reverses the inhibitory effects of norepinephrine and methylxanthines, but does not prevent the inhibitory effects of γ-aminobutyric acid or cyclic AMP (Hoffer *et al.*, 1969; Siggins *et al.*, 1969, 1971*c,d*). Nicotinate, an agent which in some systems appears to activate phosphodiesterases, reduced on microïontophoretic administration the inhibitory effects of norepinephrine and cyclic AMP (Hoffer *et al.*, 1971*b*; Siggins *et al.*, 1971*c*).

Electrical stimulation of the locus coeruleus with its afferent tracts to the cerebellum results in a decrease in the discharge rates of Purkinje cells (Siggins *et al.*, 1971*e*; Bloom *et al.*, 1972*a*; Hoffer *et al.*, 1972). The phosphodiesterase inhibitor, papaverine, potentiates the inhibitory effects of locus coeruleus stimulation. Locus coeruleus stimulation is not effective in rats that have been pretreated with agents such as reserpine or α-methyl-*p*-tyrosine that will deplete norepinephrine in presynaptic terminals of brain, or with 6-hydroxydopamine, an agent which destroys noradrenergic terminals. After 6-hydroxydopamine treatment, the spontaneous discharge rate of Purkinje cells is increased due to reductions in the frequency of long pauses in electrical activity (Hoffer *et al.*, 1971*a*). The results strongly suggest that norepinephrine, released from noradrenergic terminals of neurons originating in the locus coeruleus, regulates spontaneous electrical activity in Purkinje cells by a mechanism involving norepinephrine-elicited accumulation of cyclic AMP within the Purkinje cell. Other results are consonant with this interpretation. Thus desmethylimipramine, which inhibits presynaptic uptake of catecholamines, potentiates the inhibitory effect of norepinephrine on Purkinje cells, but has no effect in 6-hydroxydopamine-treated rats (Hoffer *et al.*, 1971*c*). Norepinephrine, tyramine, amphetamine, cyclic AMP, and methylxanthines have inhibitory effects in 6-hydroxydopamine-treated rats and in neonatal rats which have not yet established synaptic innervation of Purkinje cells (Woodward *et al.*, 1971). Prostaglandin E_1 no longer increases spontaneous discharge rates in 6-hydroxydopamine-treated rats, but still antagonizes the effects of norepinephrine (Hoffer *et al.*, 1969; Siggins *et al.*, 1971*d*). Immunofluorescent techniques for the histological assay of cyclic AMP demonstrate that topical application of norepinephrine or electrical stimulation of the locus coeruleus elicits striking increases in fluorescence of the cerebellar Purkinje cells (Siggins *et al.*, 1973). Other inhibitory agents such as glycine, serotonin, histamine, and γ-aminobutyric acid have no effect on fluorescence of Purkinje cells. It was not ascertained whether prostaglandin E_1 prevents the norepinephrine-elicited increase in fluorescence of Purkinje cells.

Inhibitory agents such as γ-aminobutyric acid, norepinephrine, cyclic AMP, and dibutyryl cyclic AMP all elicit hyperpolarization of Purkinje cells (Hoffer *et al.*, 1971*b*; Siggins *et al.*, 1971*b*). However, the latter three agents cause an increase in membrane resistance, while γ-aminobutyric acid causes a decrease in resistance. The mechanism of the change in membrane conductance elicited by cyclic AMP–dependent mechanisms is unknown. A specific phosphorylation of membrane proteins associated with ionic channels catalyzed by cyclic AMP–dependent protein kinases is an attractive hypothesis. Changes in chloride ion conductances do not appear to be involved. It should be noted that calcium ions also slow spontaneous discharge rates in Purkinje cells, while metal chelators increase discharge rates (Hoffer *et al.*, 1971*b*; Siggins *et al.*, 1971*c*).

Another laboratory, in initial studies with perhaps less definitive identification of Purkinje cells and with pentobarbital instead of halothane anesthesia (*cf.* Siggins *et al.*, 1971*a*, and discussion of Siggins *et al.*, 1971*d*), demonstrated inhibitory effects of norepinephrine but not of cyclic AMP on cerebellar Purkinje cells (Godfraind and Pumain, 1971, 1972). In these studies, glutamate was frequently used to increase spontaneous discharge rates of the Purkinje cells. A third laboratory could not confirm the inhibitory effects of cyclic AMP (Lake and Jordan, 1974), but see *Addendum.*

It is as yet unclear whether the inhibitory effects of norepinephrine on neurons in other brain regions are uniformly mediated by cyclic AMP–dependent mechanisms. In rat cerebral cortex, hippocampus, or medullary reticular formation, the inhibitory effects of norepinephrine on neuronal discharge rates are only infrequently antagonized by prostaglandin E_1 (Siggins *et al.*, 1971*d*). Norepinephrine inhibits the firing rate of a high percentage of cerebral cortical neurons in rat, cat, and guinea pig (Jordan *et al.*, 1972*a,b*; Lake *et al.*, 1972, 1973). In cat, prostaglandin antagonized the inhibitory effect of norepinephrine in nearly one-half of the cells, but was a much less efficacious antagonist in rat or guinea pig. Dibutyryl cyclic AMP had virtually no inhibitory effects on cortical neurons of these three species. Studies on potentiation of norepinephrine effects by phosphodiesterase inhibitors were difficult because of the intrinsic depressant activity of aminophylline and to a lesser extent of papaverine. The inhibitory effects of aminophylline were undiminished in 6-hydroxydopamine-treated rats, indicating that a methylxanthine-induced release of norepinephrine is not involved in this effect. Papaverine potentiated the inhibitory effects of norepinephrine in a high percentage of cells. The inhibitory effects of aminophylline were blocked in all cat cortical neurons and in the majority of rat and guinea pig neurons by prostaglandin. The inhibitory effects of norepinephrine and serotonin in cat cortical neurons were frequently prevented by "calcium antagonists" such as magnesium ions, lanthanum ions, and verapamil (Phillis *et al.*, 1973; Yarbrough *et al.*, 1974). In neurons of cat medulla oblongata, discharge rates were frequently depressed not only by norepinephrine and histamine but also by cyclic AMP (Anderson *et al.*, 1973). Cells that were excited by norepinephrine were not affected by cyclic AMP. Prostaglandin E_1 and nicotinate reduced the inhibitory effects of norepinephrine in some cells. Both the ethylenediamine salt of theophylline (aminophylline) and ethylenediamine itself were potent inhibitory agents, suggesting that effects of this salt of theophylline may not always be related to phosphodiesterase inhibition. Imidazoles inhibit firing of cortical neurons, and are known to activate phosphodiesterases, a process that should decrease rather than increase cyclic AMP levels. The inhibitory effects of a variety of imidazoles are not at all related to the potency of such compounds as *in vitro* activators of phosphodiesterases (Godfraind *et al.*, 1973). *In toto*, the various results suggest that, at least in some central neurons, norepinephrine-elicited accumulations of cyclic AMP and resultant hyperpolarizations function in inhibitory transynaptic effects.

Dopamine released from terminals originating in the substantia nigra appears to act as an inhibitory neurotransmitter in the caudate nucleus (Bloom *et al.*, 1965; Connor, 1970; York, 1972). Such effects might be mediated *via* a cyclic AMP–dependent mechanism (see *Addendum*).

In explants of fetal or newborn mouse spinal cord and cerebral cortex, cyclic AMP, its dibutyryl derivative, and caffeine temporarily restore slow wave and repetitive spike discharges that were abolished in calcium-free medium (Crain and Pollock, 1973). It was suggested that cyclic AMP is capable of mobilizing functional pools of membrane-bound calcium ions necessary in the absence of external calcium for synaptic transmission. Possible interrelationships between calcium ions and cyclic AMP as "second messengers" in a variety of tissues have been discussed (Rasmussen, 1970).

4.3.2. *Peripheral Neurons*

In sympathetic ganglia, catecholamine-elicited accumulations of cyclic AMP (see Section 3.3) appear to result in postsynaptic hyperpolarizations and hence an inhibition of neuronal transmission. For example, in rabbit superior cervical ganglion in which propagated impulses have been blocked by hexamethonium or *d*-tubocurarine, preganglionic stimulation elicits a hyperpolarization of the ganglionic neurons which is blocked by prostaglandin E_1 and potentiated by theophylline (McAfee and Greengard, 1972; Greengard and Kebabian, 1974; Kalix *et al.*, 1974). This hyperpolarization is blocked by α-antagonists. Carbachol elicits a hyperpolarization, but has no effect in the absence of calcium ions. Dopamine in the medium elicits a similar hyperpolarization which is blocked by prostaglandin E_1 and potentiated by theophylline. Cyclic AMP and its butyryl derivatives elicit a hyperpolarization, while dibutyryl cyclic GMP causes a depolarization. Cyclic GMP has no effect. Excitability of the ganglionic neuron is reduced during the period of hyperpolarization. Dopamine, theophylline, cyclic AMP and its butyryl derivatives, and cyclic GMP have no effect on axons of the cervical vagus nerve. Dibutyryl cyclic GMP, however, depolarizes the vagus nerve.

Norepinephrine elicits a hyperpolarization of ganglionic neurons of the rabbit superior cervical ganglion (Libet and Kobayashi, 1969). Both dopamine and dibutyryl cyclic AMP elicit hyperpolarization and a partial antagonism of transmission in the cat superior cervical ganglion (Machova and Kristofova, 1973). In the cat ganglion, aminophylline has both hyperpolarizing and depolarizing activities. In contrast, another group reported for the same preparation no consistent effect for dibutyryl cyclic AMP, a depressant effect for aminophylline and papaverine, and a facilatory effect for imidazole on ganglionic transmission (Varagic and Zugic, 1973).

Agents such as dopamine and norepinephrine that activate retinal adenylate cyclases (see Section 3.3) inhibit electrical activity in retinal ganglion cells (Straschill and Perwein, 1969). Dopamine is known to be released on illumination of retina (Kramer, 1971). The depolarization of the retinular cells of horseshoe crab eyes which is elicited by light is antagonized by cyclic AMP (Wulff, 1971). Cyclic AMP, theophylline, or light causes a depolarization of photoreceptor cells in horseshoe crab eyes and an increase in firing of an associated neuron (Miller *et al.*, 1971). Discussion of light-inhibited cyclic AMP– and cyclic GMP–generating systems in photoreceptors, the light and ATP (GMP) dependent formation of a heat-labile activator of photoreceptor phosphodiesterase, and the relationship of these observations to the light-elicited depolarization of photoreceptor cells, the release of dopamine, and the role of cyclic nucleotides in the visual and other sensory systems is, however, beyond the scope of this review (for further pertinent references, see Bitensky *et al.*, 1971, 1972, 1973; Bitensky and Gorman, 1972; Kurihara, 1972; Kurihara and Koyama, 1972; Miller, 1973; Pannbacker, 1973; Bensinger *et al.*, 1974).

4.3.3. Motor Neurons

A role for cyclic AMP in mechanisms involved in release of acetylcholine in neuromuscular preparations has been proposed. Thus epinephrine, dibutyryl cyclic AMP, and methylxanthines appear to increase the release of acetylcholine from the presynaptic neuronal terminal (Breckenridge *et al.*,

1967; Rasmussen and Tenenhouse, 1968; Goldberg and Singer, 1969; Varagic and Zugic, 1971; Varagic *et al.*, 1972). It has been proposed that the reduction in toxicity of *d*-tubocurarine by certain phosphodiesterase inhibitors is also related to a cyclic AMP–dependent increase in release of acetylcholine (Anttila and Vapaatalo, 1972). Adenosine, another agent which might elevate cyclic AMP levels, appears, however, to decrease release of acetylcholine in a neuromuscular preparation (Ginsborg and Hirst, 1972). Others have argued against a role of cyclic AMP in release of acetylcholine from motor neurons (Quastel and Hackett, 1971). Dibutyryl cyclic AMP has no effect on the release of radioactive acetylcholine from guinea pig cortical slices (Shimizu *et al.*, 1970*a*). A discussion of the role of cyclic AMP in release phenomena in other preparations is beyond the scope of this review. However, it might be mentioned that dibutyryl cyclic AMP and theophylline enhance the release of (nor)epinephrine from sympathetic nerves (Wooten *et al.*, 1973) and adrenal glands (Peach, 1972). Calcium ions do not appear required for such drug-elicited release. Methylxanthines may also increase release of biogenic amines in brain (see Section 4.1).

In summary, it appears that cyclic AMP may affect membrane function in a variety of ways in the central nervous system. As yet, however, a role has been firmly established only in cerebellar Purkinje cells where norepinephrine-evoked accumulations of cyclic AMP elicit a postsynaptic decrease in membrane conduction and a concomitant inhibitory hyperpolarization. Similar mechanisms, however, probably exist at other synapses. The apparent involvement of cyclic AMP in release phenomena in motor neurons and sympathetic neurons and in mobilization of calcium ions opens the possibility that similar phenomena in the central nervous system may involve cyclic AMP. Cyclic nucleotides have also been reported to effect membrane phenomena in a variety of non neuronal cells. The reversal of the reserpine-elicited block of the spontaneous activity of cardiac pacemaker cells by norepinephrine or dibutyryl cyclic AMP (Tuganowski *et al.*, 1973), the correlation of cyclic nucleotide levels with cardiac contraction cycles (Brooker, 1973; Wollenberger *et al.*, 1973), and the effects of cyclic AMP, epinephrine, and phosphodiesterase inhibitors on action potentials and membrane permeability in cardiac Purkinje fibers (Tsien *et al.*, 1972; Tsien, 1973) should be mentioned. A cyclic AMP–dependent diphosphoinositide kinase has been described (Torda, 1972*a*), and it has been proposed that activation of this enzyme plays a role in the neuronal hyperpolarization elicited by cyclic AMP (Torda, 1972*b*).

4.4. Centrally Active Drugs and Levels of Cyclic Nucleotides in Brain

Postdecapitation increases in cyclic AMP (see Section 3.1) complicate any study on the effect of psychoactive agents on levels of cyclic AMP in whole brain or in specific brain regions. Rapid freezing of animal heads partially circumvents this problem, but is not suitable for animals larger than rats. Two other rapid methods of fixing brain have been described; microwave irradiation (Schmidt *et al.*, 1972) and freeze blowing of either forebrain (Nahorski and Rogers, 1973) or whole brain (Lust *et al.*, 1973). Agents such as amphetamine and combinations of a monoamine oxidase inhibitor and dopa that increase spontaneous activity in animals had little effect on *in situ* levels of brain cyclic AMP (Paul *et al.*, 1970*a*; Ferrendelli *et al.*, 1972; Palmer *et al.*, 1972*b*; Schmidt *et al.*, 1972). β-Chloroamphetamine appeared to reduce levels of cyclic AMP. Intraperitoneal injection of dopa caused an increase in levels of cyclic AMP in rat caudate nucleus (Garelis and Neff, 1974). Central tranquilizers or depressants such as reserpine, chlorpromazine, or barbiturates either had no effect (Paul *et al.*, 1970*a*; Uzunov and Weiss, 1971; Ferrendelli *et al.*, 1972) or in the case of barbiturates reduced levels of brain cyclic AMP (Schmidt *et al.*, 1972). Chlorpromazine, desmethylimipramine, and haloperidol have been reported to increase levels of cyclic AMP in rat brain (Berndt and Schwabe, 1973). This increase was antagonized by theophylline. Ethanol, a central depressant, decreased cerebellar levels of cyclic AMP (Volicer and Gold, 1973), while chronic treatment of mice with ethanol increased cerebral levels of cyclic AMP. Phosphodiesterase inhibitors such as theophylline (a central stimulant) and papaverine (a central depressant) increased levels of brain cyclic AMP (Paul *et al.*, 1970*a*; Goldberg *et al.*, 1970). Electroconvulsive shocks caused transient large increases in cyclic AMP levels in rodent brain (Goldberg *et al.*, 1967; Sattin, 1971; Lust *et al.*, 1972). Methylxanthines, oxotremorine, and α-methyltyrosine prevented or decreased these effects. The increase in cyclic AMP elicited by hexafluorodiethyl ether in convulsant dosages was similarly antagonized by theophylline (Sattin, 1971). Another convulsant, pentylenetetrazole, had no effect on levels of cyclic AMP in rat brain (Paul *et al.*, 1970*a*).

Electroconvulsive therapy increases urinary levels of cyclic AMP (Hamadah *et al.*, 1972). Whether urinary levels reflect changes in cyclic AMP metabolism in the central nervous system is, however, not certain. A number of papers have provided data that correlate low levels of urinary cyclic AMP with depression in humans (Abdulla and Hamadah, 1970; Paul *et al.*, 1970*a,b,d*, 1971*a,b*; Cramer *et al.*, 1972*a,b*). Levels of urinary cyclic AMP reflected the extent of depression and were increased during successful therapy by electroshock treatment, antidepressants, dopa, and lithium ions. Other groups saw no correlations of urinary cyclic AMP with the affective state of manic depressive patients (Brown *et al.*, 1972; Jenner *et al.*, 1972) or of two patients with periodic catatonia (Perry *et al.*, 1973). It is possible that such urinary changes may reflect only increases in the physical activity of patients (see Robison *et al.*, 1970*a*; Paul *et al.*, 1971*b*). Levels of cyclic AMP in cerebrospinal fluid were similar in a variety of disease states, including both mania and depression (Robison *et al.*, 1970*a*; see also Cramer *et al.*, 1972*a,b*, 1973*b*). Probenecid markedly increases cerebrospinal levels of cyclic AMP in patients while having little effect on brain levels in rats (Cramer and Lindl, 1972; Cramer *et al.*, 1972*b*). The literature on cyclic AMP and cyclic GMP levels in urine and spinal fluid has been reviewed by Murad (1973).

Cyclic AMP levels in mouse forebrain were similar at low and high points of diurnal behavioral activity (Nahorski and Rogers, 1973). The increase in cyclic AMP on decapitation was, however, significantly greater at the time of peak diurnal activity. In various strains of rats, high spontaneous behavioral activity correlated with high responses of a norepinephrine-sensitive cyclic AMP–generating system in slices from midbrain–striatum and with low responses of such systems in cerebral cortical slices (Skolnick and Daly, 1974*a*).

Correlations of indicators of brain metabolic state such as levels of glycogen, phosphorylase, and glycogen synthetase with levels of cyclic AMP have as yet not been satisfactory (see Goldberg *et al.*, 1970; Paul *et al.*, 1970*a*; Rall and Gilman, 1970). Brain levels of cyclic AMP in fasted rats have been reported to be transiently elevated by an antilipolytic agent, β-pyridylcarbinol (Burkard *et al.*, 1971).

Agents such as catecholamines and prostaglandin that can increase cyclic AMP levels in brain slices have been reported to cause an increase in cyclic AMP in rat brain. Thus intravenous prostaglandin E_1 caused a transient elevation of cyclic AMP in cortex, hypothalamus, cerebellum, and brain stem (Wellman and Schwabe, 1973). Intraventricular epinephrine elicited a two- to threefold transient increase in rat brain cyclic AMP (Burkard, 1972). Norepinephrine and isoproterenol were much less effective and dopamine had only a marginal effect. Another group found no significant effect of smaller amounts of intraventricular norepinephrine on levels of rat brain cyclic AMP (Schmidt *et al.*, 1972).

The influence of drugs and other treatments on cyclic GMP levels has been studied less extensively. Levels of cyclic GMP in mouse cerebellum were increased by amphetamine, oxotremorine, and electroconvulsive shock (Ferrendelli *et al.*, 1970, 1972; Goldberg *et al.*, 1970; Lust *et al.*, 1972). Atropine, chlorpromazine, and reserpine caused a decrease in cerebellar levels. Neither atropine or chlorpromazine prevented the oxotremorine-elicited increase in cerebellum. *In vivo* administration of an inhibitor of acetylcholine esterase increased levels of cyclic GMP in mouse cerebellum (Goldberg *et al.*, 1973). Cortical levels of cyclic GMP were increased by atropine, oxotremorine, and electroconvulsive shock. Further studies on the influence of various factors on brain levels of cyclic AMP and cyclic GMP may lead to significant findings. However, important changes in cyclic nucleotide levels in specific brain regions or cell types might easily be insignificant with respect to total levels of the nucleotide.

4.5. Behavioral Effects

Effects of administration of cyclic AMP or its dibutyryl derivative in whole animals have been studied by a number of groups. In rats (Gessa *et al.*, 1970; Herman, 1973), cats (Gessa *et al.*, 1970), chickens (Asakawa and Yoshida, 1971), and goldfish (Shashoua, 1971). Intraventricular or intracerebral injection of dibutyryl cyclic AMP and less effectively of cyclic AMP elicits an increase in spontaneous motor activity. Episodes of catatonia, aggressive behaviour, and convulsions were observed in mammals. Similar sequelae were observed in mammals or chickens after intracerebral injection of dibutyryl cyclic AMP into the hypothalamus (Breckenridge and Lisk, 1969; Gessa *et al.*, 1970; Booth, 1972; Marley and Nistico, 1972) or the mesencephalic reticular formation (Gessa *et al.*, 1970). Catatonia was pronounced in cats only after intracerebral injections into the reticular formation (Gessa *et al.*, 1970). Injection into cat amygdala elicited convulsions and circling movements. Cerebellar injection elicited sleep, while no effects were seen after injection into caudate nucleus, putamen, or pallidum. The effects of dibutyryl cyclic AMP in rats were not prevented by prior administration of chlorpromazine or reserpine. It has been claimed that cyclic AMP or the dibutyryl derivative would reverse reserpine-elicited ptosis, but no details were reported (Abdulla and Hamadah, 1970). Cyclic AMP and its dibutyryl derivatives have been reported to elicit hypothermia and hyperthermia (Breckenridge and Lisk, 1969; Varagic and Beleslin, 1973) and to have effects on food and water intake (Booth, 1972; Rindi *et al.*, 1972; Sciorelli *et al.*, 1972). Intraventricular administration of dibutyryl cyclic AMP to rats shortens the narcosis elicited by amobarbital and a variety of other soporifics such as diazepam, halothane, and chloral hydrate (Cohn *et al.*, 1973). Dibutyryl cyclic AMP changes the nucleotide composition of newly formed RNA in goldfish brain (Shashoua, 1971). Topical application of dibutyryl cyclic AMP to kitten cerebral cortex elicits paroxysmal and convulsive activity and causes the appearance of transcallosally evoked responses at nonhomotopic sites, suggestive of facilitation of superficial synaptic pathways (Purpura and Shofer, 1972).

Surprisingly, in view of their polar nature, both cyclic AMP and dibutyryl cyclic AMP after intravenous or intraperitoneal administration elicit a number of sequelae which would appear to involve central mechanisms. After intraperitoneal injection, dibutyryl cyclic AMP reduces spontaneous motor activity (Henion *et al.*, 1967; Weiner and Olson, 1973) and has antianxiety properties as measured in a behavioral conflict test (Horovitz *et al.*, 1972). Intraperitoneal administration of a 6-piperidyl analogue of cyclic AMP prolongs hexobarbital-sleeping time (Vargui and Spano, 1971). Both cyclic AMP and dibutyryl cyclic AMP on intravenous administration antagonize morphine analgesia, tolerance, and dependency (Ho *et al.*, 1972, 1973*a,b*). Cyclic AMP is also effective after intracerebral injection. Drugs which might be expected to alter central levels of cyclic AMP have little effect on (theophylline) or enhance (imidazole) morphine analgesia (Contreras *et al.*, 1972). Further studies with perhaps other derivatives such as *N*-dansyl cyclic AMP (Gessa *et al.*, 1970) and 8-benzylthio-cyclic AMP will be necessary to provide further insights into the mechanisms of these pharmacological effects of cyclic AMP and their relevance to the physiological roles of cyclic AMP in the central nervous system.

5. CONCLUSION

Further studies are obviously necessary for a better understanding of the role of cyclic AMP– and cyclic GMP–dependent mechanisms in the central nervous system. The present, already voluminous literature provides many indications of important roles for cyclic AMP in (1) establishment of the synaptically integrated central nervous system, (2) regulation of synaptic efficiency and of neuronal responsiveness, (3) synthesis of neurotransmitter substances and mediation of their effects, (4) regulation of metabolic function perhaps as both an activator and an inhibitor, (5) feedback control of its own formation through activation of phosphodiesterases, and (6) interactions with calcium ions. Further insights into the precise nature and role of cyclic nucleotide mechanisms and correlations with physiological functions and with the relevant morphological entities in which cyclic AMP or cyclic GMP serves as a regulatory messenger of such functions in the central nervous system remain a challenge for the future. An *Addendum* of additional publications pertinent to the various sections of this chapter appears at the end of this volume, beginning on p. 361.

6. REFERENCES

ABDULLA, Y. H., and HAMADAH, K., 1970, 3′,5′-Cyclic adenosine monophosphate in depression and mania, *Lancet* **i:**378–381.

ABDULLA, Y. H., and MCFARLANE, E., 1972, Control of prostaglandin biosynthesis in rat brain homogenates by adenine nucleotides, *Biochem. Pharmacol.* **21:**2841–2847.

AMER, M. S., and BROWDER, H. P., 1971, Effect of quazodine on phosphodiesterase, *Proc. Soc. Exp. Biol. Med.* **136:**750–752.

AMER, M. S., GOMOLL, A. W., and MCKINNEY, G. R., 1972, Phosphodiesterase inhibition as a mechanism for the diuretic activity of 1-[tert-butylimino)methyl]-2-(3-indolyl)indoline hydrochloride (MJ-8592-1), *Res. Commun. Chem. Pathol. Pharmacol.* **4:**467–476.

ANDERSON, E. G., HAAS, H. L., and HOSLI, L., 1973, Comparison of effects of noradrenaline and histamine with cyclic AMP on brain stem neurones, *Brain Res.* **49:**471–475.

ANTTILA, P., and VAPAATALO, H., 1972, Decreased toxicity of *d*-tubocurarine after pretreatment with drugs elevating the intracellular level of c-AMP in mice, *Naunyn-Schmiedebergs Arch. Pharmacol.* **273:**175–178.

Appel, S. H., and Locher, C., 1973, Changes in synapse membrane protein phosphorylation following electroconvulsive shock, *Neurology* **23:**41Abs.

Appenzeller, O., and Palmer, G., 1972, The cyclic AMP (adenosine 3′,5′-phosphate) content of sciatic nerve: Changes after nerve crush, *Brain Res.* **42:**521–524.

Appleman, M. M., Thompson, W. J., and Russell, T. R., 1973, Cyclic nucleotide phosphodiesterases, *Advan. Cyclic Nucleotide Res.* **3:**66–98.

Asakawa, T., and Yoshida, H., 1971, Studies on the functional role of adenosine 3′,5′-monophosphate, histamine and prostaglandin E_1 in the central nervous system, *Jap. J. Pharmacol.* **21:**569–583.

Bauer, R. J., Swiatek, K. R., Robins, R. K., and Simon, L. N., 1971, Adenosine 3′,5′-cyclic monophosphate derivatives. II. Biological activity of some 8-substituted analogs, *Biochem. Biophys. Res. Commun.* **45:**526–531.

Beavo, J. A., Hardman, J. G., and Sutherland, E. W., 1970, Hydrolysis of cyclic guanosine and adenosine 3′,5′-monophosphate by rat and bovine tissues, *J. Biol. Chem.* **245:**5649–5655.

Beavo, J. A., Hardman, J. G., and Sutherland, E. W., 1971, Stimulation of adenosine 3′,5′-monophosphate hydrolysis by guanosine 3′,5′-monophosphate, *J. Biol. Chem.* **246:**3841–3846.

Beer, B., Chasin, M., Clody, D. E., Vogel, J. R., and Horovitz, Z. P., 1972, Cyclic adenosine monophosphate phosphodiesterase in brain: Effect on anxiety, *Science* **176:**428–430.

Bensinger, R. E., Fletcher, R. T., and Chader, G. J., 1974, Guanylate cyclase: Inhibition by light in retinal photoreceptors, *Science* **183:**86–87.

Berkowitz, B. A., Tarver, J. H., and Spector, S., 1970, Release of norepinephrine in the central nervous system by theophylline and caffeine, *Eur. J. Pharmacol.* **10:**64–71.

Berndt, S., and Schwabe, U., 1973, Effect of psychotropic drugs on phosphodiesterase and cyclic AMP level in rat brain *in vivo, Brain Res.* **63:**303–312.

Berti, F., Trabucchi, M., Bernareggi, V., and Fumagalli, R., 1972, The effects of prostaglandins on cyclic-AMP formation in cerebral cortex of different mammalian species, *Pharmacol. Res. Commun.* **4:**253–259.

Birnbaumer, L., 1973, Hormone-sensitive adenylyl cyclases useful models for studying hormone receptor functions in cell-free systems, *Biochim. Biophys. Acta* **300:**129–158.

Bitensky, M. W., and Gorman, R. E., 1972, Digitonin effects on photoreceptor adenylate cyclase, *Science* **175:**1363–1364.

Bitensky, M. W., Gorman, R. E., and Miller, W. H., 1971, Adenyl cyclase as a link between photon capture and changes in membrane permeability of frog photoreceptors, *Proc. Natl. Acad. Sci.* **68:**561–562.

Bitensky, M. W., Miller, W. H., Gorman, R. E., Neufeld, A. H., and Robinson, R., 1972, The role of cyclic AMP in visual excitation, *Advan. Cyclic Nucleotide Res.* **1:**317–335.

Bitensky, M. W., Miki, N., Marcus, F. R., and Keirns, J. J., 1973, The role of cyclic nucleotides in visual excitation, *Life Sci.* **13:**1451–1472.

Bloom, F. E., Costa, E., and Salmoiraghi, G. C., 1965, Anesthesia and the responsiveness of individual neurons of the caudate nucleus of the cat to acetylcholine, norepinephrine and dopamine administered by microelectrophoresis, *J. Pharmacol. Exp. Ther.* **150:**244–252.

Bloom, F. E., Hoffer, B. J., and Siggins, G. R., 1972*a*, Norepinephrine mediated cerebellar synapses: A model system for neuropsychopharmacology, *Biol. Psychiat.* **4:**157–177.

Bloom, F. E., Hoffer, B. J., Battenberg, E. R., Siggins, G. R., Steiner, A. L., Parker, C. W., and Wedner, H. J., 1972*b*, Adenosine 3′,5′-monophosphate is localized in cerebellar neurons: Immunofluorescence evidence, *Science* **177:**436–438.

Bloom, F. E., Hoffer, B. J., Siggins, G. R., Burker, J. L., and Nicoll, R. A., 1972*c*, Effects of serotonin on central neurons: Microiontophoretic administration, *Fed. Proc.* **31:**97–106.

Blume, A. J., Dalton, C., and Sheppard, H., 1973, Adenosine-mediated elevation of cyclic 3′:5′-adenosine monophosphate concentrations in cultured mouse neuroblastoma cells, *Proc. Natl. Acad. Sci.* **70:**3099–3102.

BOEHME, E., 1970, Guanyl Cyclase Bildung von Guanosine-3′,5′-monophosphat in Niere und anderen Geweben der Ratte, *Eur. J. Biochem.* **14:**422–429.

BOOTH, D. A., 1972, Unlearned and learned effects of intrahypothalamic cyclic AMP injection on feeding, *Nature New Biol.* **237:**222–224.

BRADHAM, L. S., 1972, Comparison of the effects of Ca^{2+} and Mg^{2+} on the adenyl cyclase of beef brain, *Biochim. Biophys. Acta* **276:**434–443.

BRADHAM, L. S., HOLT, D. A., and SIMS, M., 1970, The effect of Ca^{2+} on the adenyl cyclase of calf brain, *Biochim. Biophys. Acta* **201:**250–260.

BRAY, J. J., KON, C. M., and BRECKENRIDGE, B. M., 1971, Adenyl cyclase cyclic nucleotide phosphodiesterase and axoplasmic flow, *Brain Res.* **26:**385–394.

BRECKENRIDGE, B. M., 1964, The measurement of cyclic adenylate in tissues, *Proc. Natl. Acad. Sci.* **57:**1580–1586.

BRECKENRIDGE, B. M., and JOHNSTON, R. E., 1969, Cyclic 3′,5′-nucleotide phosphodiesterase in brain, *J. Histochem. Cytochem.* **17:**505–511.

BRECKENRIDGE, B. M., and LISK, R. D., 1969, Cyclic adenylate and hypothalamic regulatory functions, *Proc. Soc. Exp. Biol. Med.* **131:**934–935.

BRECKENRIDGE, B. M., BURN, J. H., and MATSCHINSKY, F. M., 1967, Theophylline, epinephrine, and neostigmine facilitation of neuromuscular transmission, *Proc. Natl. Acad. Sci.* **57:**1893–1897.

BROOKER, G., 1973, Oscillation of cyclic adenosine monophosphate concentration during the myocardial contraction cycle, *Science* **182:**933–934.

BROOKER, G., THOMAS, L. J., JR., and APPLEMAN, M. M., 1968, The assay of adenosine 3′,5′-cyclic monophosphate and guanosine 3′,5′-cyclic monophosphate in biological materials by enzymatic radioisotopic displacement, *Biochemistry* **7:**4177–4181.

BROWN, B. L., SALWAY, J. G., ALBANO, J. D. M., HULLIN, R. P., and EKINS, R. P., 1972, Urinary excretion of cyclic AMP and manic-depressive psychosis, *Brit. J. Psychiat.* **120:**405–408.

BROWN, J. H., and MAKMAN, M. H., 1972, Stimulation by dopamine of adenylate cyclase in retinal homogenates and of adenosine-3′:5′-cyclic monophosphate formation in intact retina, *Proc. Natl. Acad. Sci.* **69:**539–543.

BROWN, J. H., and MAKMAN, M. H., 1973, Influence of neuroleptic drugs and apomorphine on the dopamine-sensitive adenylate cyclase of retina, *J. Neurochem.* **21:**477–479.

BROWNING, E. T., GROPP, V. E., JR., and KON, C., 1974*a*, Papaverine, a potent inhibitor of respiration in C–6 astrocytoma cells, *Mol. Pharmacol.* **10:**175–181.

BROWNING, E. T., SCHWARTZ, J. P., and BRECKENRIDGE, B. M., 1974*b*, Norepinephrine-sensitive properties of C–6 astrocytoma cells, *Mol. Pharmacol.* **10:**162–174.

BURKARD, W. P., 1972, Catecholamine induced increase of cyclic adenosine 3′,5′-monophosphate in rat brain *in vivo*, *J. Neurochem.* **19:**2615–2619.

BURKARD, W. P., and BARTHOLINI, G., 1973, Possible influence of endogenous cyclic AMP on serotonin and dopamine turnover in rat brain *in vivo*, *Experientia* **29:**762Abs.

BURKARD, W. P., and GEY, K. F., 1968, Adenyl Cyclase im Rattenhirn, *Helv. Physiol. Acta* **26:**197–198.

BURKARD, W. P., LENGSFELD, H., and GEY, K. F., 1971, Cyclic adenosine 3′,5′-monophosphate and adenylcyclase in liver, adipose tissue and brain of rats treated with α-pyridylcarbinol, *Biochem. Pharmacol.* **20:**23–28.

CAMPBELL, M. T., and OLIVER, I. T., 1972, 3′:5′-Cyclic nucleotide phosphodiesterases in rat tissue, *Eur. J. Biochem.* **28:**30–37.

CEDAR, H., and SCHWARTZ, J. H., 1972, Cyclic adenosine monophosphate in the nervous system of *Aplysia californica*. II. Effect of serotonin and dopamine, *J. Gen. Physiol.* **60:**570–587.

CEDAR, H., KANDEL, E. R., and SCHWARTZ, J. H., 1972, Cyclic adenosine monophosphate in the nervous system of *Aplysia californica*. I. Increased synthesis in response to synaptic stimulation, *J. Gen. Physiol.* **60:**558–569.

CEHOVIC, G., POSTERNAK, T., and CHAROLLAIS, E., 1972, A study of the biological activity and resistance to phosphodiesterase of some derivatives and analogues of cyclic AMP, *Advan. Cyclic Nucleotide Res.* **1:**521–546.

CHADER, G. J., 1971, Hormonal effects on the neural retina: Induction of glutamine synthetase by cyclic-3′,5′-AMP, *Biochem. Biophys. Res. Commun.* **43:**1102–1105.

CHASIN, M., RIVKIN, I., MAMRAK, F., SAMANIEGO, G., and HESS, S. M., 1971, α- and β-Adrenergic receptors as mediators of accumulation of cyclic adenosine 3′,5′-monophosphate in specific areas of guinea pig brain, *J. Biol. Chem.* **246:**3037–3041.

CHASIN, M., HARRIS, D. W., PHILLIPS, M. B., and HESS, S. M., 1972, 1-Ethyl-4(isopropylidenehydrazolo-(3,4*b*)-pyridine-5-carboxylic acid, ethyl ester, hydrochloride (SQ 20009)—A potent new inhibitor of cyclic 3′,5′-nucleotide phosphodiesterases, *Biochem. Pharmacol.* **21:**2443–2450.

CHASIN, M., MAMRAK, F., SAMANIEGO, S. G., and HESS, S. M., 1973, Characteristics of the catecholamine and histamine receptor sites mediating accumulation of cyclic adenosine 3′,5′-monophosphate in guinea pig brain, *J. Neurochem.* **21:**1415–1427.

CHASIN, M., MAMRAK, F., and SAMANIEGO, S. G., 1974, Preparation and properties of a cell-free, hormonally responsive adenylate cyclase from guinea pig brain, *J. Neurochem.* **22:**1031–1038.

CHEUNG, W. Y., 1966, Inhibition of cyclic nucleotide phosphodiesterase by adenosine 5′-triphosphate and inorganic pyrophosphate, *Biochem. Biophys. Res. Commun.* **23:**214–219.

CHEUNG, W. Y., 1967*a*, Properties of cyclic 3′,5′-nucleotide phosphodiesterase from rat brain, *Biochemistry* **5:**1079–1087.

CHEUNG, W. Y., 1967*b*, Cyclic 3′,5′-nucleotide phosphodiesterase: Pronounced stimulation by snake venom, *Biochem. Biophys. Res. Commun.* **29:**478–482.

CHEUNG, W. Y., 1969, Cyclic 3′,5′-nucleotide phosphodiesterase preparation of a partially inactive enzyme and its subsequent stimulation by snake venom, *Biochim. Biophys. Acta* **191:**303–315.

CHEUNG, W. Y., 1970, Cyclic nucleotide phosphodiesterase, *Advan. Biochem. Psychopharmacol.* **3:**51–65.

CHEUNG, W. Y., 1971*a*, Cyclic 3′,5′-nucleotide phosphodiesterase effect of divalent cations, *Biochim. Biophys. Acta* **242:**395–409.

CHEUNG, W. Y., 1971*b*, Cyclic 3′,5′-nucleotide phosphodiesterase: Evidence for and properties of a protein activator, *J. Biol. Chem.* **246:**2859–2869.

CHEUNG, W. Y., and SALGANICOFF, L., 1967, Cyclic 3′,5′-nucleotide phosphodiesterase: Localization and latent activity in rat brain, *Nature* **214:**90–91.

CHOU, W. S., HO, A. K. S., and LOH, H. H., 1971*a*, Effect of acute and chronic morphine and norepinephrine on brain adenyl cyclase activity, *Proc. West. Pharmacol. Soc.* **14:**42–46.

CHOU, W. S., HO, A. K. S., and LOH, H. H., 1971*b*, Neurohormones on brain adenyl cyclase activity *in vivo, Nature New Biol.* **233:**280–281.

CLARK, A. G., JOVIC, R., ORNELLAS, M. R., and WELLER, M., 1972, Brain microsomal protein kinase in the chronically morphinized rat, *Biochem. Pharmacol.* **21:**1989–1990.

CLARK, R. B., and PERKINS, J. P., 1971, Regulation of adenosine 3′:5′-cyclic monophosphate concentration in cultured human astrocytoma cells by catecholamines and histamine, *Proc. Natl. Acad. Sci.* **68:**2757–2760.

CLARK, R. B., SU, Y.-F., GROSS, R., and PERKINS, J. P., 1974, Regulation of adenosine 3′,5′-monophosphate content in human astrocytoma cells by adenosine and the adenine nucleotides, *J. Biol. Chem.* **249:**5296–5303.

COHEN, K. L., and BITENSKY, M. W., 1969, Inhibitory effects of alloxan on mammalian adenyl cyclase, *J. Pharmacol. Exp. Ther.* **169:**80–86.

COHN, M. L., YAMAOKA, H., TAYLOR, F. H., and KRAYNACK, B., 1973, Action of intracerebroventricular dibutyryl cyclic AMP on amobarbital anaesthesia in rats, *Neuropharmacology* **12:**401–405.

Collier, H. O. J., and Roy, A. C., 1974, Morphine-like drugs inhibit the stimulation by E prostaglandins of cyclic AMP formation by rat brain homogenates, *Nature* **248:**24–27.

Connor, J. D., 1970, Caudate nucleus neurones; correlation of the effects of substantia nigra stimulation with iontophoretic dopamine, *J. Physiol.* **208:**691–703.

Contreras, E., Castillo, S., and Quijada, L., 1972, Effect of drugs that modify 3′,5′-AMP concentrations on morphine analgesia, *J. Pharm. Pharmacol.* **24:**65–66.

Corrodi, H., Fuxé, K., and Jonsson, G., 1972, Effects of caffeine on central monoamine neurons, *J. Pharm. Pharmacol.* **24:**155–158.

Crain, S. M., and Pollock, E. D., 1973, Restorative effects of cyclic AMP on complex bioelectric activities of cultured fetal rodent CNS tissues after acute Ca^{++} deprivation, *J. Neurobiol.* **4:**321–342.

Cramer, H., and Lindl, T., 1972, Probenecid inhibits efflux of adenosine 3′,5′-monophosphate (cAMP) from cerebrospinal fluid (CSF) in the rat, *Psychopharmacologia* **26:**49Abs.

Cramer, H., Paul, M. I., Silbergeld, S., and Forn, J., 1971, Determination of regional distribution of adenosine 3′,5′-monophosphate in rat brain, *J. Neurochem.* **18:**1605–1608.

Cramer, H., Ng, L. K. Y., and Chase, T. N., 1972*a*, Effect of probenecid on levels of cyclic AMP in human cerebrospinal fluid, *J. Neurochem.* **19:**1601–1602.

Cramer, H., Goodwin, F. K., Post, R. M., and Bunney, W. E., Jr., 1972*b*, Effects of probenecid and exercise on cerebrospinal-fluid cyclic AMP in affective illness, *Lancet* **i:**1346–1347.

Cramer, H., Johnson, D. G., Hanbauer, I., Silberstein, S. D., and Kopin, I. J., 1973*a*, Accumulation of adenosine 3′,5′-monophosphate induced by catecholamines in the rat superior cervical ganglion *in vitro*, *Brain Res.* **53:**97–104.

Cramer, H., Ng, L. K. Y., and Chase, T. N., 1973*b*, Adenosine 3′,5′-monophosphate in cerebrospinal fluid. Effect of drugs and neurologic disease, *Arch. Neurol.* **29:**197–199.

Dalton, C., Crowley, H. J., Sheppard, H., and Schallek, W., 1974, Regional cyclic nucleotide phosphodiesterase activity in cat central nervous system: Effects of benzodiazepines, *Proc. Soc. Exp. Biol. Med.* **145:**407–410.

Deguchi, T., and Axelrod, J., 1973, Superinduction of serotonin *N*-acetyltransferase and supersensitivity of adenyl cyclase to catecholamines in denervated pineal gland, *Mol. Pharmacol.* **9:**612–618.

De Robertis, E., Arnaiz, G. R. D.-L., Butcher, R. W., and Sutherland, E. W., 1967, Subcellular distribution of adenyl cyclase and cyclic phosphodiesterase in rat brain cortex, *J. Biol. Chem.* **242:**3487–3493.

Dittmann, J., and Herrmann, H.-D., 1970, An action of adenosine 3′,5′-monophosphate on glucose metabolism of rabbit brain slices, *Experientia* **26:**133–134.

Ditzion, B. R., Paul, M. I., and Pauk, G. L., 1970, Measurement of adenosine 3′,5′-monophosphate (cyclic AMP) in brain, *Pharmacology* **3:**25–31.

Dousa, T., and Hechter, O., 1970, Lithium and brain adenyl cyclase, *Lancet* **i:**834–835.

Drummond, G. I., and Perrott-Yee, S., 1961, Enzymatic hydrolysis of adenosine 3′,5′-phosphoric acid, *J. Biol. Chem.* **236:**1126–1129.

Drummond, G. I., and Powell, C. A., 1970, Analogues of adenosine 3′,5′-cyclic phosphate as activators of phosphorylase b kinase and as substrates for cyclic 3′,5′-nucleotide phosphodiesterase, *Mol. Pharmacol.* **6:**24–30.

Ebadi, M. S., Weiss, B., and Costa, E., 1971*a*, Microassay of adenosine 3′,5′-monophosphate (cyclic AMP) in brain and other tissues by the luciferin-luciferase system, *J. Neurochem.* **18:**183–192.

Ebadi, M. S., Weiss, B., and Costa, E., 1971*b*, Distribution of cyclic adenosine monophosphate in rat brain, *Arch. Neurol.* **24:**353–357.

Erwin, V. G., 1969, Enhancement of brain glutamate dehydrogenase activity and glutamate oxidation by adenine nucleotides, *Mol. Pharmacol.* **5:**615–621.

FARBER, D. B., and LOLLEY, R. N., 1973, Proteins in the degenerative retina of C3H mice: Deficiency of a cyclic nucleotide phosphodiesterase and opsin, *J. Neurochem.* **21:**817–828.

FERRENDELLI, J. A., STEINER, A. L., MCDOUGAL, D. B., JR., and KIPNIS, D. M., 1970, The effect of oxotremorine and atropine on cGMP and cAMP levels in mouse cerebral cortex and cerebellum, *Biochem. Biophys. Res. Commun.* **41:**1061–1067.

FERRENDELLI, J. A., KINSCHERF, D. A., and KIPNIS, D. M., 1972, Effects of amphetamine, chlorpromazine and reserpine on cyclic GMP and cyclic AMP levels in mouse cerebellum, *Biochem. Biophys. Res. Commun.* **46:**2114–2120.

FERRENDELLI, J. A., KINSCHERF, D. A., and CHANG, M. M., 1973*a*, Regulation of levels of guanosine cyclic 3′,5′-monophosphate in the central nervous system: Effects of depolarizing agents, *Mol. Pharmacol.* **9:**445–454.

FERRENDELLI, J. A., JOHNSON, E. M., JR., CHANG, M.-M., and NEEDLEMAN, P., 1973*b*, Inhibition of brain adenylate cyclase by ethacrynic acid and dithiobisnitrobenzoic acid, *Biochem. Pharmacol.* **22:**3133–3136.

FERRENDELLI, J. A., CHANG, M. M., and KINSCHERF, D. A., 1974, Elevation of cyclic GMP levels in central nervous system by excitatory and inhibitory amino acids, *J. Neurochem.* **22:**535–540.

FERTEL, R., UZUNOV, P., and WEISS, B., 1973, Selective activation and inhibition of the multiple forms of cyclic 3′,5′-AMP phosphodiesterase of rat brain, *Fed. Proc.* **32:**679Abs.

FLORENDO, N. T., BARRNETT, R. J., and GREENGARD, P., 1971, Cyclic 3′,5′-nucleotide phosphodiesterase: Cytochemical localization in cerebral cortex, *Science* **173:**745–747.

FORN, J., and KRISHNA, G., 1971, Effect of norepinephrine, histamine and other drugs on cyclic 3′,5′-AMP formation in brain slices of various animal species, *Pharmacology* **5:**193–204.

FORN, J., and VALDECASAS, F. G., 1971, Effects of lithium on brain adenyl cyclase activity, *Biochem. Pharmacol.* **20:**2773–2779.

FORN, J., TAGLIAMONTE, A., TAGLIAMONTE, P., and GESSA, G. L., 1972, Stimulation by dibutyryl cyclic AMP of serotonin synthesis and tryptophan transport in brain slices, *Nature New Biol.* **237:**245–247.

FRAZIER, W. A., OHLENDORF, C., FORREST, B., ALOE, L., JOHNSON, E. M., FERRENDELLI, J. A., and BRADSHAW, R. A., 1973, Mechanism of action of nerve growth factor and cyclic AMP on neurite outgrowth in embryonic chick sensory ganglia: Demonstration of independent pathways of stimulation, *Proc. Natl. Acad. Sci.* **70:**2448–2452.

FRENCH, S. W., and PALMER, D. S., 1973, Adrenergic supersensitivity during ethanol withdrawal in the rat, *Res. Commun. Chem. Pathol. Pharmacol.* **6:**651–662.

FUMAGALLI, R., BERNAREGGI, V., BERTI, F., and TRABUCCHI, M., 1971, Cyclic AMP formation in human brain: An *in vitro* stimulation by neurotransmitters, *Life Sci.* **10(I):**1111–1115.

FURLANUT, M., CARPENEDO, F., and FERRARI, M., 1973, Effects of some isoquinoline compounds and certain derivatives on brain phosphodiesterase activity, *Biochem. Pharmacol.* **22:**2642–2644.

FURMANSKI, P., SILVERMAN, D. J., and LUBIN, M., 1971, Expression of differentiated functions in mouse neuroblastoma mediated by dibutyryl-cyclic adenosine monophosphate, *Nature* **233:**413–415.

GABALLAH, S., and POPOFF, C., 1971*a*, Cyclic 3′,5′-nucleotide phosphodiesterase in nerve endings of developing rat brain, *Brain Res.* **25:**220–222.

GABALLAH, S., and POPOFF, C., 1971*b*, Localization of adenosine 3′,5′-monophosphate-dependent protein kinase in brain, *J. Neurochem.* **18:**1795–1797.

GABALLAH, S., POPOFF, C., and SOOKNANDAN, G., 1971, Changes in cyclic 3′,5′-adenosine monophosphate–dependent protein kinase levels in brain development, *Brain Res.* **31:**229–232.

GARELIS, E., and NEFF, N. H., 1974, Cyclic adenosine monophosphate: Selective increase in caudate nucleus after administration of L-dopa, *Science* **183:**532–533.

GESSA, G. L., KRISHNA, G., FORN, J., TAGLIAMONTE, A., and BRODIE, B. B., 1970, Behavioral and vegetative effects produced by dibutyryl cyclic AMP injected into different areas of the brain, *Advan. Biochem. Psychopharmacol.* **3:**371–381.

GILLESPIE, E., 1971, Colchicine binding in tissue slices: Decrease by calcium and biphasic effect of adenosine 3′,5′-monophosphate, *J. Cell Biol.* **50:**544–549.

GILMAN, A. G., and MINNA, J. D., 1973, Expression of genes for metabolism of cyclic adenosine 3′:5′-monophosphate in somatic cells. I. Responses to catecholamines in parental and hybrid cells, *J. Biol. Chem.* **248:**6610–6617.

GILMAN, A. G., and NIRENBERG, M., 1971*a*, Effect of catecholamines on the adenosine 3′-5′-cyclic monophosphate concentrations of clonal satellite cells of neurons, *Proc. Natl. Acad. Sci.* **68:**2165–2168.

GILMAN, A. G., and NIRENBERG, M., 1971*b*, Effect of catecholamines on the adenosine monophosphate metabolism in cultured neuroblastoma cells, *Nature* **234:**356–358.

GILMAN, A. G., and SCHRIER, B. K., 1972, Adenosine cyclic 3′,5′-monophosphate in fetal rat brain cell cultures, *Mol. Pharmacol.* **8:**410–416.

GINSBORG, B. L., and HIRST, G. D., 1972, The effect of adenosine on the release of the transmitter from the phrenic nerve of the rat, *J. Physiol.* **224:**629–645.

GLICK, N. B., and QUASTEL, J. H., 1972, Effects of cerebral stimuli on adenine incorporation into nucleotides and RNA in brain slices from the rat, *Canad. J. Biochem.* **50:**672–683.

GODFRAIND, J. M., and PUMAIN, R., 1971, Cyclic adenosine monophosphate and norepinephrine: Effect on Purkinje cells in rat cerebellar cortex, *Science* **174:**1257–1258.

GODFRAIND, J. M., and PUMAIN, R., 1972, Cyclic-AMP and noradrenaline iontophoretic release on rat cerebellar Purkinje neurons, *Arch. Int. Pharmacodyn. Ther. Suppl.* **196:**131–132.

GODFRAIND, J. M., KRNJEVIĆ, K., MARETIC, H., and PUMAIN, R., 1973, Inhibition of cortical neurons by imidazole and some derivatives, *Canad. J. Physiol. Pharmacol.* **51:**790–797.

GOLDBERG, A. L., and SINGER, J. J., 1969, Evidence for a role of cyclic AMP in neuromuscular transmission, *Proc. Natl. Acad. Sci.* **64:**134–141.

GOLDBERG, N. D., and O'TOOLE, A. G., 1969, The properties of glycogen synthetase and regulation of glycogen biosynthesis in rat brain, *J. Biol. Chem.* **244:**3053–3061.

GOLDBERG, N. D., LARNER, J., SASKO, H., and O'TOOLE, A. G., 1967, Enzymatic analysis of cyclic 3′,5′-AMP in mammalian tissues and urine, *Anal. Biochem.* **28:**523–544.

GOLDBERG, N. D., DIETZ, S. B., and O'TOOLE, A., 1969, Cyclic guanosine 3′,5′-monophosphate in mammalian tissue and urine, *J. Biol. Chem.* **244:**4458–4466.

GOLDBERG, N. D., LUST, W. D., O'DEA, R. F., WEI, S., and O'TOOLE, A. G., 1970, A role of cyclic nucleotides in brain metabolism, *Advan. Biochem. Psychopharmacol.* **3:**67–87.

GOLDBERG, N. D., O'DEA, R. F., and HADDOX, M. K., 1973, Cyclic GMP, *Advan. Cyclic Nucleotide Res.* **3:**155–223.

GOLDFINE, I. D., PERLMAN, R., and ROTH, J., 1971, Inhibition of cyclic 3′,5′-AMP phosphodiesterase in islet cells and other tissues by tolbutamide, *Nature* **234:**295–296.

GOLDSTEIN, M., ANAGNOSTE, B., and SHIRRON, C., 1973, The effect of trivastal, haloperidol and dibutyryl cyclic AMP on [^{14}C]dopamine synthesis in rat striatum, *J. Pharm. Pharmacol.* **25:**348–351.

GOODMAN, D. B. P., RASMUSSEN, H., DIBELLA, F., and GUTHROW, C. E., JR., 1970, Cyclic adenosine 3′,5′-monophosphate-stimulated phosphorylation of isolated neurotubule subunits, *Proc. Natl. Acad. Sci.* **67:**652–659.

GOODMAN, R., OESCH, F., and THOENEN, H., 1974, Changes in enzyme patterns produced by high potassium concentrations and dibutyryl cyclic AMP in organ cultures of sympathetic ganglia, *J. Neurochem.* **23:**369–378.

GORODIS, and MORGAN, 1973, Guanyl cyclase in rat brain subcellular fractions, *FEBS Lett.* **34:**71–73.

GREENGARD, P., and KUO, J. F., 1970, On the mechanism of action of cyclic AMP, *Advan. Biochem. Psychopharmacol.* **3:**287–306.

GREENGARD, P., and KEBABIAN, J. W., 1974, Role of cyclic AMP in synaptic transmission in the mammalian peripheral nervous system, *Fed. Proc.* **33:**1059–1067.

GUNAGA, K. P., and MENON, K. M. J., 1973, Effect of catecholamines and ovarian hormones on cyclic AMP accumulation in rat hypothalamus, *Biochem. Biophys. Res. Commun.* **54:**440–448.

HAAS, D. C., HIER, D. B., ARNASON, B. G. W., and YOUNG, M., 1972, On a possible relationship of cyclic AMP to the mechanisms of action of nerve growth factor, *Proc. Soc. Exp. Biol. Med.* **140:**45–47.

HAMADAH, K., HOLMES, H., BARKER, G. B., HARTMAN, G. C., and PARKE, D. V. W., 1972, Effect of electric convulsion therapy on urinary excretion of 3′,5′-cyclic adenosine monophosphate, *Brit. Med. J.* **19:**439–441.

HAMPRECHT, B., and SCHULTZ, J., 1973*a*, Stimulation of prostaglandin E_1 of adenosine 3′,5′-cyclic monophosphate formation in neuroblastoma cells in the presence of phosphodiesterase inhibitors, *FEBS Letters* **34:**85–89.

HAMPRECHT, B., and SCHULTZ, J., 1973*b*, Influence of norepinephrine, prostaglandin E_1 and inhibitors of phosphodiesterase activity on levels of adenosine 3′:5′-cyclic monophosphate in somatic cell hybrids, *Hoppe-Seylers Z. Physiol. Chem.* **354:**1633–1641.

HAMPRECHT, B., JAFFE, B. M., and PHILPOTT, G. W., 1973, Prostaglandin production by neuroblastoma, glioma and fibroblast cell lines, stimulation by N6,O2′-dibutyryl adenosine 3′:5′-cyclic monophosphate, *FEBS Letters* **36:**193–198.

HARDMAN, J. G., and SUTHERLAND, E. W., 1969, Guanyl cyclase, an enzyme catalyzing the formation of guanosine 3′,5′-monophosphate from guanosine triphosphate, *J. Biol. Chem.* **244:**6363–6370.

HARRIS, D. H., CHASIN, M., PHILLIPS, M. B., GOLDENBERG, H., SAMANIEGO, S., and HESS, S. M., 1973, Effect of cyclic nucleotides on activity of cyclic 3′,5′-adenosine monophosphate phosphodiesterase, *Biochem. Pharmacol.* **22:**221–228.

HELLER, I. H., and MCILWAIN, H., 1973, Release of [^{14}C]adenine derivatives from isolated subsystems of the guinea pig brain: Actions of electrical stimulation and of papaverine, *Brain Res.* **53:**105–116.

HENION, W. F., SUTHERLAND, E. W., and POSTERNAK, T., 1967, Effects of derivatives of adenosine 3′,5′-phosphate on liver slices and intact animals, *Biochim. Biophys. Acta* **148:**106–113.

HERMAN, Z. S., 1973, Behavioral effects of dibutyryl cyclic 3′,5′-AMP, noradrenaline and cyclic 3′,5′-AMP in rats, *Neuropharmacology* **12:**705–709.

HERTZ, L., 1966, Neuroglial localization of potassium and sodium effects on respiration in brain, *J. Neurochem.* **13:**1373–1387.

HETENYI, G., JR., and SINGHAL, P. L., 1973, Effect of insulin on cerebral adenyl cyclase and phosphodiesterase, *Hormone Metab. Res.* **5:**139.

HIER, D. B., ARNASON, B. G. W., and YOUNG, M., 1972, Studies on the mechanism of action of nerve growth factor, *Proc. Natl. Acad. Sci.* **69:**2268–2272.

HIER, D. B., ARNASON, B. G. W., and YOUNG, M., 1973, Nerve growth factor: Relationship to the cyclic AMP system of sensory ganglia, *Science* **182:**79–81.

HO, I. K., LOH, H. H., and WAY, E. L., 1972, Effect of cyclic AMP on morphine analgesia tolerance and physical dependence, *Nature* **238:**397–398.

HO, I. K., LOH, H. H., and WAY, E. L., 1973*a*, Effects of cyclic 3′,5′-adenosine monophosphate on morphine tolerance and physical dependence, *J. Pharmacol. Exp. Ther.* **185:**347–357.

HO, I. K., LOH, H. H., and WAY, E. L., 1973*b*, Cyclic adenosine monophosphate antagonism of morphine analgesia, *J. Pharmacol. Exp. Ther.* **185:**336–346.

HOFFER, B. J., SIGGINS, G. R., and BLOOM, F. E., 1969, Prostaglandins E_1 and E_2 antagonize norepinephrine effects on cerebellar Purkinje cells: Microelectrophoretic study, *Science* **166:**1418–1420.

HOFFER, B. J., SIGGINS, G. R., and BLOOM, F. E., 1970, Possible cyclic AMP–mediated adrenergic synapses to rat cerebellar Purkinje cells: Combined structural, physiological, and pharmacological analyses, *Advan. Biochem. Psychopharmacol.* **3:**349–370.

HOFFER, B. J., SIGGINS, G. R., WOODWARD, D. J., and BLOOM, F. E., 1971*a*, Spontaneous discharge of Purkinje neurons after destruction of catecholamine-containing afferents by 6-hydroxydopamine, *Brain Res.* **30:**425–430.

HOFFER, B. J., SIGGINS, G. R., OLIVER, A. P., and BLOOM, F. E., 1971*b*, Cyclic AMP mediation of norepinephrine inhibition in rat cerebellar cortex: A unique class of synaptic responses, *Ann. N.Y. Acad. Sci.* **185:**531–549.

HOFFER, B. J., SIGGINS, G. R., and BLOOM, F. E., 1971*c*, Studies on norepinephrine-containing afferents of Purkinje cells of rat cerebellum. II. Sensitivity of Purkinje cells to norepinephrine and related substances administered by microiontophoresis, *Brain Res.* **25:**523–534.

HOFFER, B. J., SIGGINS, G. R., OLIVER, A. P., and BLOOM, F. E., 1972, Cyclic AMP–mediated adrenergic synapses to cerebellar Purkinje cells, *Advan. Cyclic Nucleotide Res.* **1:**411–423.

HOFMANN, F., and SOLD, G., 1972, A protein kinase activity from rat cerebellum stimulated by guanosine-3′:5′-monophosphate, *Biochem. Biophys. Res. Commun.* **49:**1100–1107.

HOMMES, F. A., and BEERE, A., 1971, The development of adenyl cyclase in rat liver, kidney, brain and skeletal muscle, *Biochim. Biophys. Acta* **237:**296–300.

HONDA, F., and IMAMURA, H., 1968, Inhibition of cyclic 3′,5′-nucleotide phosphodiesterase by phenothiazine and reserpine derivatives, *Biochim. Biophys. Acta* **161:**267–269.

HOROVITZ, Z. P., BEER,B., CLODY, D. E., VOGEL, J. R., and CHASIN, M., 1972, Cyclic AMP and anxiety, *Psychosomatics* **13:**85–92.

HUANG, M., and DALY, J. W., 1972, Accumulation of cyclic adenosine monophosphate in incubated slices of brain tissue. 1. Structure–activity relationships of agonists and antagonists of biogenic amines and of tricyclic tranquilizers and antidepressants, *J. Med. Chem.* **15:**458–462.

HUANG, M., and DALY, J. W., 1974*a*, Adenosine-elicited accumulation of cyclic AMP in brain slices: Potentiation by agents which inhibit uptake of adenosine, *Life Sci.* **14:**489–503.

HUANG, M., and DALY, J. W., 1974*b*, Interrelationships among levels of ATP, adenosine and cyclic AMP in incubated slices of guinea pig cerebral cortex: Effect of depolarizing agents, psychotropic drugs and metabolic inhibitors, *J. Neurochem.*, **23:**393–404.

HUANG, M., SHIMIZU, H., and DALY, J., 1971, Regulation of adenosine cyclic 3′,5′-phosphate formation in cerebral cortical slices: Interaction among norepinephrine, histamine, serotonin, *Mol. Pharmacol.* **7:**155–162.

HUANG, M., SHIMIZU, H., and DALY, J. W., 1972, Accumulation of cyclic adenosine monophosphate in incubated slices of brain tissue. 2. Effects of depolarizing agents, membrane stabilizers, phosphodiesterase inhibitors, and adenosine analogs, *J. Med. Chem.* **15:**462–466.

HUANG, M., GRUENSTEIN, E., and DALY, J. W., 1973*a*, Depolarization-evoked accumulation of cyclic AMP in brain slices: Inhibition by exogenous adenosine deaminase, *Biochim. Biophys. Acta* **329:**147–151.

HUANG, M., HO, A. K. S., and DALY, J. W., 1973*b*, Accumulation of adenosine cyclic 3′,5′-monophosphate in rat cerebral cortical slices: Stimulatory effect of alpha and beta adrenergic agents after treatment with 6-hydroxydopamine, 2,3,5-trihydroxyphenethylamine and dihydroxytryptamines, *Mol. Pharmacol.* **9:**711–717.

INOUE, Y., YAMAMURA, H., and NISHIZUKA, Y., 1973, Protamine kinase independent of adenosine 3′,5′-monophosphate from rat brain cytosol, *Biochem. Biophys. Res. Commun.* **50:**228–236.

ISHIKAWA, E., ISHIKAWA, S., DAVIS, J. W., and SUTHERLAND, E. W., 1969, Determination of guanosine 3′,5′-monophosphate in tissues and of guanyl cyclase in rat intestine, *J. Biol. Chem.* **244:**6371–6376.

ISRÄEL, M. A., KIMURA, H., and KURIYAMA, K., 1972, Changes in activity and hormonal sensitivity of brain adenyl cyclase following chronic ethanol administration, *Experientia* **28:**1322–1323.

IWANGOFF, P., and ENZ, A., 1971, The effect of dihydroergotamine on the phosphodiesterase activity of cat grey matter, *Experientia* **27:**1258–1259.

IWANGOFF, P., and ENZ, A., 1972, The influence of various dihydroergotamine analogues on cyclic adenosine-3′,5′-monophosphate phosphodiesterase in the grey matter of cat brain *in vitro, Agents Actions* **2:**223–230.

JANIEC, W., TRZECIAK, H., and HERMAN, Z., 1970, The influence of adrenaline and optical isomers of INPEA on the adenyl cyclase activity in brain hemispheres of rats *in vitro, Arch. Int. Pharmacodyn.* **185:**254–258.

JARD, S., PREMONT, J., and BENDA, P., 1972, Adenylate cyclase, phosphodiesterases and protein kinase of rat glial cells in culture, *FEBS Letters* **26:**344–348.

JASTORFF, B., and BAR, H.-B., 1973, Effects of 5′amido analogues of adenosine 3′,5′-monophosphate and adenosine 3:5′-monophosphothioate on protein kinase, binding protein and phosphodiesterases, *Eur. J. Biochem.* **37:**497–504.

JENNER, F. A., SAMPSON, G. A., THOMPSON, E. A., SOMERVILLE, A. R., BEARD, N. A., and SMITH, A. A., 1972, Manic-depressive psychosis and urinary excretion of cyclic AMP, *Brit. J. Psychiat.* **121:**236–237.

JOHNSON, E. M., MAENO, H., and GREENGARD, P., 1971, Phosphorylation of endogenous protein of rat brain by a cyclic adenosine 3′,5′-monophosphate–dependent protein kinase, *J. Biol. Chem.* **246:**7731–7739.

JOHNSON, E. M., UEDA, T., MAENO, H., and GREENGARD, P., 1972, Adenosine 3′,5-monophosphate–dependent phosphorylation of a specific protein in synaptic membrane fractions from rat cerebrum, *J. Biol. Chem.* **247:**5650–5652.

JOHNSON, G. A., BOUKMA, S. J., LAHTI, R. A., and MATHEWS, J., 1973, Cyclic AMP and phosphodiesterase in synaptic vesicles from mouse brain, *J. Neurochem.* **20:**1387–1392.

JOHNSON, R. A., and SUTHERLAND, E. W., 1973, Detergent-dispersed adenylate cyclase from rat brain: Effects of fluoride, cations and chelators, *J. Biol. Chem.* **248:**5114–5121.

JOHNSTON, G. A. R., and BALCAR, V. J., 1973, High affinity uptake of cyclic AMP in rat brain slices, *Brain Res.* **59:**451–453.

JONES, G. H., MURTHY, D. V. K., TEGG, D., GOLLING, R., and MOFFATT, J. G., 1973, Analogs of adenosine 3′,5′-cyclic phosphate. II. Synthesis and enzymatic activity of derivatives of 1,N^6-ethanoadenosine 3′,5′-cyclic phosphate, *Biochem. Biophys. Res. Commun.* **53:**1338–1343.

JORDAN, L. M., LAKE, N., and PHILLIS, J. W., 1972*a*, Mechanism of noradrenaline depression of cortical neurones: A species comparison, *Eur. J. Pharmacol.* **20:**381–384.

JORDAN, L. M., LAKE, N., and PHILLIS, J. W., 1972*b*, Noradrenaline excitation of cortical neurones: A reply, *J. Pharm. Pharmacol.* **24:**739–741.

KAKIUCHI, S., and RALL, T. W., 1968*a*, Studies on adenosine 3′,5′-phosphate in rabbit cerebral cortex, *Mol. Pharmacol.* **4:**379–388.

KAKIUCHI, S., and RALL, T. W., 1968*b*, The influence of chemical agents on the accumulation of adenosine 3′,5′-phosphate in slices of rabbit cerebellum, *Mol. Pharmacol.* **4:**367–378.

KAKIUCHI, S., and YAMAZAKI, R., 1970*a*, Calcium dependent phosphodiesterase activity and its activating factor (PAF) from brain: Studies on cyclic 3′,5′-nucleotide phosphodiesterase, *Biochem. Biophys. Res. Commun.* **41:**1104–1110.

KAKUICHI, S., and YAMAZAKI, R., 1970*b*, Properties of a heat-stable phosphodiesterase activating factor isolated from brain extract. II. Studies on cyclic 3′,5′ nucleotide phosphodiesterases, *Proc. Jap. Acad.* **46:**587–592.

KAKIUCHI, S., and YAMAZAKI, R., 1970*c*, Stimulation of the activity of cyclic 3′,5′-nucleotide phosphodiesterase by calcium ion, *Proc. Jap. Acad.* **46:**387–392.

KAKIUCHI, S., RALL, T. W., and MCILWAIN, H., 1969, The effect of electrical stimulation upon the accumulation of adenosine 3′,5′-phosphate in isolated cerebral tissue, *J. Neurochem.* **16:**485–491.

KAKIUCHI, S., YAMAZAKI, R., and TESHIMA, Y., 1971, Cyclic 3′,5′-nucleotide phosphodiesterase. IV. Two enzymes with different properties from brain, *Biochem. Biophys. Res. Commun.* **42:**968–974.

KAKIUCHI, S., YAMAZAKI, R., and TESHIMA, Y., 1972, Regulation of brain phosphodiesterase activity: Ca^{++} plus Mg^{++}-dependent phosphodiesterase and its activating factor from rat brain, *Advan. Cyclic Nucleotide Res.* **1:**455–477.

KAKIUCHI, S., YAMAZAKI, R., TESHIMA, Y., and UENISHI, K., 1973, Regulation of nucleotide cyclic 3′:5′-monophosphate phosphodiesterase activity from rat brain by a modulator and Ca^{2+}, *Proc. Natl. Acad. Sci.* **70:**3526–3535.

KALISKER, A., RUTLEDGE, C. O., and PERKINS, J. P., 1973, Effect of nerve degeneration by 6-hydroxydopamine on catecholamine-stimulated adenosine 3′,5′-monophosphate formation in rat cerebral cortex, *Mol. Pharmacol.* **9:**619–629.

KALIX, P., MCAFEE, D., SCHORDERET, M., and GREENGARD, P., 1974, Pharmacological analysis of synaptically mediated increase in cyclic adenosine monophosphate in rabbit superior cervical ganglion, *J. Pharmacol. Exp. Ther.* **188:**676–687.

KATZ, S., and TENENHOUSE, A., 1973*a*, The relationship of adenyl cyclase to the activity of other ATP utilizing enzymes and phosphodiesterase in preparations of rat brain, mechanism of stimulation of cyclic AMP accumulation by NaF, *Brit. J. Pharmacol.* **48:**505–515.

KATZ, S., and TENENHOUSE, A., 1973*b*, The relationship of adenyl cyclase to the activity of other ATP utilizing enzymes and phosphodiesterase in preparations of rat brain: Mechanism of stimulation of cyclic AMP accumulation by adrenaline, ouabain and Mg^{++}, *Brit. J. Pharmacol.* **48:**516–526.

KAUFFMAN, F. C., HARKONEN, M. H. A., and JOHNSON, E. C., 1972, Adenyl cyclase and phosphodiesterase activity in cerebral cortex of normal and undernourished neonatal rats, *Life Sci.* **11(II):**613–621.

KEBABIAN, J. W., and GREENGARD, P., 1971, Dopamine-sensitive adenyl cyclase: Possible role in synaptic transmission, *Science* **174:**1346–1349.

KEBABIAN, J. W., PETZOLD, G. L., and GREENGARD, P., 1972, Dopamine-sensitive adenylate cyclase in caudate nucleus of rat brain and its similarity to the "dopamine receptor," *Proc. Natl. Acad. Sci.* **69:**2145–2149.

KEEN, P., and MCLEAN, W. G., 1972*a*, Effect of dibutyryl cyclic-AMP on levels of dopamine-β-hydroxylase in isolated superior cervical ganglia, *Naunyn-Schmiedebergs Arch. Pharmacol.* **275:**465–469.

KEEN, P., and MCLEAN, W. G., 1972*b*, The effect of N^6,$O^{2'}$-dibutyryl adenosine 3′:5′-cyclic monophosphate on noradrenaline synthesis in isolated superior cervical ganglia, *Brit. J. Pharmacol.* **46:**529–530.

KIRKLAND, W. L., and BURTON, P. R., 1972, Cyclic adenosine monophosphate–mediated stabilization of mouse neuroblastoma cell neurite microtubules exposed to low temperature, *Nature New Biol.* **240:**205–207.

KLAINER, L. M., CHI, Y.-M., FREIDBERG, S. L., RALL, T. W., and SUTHERLAND, E. W., 1962, IV. The effects of neurohormones on the formation of adenosine 3′,5′-phosphate by preparations from brain and other tissues, *J. Biol. Chem.* **237:**1239–1243.

KLEIN, D. C., YUWILER, A., WELLER, J. L., and PLOTKIN, S., 1973, Postsynaptic adrenergic-cyclic AMP control of the serotonin content of cultured rat pineal glands, *J. Neurochem.* **21:**1261–1271.

KODAMA, T., MATSUKADO, Y., SUZUKI, T., TANAKA, S., and SHIMIZU, H., 1971, Stimulated formation of adenosine 3′,5′-monophosphate by desipramine in brain slices, *Biochim. Biophys. Acta* **252:**165–170.

KODAMA, T., MATSUKADO, Y., and SHIMIZU, H., 1973, The cyclic AMP system of human brain, *Brain Res.* **50:**135–146.

KOHRMAN, A. F., 1973, Patterns of development of adenyl cyclase activity and norepinephrine responsiveness in the rat, *Pediat. Res.* **7:**575–581.

KRAMER, S. G., 1971, Dopamine: A retinal neurotransmitter. I. Retinal uptake, storage and light stimulated release of H3-dopamine *in vivo*, *Invest. Ophthalmol.* **10:**438–452.

KRISHNA, G., FORN, J., VOIGHT, K., PAUL, M., and GESSA, G. L., 1970, Dynamic aspects of neurohormonal control of cyclic 3′,5′-AMP synthesis in brain, *Advan. Biochem. Psychopharmacol.* **3:**155–172.

KUEHL, F. A., JR., HUMES, J. L., CIRILLO, V. J., and HAM, E. A., 1972, Cyclic AMP and prostaglandins in hormone action, *Advan. Cyclic Nucleotide Res.* **1**:493–502.

KUO, J. F., and GREENGARD, P., 1969*a*, Cyclic nucleotide–dependent protein kinases. IV. Widespread occurrence of adenosine 3′,5′-monophosphate dependent protein kinase in various tissues and phyla of the animal kingdom, *Proc. Natl. Acad. Sci.* **64**:1349–1355.

KUO, J. F., and GREENGARD, P., 1969*b*, Adenosine 3′,5-monophosphate–dependent protein kinase from brain, *Science* **165**:63–65.

KUO, J. F., and GREENGARD, P., 1970*a*, Stimulation of adenosine 3′,5′-monophosphate–dependent and guanosine 3′,5′-monophosphate–dependent protein kinases by some analogs of adenosine 3′,5′-monophosphate, *Biochem. Biophys. Res. Commun.* **40**:1032–1038.

KUO, J. F., and GREENGARD, P., 1970*b*, Cyclic nucleotide–dependent protein kinases. VII. Comparison of various histones as substrates for adenosine 3′,5′-monophosphate–dependent and guanosine 3′,5′-monophosphate–dependent protein kinases, *Biochim. Biophys. Acta* **212**:434–440.

KUO, J. F., and GREENGARD, P., 1973, Stimulation of cyclic GMP dependent protein kinase by a protein fraction which inhibits cyclic AMP–dependent protein kinases, *Fed. Proc.* **30**:1089Abs.

KUO, J. F., KRUEGER, B. K., SANES, J. R., and GREENGARD, P., 1970, Cyclic nucleotide–dependent protein kinases. V. Preparation and properties of adenosine 3′,5′-monophosphate–dependent protein kinase from various bovine tissues, *Biochim. Biophys. Acta* **212**:79–91.

KUO, J.-F., LEE, T.-P., REYES, P. L., WALTON, K. G., DONNELLY, T. E., JR., and GREENGARD, P., 1972, Cyclic nucleotide–dependent protein kinases. X. An assay method for the measurement of guanosine 3′,5′-monophosphate in various biological materials and a study of agents regulating its levels in heart and brain, *J. Biol. Chem.* **247**:16–22.

KUO, W.-N., and KUO, J. F., 1973, Accumulation of cyclic GMP and cyclic AMP levels in rat lung and other tissues by various agents as determined by double-prelabeling with radioactive guanine and adenine, *Fed. Proc.* **32**:773Abs.

KURIHARA, K., 1972, Inhibition of cyclic 3′,5′-nucleotide phosphodiesterase in bovine taste papillae by bitter taste stimuli, *FEBS Letters* **27**:279–281.

KURIHARA, K., and KOYAMA, N., 1972, High activity of adenyl cyclase in olfactory and gustatory organs, *Biochem. Biophys. Res. Commun.* **48**:30–34.

KURIYAMA, K., and ISRÄEL, M. A., 1973, Effect of ethanol administration on cyclic 3′,5′-adenosine monophosphate metabolism in brain, *Biochem. Pharmacol.* **22**:2919–2922.

KURODA, Y., and MCILWAIN, H., 1973, Subcellular localization of [^{14}C]adenine derivatives newly-formed in cerebral tissues and the effects of electrical excitation, *J. Neurochem.* **21**:889–900.

LAKE, N., and JORDAN, L. M., 1974, Failure to confirm cyclic-AMP as second messenger for norepinephrine in rat cerebellum, *Science* **183**:663–664.

LAKE, N., JORDAN, L. M., and PHILLIS, J. W., 1972, Mechanism of noradrenaline action in cat cerebral cortex, *Nature New Biol.* **240**:249–250.

LAKE, N., JORDAN, L. M., and PHILLIS, J. W., 1973, Evidence against cyclic adenosine 3′,5′-monophosphate (AMP) mediation of noradrenaline depression of cerebral cortical neurons, *Brain Res.* **60**:411–421.

LEE, C.-J., and DUBOS, R., 1972, Lasting biological effects of early environmental influences. VII. Metabolism of adenosine 3′,5′-monophosphate in mice exposed to early environmental stress, *J. Exp. Med.* **135**:220–234.

LEE, T.-P., KUO, J. F., and GREENGARD, P., 1972, Role of muscarinic cholinergic receptors in regulation of guanosine 3′,5′-cyclic monophosphate content in mammalian brain, heart muscle, and intestinal smooth muscle, *Proc. Natl. Acad. Sci.* **69**:3287–3291.

LEONARD, B. E., 1972, Effect of phentolamine on the increase in brain glycolysis following the intraventricular administration of dibutyryl-3/,5′-cyclic adenosine monophosphate and sodium fluoride to mice, *Biochem. Pharmacol.* **21:**115–117.

LIBET, B., and KOBAYASHI, H., 1969, Generation of adrenergic and cholinergic potentials in sympathetic ganglion cells, *Science* **164:**1530–1532.

LIM, R., and MITSUNOBU, K., 1972, Effect of dibutyryl cyclic AMP on nucleic acid and protein synthesis in neuronal and glial tumor cells, *Life Sci.* **11(II):**1063–1070.

LIM, R., MITSUNOBU, K., and LI, W. K. P., 1973, Maturation-stimulation effect of brain extract and dibutyryl cyclic AMP on dissociated embryonic brain cells in culture, *Exp. Cell. Res.* **79:**243–246.

LINDL, T., and CRAMER, H., 1974, Formation, accumulation and release of adenosine 3′,5′-monophosphate induced by histamine in the superior cervical ganglion of the rat *in vitro, Biochim. Biophys. Acta,* **343:**182–191.

LUST, W. D., and PASSONNEAU, J. V., 1973, Cyclic adenosine monophosphate, metabolites, and phosphorylase in neural tissue: A comparison of methods of fixation, *Science* **181:**280–282.

LUST, W. D., PASSONNEAU, J. V., and GOLDBERG, N. D., 1972, Reciprocal changes in 3′,5′-cAMP (cAMP) and 3′,5′-cGMP (cGMP) following electroconvulsive shock, *Fed. Proc.* **31:**555Abs.

MACHOVA, J., and KRISTOFOVA, A., 1973, The effect of dibutyryl cyclic AMP, dopamine and aminophylline on ganglionic surface potential and transmission, *Life Sci.* **13:**525–535.

MACINTYRE, E. H., WINTERSGILL, C. J., PERKINS, J. P., and VATTER, A. E., 1972, The responses in culture of human tumour astrocytes and neuroblasts to $N^6,O^{2'}$-dibutyryl adenosine 3′,5′-monophosphoric acid, *J. Cell Sci.* **11:**639–667.

MACKAY, A. V. P., and IVERSEN, L. L., 1972, Increased tyrosine hydroxylase activity of sympathetic ganglia cultured in the presence of dibutyryl cyclic AMP, *Brain Res.* **48:**424–426.

MAENO, H., and GREENGARD, P., 1972, Phosphoprotein phosphates from rat cerebral cortex, *J. Biol. Chem.* **247:**3269–3277.

MAENO, H., JOHNSON, E. M., and GREENGARD, P., 1971, Subcellular distribution of adenosine 3′,5′-monophosphate–dependent protein kinase in rat brain, *J. Biol. Chem.* **246:**134–142.

MANDEL, L. R., 1971, Inhibition of cyclic 3′,5′-adenosine monophosphate phosphodiesterase by substituted imidazopyrazines, *Biochem. Pharmacol.* **20:**3413–3421.

MARLEY, E., and NISTICO, G., 1972, Effects of catecholamines and adenosine derivatives given into the brain of fowls, *Brit. J. Pharmacol.* **46:**619–636.

MCAFEE, D. A., and GREENGARD, P., 1972, Adenosine 3′,5′-monophosphate: Electrophysiological evidence for a role in synaptic transmission, *Science* **178:**310–312.

MCAFEE, D. A., SCHORDERET, M., and GREENGARD, P., 1971, Adenosine 3′,5′-monophosphate in nervous tissue: Increase associated with synaptic transmission, *Science* **171:**1156–1158.

MCCUNE, R. W., GILL, T. H., VON HUNGEN, K., and ROBERTS, S., 1971, Catecholamine-sensitive adenyl cyclase in cell-free preparations from rat cerebral cortex, *Life Sci.* **10(II):**443–450.

MCILWAIN, H., 1972, Regulatory significance of the release and action of adenine derivatives in cerebral systems, *Biochem. Soc. Symp.* **36:**69–85.

MCKENZIE, S. G., and BAR, H. P., 1973, On the mechanism of adenyl cyclase inhibition by adenosine, *Canad. J. Physiol. Pharmacol.* **51:**190–196.

MCNEILL, J. H., LEE, C.-Y., and MUSCHEK, L. D., 1972, The effect of phentolamine and other drugs on rat brain phosphodiesterase, *Canad. J. Physiol. Pharmacol.* **50:**840–849.

MEYER, R. B., SHUMAN, D. A., ROBINS, R. K., BAUER, R. J., DIMMITT, M. K., and SIMON, L. N., 1972, Synthesis and biological activity of several 6-substituted 9-β-D-ribofuranosyl purine 3′,5′-cyclic phosphates, *Biochemistry* **11:**2704–2709.

MEYER, R. B., SHUMAN, D. A., ROBINS, R. K., MILLER, J. P., and SIMON, L. N., 1973, Synthesis and enzymic studies of 5′-aminoimidazole and *N*-1 and N^6-substituted adenine ribonucleotide cyclic 3′,5′-phosphates prepared from adenosine cyclic 3′,5′-phosphate, *J. Med. Chem.* **16:**1319–1323.

MIKI, N., and YOSHIDA, H., 1972, Purification and properties of cyclic AMP phosphodiesterase from rat brain, *Biochim. Biophys. Acta* **268:**166–174.

MILLER, J. P., SHUMAN, D. A., SCHOLTEN, M. B., DIMMITT, M. K., STEWART, C. M., KHWAJA, T. A., ROBINS, R. K., and SIMON, L. N., 1973*a*, Synthesis and biological activity of some 2′ derivatives of adenosine 3′,5′-cyclic phosphate, *Biochemistry* **12:**1010–1015.

MILLER, J. P., BOSWELL, K. H., MUNEYAMA, K., SIMON, L. N., ROBINS, R. K., and SHUMAN, D. A., 1973*b*, Synthesis and biochemical studies of various 8-substituted derivatives of guanosine 3′,5′-cyclic phosphate, inosine 3′,5′-cyclic phosphate, and xanthosine 3′,5′-cyclic phosphate, *Biochemistry* **12:**5310–5319.

MILLER, H., 1973, Cyclic nucleotides and photoreception, *Exp. Eye Res.* **16:**357–363.

MILLER, W. H., GORMAN, R. E., and BITENSKY, M. W., 1971, Cyclic adenosine monophosphate: Function in photoreceptors, *Science* **174:**295–297.

MINNA, J. D., and GILMAN, A. G., 1973, Expression of genes for metabolism of cyclic adenosine 3′:5′-monophosphate in somatic cells. II. Effects of prostaglandin E_1 and theophylline on parental and hybrid cells, *J. Biol. Chem.* **248:**6618–6625.

MIYAMOTO, E., KUO, J. F., and GREENGARD, P., 1969*a*, Adenosine 3′,5′-monophosphate–dependent protein kinase from brain, *Science* **165:**63–65.

MIYAMOTO, E., KUO, J. F., and GREENGARD, P., 1969*b*, Cyclic nucleotide–dependent protein kinases: I. Purification and properties of adenosine 3′,5′-monophosphate–dependent protein kinase from bovine brain, *J. Biol. Chem.* **244:**6395–6402.

MIYAMOTO, E., PETZOLD, G. L., HARRIS, J. S., and GREENGARD, P., 1971, Dissociation and concomitant activation of adenosine 3′,5′-monophosphate–dependent protein kinase by histone, *Biochem. Biophys. Res. Commun.* **44:**305–312.

MIZON, J., SHANDRANI, E., and MIZON, C., 1971, Détermination de l'activite inhibitrice de quelques nouvelles théophyllines substituées sur la phosphodiestérase spécifique des nucléotides cycliques, *Thérapie* **26:**911–917.

MONARD, D., SOLOMON, F., RENTSCH, M., and GYSIN, R., 1973, Glia-induced morphological differentiation in neuroblastoma cells, *Proc. Natl. Acad. Sci.* **70:**1894–1897.

MONN, E., and CHRISTIANSEN, R. O., 1971, Adenosine 3′,5′-monophosphate phosphate phosphodiesterases: Multiple molecular forms, *Science* **173:**540–541.

MRSULJA, B. B., 1972*a*, The influence of some biogenic amines and cyclic *N*-2-*O*-dibutyryl-adenosine-3′-5′-monophosphate on glycogen content in rat brain slices, *Experientia* **28:**1067.

MRSULJA, B. R., 1972*b*, The influence of propranolol and dibenzyline on glycogenolytic effects of some biogenic amines in rat brain slices, *Experientia* **28:**1072–1073.

MUNEYAMA, K., BAUER, R. J., SHUMAN, D. A., ROBINS, R. K., and SIMON, L. N., 1971, Chemical synthesis and biological activity of 8-substituted adenosine 3′,5′-cyclic monophosphate derivatives, *Biochemistry* **10:**2390–2395.

MURAD, F., 1973, Clinical studies and applications of cyclic nucleotides, *Advan. Cyclic Nucleotide Res.* **3:**355–383.

MURRAY, A. W., and FROSCIO, M., 1971, Cyclic adenosine 3′,5′-monophosphate and microtubule function: Specific interaction of the phosphorylated protein subunits with a soluble brain component, *Biochem. Biophys. Res. Commun.* **44:**1089–1095.

NAHORSKI, S. R., and ROGERS, K. J., 1973, The adenosine 3′,5′-monophosphate content of brain tissue obtained by an ultra-rapid freezing technique, *Brain Res.* **51:**332–336.

NAHORSKI, S. R., ROGERS, K. J., and PINNS, J., 1973, Cerebral phosphodiesterase and dopamine receptor, *J. Pharm. Pharmacol.* **25:**912–913.

NAITO, K., and KURIYAMA, K., 1973, Effect of morphine administration on adenyl cyclase and 3′,5′-cyclic nucleotide phosphodiesterase activities in the brain, *Jap. J. Pharmacol.* **23:**274–276.

NATHANSON, J. A., and GREENGARD, P., 1973, Octopamine-sensitive adenylate cyclase: Evidence for a biological role of octopamine in nervous tissue, *Science* **180:**308–310.

NEWBURGH, R. W., and ROSENBERG, R. N., 1972, Effect of norepinephrine on glucose metabolism in glioblastoma and neuroblastoma cells in cell culture, *Proc. Natl. Acad. Sci.* **69:**1677–1680.

OPLER, L. A., and MAKMAN, M. H., 1972, Mediation by cyclic AMP of hormone-stimulated glycogenolysis in cultured rat astrocytoma cells, *Biochem. Biophys. Res. Commun.* **46:**1140–1145.

OTTEN, U., OESCH, F., and THOENEN, H., 1973, Dissociation between changes in cyclic AMP and subsequent induction of tyrosine hydroxylase in rat superior cervical ganglion and adrenal medulla, *Naunyn-Schmiedebergs Arch. Pharmacol.* **280:**129–140.

OTTEN, U., MUELLER, R. A., OESCH, F., and THOENEN, H., 1974, Location of an isoproterenol-responsive cyclic AMP-pool in adrenergic nerve cell bodies and its relationship to tyrosine hydroxylase induction, *Proc. Natl. Acad. Sci.* **71:**2217–2221.

PALMER, G. C., 1972, Increased cyclic AMP response to norepinephrine in the rat brain following 6-hydroxydopamine, *Neuropharmacology* **11:**145–149.

PALMER, G. C., 1973*a*, Adenyl cyclase in neuronal and glial-enriched fractions from rat and rabbit brain, *Res. Commun. Chem. Pathol. Pharmacol.* **5:**603–613.

PALMER, G. C., 1973*b*, Influence of amphetamines, protriptyline and pargyline on the time course of the norepinephrine-induced accumulation of cyclic AMP in rat brain, *Life Sci.* **12(II):**345–355.

PALMER, G. C., and BURKS, T. F., 1971, Central and peripheral adrenergic blocking actions of LSD and BOL, *Eur. J. Pharmacol.* **16:**113–116.

PALMER, G. C., ROBISON, G. A., and SULSER, F., 1971, Modification by psychotropic drugs of the cyclic adenosine monophosphate response to norepinephrine in rat brain, *Biochem. Pharmacol.* **20:**236–239.

PALMER, G. C., SCHMIDT, M. J., and ROBISON, G. A., 1972*a*, Development and characteristics of the histamine-induced accumulation of cyclic AMP in the rabbit cerebral cortex, *J. Neurochem.* **19:**2251–2256.

PALMER, G. C., ROBISON, G. A., MANIAN, A. A., and SULSER, F., 1972*b*, Modification by psychotropic drugs of the cyclic AMP response to norepinephrine in the rat brain *in vitro*, *Psychopharmacologia* **23:**201–211.

PALMER, G. C., SULSER, F., and ROBISON, G. A., 1973, Effects of neurohumoral and adrenergic agents on cyclic AMP levels in various areas of the rat brain *in vitro*, *Neuropharmacology* **12:**327–337.

PANNBACKER, R. G., 1973, Control of guanylate cyclase activity in the rod outer segment, *Science* **182:**1138–1139.

PANNBACKER, R. G., FLEISCHMAN, D. E., and REED, D. W., 1972, Cyclic nucleotide phosphodiesterase: High activity in a mammalian photoreceptor, *Science* **175:**757–758.

PAUL, M. I., PAUK, G. L., and DITZION, B. R., 1970*a*, The effect of centrally acting drugs on the concentration of brain adenosine 3′,5′-monophosphate, *Pharmacology* **3:**148–154.

PAUL, M. I., DITZION, B. R., PAUK, G. L., and JANOWSKY, D. S., 1970*b*, Urinary adenosine 3′,5′-monophosphate excretion in affective disorders, *Am. J. Psychiat.* **126:**1493–1497.

PAUL, M. I., CRAMER, H., and GOODWIN, F. K., 1970*c*, Urinary cyclic AMP in affective illness, *Lancet* **i:**996.

PAUL, M. I., DITZION, B. R., and JANOWSKY, D. S., 1970*d*, Affective illness and cyclic-AMP excretion, *Lancet* **i:**88.

PAUL, M. I., CRAMER, H., and GOODWIN, F. K., 1971*a*, Urinary cyclic AMP excretion in depression and mania, *Arch. Gen. Psychiat.* **24:**327–333.

PAUL, M. I., CRAMER, H., and BUNNEY, W. E., JR., 1971*b*, Urinary adenosine 3′,5′-monophosphate in the switch process from depression to mania, *Science* **171:**300–303.

PEACH, M. J., 1972, Stimulation of release of adrenal catecholamine by adenosine 3′:5′-cyclic monophosphate and theophylline in the absence of extracellular Ca^{2+}, *Proc. Natl. Acad. Sci.* **69:**834–836.

PERKINS, J. P., 1973, Adenyl cyclase, *Advan. Cyclic Nucleotide Res.* **3:**1–64.

PERKINS, J. P., and MOORE, M. M., 1971, Adenyl cyclase of rat cerebral cortex, *J. Biol. Chem.* **246:**62–68.

PERKINS, J. P., and MOORE, M. M., 1973*a*, Characterization of the adrenergic receptors mediating a rise in cyclic 3′,5′-adenosine monophosphate in rat cerebral cortex, *J. Pharmacol. Exp. Ther.* **185:**371–378.

PERKINS, J. P., and MOORE, M., 1973*b*, Regulation of the adenosine cyclic 3′,5′-monophosphate content of rat cerebral cortex: Ontogenetic development of the responsiveness to catecholamines and adenosine, *Mol. Pharmacol.* **9:**774–782.

PERKINS, J. P., MACINTYRE, E. H., RILEY, W. D., and CLARK, R. B., 1971, Adenyl cyclase, phosphodiesterase and cyclic AMP dependent protein kinase of malignant glial cells in culture, *Life Sci.* **10(I):**1069–1080.

PERRY, T. L., HEMMINGS, S., DRUMMOND, G. I., HANSEN, S., and GJESSING, L. R., 1973, Urinary cyclic AMP in periodic catatonia, *Am. J. Psychiat.* **130:**927–929.

PHILLIS, J. W., LAKE, N., and YARBROUGH, G., 1973, Calcium mediation of the inhibitory effects of biogenic amines on cerebral cortical neurones, *Brain Res.* **53:**465–469.

PICHARD, A.-L., HANOUNE, J., and KAPLAN, J.-C., 1972, Human brain and platelet cyclic adenosine 3′,5′-monophosphate phosphodiesterases: Different response to drugs, *Biochim. Biophys. Acta* **279:**217–220.

PICHICHERO, M., BEER, B., and CLODY, D. E., 1973, Effects of dibutyryl cyclic AMP on restoration of function of damaged sciatic nerve in rats, *Science* **182:**724–725.

POECH, G., and KUKOVETZ, W. R., 1971, Papaverine-induced inhibition of phosphodiesterase activity in various mammalian tissues, *Life Sci.* **10(I):**133–144.

PRASAD, K. N., 1972*a*, Neuroblastoma clone: Prostaglandin versus dibutyryl cyclic AMP, 8-benzylthio-cyclic AMP, phosphodiesterase inhibitors and x-rays, *Proc. Soc. Exp. Biol. Med.* **140:**126–129.

PRASAD, K. N., 1972*b*, Morphological differentiation induced by prostaglandin in mouse neuroblastoma cells in culture, *Nature New Biol.* **236:**49–52.

PRASAD, K. N., 1972*c*, Cyclic AMP–induced differentiated mouse neuroblastoma cells lose tumourgenic characteristics, *Cytobios* **6:**163–166.

PRASAD, K. N., and HSIE, A. W., 1971, Morphologic differentiation of urine neuroblastoma cells induced *in vitro* by dibutyryl adenosine 3′:5′-cyclic monophosphate, *Nature New Biol.* **233:**141–142.

PRASAD, K. N., and KUMAR, S., 1973, Cyclic 3′,5′-phosphodiesterase activity during cyclic AMP–induced differentiation of neuroblastoma cells in culture, *Proc. Soc. Exp. Biol. Med.* **142:**406–409.

PRASAD, K. N., and MANDAL, B., 1972, Catechol-*O*-methyl-transferase activity in dibutyryl cyclic AMP, prostaglandin and x-ray-induced differentiated neuroblastoma cell culture, *Exp. Cell Res.* **74:**532–534.

PRASAD, K. N., and MANDAL, B., 1973, Choline acetyltransferase level in cyclic AMP and X-ray induced morphologically differentiated neuroblastoma cells in culture, *Cytobios* **8:**75–80.

PRASAD, K. N., and SHEPPARD, J. R., 1972*a*, Neuroblastoma cell culture: Membrane changes during cyclic AMP–induced morphological differentiation, *Proc. Soc. Exp. Biol. Med.* **141:**240–243.

PRASAD, K. N., and SHEPPARD, J. R., 1972*b*, Inhibitors of cyclic-nucleotide phosphodiesterase induce morphological differentiation of mouse neuroblastoma cell culture, *Exp. Cell. Res.* **73:**436–440.

PRASAD, K. N., and VERNADAKIS, A., 1972, Morphological and biochemical study in x-ray and dibutyryl cyclic AMP–induced differentiated neuroblastoma cells, *Exp. Cell Res.* **70:**27–32.

PRASAD, K. N., WAYMIRE, J. C., and WEINER, N., 1972, A further study on the morphology and biochemistry of X-ray and dibutyryl cyclic AMP–induced differentiated neuroblastoma cells in culture, *Exp. Cell Res.* **74:**110–114.

PRASAD, K. N., MANDAL, B., WAYMIRE, J. C., LEES, G. J., VERNADAKIS, A., and WEINER, N., 1973*a*, Basal level of neurotransmitter synthesizing enzymes and effect of cyclic AMP agents on the morphological differentiation of isolated neuroblastoma clones, *Nature New Biol.* **241:**117–119.

PRASAD, K. N., GILMER, K., and KUMAR, S., 1973*b*, Morphologically "differentiated" mouse neuroblastoma cells induced by noncyclic AMP agents: Levels of cyclic AMP, nucleic acid and protein, *Proc. Soc. Exp. Biol. Med.* **143:**1168–1171.

PULL, I., and MCILWAIN, H., 1972*a*, Adenine derivatives as neurohumoral agents in the brain: The quantities liberated on excitation of superfused cerebral tissues, *Biochem. J.* **130:**975–981.

PULL, I., and MCILWAIN, H., 1972*b*, Metabolism of [^{14}C]adenine and derivatives by cerebral tissues, superfused and electrically stimulated, *Biochem. J.* **126:**965–973.

PULL, I., and MCILWAIN, H., 1973, Output of [^{14}C]adenine nucleotides and their derivatives from cerebral tissues: Tetrodotoxin-resistant and calcium ion–requiring components, *Biochem. J.* **136:**893–901.

PURPURA, D. P., and SHOFER, R. J., 1972, Excitatory action of dibutyryl cyclic adenosine monophosphate on immature cerebral cortex, *Brain Res.* **38:**179–181.

QUASTEL, D. M. J., and HACKETT, J. T., 1971, Quantal release of acetylcholine at the neuromuscular junction is not mediated by cyclic 3′,5′adenosine monophosphate, *Fed. Proc.* **30:**557Abs.

RALL, T. W., and SATTIN, A., 1970, Factors influencing the accumulation of cyclic AMP in brain *Res. Prog. Bull.* **8(3):**221–317.

RALL, T. W., and SATTIN, A., 1970, Factors influencing the accumulation of cyclic AMP in brain tissue, *Advan. Biochem. Psychopharmacol.* **3:**113–133.

RAMSDEN, E. N., 1970, Cyclic AMP in depression and mania, *Lancet* **ii:**108.

RAPPAPORT, L., LETERRIER, J. F., and NUNEZ, J., 1972, Non phosphorylation *in vitro* of the 6S tubulin from brain and thyroid tissue, *FEBS Letters* **26:**349–352.

RASMUSSEN, H., 1970, Cell communication, calcium ion, and cyclic adenosine monophosphate, *Science* **170:**404–412.

RASMUSSEN, H., and TENENHOUSE, A., 1968, Cyclic adenosine monophosphate, Ca^{++} and membranes, *Proc. Natl. Acad. Sci.* **59:**1364–1370.

REDDINGTON, M., RODNIGHT, R., and WILLIAMS, M., 1973, Turnover of protein-bound serine phosphate in respiring slices of guinea-pig cerebral cortex, *Biochem. J.* **132:**475–482.

RICHELSON, E., 1973, Stimulation of tyrosine hydroxylase activity in an adrenergic clone of mouse neuroblastoma by dibutyryl cyclic AMP, *Nature New Biol.* **242:**175–176.

RIGBERG, M., VACIK, J. P., and SHELVER, W. H., 1969, Utilization of radiometric analysis for measurement of activation of adenyl cyclase by sympathomimetic amines, *J. Pharmaceut. Sci.* **58:**358–359.

RINDI, G., SCIORELLI, G., POLONI, M., and ACANFORA, F., 1972, Induction of ingestive responses by cAMP applied into the rat hypothalamus, *Experientia* **28:**1047–1049.

ROBERTS, E., and SIMONSEN, D. G., 1970, Some properties of cyclic 3′,5′-nucleotide phosphodiesterase of mouse brain: Effects of imidazole-4-acetic acid, chlorpromazine, cyclic 3′,5′-GMP, and other substances, *Brain Res.* **24:**91–111.

ROBISON, G. A., COPPER, A. J., WHYBROW, P. C., and PRANGE, A. J., 1970*a*, Cyclic AMP in affective disorders, *Lancet* **ii:**1028–1029.

ROBISON, G. A., SCHMIDT, M. J., and SUTHERLAND, E. W., 1970*b*, On the development and properties of the brain adenyl cyclase system, *Advan. Biochem. Psychopharmacol.* **3:**11–30.

ROISEN, F. J., and MURPHY, R. A., 1973, Neurite development *in vitro*. II. The role of microfilaments and microtubules in dibutyryl adenosine 3′,5′-cyclic monophosphate and nerve-growth-factor stimulated maturation, *J. Neurobiol.* **4:**397–417.

ROISEN, F. J., MURPHY, R. A., RICHICHERO, M. E., and BRADEN, W. G., 1972*a*, Cyclic adenosine monophosphate stimulation of axonal elongation, *Science* **175:**73–74.

ROISEN, F. J., MURPHY, R. A., and BRADEN, W. G., 1972*b*, Neurite development *in vitro*. I. The effects of adenosine 3′,5′-cyclic monophosphate (cyclic AMP), *J. Neurobiol.* **4:**347–368.

ROISEN, F. J., MURPHY, R. A., and BRADEN, W. G., 1972*c*, Dibutyryl cyclic adenosine monophosphate stimulation of colcemid-inhibited axonal elongation, *Science* **177:**809–811.

ROISEN, F. J., MURPHY, R. A., and BRADEN, W. G., 1972*d*, Neurite development *in vitro*. I. The effects of adenosine 3′5′-cyclic monophosphate (cyclic AMP), *J. Neurobiol.* **3:**347–368.

ROJAKOVICK, A. S., and MARCH, R. B., 1972, The activation and inhibition of adenyl cyclase from the brain of the Madagascar cockroach (*Gromphadorhina portentosa*), *Comp. Biochem. Physiol.* **43B:**209–215.

RUSSELL, J. R., THOMPSON, W. J., SCHNEIDER, F. W., and APPLEMAN, M. M., 1972, 3′:5′-Cyclic monophosphate phosphodiesterase: Negative cooperativity, *Proc. Natl. Acad. Sci.* **69:**1791–1795.

SATTIN, A., 1971, Increase in the content of adenosine 3′,5′-monophosphate in mouse forebrain during seizures and prevention of the increase by methylxanthines, *J. Neurochem.* **18:**1087–1096.

SATTIN, A., and RALL, T. W., 1970, The effect of adenosine and adenine nucleotides on the cyclic adenosine 3′,5′-phosphate content of guinea pig cerebral cortex slices, *Mol. Pharmacol.* **6:**13–23.

SCHIMMER, B. P., 1971, Effects of catecholamines and monovalent cations on adenylate cyclase activity in cultured glial tumor cells, *Biochem. Biophys. Acta* **252:**567–573.

SCHIMMER, B. P., 1973, Influence of Li^+ on epinephrine-stimulated adenylate cyclase activity in cultured glial tumor cells, *Biochim. Biophys. Acta* **326:**186–192.

SCHMIDT, M. J., and ROBISON, G. A., 1971, The effect of norepinephrine on cyclic AMP levels in discrete regions of the developing rabbit brain, *Life Sci.* **10(I):**459–464.

SCHMIDT, M. J., and ROBISON, G. A., 1972, The effect of neonatal thyroidectomy on the development of the adenosine 3′,5′-monophosphate system in the rat brain, *J. Neurochem.* **19:**937–947.

SCHMIDT, M. J., and SOKOLOFF, L., 1973, Activity of cyclic AMP–dependent microsomal protein kinase and phsphorylation of ribosomal protein in rat brain during postnatal development, *J. Neurochem.* **21:**1193–1205.

SCHMIDT, M. J., PALMER, E. C., DETTBARN, W.-D., and ROBISON, G. A., 1970, Cyclic AMP and adenyl cyclase in the developing rat brain, *Develop. Psychobiol.* **3:**53–67.

SCHMIDT, M. J., SCHMIDT, D. E., and ROBISON, G. A., 1971, Cyclic adenosine monophosphate in brain areas: Microwave irradiation as a means of tissue fixation, *Science* **173:**1142–1143.

SCHMIDT, M. J., HOPKINS, J. T., SCHMIDT, D. E., and ROBISON, G. A., 1972, Cyclic AMP in brain areas: Effects of amphetamine and norepinephrine assessed through the use of microwave radiation as a means of tissue fixation, *Brain Res.* **42:**465–477.

SCHMIDT, S. Y., and LOLLEY, R. N., 1973, Cyclic-nucleotide phosphodiesterase: An early defect in inherited retinal degeneration in C3H mice, *J. Cell Biol.* **57:**117–123.

SCHRIER, B. K., and GILMAN, A. G., 1973, Elevation of cyclic AMP content of rat brain cell cultures by adenosine, *Fed. Proc.* **32:**680Abs.

SCHRIER, B. K., and SHAPIRO, D. L., 1973, Effects of N^6-monobutyryl-cyclic AMP on glutamate decarboxylase activity in fetal rat brain cells and glial tumor cells in culture, *Exp. Cell Res.* **80:**459–465.

SCHORDERET, M., MCAFEE, D. A., and GREENGARD, P., 1972, Cyclic AMP as a possible mediator of adrenergic transmission in sympathetic ganglia, *Advan. Cyclic Nucleotide Res.* **1:**337–356.

SCHULTZ, J., 1974*a*, Adenosine 3′,5′-monophosphate in guinea pig cerebral cortical slices: Effect of benzodiazepines, *J. Neurochem.*, **22:**685–690

SCHULTZ, J., 1974*b*, Inhibition of 3′,5′-nucleotide phosphodiesterase in guinea pig cerebral cortical slices, *Arch. Biochem. Biophys.* **163:**15–20.

SCHULTZ, J. and DALY, J. W., 1973*a*, Cyclic adenosine 3′,5′-monophosphate in guinea pig cerebral cortical slices. I. Formation of cyclic adenosine 3′,5′-monophosphate from endogenous adenosine triphosphate and from radioactive adenosine triphosphate formed during a prior incubation with radioactive adenine, *J. Biol. Chem.* **248:**843–852.

SCHULTZ, J., and DALY, J. W., 1973*b*, Cyclic adenosine 3′,5′-monophosphate in guinea pig cerebral cortical slices. II. The role of phosphodiesterase activity in the regulation of levels of cyclic adenosine 3′,5′-monophosphate, *J. Biol. Chem.* **248:**853–859.

SCHULTZ, J., and DALY, J. W., 1973*c*, Cyclic adenosine 3′,5′-monophosphate in guinea pig cerebral cortical slices. III. Formation, degradation, and reformation of cyclic adenosine 3′,5′-monophosphate during sequential stimulations by biogenic amines and adenosine, *J. Biol. Chem.* **248:**860–866.

SCHULTZ, J., and DALY, J. W., 1973*d*, Adenosine 3′,5′-monophosphate in guinea pig cerebral cortical slices: Effects of α- and β-adrenergic agents, histamine, serotonin and adenosine, *J. Neurochem.* **21:**573–579.

SCHULTZ, J., and DALY, J. W., 1973*e*, Accumulation of cyclic adenosine 3′,5′-monophosphate in cerebral cortical slices from rat and mouse stimulatory effect of α- and β-adrenergic agents and adenosine, *J. Neurochem.* **21:**1319–1326.

SCHULTZ, J., and HAMPRECHT, B., 1973, Adenosine 3′,5′-monophosphate in cultured neuroblastoma cells: Effect of adenosine, phosphodiesterase inhibitors and benzazepines, *Naunyn-Schmiedebergs Arch. Pharmacol.* **278:**215–225.

SCHULTZ, J., HAMPRECHT, B., and DALY, J. W., 1972, Accumulation of adenosine 3′:5′-cyclic monophosphate in clonal glial cells: Labeling of intracellular adenine nucleotides with radioactive adenine, *Proc. Natl. Acad. Sci.* **69:**1266–1270.

SCHWARTZ, J. P., MORRIS, N. R., and BRECKENRIDGE, B. M., 1973, Adenosine 3′,5′-monophosphate in glial tumor cells, *J. Biol. Chem.* **248:**2699–2704.

SCIORELLI, G., POLONI, M., and RINDI, G., 1972, Evidence for cholinergic mediation of ingestive responses elicited by dibutyryl-adenosine-3′,5′-monophosphate in rat hypothalamus, *Brain Res.* **48:**427–431.

SEEDS, N. W., and GILMAN, A. G., 1971, Norepinephrine stimulated increase of cyclic AMP levels in developing mouse brain cell cultures, *Science* **174:**292.

SHANTA, T. R., WOODS, W. D., WAITZMAN, M. B., and BOURNE, G. H., 1966, Histochemical method for localization of cyclic 3′,5′-nucleotide phosphodiesterase, *Histochemie* **7:**177–190.

SHAPIRO, D. L., 1973, Morphological and biochemical alterations in fetal rat brain cells cultured in the presence of monobutyryl cyclic AMP, *Nature* **241:**203–204.

SHASHOUA, V. E., 1971, Dibutyryl adenosine cyclic 3′:5′-monophosphate effects on goldfish behavior and brain RNA metabolism, *Proc. Natl. Acad. Sci.* **68:**2835–2838.

SHEPPARD, H., and WIGGAN, G., 1971, Different sensitivities of the phosphodiesterases (adenosine-3′,5′-cyclic phosphate 3′-phosphohydrolase) of dog cerebral cortex and erythrocytes to inhibition by synthetic agents and cold, *Biochem. Pharmacol.* **20:**2128–2130.

SHEPPARD, H., WIGGAN, G., and TSIEN, W. H., 1972, Structure–activity relationships for inhibitors of phosphodiesterase from erythrocytes and other tissues, *Advan. Cyclic Nucleotide Res.* **1:**103–112.

SHEPPARD, J. R., and PRASAD, K. N., 1973, Cyclic AMP levels and the morphological differentiation of mouse neuroblastoma cells, *Life Sci.* **12:**431–439.

SHIMIZU, H., and DALY, J., 1970, Formation of cyclic adenosine 3′,5′-monophosphate from adenosine in brain slices, *Biochim. Biophys. Acta* **222:**465–473.

SHIMIZU, H., and DALY, J. W., 1972*a*, Methods for the measurement of cyclic AMP in brain, in: *Methods in Neurochemistry*, Vol. 2 (R. Fried, ed.), pp. 147–168, Marcel Dekker, New York.

SHIMIZU, H., and DALY, J. W., 1972*b*, Effect of depolarizing agents on accumulation of cyclic adenosine 3′,5′-monophosphate in cerebral cortical slices, *Eur. J. Pharmacol.* **17:**240–252.

SHIMIZU, H., and OKAYAMA, H., 1973, An ATP pool associated with adenyl cyclase of brain tissue, *J. Neurochem.* **20:**1279–1283.

SHIMIZU, H., DALY, J. W., and CREVELING, C. R., 1969, A radioisotopic method for measuring the formation of adenosine 3′,5′-cyclic monophosphate in incubated slices of brain, *J. Neurochem.* **16:**1609–1619.

SHIMIZU, H., CREVELING., C. R., and DALY, J., 1970*a*, Stimulated formation of adenosine 3′,5′-cyclic phosphate in cerebral cortex: Synergism between electrical activity and biogenic amines, *Proc. Natl. Acad. Sci.* **65:**1033–1040.

SHIMIZU, H., CREVELING, C. R., and DALY, J. W., 1970*b*, Cyclic adenosine 3′,5′-monophosphate formation in brain slices: Stimulation by batrachotoxin, ouabain, veratridine, and potassium ions, *Mol. Pharmacol.* **6:**184–188.

SHIMIZU, H., CREVELING, C. R., and DALY, J. W., 1970*c*, The effect of histamines and other compounds on the formation of adenosine 3′,5′-monophosphate in slices from cerebral cortex, *J. Neurochem.* **17:**441–444.

SHIMIZU, H., CREVELING, C. R., and DALY, J. W., 1970*d*, Effect of membrane depolarization and biogenic amines on the formation of cyclic AMP in incubated brain slices, *Advan. Biochem. Psychopharmacol.* **3:**135–154.

SHIMIZU, H., TANAKA, S., SUZUKI, T., and MATSUKADO, Y., 1971, The response of human cerebrum adenyl cyclase to biogenic amines, *J. Neurochem.* **18:**1157–1161.

SHIMIZU, H., TANAKA, S., and KODAMA, T., 1972, Adenosine kinase of mammalian brain: Partial purification and its role for the uptake of adenosine, *J. Neurochem.* **19:**687–698.

SHIMIZU, H., TAKENOSHITA, M., HUANG, M., and DALY, J. W., 1973, Accumulation of adenosine 3′,5′-monophosphate in brain slices: Interaction of local anaesthetics and depolarizing agents, *J. Neurochem.* **20:**91–95.

SIGGINS, G. R., HOFFER, B. J., and BLOOM, F. E., 1969, Cyclic adenosine monophosphate: Possible mediator for norepinephrine effects on cerebellar Purkinje cells, *Science* **165:**1018–1020.

SIGGINS, G. B., HOFFER, B. J., and BLOOM, F. E., 1971*a*, Cyclic adenosine monophosphate and norepinephrine: Effect on Purkinje cells in rat cerebellar cortex, *Science* **174:**1258–1259.

SIGGINS, G. R., OLIVER, A. P., HOFFER, B. J., and BLOOM, F. E., 1971*b*, Cyclic adenosine monophosphate and norepinephrine: Effects on transmembrane properties of cerebellar Purkinje cells, *Science* **171:**192–194.

SIGGINS, G. R., HOFFER, B. J., and BLOOM, F. E., 1971*c*, Studies on norepinephrine-containing afferents to Purkinje cells of rat cerebellum. III. Evidence for mediation of norepinephrine effects by cyclic 3′,5′-adenosine monophosphate, *Brain Res.* **25:**535–553.

SIGGINS, G., HOFFER, B., and BLOOM, F., 1971*d*, Prostaglandin–norepinephrine interactions in brain: Microelectrophoretic and histochemical correlates, *Ann. N.Y. Acad. Sci.* **180:**302–323.

SIGGINS, G. R., HOFFER, B. J., OLIVER, A. P., and BLOOM, F. E., 1971*e*, Activation of a central noradrenergic projection to cerebellum, *Nature* **233:**481–483.

SIGGINS, G. R., BATTENBERG, E. F., HOFFER, B. J., and BLOOM, F. E., 1973, Noradrenergic stimulation of cyclic adenosine monophosphate in rat Purkinje neurons: An immunocytochemical study, *Science* **179:**585–588.

SILBERSTEIN, S. D., BRIMIJOIN, S., MOLINOFF, P. B., and LEMBERGER, L., 1972, Induction of dopamine-β-hydroxylase in rat superior ganglia in organ culture, *J. Neurochem.* **19:**919–921.

SIMANTOV, R., and SACHS, L., 1972, Enzyme regulation in neuroblastoma cells: Selection of clones with low acetyl-cholinesterase activity and the independent control of acetylcholinesterase and choline-*O*-acetyltransferase, *Eur. J. Biochem.* **30:**123–129.

SIMANTOV, R., and SACHS, L., 1973, Regulation of acetylcholine receptors in relation to acetylcholinesterase in neuroblastoma cells, *Proc. Natl. Acad. Sci.* **70:**2902–2905.

SIMON, L. N., SHUMAN, D. A., and ROBINS, R. K., 1973, The chemistry and biological properties of nucleotides related to nucleoside 3′,5′-cyclic phosphates, *Advan. Cyclic Nucleotide Res.* **3:**225–353.

SINGHAL, R. L., LAFRENIERE, R., and LING, G. M., 1973, Cerebrocortical adenyl cyclase activity following neonatal thyroid hormone deficiency, *Int. J. Clin. Pharmacol. Ther. Toxicol.* **8:**1–4.

SKOLNICK, P., and DALY, J. W., 1974*a*, Norepinephrine-elicited accumulation of adenosine 3′,5′-monophosphate in brain slices: Relationship to spontaneous behavioral activity and levels of brain tyrosine hydroxylase in several rat strains, *Science* **184:**175–177.

SKOLNICK, P., and DALY, J. W., 1974*b*, The accumulation of adenosine 3′,5′-monophosphate in cerebral cortical slices of the quaking mouse, a neurologic mutant, *Brain Res.*, **73:**513–525.

SKOLNICK, P., and DALY, J. W., 1975, Functional compartments of adenine nucleotides serving as precursors of adenosine 3′,5′-monophosphate in mouse cerebral cortex, *J. Neurochem.* **24:**451–456.

SKOLNICK, P., HUANG, M., DALY, J., and HOFFER, B., 1973, Accumulation of adenosine 3′,5′-monophosphate in incubated slices from discrete regions of squirrel monkey cerebral cortex: Effect of norepinephrine, serotonin and adenosine, *J. Neurochem.* **21:**237–240.

SOIFER, D., LASZLO, A. H., and SCOTTO, J. M., 1972, Enzymatic activity in tubulin preparations. I. Intrinsic protein kinase activity in lyophilized preparations of tubulin from porcine brain, *Biochim. Biophys. Acta* **271:**182–192.

SOMERVILLE, A. R., and SMITH, A. A., 1972, The effects of propranolol and electrical stimulation on the cyclic 3′,5′-AMP content of isolated cerebral tissue, *J. Neurochem.* **19:**2003–2006.

STEINER, A. L., PARKER, C. W., and KIPNIS, D. M., 1970, The measurement of cyclic nucleotides by radioimmunoassay, *Advan. Biochem. Psychopharmacol.* **3:**89–112.

STEINER, A. L., FERRENDELLI, J. A., and KIPNIS, D. M., 1972, Radioimmunoassay for cyclic nucleotides. III. Effect of ischemia, changes during development and regional distribution of adenosine 3′,5′-monophosphate and guanosine 3′,5′-monophosphate in mouse brain, *J. Biol. Chem.* **247:**1121–1124.

STRASCHILL, M., and PERWEIN, J., 1969, The inhibition of retinal ganglion cells by catecholamines and γ-aminobutyric acid, *Pfluegers Arch.* **312:**45–54.

SWISLOCKI, N. I., and TIERNEY, J., 1973, Solubilization, stabilization, and partial purification of brain adenylate cyclase from rat, *Biochemistry* **12:**1862–1866.

TAGLIAMONTE, A., TAGLIAMONTE, P., FORN, J., PEREZ-CRUET, J., KRISHNA, G., and GESSA, G. L., 1971*a*, Stimulation of brain serotonin synthesis by dibutyryl-cyclic AMP in rats, *J. Neurochem.* **18:**1191–1196.

TAGLIAMONTE, A., TAGLIAMONTE, P., PEREZ-CRUET, J., and GESSA, G. L., 1971*b*, Increase of brain tryptophan caused by drugs that stimulate serotonin synthesis, *Nature New Biol.* **229:**125–126.

TAGLIAMONTE, A., TAGLIAMONTE, P., PEREZ-CRUET, J., STERN, A., and GESSA, G. L., 1971*c*, Effect of psychotropic drugs on tryptophan concentration in the rat brain, *J. Pharmacol. Exp. Ther.* **177:**475–480.

TAKAGAKI, G., 1972, Control of aerobic glycolysis in guinea-pig cerebral cortex slices, *J. Neurochem.* **19:**1737–1751.

THOMPSON, W. J., and APPLEMAN, M. M., 1971*a*, Characterizations of cyclic nucleotide phosphodiesterases of rat tissues, *J. Biol. Chem.* **246:**3145–3150.

THOMPSON, W. J., and APPLEMAN, M. M., 1971*b*, Multiple cyclic nucleotide phosphodiesterase activities from rat brain, *Biochemistry* **10:**311–316.

THOMPSON, W. J., and APPLEMAN, M. M., 1971*c*, Cyclic nucleotide phosphodiesterase and cyclic AMP, *Ann. N.Y. Acad. Sci.* **185:**36–41.

TORDA, C., 1972*a*, Cyclic AMP–dependent diphosphoinositide kinase, *Biochim. Biophys. Acta* **286:**389–395.

TORDA, C., 1972*b*, Hyperpolarization by cyclic AMP (activation of diphosphoinositide kinase), *Experientia* **28:**1438–1439.

TSIEN, R. W., 1973, Adrenaline-like effects of intracellular iontophoresis of cyclic AMP in cardiac Purkinje fibres, *Nature New Biol.* **245:**120–122.

TSIEN, R. W., GILES, W., and GREENGARD, P., 1972, Cyclic AMP mediates the effects of adrenaline on cardiac Purkinje fibers, *Nature New Biol.* **240:**181–183.

TUGANOWSKI, W., KRAUSE, M., and KOREZAK, K., 1973, The effect of dibutyryl 3′,5′-cyclic AMP on the cardiac pacemaker, arrested with reserpine and α-methyltyrosine, *Naunyn-Schmiedebergs Arch. Pharmacol.* **280:**63–70.

UEDA, T., MAENO, H., and GREENGARD, P., 1973, Regulation of endogenous phsophorylation of specific proteins in synaptic membrane fractions from rat brain by adenosine 3′:5′-monophosphate, *J. Biol. Chem.* **248:**8295–8305.

UZUNOV, P., and WEISS, B., 1971, Effects of phenothiazine tranquilizers on the cyclic 3′,5′-adenosine monophosphate system of rat brain, *Neuropharmacology* **10:**697–708.

UZUNOV, P., and WEISS, B., 1972, Separation of multiple molecular forms of cyclic adenosine 3′,5′-monophosphate phosphodiesterase in rat cerebellum by polyacrylamide gel electrophoresis, *Biochim. Biophys. Acta* **284:**220–226.

UZUNOV, P., SHEIN, H. M., and WEISS, B., 1973, Cyclic AMP phosphodiesterase in cloned astrocytoma cells: Norepinephrine induces a specific enzyme form, *Science* **180:**304–306.

VARAGIC, V. M., and BELESLIN, D. B., 1973, The effect of cyclic *N*-2-*O*-dibutyryladenosine-3′,5′-monophosphate, adenosine triphosphate and butyrate on the body temperatures of conscious cats, *Brain Res.* **57:**252–254.

VARAGIC, V. M., and ZUGIC, M., 1971, Interactions of xanthine derivatives, catecholamines and glucose-6-phosphate on the isolated phrenic nerve diaphragm preparation of the rat, *Pharmacology* **5:**275–286.

VARAGIC, V. M., and ZUGIC, M., 1973, The effect of N^6-2′-*O*-dibutyryl 3′,5′-cyclic adenosine monophosphate, imidazole and aminophylline on ganglionic transmission in the superior cervical ganglion of the cat, *Brit. J. Pharmacol.* **49:**407–414.

VARAGIC, V. M., ZUGIC, M., and MRSULJA, B. B., 1972, The effect of cyclic *N*-2-*O*-dibutyryl-adenosine-3′,5′-monophosphate on neuromuscular transmission and concentration of glycogen in the isolated phrenic nerve–diaphragm preparation of the rat, *Experientia* **28:**305–306.

VARGUI, L., and SPANO, P. F., 1971, Some central effects of a new derivative of cyclic 3′,5′-adenosine monophosphate, *Naunyn-Schmiedebergs Arch. Pharmacol.* **269:**410Abs.

VERNIKOS-DANELLIS, J., and HARRIS, C. G., III, 1968, The effect of *in vitro* and *in vivo* caffeine, theophylline and hydrocortisone on the phosphodiesterase activity of the pituitary, median eminence, heart and cerebral cortex of the rat, *Proc. Soc. Exp. Biol. Med.* **128:**1016–1021.

VOLICER, L., and GOLD, B. I., 1973, Effect of ethanol on cyclic AMP levels in the rat brain, *Life Sci.* **13:**269–280.

VON HUNGEN, K., and ROBERTS, S., 1973*a*, Adenylate-cyclase receptors for adrenergic neurotransmitters in rat cerebral cortex, *Eur. J. Biochem.* **36:**391–401.

VON HUNGEN, K., and ROBERTS, S., 1973*b*, Catecholamine and Ca^{2+} activation of adenylate cyclase systems in synaptosomal fractions from rat cerebral cortex, *Nature New Biol.* **242:**58–60.

WALDECK, B., 1971, Some effects of caffeine and aminophylline on the turnover of catecholamines in the brain, *J. Pharm. Pharmacol.* **23:**824–830.

WALINDER, O., 1972, Calf brain phosvitin kinase: Purification of the kinase associated with a phosphate-incorporating protein, *Biochim. Biophys. Acta* **258:**411–421.

WALKER, J. B., and WALKER, J. P., 1973*a*, Neurohumoral regulation of adenylate cyclase activity in rat striatum, *Brain Res.* **54:**386–390.

WALKER, J. B., and WALKER, J. P., 1973*b*, Properties of adenylate cyclase from senescent rat brain, *Brain Res.* **54:**391–396.

WALKER, J. E., LEWIN, E., SHEPPARD, J. R., and CROMWELL, R., 1973, Enzymatic regulation of adenosine 3′,5′-monophosphate (cyclic AMP) in the freezing epileptogenic lesion of rat brain and in homologous contralateral cortex, *J. Neurochem.* **21:**79–85.

WALSH, D. A., ASHBY, C. D., GONZALEZ, C., CALKINS, D., FISCHER, E. H., and KREBS, E. G., 1971, Purification and characterization of a protein inhibitor of adenosine 3′,5′-monophosphate–dependet protein kinases, *J. Biol. Chem.* **246:**1977–1985.

WAYMIRE, J. C., WAINER, N., and PRASAD, K. N., 1972, Regulation of tyrosine hydroxylase activity in cultured mouse neuroblastoma cells: Elevation induced by analogs of adenosine 3':5'-cyclic monophosphate, *Proc. Natl. Acad. Sci.* **69:**2241–2245.

WEINER, M., and OLSON, J. W., 1973, The behavioral effects of dibutyryl cyclic AMP in mice, *Life* Sci. **12:**345–356.

WEINRYB, I., CHASIN, M., FREE, C. A., HARRIS, D. N., GOLDENBERG, H., MICHEL, I. M., PAIK, V. S., PHILLIPS, M., SAMANIEGO, S., and HESS, S. M., 1972, Effects of therapeutic agents on cyclic AMP metabolism *in vitro, J. Pharm. Sci.* **61:**1556–1567.

WEISS, B., 1969, Effects of environmental lighting and chronic denervation on the activation of adenyl cyclase of rat pineal gland by norepinephrine and sodium fluoride, *J. Pharmacol. Exp. Ther.* **168:**146–152.

WEISS, B., 1971, Ontogenetic development of adenyl cyclase and phosphodiesterase in rat brain, *J. Neurochem.* **18:**469–477.

WEISS, B., 1972, Psychopharmacological agents and the cyclic AMP system of rat brain, *Advan. Cyclic Nucleotide Res.* **1:**435–453.

WEISS, B., and COSTA, E., 1967, Adenyl cyclase activity in rat pineal gland: Effects of chronic denervation and norepinephrine, *Science* **156:**1750–1752.

WEISS, B., and COSTA, E., 1968, Regional and subcellular distribution of adenyl cyclase and 3',5'-cyclic nucleotide phosphodiesterase in brain and pineal gland, *Biochem. Pharmacol.* **17:**2107–2116.

WEISS, B., and STRADA, S. J., 1972, Neuroendocrine control of the cyclic AMP system of brain and pineal gland, *Advan. Cyclic Nucleotide Res.* **1:**357–374.

WEISS, B., SHEIN, H. M., and SNYDER, R., 1971, Adenylate cyclase and phosphodiesterase activity of normal and SV_{40} virus transformed hamster astrocytes in cell culture, *Life Sci.* **10(I):**1253–1260.

WELLER, M., and RODNIGHT, R., 1970, Stimulation by cyclic AMP of intrinsic protein kinase activity in ox brain membrane preparation, *Nature* **225:**187–188.

WELLER, M., and RODNIGHT, R., 1971, Turnover of proten-bound phosphorylserine in membrane preparations of ox brain catalyzed by intrinsic kinase and phosphatase activity, *Biochem. J.* **124:**393–406.

WELLER, M., and RODNIGHT, R., 1973, Protein kinase activity in membrane preparations from ox brain: Stimulation of intrinsic activity by adenosine 3':5'-cyclic monophosphate, *Biochem. J.* **132:**483–492.

WELLER, M., RODNIGHT, R., and CARRERA, D., 1972, Determination of adenosine 3',5'-cyclic monophosphate in cerebral tissues by saturation analysis: Assessment of a method using a binding protein from ox muscle, *Biochem. J.* **129:**113–121.

WELLMANN, W., and SCHWABE, U., 1973, Effects of prostaglandins E_1, E_2 and $F_{2\alpha}$ on cyclic AMP levels in brain *in vivo, Brain Res.* **59:**371–378.

WERNER, I., PETERSON, G. R., and SHUSTER, L., 1971, Choline acetyltransferase and acetylcholine esterase in cultured brain cells from chick embryos, *J. Neurochem.* **18:**141–151.

WHITE, A. A., and AURBACH, G. D., 1969, Detection of guanyl cyclase in mammalian tissues, *Biochim. Biophys. Acta* **191:**686.

WILLIAMS, R. H., LITTLE, S. A., and ENSINCK, J. W., 1969, Adenyl cyclase and phosphodiesterase activities in brain areas of man, monkey and rat, *Am. J. Med. Sci.* **258:**190–202.

WILLIAMS, R. H., LITTLE, S. A., BEUG, A. G., and ENSINCK, J. W., 1971, Cyclic nucleotide phosphodiesterase activity in man, monkey, and rat, *Metab. Clin. Exp.* **20:**743–748.

WOLLENBERGER, A., BABSKII, E. B., KRAUSE, E.-G., GENZ, S., BLOHM, D., and BOGDANOVA, E. V., 1973, Cyclic changes in levels of cyclic AMP and cyclic GMP in frog myocardium during the cardiac cycle, *Biochem. Biophys. Res. Commun.* **55:**446–452.

WOODWARD, D. J., HOFFER, B. J., SIGGINS, G. R., and BLOOM, F. E., 1971, The ontogenetic development of synaptic junctions, synaptic activation and responsiveness to neurotransmitter substances, in rat cerebellar Purkinje cells, *Brain Res.* **34:**73–97.

WOOTEN, G. F., THOA, N. B., KOPIN, I. J., and AXELROD, J., 1973, Enhanced release of dopamine-β-hydroxylase and norepinephrine from sympathetic nerves by dibutyryl cyclic adenosine monophosphate and theophylline, *Mol. Pharmacol.* **9:**178–183.

WULFF, V. J., 1971, The effect of cyclic AMP on *Limulus* lateral eye retinular cells, *Vision Res.* **11:**1493–1495.

YAMAMOTO, M., and MASSEY, K. L., 1969, Cyclic 3′,5′-nucleotide phosphodiesterase of fish (*Salmo gairdnerii*) brain, *Comp. Biochem. Physiol.* **30:**941–954.

YARBROUGH, G. G., LAKE, N., and PHILLIS, J. W., 1974, Calcium antagonism and its effect on the inhibitory actions of biogenic amines on cerebral cortical neurones, *Brain Res.* **67:**77–88.

YORK, D. H., 1972, Dopamine receptor blockade: A central action of chlorpromazine on striatal neurones, *Brain Res.* **37:**91–99.

ZANELLA, J., JR., and RALL, T. W., 1973, Evaluation of electrical pulses and elevated levels of potassium ions as stimulants of adenosine 3′,5′-monophosphate (cyclic AMP) accumulation in guinea-pig brain, *J. Pharmacol. Exp. Ther.* **186:**241–251.

3

PURINERGIC TRANSMISSION

G. Burnstock

1. INTRODUCTION

It is now well established that there are intramural inhibitory neurons which are neither adrenergic nor cholinergic in the gastrointestinal tract of a wide range of vertebrate species (see Burnstock, 1969, 1972; Campbell, 1970; Furness and Costa, 1973). Evidence that these inhibitory responses are *not* due to adrenergic nerves is conclusive. Relaxation of intestine produced by stimulation of perivascular sympathetic nerves is prevented by low concentrations of α- and β-adrenoceptor antagonists or by adrenergic neuron blocking drugs, without affecting the inhibitory responses to transmural stimulation. Inhibitory junction potentials and relaxations in response to transmural stimulation are unimpaired in the guinea pig colon after degeneration of sympathetic adrenergic nerves (see Fig. 3). Relaxation of the guinea pig taenia coli in response to transmural stimulation or nicotine persists in organ cultures and in anterior eye chamber transplants after all adrenergic nerves have disappeared. Transmission from intrinsic inhibitory neurons has been recorded in avian gizzard and mammalian anal sphincter, which are *contracted* by catecholamines. Most recently, inhibitory nerve-mediated responses were demonstrated in developing fetal rabbit intestine before adrenergic nerves appeared (Gershon and Thompson, 1973).

Evidence has been presented which suggests that the principal active substance released by these inhibitory nerves is a purine nucleotide, probably ATP (see Burnstock, 1972, and Section 6); they have therefore been termed "purinergic" (Burnstock, 1971).

G. Burnstock ● Department of Anatomy and Embryology, University College London, London, WC1E 6BT

Knowledge of purinergic neurons is in its infancy, in contrast to the voluminous literature on the biochemistry, electrophysiology, and pharmacology of transmission and morphology of adrenergic and cholinergic nerves. Nevertheless, certain features of purinergic nerves are already clearly established, and by analogy with the pathways known for cholinergic and adrenergic systems a tentative model of the synthesis, storage, release, and inactivation of ATP during purinergic nerve transmission was proposed (Burnstock, 1972) (Fig. 1). This model has provided a framework and stimulus for further studies, and since its presentation there have been an increasing number of publications in the field: the possibility that purinergic nerves supply various organs, including the trachea, seminal vesicle, esophagus, bladder, uterus, various blood vessels, lung, and the CNS, as well as the gastrointestinal tract has been recognized (see Section 2); knowledge of the structure (see Section 3), electrophysiology (see Section 4), and physiological roles of purinergic nerves (see Section 5) has been extended; further evidence consistent with the hypothesis that ATP is the neurotransmitter released from purinergic nerves has been presented (see Section 6); and the search for drugs which potentiate or block purinergic transmission has been continued (see Section 7). There is growing interest in the clinical implications of the purinergic nerve hypothesis (see editorials by Christensen, 1971; McIntyre, 1973). The role of ATP in regulation of blood flow in

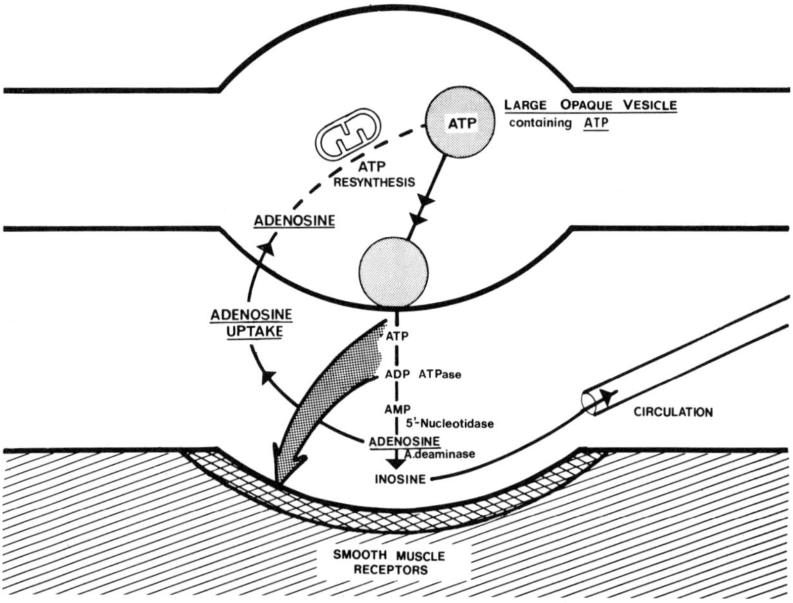

FIG. 1. Schematic representation of synthesis, storage, release, and inactivation of ATP at the purinergic neuromuscular junction. From Burnstock (1972).

skeletal muscle, kidney, and heart (see Section 2.4) and in storage and release of amines from chromaffin and mast cells (see Section 2.3), of hormones from the hypothalamic–pituitary adrenal axis (Geschwind, 1970; Unsicker, 1973*a*; Cook *et al.*, 1974), and of acetylcholine (ACh) from cholinergic nerves (see Sections 6.2 and 8) is also attracting attention.

2. DISTRIBUTION OF PURINERGIC NERVES

The presence of nonadrenergic, noncholinergic nerves is indicated if nerve-mediated responses to stimulation of either extrinsic or intrinsic nerve fibers remain in the presence of atropine and adrenergic neuron or adrenoceptor blocking agents or after sympathetic denervation, and if this response is blocked by a low concentration of tetrodotoxin. A combination of various features can be used to test whether these nerves are purinergic (see later sections for details), including: (1) the identification of ATP (with luminometry, Paddle and Burnstock, 1974) or the breakdown products of ATP (with chromatography, Burnstock *et al.*, 1970) in the perfusate of nerve-stimulated organs; (2) the detection of labeled nucleotide in the perfusate of nerve-stimulated organs following incubation in tritium-labeled adenosine (with liquid scintillometry, Su *et al.*, 1971); (3) the presence of nerve profiles containing a predominance of "large opaque vesicles" (LOV), particularly after short-term "loading" and long-term "degeneration" of adrenergic nerves with 6-hydroxydopamine (6-OHDA) (with electron microscopy, Burnstock, 1975); (4) the response of tissue to low concentrations of ATP which mimic in both kind (contraction or relaxation or a combination) and time course the response to nonadrenergic, noncholinergic nerve stimulation (Burnstock *et al.*, 1972*a,b*); (5) the presence of high concentrations of enzymes that break down ATP, such as Mg^{2+}-activated ATPase, 5′-nucleotidase, and adenosine deaminase (with cytochemistry and histochemistry, see Burnstock, 1972); (6) the recording of inhibitory junction potentials in smooth muscle cells during stimulation of the nerves which are comparable in form and properties to those established for purinergic nerves in the intestine and stomach (with electrophysiology, Bennett *et al.*,1966*b*; Tomita and Watanabe, 1973); (7) potentiation of the nerve-mediated response by dipyridamole (Satchell *et al.*, 1972) or blockade by imidazoline compounds such as antazoline and phentolamine (Satchell *et al.*, 1973), by quinidine (Burnstock *et al.*, 1970), or by 2-2′-pyridylisatogen (Hooper *et al.*, 1974) (although the results of pharmacological experiments with these blocking agents must be interpreted with care since they do not appear to be specific blockers of purinergic nerves); (8) reinnervation of the organ by nonadrenergic, noncholinergic nerves when transplanted into the anterior chamber of the eye (see Burnstock *et al.*, 1971).

2.1. Gastrointestinal Tract

Evidence for the distribution of purinergic nerves in the gastrointestinal tract (see Fig. 4) was reviewed previously (Burnstock, 1972). Therefore, emphasis will be placed on the contributions from more recent publications.

2.1.1. *Stomach*

Evidence is now available that there is purinergic inhibitory nervous control of the vertebrate stomach (Lock and Weber, 1971; see Burnstock, 1972, and Abrahamsson, 1973). The cell bodies of these neurons appear to be located in Auerbach's plexus and many, if not all, are controlled by preganglionic parasympathetic nerves running in the vagal trunks. Concentrations of adrenoceptor or adrenergic neuron blocking drugs which abolish the response to sympathetic (adrenergic) nerve stimulation do not block the inhibitory responses to vagal stimulation or reflex relaxation of the stomach. The frequency of stimulation of vagal inhibitory fibers that gives maximal responses is low (about 5–10 Hz) compared to stimulation frequences of 30 Hz or more required for maximal responses to sympathetic nerve stimulation.

Most preganglionic terminals on purinergic neurons appear to be cholinergic, since the inhibitory responses resulting from stimulation of the vagus nerves or from vago-vagal reflexes are blocked by nicotinic ganglion blocking agents (Ohga *et al.*, 1970; Abrahamsson, 1973). However, there appears to be a small component of hexamethonium-resistant vagal inhibition, possibly due to the presence of tryptaminergic synapses in the vagal pathway (Bülbring and Gershon, 1967; Beani *et al.*, 1971; Nakazato and Ohga, 1971; Lock and Weber, 1971), or to the presence of a small component of postganglionic, nonadrenergic inhibitory fibers in the vagus nerves, which may or may not be purinergic.

2.1.2. *Esophagus*

Purinergic nerves have been implicated in reflex relaxation of the esophago-gastric junction (Code and Schlegel, 1968) and in esophageal peristalsis in man (Dimarino and Cohen, 1974). Inhibitory junction potentials (IJPs) have been recorded in cat esophagus (Diamant, 1973). Stimulation of longitudinal and mucosal muscle strips from the esophagus of the opossum revealed both cholinergic excitatory responses and rebound contraction mediated by nonadrenergic inhibitory nerves (Lund and Christensen, 1969; Weisbrodt and Christensen, 1972). A hyoscine-resistant contraction of the isolated esophagus of the chicken in response to stimulation of the parasympathetic nerves has also been described (Hassan, 1969; Bartlet, 1972; see also Roman and Car, 1967). These responses were not blocked by bretylium or hexamethonium, but were abolished by nerve section, implying that there is a noncholinergic, nonadrenergic postganglionic component in the vagal pathway.

2.1.3. Small Intestine

Purinergic nerves have been demonstrated in the small intestine of a variety of mammalian species, including guinea pig, mouse, rat, rabbit, cat, and man (see Burnstock, 1972, for earlier references, and Weston, 1971; Biber and Fara, 1973; Bennett and Stockley, 1973; Furness and Costa, 1973; Gershon and Thompson, 1973; Hirst and McKirdy, 1974).

Most of the terminal regions of purinergic neurons in the mammalian small intestine appear to supply the circular muscle coat; few fibers, if any, supply muscle cells in the longitudinal coat (Hirst and McKirdy, 1974). It seems unlikely that the purinergic inhibitory neurons in the small intestine have extrinsic nerve connections, but rather that they are controlled by intramural cholinergic neurons (see Burnstock and Costa, 1973; Furness and Costa, 1973; Hirst and McKirdy, 1974). The axons of purinergic inhibitory neurons extend for about 1.5 cm in an anal direction before becoming varicose and entering the circular muscle coat (Hirst and McKirdy, 1974).

Noncholinergic, nonadrenergic *excitatory* nerves have also been shown to supply the small intestine of a number of vertebrate species (see Burnstock, 1972; Furness and Costa, 1973). Whether some or all of these excitatory nerves are purinergic or whether they are nerves releasing another neurotransmitter substance has not yet been clearly resolved (see Section 7.1).

2.1.4. Large Intestine

Purinergic responses to transmural stimulation have been demonstrated in the large intestine of guinea-pig, pig, chimpanzee, dog, rabbit, mouse, rat, Mongolian gerbil, and man, as well as in the guinea pig taenia coli (see Campbell, 1970; Rikimaru *et al.*, 1971*a*; Burnstock, 1972; Tomita, 1972; Stockley and Bennett, 1973). Purinergic nerves have also been shown to supply the internal anal sphincter of monkey, guinea pig, and cat (Rayner, 1970; Garrett and Howard, 1972; Costa and Furness, 1973). The sacral parasympathetic (pelvic) nerves do not mediate the purinergic inhibitory responses of the large intestine, except for a short segment of the distal rectum (Julé and Gonella, 1972; Furness and Costa, 1973). Terminals of intramural cholinergic neurons appear to be located on purinergic neurons. Experiments carried out by Ito and Kuriyama (1973) have shown that branches of purinergic nerves which arise from Auerbach's plexus beneath the taenia coli of guinea pig spread from one taenia coli to the next, a width of about 3 cm. The nonadrenergic inhibitory responses demonstrated in muscle taken from human large intestine were not seen in aganglionic bowel taken from patients with Hirschsprung's disease or in aganglionic megacolon of piebald-lethal mice (Webster, 1974).

Primary, noncholinergic *contraction* to nerve stimulation has been observed in the proximal colon of the guinea pig and in the distal colon of the cat, dog, and man (see Burnstock, 1972; Furness and Costa, 1973; Stockley and Bennett, 1973). It seems likely that some of the hyoscine-resistant contractions in the distal colon are secondary rebound contractions following the stimulation of intrinsic inhibitory nerves. There is some evidence that in the cat and dog these excitatory nerves are controlled by fibers running in the pelvic nerves, while in the guinea pig they are activated largely by fibers in the perivascular nerves. Noncholinergic, nonadrenergic excitatory nerves have also been demonstrated in the large intestine of amphibians, reptiles, and birds (see Section 8).

2.2. Lung and Trachea

2.2.1. Lung

There is good evidence that purinergic inhibitory nerves supply smooth muscles in the lung of amphibians (Campbell, 1971; Robinson *et al.*, 1971) and reptiles (Berger, 1973). Relaxation of lung musculature in response to stimulation of the vagus nerves is unaffected by adrenergic neuron and cholinergic blocking agents. This response persists after destruction of adrenergic nerves with 6-OHDA, as do nerve profiles containing a predominance of LOV (Robinson *et al.*, 1971). ATP causes relaxation of the frog lung (Meves, 1953). Bronchodilator responses to vagal stimulation have been reported in mammals (Widdicombe, 1963) and adenosine and AMP dilate the bronchioles (Bennett and Drury, 1931). More recently, nerve profiles with a predominance of LOV have been described in the primary bronchioles of the chicken lung (Cook and King, 1970) and in the alveolar ducts and sacs of mouse lung (Hung *et al.*, 1972).

2.2.2. Trachea

Evidence has been presented for the existence of noncholinergic, nonadrenergic inhibitory nerves in the guinea pig trachea (Coleman, 1973; Coburn and Tomita, 1973; Coleman and Levy, 1974). The thoracic segment contains mostly (or possibly all) nonadrenergic nerves, while the cervical segments of the trachea also contain some adrenergic nerves. The response to stimulation of the nonadrenergic nerves was blocked by tetrodotoxin but was unaffected by guanethidine, bretylium, or propranolol or after sympathetic nerve function had been abolished with 6-OHDA, reserpine, or syrosingopine. Experiments undertaken to characterize the transmitter showed that it was unlikely to be histamine, 5-hydroxytryptamine (5-HT), a prostaglandin, or cyclic 3′,5′-AMP. However, since dipyridamole potentiated the nerve-mediated response and unmasked an inhibitory response to exogenously applied ATP (Coleman, 1973; Kinnaird, personal communication), and since maximal relaxation is elicited at low stimulation frequencies (Coburn and Tomita, 1973), it seems likely that the nonadrenergic inhibitory nerves supplying the trachea are comparable to the purinergic nerves in the gastrointestinal tract.

2.3. Vascular System

While vasoconstriction is usually mediated by norepinephrine (NE) released from adrenergic nerves, the mechanism of vasodilatation is less well understood. Several different substances including ACh, histamine, NE which acts on β-adrenoceptors, bradykinin, prostaglandins, and angiotensin have been implicated in different parts of the vascular system. However, these substances do not seem to explain adequately some reports of vasodilatation, and the possibility that purinergic nerves might be involved has also been considered (see Burnstock, 1972; Su, 1975).

Strong evidence has been presented for the existence of nonadrenergic, noncholinergic inhibitory fibers to the portal vein of the rabbit (Hughes and Vane, 1967, 1970). The inhibitory responses induced by either electrical stimulation or nicotine are blocked by tetrodotoxin and mimicked by the direct action of ATP. Thus they appear to fit into the pattern already established for purinergic nerves in the gut, but the possibility that vasodilatation is the result of ATP released during antidromic stimulation of sensory nerves cannot be discounted (Holton, 1959).

There have been many reports of vasodilatation of skin vessels, either by reflex or in response to nerve stimulation, which is not wholly abolished by atropine (see Haddy and Scott, 1968). Intra-arterial infusion of adenyl compounds leads to increased flow rates and vascular dilatation of rabbit ear, cat hind limb, human finger, ear, hand, and forearm. Similarly, adenyl compounds cause a fall in perfusion pressure in isolated preparations of rabbit ear and dog fore and hind legs. Kiernan (1972*b*) has suggested that ATP released from nerves during the axonal reflex produces vasodilatation of skin vessels by releasing histamine from mast cells in the vicinity. Certainly there is increasing evidence that ATP is the only putative transmitter capable of releasing histamine and 5-HT from mast cells in skin, peritoneum, and lung (Bloom *et al.*, 1970; Ichikawa *et al.*, 1972; Johansen and Chakravarty, 1972; Kiernan, 1972*a*). ATP has been found in the venous effluent from the rabbit ear during stimulation of the great auricular nerve (Holton, 1959). Purine nucleotides cause vasodilatation of prevenous resistance vessels in the dog paw, and these have also been considered, among a variety of other substances, as possible mediators of the noncholinergic, nonadrenergic dilator system which supplies them (Ballard *et al.*, 1970).

It is well known that skeletal muscle contraction is accompanied or followed by vasodilatation, which in fast muscles is sufficient to produce an eightfold increase in blood flow (Hilton *et al.*, 1970). A similar vasodilatation is common in stress situations and during fainting (Shepherd, 1963). Several agents have been considered as the mediator of this vasodilatation, including adenine nucleotides, particularly ATP, although it seems unlikely that this is being released from nerves (see Burnstock, 1972; Forrester, 1972; Forrester and Hassan, 1973; Tominaga *et al.*, 1973; Weissel *et al.*, 1973). It was estimated that 7.5–10.5 μg ATP/min (or 14–20 nmol ATP/min) was released into the venous effluent from human forearm muscle during exercise, which induced a threefold increase in blood flow; this compares with 16 μg ATP/min required to produce a comparable increase in blood flow when ATP is infused interarterially into the forearm (Forrester, 1972).

ATP- and adenosine-induced vasodilatation in the coronary artery has been studied extensively because of its possible implication in coronary occlusion and relevance to the treatment of angina pectoris (see Burnstock, 1972; Schnaar and Sparks, 1972; Olsson *et al.*, 1972; Moir and Downs, 1972; Stein, 1973). Most workers found ATP and ADP to be the most potent adenyl compounds on coronary vessel musculature; AMP, adenosine, and cyclic AMP are from one-fourth to one-third as potent as ATP, while adenine, hypoxanthine, guanine, cytosine, and uracil are either inactive or of very low potency. This order of potency of the adenyl compounds is comparable to that observed in preparations of purinergically innervated gut. It has been proposed that adenosine plays a physiological role in the regulation of blood flow in the coronary arteries (Berne, 1964; Rubio *et al.*, 1969; Berne *et al.*, 1971). Adenosine appears in coronary sinus blood during reactive hyperemia in the blood-perfused dog heart, and the assumption has been made that it originates in the cardiac muscle. It is clear that extrinsic nerves supplying the heart are not responsible for such a regulatory process, but the possibility of intramural nerves (see Hibbs and Ellison, 1973) being involved has not yet been investigated. In recent experiments in our laboratory using the sensitive luciferin–luciferase firefly technique (luminometry) (Paddle and Burnstock, 1974), a two- to sevenfold increase in ATP has been observed in the coronary outflow during reactive hyperemia induced by hypoxia. Only 1% of ATP introduced into the coronary system was collected in the outflow, most of it being broken down to adenosine during its passage. This probably accounts for the earlier impression that adenosine rather than ATP was being released during reactive hyperemia, together with the suggestion that adenosine but not ATP can pass readily across cell membranes (Glynn, 1957; Wiedmeier *et al.*, 1972). However, it is well known that ATP is considerably more effective than adenosine in producing vasodilatation of coronary vessels, so the possibility that ATP rather than adenosine is the physiological regulator of coronary blood flow must now be considered. Whether the source of the ATP is anoxic cardiac muscle or nerves must also be carefully examined.

Nonadrenergic, noncholinergic nerve-mediated vasodilatation of intestinal vessels has been reported during reflex activity (Hultén, 1969; Biber *et al.*, 1971) and after periarterial mesenteric nerve stimulation following adrenergic neuron blockade (Ross, 1973). It is not yet clear whether these nerves are purinergic, although vasodilatation of mesenteric and intestinal vessels is produced by adenyl compounds (see Burnstock, 1972), in many cases with doses lower than those required to relax the intestine.

Following blockade of the adrenergic constrictor nerves to guinea pig uterine arteries, a dilatation was revealed which was associated with hyperpolarization and was resistant to hyoscine (Bell, 1968, 1969). The transmitter responsible for this response remains obscure, but the pharmacological findings suggest that it is not histamine, 5-HT, or a catecholamine that stimulates β-receptors.

Adenyl compounds have been reported to have variable and inconsistent effects on net blood flow through the kidney (see Burnstock, 1972; Hashimoto and Kokubun, 1972; Gaál *et al.*, 1972). If adenine nucleotides have a physiological role in the regulation of blood flow through the renal vascular bed, ATP would be the logical candidate, because it is the only one that consistently produces vasodilatation on intraarterial administration and is more potent than AMP or adenosine. AMP appears in the renal venous effluent after release of renal artery occlusion and during both autoregulation and reactive hyperemia. Additional support for nucleotide participation in renal blood flow regulation is that the spontaneous disappearance of autoregulation in the dog kidney can be restored with dipyridamole (Ono *et al.*, 1966), an agent that potentiates the effects of adenine nucleotides and purinergic nerve stimulation in the gut (Satchell *et al.*, 1972).

Stimulation of the chorda tympani produces vasodilatation of the vessels of the salivary gland, which is not abolished by atropine in concentrations that prevent salivary secretion (Heidenhain, 1872; Darke and Smaje, 1973). Perhaps the most popular contender for the vasodilator agent has been bradykinin (Hilton and Lewis, 1957), although this has recently been seriously questioned (Schachter *et al.*, 1973).

There is evidence that the parasympathetic fibers which control the vessels concerned with erection of the penis of dogs are neither adrenergic nor cholinergic (Dorr and Brody, 1967).

2.4. Urinogenital System

2.4.1. Urinary Bladder

The pelvic nerves provide excitatory control of the urinary bladder and it was assumed for many years that this was mediated by classical cholinergic nerves, even though most of the response was resistant to blockade by atropine (Langley and Anderson, 1895). "Atropine resistance" to the excitatory autonomic nerves supplying the bladder appears to be a characteristic feature throughout vertebrates (see Section 8). One explanation is that the ACh receptors at the neuromuscular junctions are inaccessible to atropine; another is that atropine is displaced from the receptors competitively by high local concentrations of ACh. Another explanation for atropine resistance, favored by most recent workers in the field, is that the majority of the excitatory nerves supplying the bladder are noncholinergic. ATP (but not ACh) closely mimics the response to noncholinergic excitatory nerve stimulation in terms of its rates of both onset and decline (Buchthal and Kahlson, 1944; Matsumura *et al.*, 1968; Ambache and Zar, 1970) and has been proposed as the transmitter released by these nerves (Dumsday, 1971; Burnstock *et al.*, 1972*b*). As in the gut, the sensitivity of the bladder is greatest to ATP; ADP and AMP appear to have one-tenth and 1/200 of the potency, respectively (Ambache and Zar, 1970); cyclic AMP and *S*-adenosylmethionine are inactive. Further evidence for a purinergic nerve supply to the bladder comes from experiments in which the excitatory responses of the guinea pig bladder to both pelvic nerve stimulation and ATP were abolished by quinidine, without blocking the excitatory response to applied ACh (Burnstock *et al.*, 1972*b*). 5-HT, bradykinin, histamine, and catecholamine do not appear to be excitatory neurotransmitters in the bladder (Edvardsen, 1968; Ambache and Zar, 1970; Burnstock *et al.*, 1972*b*).

2.4.2. Reproductive Organs

a. Retractor Penis. Parasympathetic inhibitory fibers to the dog retractor penis which are neither adrenergic nor cholinergic have been described and compared to those known in the gut (Luduena and Grigas, 1966). However ATP does not appear to be the transmitter (Luduena and Grigas, 1972).

b. Uterus. Adenyl compounds cause contraction of the uterine smooth muscle of most species (see Burnstock, 1972). ATP was most potent AMP less so, and adenosine least potent. IMP had about one-tenth the potency of AMP, while adenine and hypoxanthine were inactive. Barsoum and Gaddum (1935) found that adenosine caused relaxation of the uteri of dogs, cats and rabbits, but Arulappu (1967) distinguished both excitatory and inhibitory receptors to adenosine in uterine muscle and showed selective block with phenothiazine and quinidine, respectively. Hervonen (1973) demonstrated nerve profiles containing a predominance of LOV in the rabbit uterus.

c. Seminal Vesicle. Evidence has been presented recently that ATP is a neurotransmitter in guinea pig seminal vesicle (Nakanishi and Takeda, 1972, 1973). The nonadrenergic, noncholinergic excitatory responses of the seminal vesicle to stimulation of the hypogastric nerve are closely mimicked by exogenously applied ATP.

2.5. Eye

Although there is no direct evidence for purinergic innervation of structures in the eye, some indirect evidence comes from a study of the reinnervation of ganglion-free transplants of guinea pig taenia coli into the anterior chamber of the eye (Burnstock *et al.*, 1971). As with other transplants of autonomically innervated smooth muscle into the anterior eye chamber (Malmfors and Olson, 1970; Malmfors *et al.*, 1971) the nerves in the transplant degenerate during the first day or two after transplantation. Nerves which normally supply the eye begin to reinnervate the transplant after about 1 wk and by 2–4 wk transmission is reestablished.

A surprising result of the reinnervation of transplants of taenia coli was that, in addition to adrenergic and cholinergic nerves, there was physiological and pharmacological evidence for reinnervation by purinergic nerves (Burnstock *et al.*, 1971). This result suggests that purinergic nerves are normally present supplying some structures in the eye. It is conceivable that the nonadrenergic inhibition seen in the taenia transplants might be due to antidromic stimulation of ocular sensory fibers which have penetrated the transplant. These might release ATP, as is reported in vascular smooth muscle (Holton, 1959) or prostaglandins, as is reported for the trigeminal sensory fibers in the iris (Ambache, 1957; Änggård and Samuelsson, 1964; Bergström *et al.*, 1968). However, it seems unlikely that the nonadrenergic response is due to sensory nerves growing into the taenia transplants in view of the close similarity of the inhibitory responses in transplanted taenia to those recorded in control tissue where they have been shown not to be due to sensory nerves (Burnstock *et al.*, 1966, 1971). It has been suggested that the fall in intraocular pressure and hyperemia of the iris in the rabbit eye following degeneration of the adrenergic nerve supply are due to the release of a nonadrenergic, noncholinergic transmitter substance (Treister and Bárány, 1970), probably from nerves of parasympathetic origin (Uusitalo and Palkama, 1971).

2.6. CNS

Since the purinergic nerve hypothesis was proposed in relation to the autonomic nervous system, there has been considerable interest in exploring the possibility that purinergic nerves are also present in the CNS.

Pull and McIlwain (1972*a,b,* 1973) have demonstrated the release of adenine nucleotides and their derivatives from superfused guinea pig neocortex subjected to field stimulation *in vitro.* Subsequently, Heller and McIlwain (1973) showed release of labeled nucleotides from isolated superior colliculus and lateral geniculate body incubated in [^{14}C]adenine and stimulated through an incoming optic tract, but not from preparations of piriform cortex stimulated through the lateral olfactory tract. McIlwain and his colleagues discussed their results in terms of a neurohumoral role for adenine derivatives in the brain. The amount of adenine derivatives (including adenine nucleotides, adenosine, inosine, and hypoxanthine) yielded to superfusates on excitation was estimated as 3–7 pmol/g tissue/stimulating pulse (Pull and McIlwain, 1972*b*). This compares with 6 pmol/g neural tissue/stimulating pulse calculated for release of ATP from toad stomach during stimulation of purinergic nerves (Burnstock *et al.*, 1970). Small amounts of adenosine or ATP applied to some regions of the brain *in situ* have electrophysiological, biochemical, and behavioral effects (Dale, 1935; Emmelin and Feldberg, 1948; Babskii and Malkiman, 1950; Feldberg and Sherwood, 1954; Galindo *et al.*, 1967; McLennan, 1970; Shneour and Hansen, 1971; Marley and Nistico, 1972; Phillis *et al.*, 1975), and in isolated tissues adenosine increases cyclic AMP content (see below). Inosine and hypoxanthine did not have these actions. Release of adenine nucleotides on excitation requires Ca^{2+} and is partly inhibited by tetrodotoxin (Pull and McIlwain, 1973). Synaptosomes take up [^{14}C]adenosine and show augmented output of ^{14}C derivatives on electrical stimulation (Kuroda and McIlwain, 1973).

Shimizu and his colleagues (see Shimizu, 1973; Shimizu and Okayama, 1973) support the view that purinergic nerves occur in the brain. They have found a specific adenosine-sensitive adenylate cyclase in the cerebrum of several mammalian species, including man, which is not present in other tissues. Release of label from slices of guinea pig cerebrum prelabeled with [^{14}C]adenine was blocked with tetrodotoxin, and was taken as evidence that release probably occurred from neuronal rather than glial cells. Although the stored form of neurotransmitter in the brain appears to be ATP, adenosine, ADP, and AMP are as effective as ATP as a stimulatory effector of brain adenyl cyclase. Shimizu suggests that ATP in purinergic nerves of the brain is metabolized to AMP during nerve stimulation or membrane depolarization and further converted by 5′-nucleotidase to adenosine before release.

Cyclic AMP is also being considered in relation to nerve transmission in the brain (see Daly, Chapter 2 of this volume). Cyclic AMP and phosphodiesterase have been demonstrated in isolated synaptic vesicles from presynaptic nerve endings in mouse brain (Boukma *et al.*, 1973), and Wooten *et al.* (1973) have suggested that cyclic 3′,5′-AMP may have a role in release, acting either in parallel with calcium or indirectly by mobilizing intracellular, bound calcium. However, most workers regard cyclic AMP accumulation in the brain as the result of the postsynaptic action of adenosine, catecholamines, serotonin, or histamine on adenylate cyclase receptors (Kakiuchi *et al.*, 1969; Rall and Sattin, 1970; Hoffer *et al.*, 1970; Sattin and Rall, 1970; Shimizu *et al.*, 1970, 1971; Forn and Krishna, 1971; Fumagalli *et al.*, 1971; Marx, 1972; Shimizu and Daly, 1970; Kodama *et al.*, 1973; Schultz and Daly, 1973*a,b*; Skolnick *et al.*, 1973; Huang and Daly, 1974; Huang *et al.*, 1972). Mouse neuroblastoma cells appear to offer a model system for investigation of the mechanism by which the cyclic AMP content of nerve cells responds to exogenous adenosine and of the effect of these responses on nerve function (Blume *et al.*, 1973). The response of the cyclic AMP-generating system to putative neurotransmitters differs between discrete functional regions of the cerebral cortex (Skolnick *et al.*, 1973).

The possibility that purinergic nerve components occur in the spinal cord has not yet been specifically investigated. However, parts of the cord have been shown to be sensitive to ATP (Buchthal *et al.*, 1947) and nerve profiles of small unmyelinated axons have been described in the outer margins of the substantia gelatinosa of the cat and dog spinal cord which contain a predominance of LOV, 750–1500 Å in diameter (Ralston, 1968; Westman and Bowsher, 1971; Bodian, 1972; Duncan and Morales, 1973*a,b*). These are comparable to those seen in purinergic nerve profiles in the gastrointestinal tract and lung (see Section 3). Similar profiles have been seen in the subnucleus caudalis of the trigeminal nerve (Kerr, 1970). These nerve profiles do not appear to be the same as those containing "large granular vesicles" in regions of the brain known to contain high levels of catecholamine (see Hökfelt, 1967; Bloom and Aghajanian, 1968) and therefore may be of particular interest in relation to the question of the origin of noncholinergic, nonadrenergic nerves supplying some regions of the intestine and some blood vessels (see Sections 2.1 and 2.4). According to Duncan and Morales (1973*b*), the origin of most of these nerve profiles in the substantia gelatinosa is in small neurons in the immediate vicinity of the axon terminals, but some dorsal root ganglion cells may also contribute. High levels of 5′-nucleotidase have been demonstrated histochemically in the substantia gelatinosa of mouse spinal cord (Suran, 1974).

3. FINE STRUCTURE AND HISTOCHEMISTRY OF PURINERGIC NERVES

3.1. Fine Structure of Purinergic Nerves

Purinergic nerve profiles are characterized by a predominance of large vesicles, termed "large opaque vesicles" (LOV) in order to distinguish them from the "large granular vesicles" (LGV) found in small numbers (3–5%) in most adrenergic and cholinergic nerves (Robinson *et al.*, 1971; Burnstock

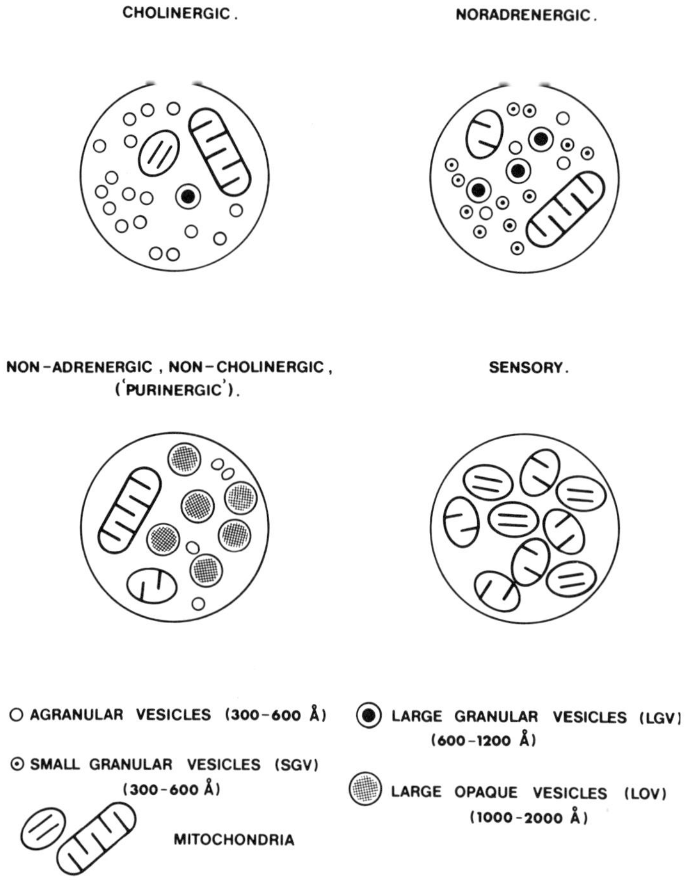

FIG. 2. Diagrammatic representation of sections through the terminal varicosities of autonomic nerves. Modified from Burnstock and Iwayama (1971).

and Iwayama, 1971; Burnstock, 1972) (Fig. 2). Purinergic nerve profiles sometimes also contain a few small oblate or spherical profiles with electron-transparent cores, as well as mitochondria. LOV differ from LGV in the following ways: (1) LOV are larger (800–2000 Å) than LGV (600–1200 Å); (2) while LGV are characterized by a well-defined electron-transparent halo between the granular core and the vesicle membrane, LOV do not have a prominent halo, although there appears to be some fixation and species variation in this respect; (3) the granular matrix in LOV is usually less dense than the granular core of LGV; (4) LGV are at first "loaded," then depleted and destroyed by 6-OHDA, while LOV are unaffected (see also Baumgarten *et al.*, 1970). LOV are not affected by catecholamine-depleting drugs, such as reserpine, metariminol, and guanethidine, nor are they labeled autoradiographically with catecholamines (Taxi and Droz, 1967). It has been shown recently that redback spider venom destroys LOV in purinergic nerve profiles in the guinea pig ileum and that this is associated with abolition of the inhibitory junction potentials (Einhorn, Hamilton, and Hirst, personal communication).

Many nerve profiles of this kind have been seen in the alimentary tract of a number of vertebrate species (see Burnstock, 1972, for earlier references; Baumgarten *et al.*, 1970; Pick, 1970; Tafuri and Maria, 1970; Burnstock and Iwayama, 1971; Gabella, 1972; Duchon *et al.*, 1973).

Identification of purinergic nerve profiles in the gastrointestinal tract is complicated because there appear to be two types of adrenergic axon (Dermietzel, 1971; Burnstock and Iwayama, 1971; Gabella, 1972; Furness and Costa, 1974). One type contains a predominance of small granular vesicles (300–700 Å in diameter) and is characteristic of adrenergic neurons in other parts of the body; these profiles are always seen in relation to blood vessels but are relatively rarely found in the muscle coats, except in some regions of the small intestine of rats and guinea pigs (Nagasawa and Mito, 1967; Gabella, 1970, 1972). The other type of adrenergic axon profile contains a predominance of LGV (500–1100 Å in diameter); these profiles have been seen in the stomach, upper small intestine, and colon, but not in the ileum of most species of mammals (Tafuri, 1964; Honjin *et al.*, 1965; Baumgarten *et al.*, 1970). These profiles can usually be distinguished from purinergic axons by examination of the size of the vesicle and the prominence of the halo between the granular core and vesicle membrane, but the surest method of identification is to use 5- or 6-OHDA as a marker (Baumgarten *et al.*, 1970; Gabella, 1971).

Profiles with a predominance of LOV have recently been observed in a variety of organs other than the gut in a wide range of species and open up the possibility that these organs may be supplied by purinergic nerves, although it must be recognized that morphological criteria alone are not sufficient to establish their presence. They have been observed in the lungs of toad (Robinson *et al.*, 1971), mouse (Hung *et al.*, 1972), chicken (Cook and King, 1970), and rabbit (Lauweryns *et al.*, 1973); the parathyroid gland (Unsicker, 1971; Altenähr, 1971); the avian adrenal gland (Unsicker, 1973*a*); enlarged axons of the area postrema (Ishii and Nakamura, 1972); the substantia gelatinosa of the spinal cord (Duncan and Morales, 1973*a,b*); amphibian sympathetic ganglia (Uchizono and Ohsawa, 1973); the testis of the immature tortoise (Unsicker, 1973*b*); and rabbit uterus, where they were unaffected by 6-OHDA (Hervonen, 1973). Profiles resembling purinergic nerves have also been described in hagfish red muscle fibers, although it has been suggested that these may be adrenergic (Korneliussen, 1973), dogfish myotomal muscle (Bone, 1972), and frog toe muscles (Osborne, 1971). The α-granules seen in platelets bear a close similarity to LOV and it is interesting that they disappear in association with the appearance of platelet nucleotides and calcium in the surrounding medium (Droller, 1973).

3.2. Histochemical Approaches to Localization of Purinergic Nerves

The distribution of enzymes which can degrade ATP and its derivatives is of interest because it might lead to the development of a histochemical method for identifying purinergic nerves. The role of these enzymes in purinergic transmission is considered in the model proposed in Fig. 1. Many enzymes with a wide variation in specificity can act to hydrolyze ATP. These include nonspecific alkaline phosphatases, polyphosphatases, nucleoside triphosphatases, and specific adenosine triphosphatases. Intracellular, as well as extracellular, localization of these enzymes should be considered in relation to the transmitter inactivation mechanism.

Although an extensive literature now exists describing adenosine triphosphatase (ATPase) localization in different tissues, any general correlation of the published work at this stage is complicated by variations in experimental conditions and species variation. The specificity of histochemical staining methods for ATPases has also been questioned, and this must be borne in mind when considering the reports of ATPase activity localized histochemically in a number of autonomically innervated tissues (see Burnstock, 1972). There seems to be some general agreement that ATPase activity in intestine and in some blood vessels differs from its activity in other tissues in that the staining is more intense and is not easily inhibited by the ATPase inhibitor, *p*-chloromercuribenzoate. In the circular muscle coat of the intestine, where, unlike the longitudinal coat, there are many close (150–200 Å) neuromuscular junctions (see Burnstock, 1970), ATPase has been shown to be localized in plasmalemmal vesicles in the smooth muscle membrane (Rostgaard and Barrnett, 1964; Lane, 1967). This might be significant in view of the abundance of plasmalemmal vesicles which are characteristic of the smooth muscle membrane adjacent to axons containing LOV at close neuromuscular junctions in the circular muscle of the colon and rectum (Nagasawa and Mito, 1967; Burnstock and Iwayama, 1971).

While the histochemical demonstration of 5′-nucleotidase has escaped the controversy that has surrounded the localization of ATPase, it does not appear to offer a promising method for localizing purinergic nerves (see Burnstock, 1972). The levels of 5′-nucleotidase vary greatly in different species (Reis, 1937, 1951; Freiman *et al.*, 1961; Borgers, 1971; Nakatsu and Drummond, 1972; Rubio *et al.*, 1973). High activity of 5′-nucleotidase has been reported in many smooth muscles, but less in cardiac or skeletal muscle of most vertebrate species. 5′-Nucleotidase activity was reported to be high in the longitudinal muscle of the intestine of the dog and in the outer layer of the circular muscle (Freiman *et al.*, 1961).

The recent synthesis of highly fluorescent ATP analogues (Secrist *et al.*, 1972; Yip and Tsou, 1973; Dutta *et al.*, 1973) provides an exciting possibility for the development of a fluorescence histochemical method for the detection of purinergic nerves. Immunofluorescence methods may also be applicable (see Bloom *et al.*, 1972). At the electron microscopic level, it may be possible to examine whether ATP is contained in LOV by using autoradiographic methods in a comparable way to those used for localization of labeled NA in adrenergic nerves (Wolfe *et al.*, 1962; Taxi and Droz, 1966; Devine and Simpson, 1968) and of other suspected neurotransmitters (Ehinger and Falck, 1971; Hösli and Hösli, 1972). However, autoradiographic localization of a diffusable substance like ATP may present serious difficulties (see Roth and Stumpf, 1969; Rogers, 1973).

4. ELECTROPHYSIOLOGY OF PURINERGIC TRANSMISSION

Most studies of the electrophysiology of purinergic nerve transmission have been carried out on the taenia coli of the guinea pig (see Bennett and Burnstock, 1968; Holman, 1970; Tomita, 1972; Tomita and Watanabe, 1973), but inhibitory junction potentials have also been recorded in the longitudinal muscle (Kuriyama *et al.*, 1967; Hidaka and Kuriyama, 1969) and circular muscle (Hirst and McKirdy, 1974) of guinea pig ileum and jejunum, circular muscle of guinea pig caecum (Ito and Kuriyama, 1973), longitudinal and circular muscle of the guinea pig and rabbit colon (Furness, 1969*a,b*; Julé and Gonella, 1972; Small, 1972), chicken and pigeon gizzard (Bennett, 1969*a,b,* 1970), guinea pig stomach (Kuriyama *et al.*, 1970; Beani *et al.*, 1971; Beck and Osa, 1971), cat esophagus (Diamant, 1973), guinea pig internal anal sphincter (Costa and Furness, 1973), and pig and sheep intestine (Furness, unpublished observations).

4.1. Inhibitory Junction Potentials

Stimulation of intramural purinergic nerves with single pulses of short duration (less than 0.3 ms) produces transient hyperpolarizations or inhibitory junction potentials (IJPs) of up to 25 mV in single smooth muscle cells of the gut (see Fig. 3a). IJPs have also been recorded in the stomach in response to stimulation of vagal nerves (Bennett, 1969*b*, 1970; Beani *et al.*, 1971). IJPs are unaffected by adrenergic neuron blocking agents or sympathetic denervation, but are abolished by tetrodotoxin.

Repetitive stimulation of purinergic nerves results in summation of individual IJPs and prolonged hyperpolarization of up to 50 mV (Fig. 3b,c,d). There may be some facilitation of the first two or three IJPs in a train (Furness, 1969*a*). The amplitude of IJPs in response to single stimuli can be graded with increasing strength of stimulation up to a maximum of about

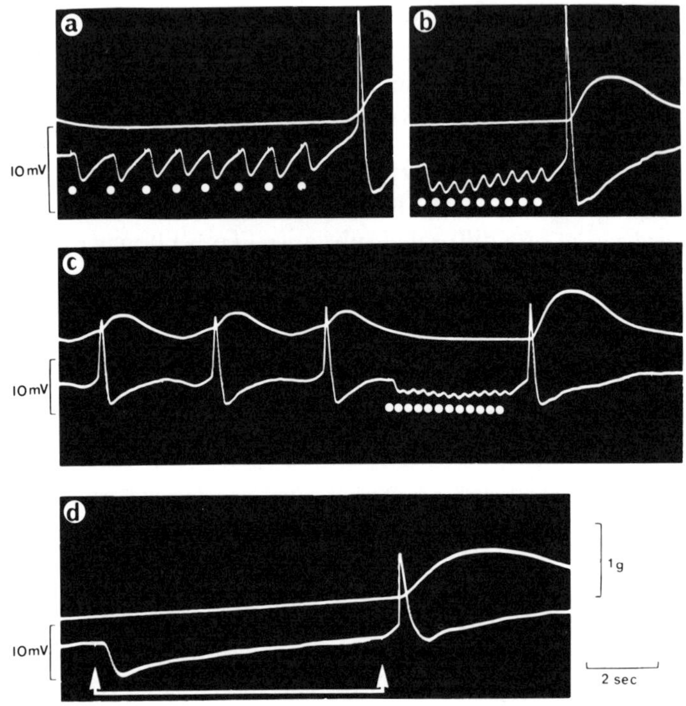

FIG. 3. Inhibitory junction potentials (IJPs) recorded in smooth muscle of the atropinized guinea-pig taenia coli in response to transmural stimulation of the intramural nerves remaining following degeneration of the adrenergic nerves by treatment of the animal with 6-hydroxydopamine (250 mg/kg intraperitoneally for 2 successive days) 7 days previously. Upper trace, mechanical record. Lower trace, changes in membrane potential recorded with a sucrose-gap method (Burnstock and Straub, 1958). The junction potentials recorded with this method are qualitatively, but not quantitatively, similar to those recorded with intracellular microelectrodes. (a) Responses to low-frequency stimulation (1/s). Note the long latency and slow time course of individual IJPs, and rebound excitation (spike and contraction) following cessation of stimulation. (b) Response to a stimulation frequency of 3/s. Note summation of individual IJPs and rebound contraction. (c) Response of a spontaneously active preparation to stimulation at 4/s. Note that the hyperpolarization maintained during repetitive stimulation raises the membrane potential beyond the zone of spontaneous initiation of action potentials and leads to relaxation. Rebound contraction follows cessation of stimulation. (d) Responses to high-frequency stimulation (30/s). Note that individual IJPs fuse and are represented by a maintained hyperpolarization followed by depolarization and rebound excitation on cessation of stimulation. From Burnstock (1972).

25 mV, whereas the maximum amplitude reached during repetitive stimulation is about 50 mV. The time taken to reach maximum hyperpolarization during repetitive stimulation at 10 Hz or more is slightly shorter than that of the rise time of a single IJP; when maximum hyperpolarization is reached, the response begins to decay in spite of continuing stimulation. At stimulation frequencies of 30 Hz or more, relaxation is rarely maintained for more

than about 15 s, and even at 5–10 Hz (Burnstock *et al.*, 1966) it begins to weaken after more than 20–30 s.

The latency of the IJP in response to postganglionic stimulation of the intramural purinergic nerves in the gut of various species is long (about 45–80 ms) relative to the latencies of adrenergic excitatory junction potentials (EJPs) recorded in nonintestinal smooth muscle (about 6–20 ms). This long latency, however, appears to be comparable to that of cholinergic EJPs recorded in smooth muscle. In the taenia coli, measurements of the increase in latency of the IJP at increasing distances between stimulating and recording electrodes implied a conduction velocity of 10–20 cm/s in the terminal regions of purinergic nerves (Bülbring and Tomita, 1967). This is consistent with a mean velocity of 16 cm/s measured for purinergic nerves supplying the circular muscle coat of the guinea pig caecum (Ito and Kuriyama, 1973).

The time course of the IJP appears to be comparable with or perhaps slightly longer than that of cholinergic EJPs recorded in the gut, but considerably longer than that of some adrenergic EJPs (see Table 1). The rise time of the IJP is about 150–250 ms; the decay time to half maximum is 200–400 ms and is approximately exponential, while the total duration of the IJP is of the order of 1 s. Since the maximum rate of spontaneously firing action potentials in the taenia coli is about 1 Hz (Burnstock, 1958; Holman, 1958; Jenkinson and Morton, 1965), an IJP lasting for about 1 s would be necessary to inhibit spike initiation and bring about relaxation.

Spontaneous hyperpolarizations with about the same time course and amplitude as IJPs have been observed on rare occasions in mammalian preparations (Bennett *et al.*, 1966*b*; Furness, 1969*a*) and appear in trains in the longitudinal coat of carp stomach (Ito and Kuriyama, 1971). They may represent the spontaneous release of packages of transmitter from terminal regions of nerves, but it seems more likely that they are the result of nerve impulses generated spontaneously in purinergic neurons in the myenteric ganglia. Regular spontaneous activity of circular muscle cells of the caecum following inhibition of purinergic inhibitory nerve activity with tetrodotoxin was considered to support this view (Ito and Kuriyama, 1973). It is interesting in this respect that bursts of spontaneous electrical activity have been recorded from single ganglion cells in Auerbach's plexus (Yokoyama, 1966; Wood, 1970, 1973; Ohkawa and Prosser, 1972).

A characteristic feature of the responses to stimulation of purinergic nerves is the rebound excitation which follows the main inhibitory response (Burnstock *et al.*, 1963; Bennett, 1966*a*; Campbell, 1966; Furness, 1971; Wood and Marsh, 1973). Rebound excitation usually occurs at the end of stimulation, but may also "break through" during a period of repetitive stimulation, especially at high frequency. The electrical activity associated with rebound contractions consists of depolarization following cessation of the hyperpolarization produced by purinergic inhibitory nerve stimulation

TABLE 1

Comparison of the Latency and Time Course of Junction Potentials in Response to Stimulation of Postganglionic Nerves

	Preparation	Minimum latency (ms)	Rise time (ms)	Total duration (ms)	Reference
Inhibitory junction potentials (purinergic)	Guinea pig taenia coli	80	200–500	1000	Bennett *et al.* (1966*b*)
		140	200–300		Bülbring and Tomita (1967)
	Rabbit colon	80	150–250	800–1200	Furness (1969*a*)
	Guinea pig colon	45	150–250	800–1300	Furness (1969*a*)
	Chick and pigeon gizzard	70	150–250	500–1500	Bennett (1969*b*)
	Guinea pig jejunum	50	120–280	1000	Kuriyama *et al.* (1967)
	Guinea pig stomach	150[a]	200–300	1000–1800	Beani *et al.* (1971)
Excitatory junction potentials (cholinergic)	Rabbit colon	220	~250	~600	Gillespie (1968)
	Guinea pig colon	15	150–200	400–700	Furness (1971)
	Guinea pig taenia coli	100	100–200	500–800	Bennett (1966*a*)
	Chick esophagus	90	150–250	600–1200	Ohashi (1971)
	Pigeon gizzard (anoxic)	70		430–900	Bennett (1969*b*)
	Guinea pig jejunum	20			Hidaka and Kuriyama (1969)
	Guinea pig stomach	150[a]	200	400–500	Beani *et al.* (1971)
Excitatory junction potentials (adrenergic)	Guinea pig vas deferens	20[a]	15–20 (half rise time)	1000	Burnstock and Holman (1961)
		6	40	500	Kuriyama (1963)
	Mouse vas deferens	10	10–20	100–250	Holman (1970)
		5	28–34		Furness (1970)
	Cat nictitating membrane	20	50–80	500	Eccles and Magladery (1937)
	Rabbit ear and mesenteric arteries	12	70–100	500–1000	Speden (1967)
	Guinea pig uterine artery	20		900–1000	Bell (1969)
End-plate potential	Rat skeletal neuromuscular junction	0·2	0·6	2–3	Boyd and Martin (1956)

[a]These figures for the latency of junction potentials were recorded following preganglionic stimulation.

(see Fig. 3d). The membrane potential usually depolarizes beyond its original level, with the result that the frequency of spike discharge, and therefore contraction, is greater than that seen before nerve stimulation. In preparations where there are no spontaneous spikes and associated contractions, stimulation of the inhibitory purinergic nerves still produces hyperpolarization. Since this is followed by rebound depolarization and subsequent initiation of spike activity, the result is to produce contraction rather than relaxation. The mechanism of rebound excitation is not understood.

4.2. Postsynaptic Action of Transmitter

Tomita and Watanabe (1973) showed that while hyperpolarization of smooth muscle cells in guinea pig taenia coli produced by sympathetic nerve stimulation and exogenously applied NE is due to an increase of both K^+ and Cl^- conductance, the hyperpolarization produced by purinergic nerves and exogenously applied ATP is due to a specific increase in K conductance. This result confirmed the earlier reports of the ionic basis of the IJP (Bennett *et al.*, 1963; Tomita, 1972) and was taken as support for the purinergic nerve hypothesis. Low $[Ca]_0$ and high $[Mg]_0$ have been reported to have no effect on the IJP (Hidaka and Kuriyama, 1969); this surprising observation needs further exploration.

4.3. Interaction of Purinergic with Cholinergic and Adrenergic Responses in Single Cells

In the absence of specific blocking agents, the response of most smooth muscle cells of the taenia coli to transmural stimulation appears to be a mixture of inhibitory and excitatory junction potentials. It is interesting that "multiaxonal junctions," where groups of up to seven axons lie in close apposition with single muscle cells, have been described in the circular coat of the intestine (Brettschneider, 1962; Rogers and Burnstock, 1966). Only small groups of cells are encountered which receive a predominantly cholinergic excitatory innervation (Bennett, 1966*b*). Occasionally, cells are found which respond to transmural stimulation with a diphasic response consisting of depolarization followed by hyperpolarization. In the presence of atropine, IJPs can be seen in the majority of cells (Bennett *et al.*, 1966*b*).

Stimulation of the pelvic nerves in rabbit and guinea pig evokes EJPs in most cells of the longitudinal muscle coat of the colon (Gillespie, 1962, 1968; Furness, 1969*a*), but transmural stimulation produces EJPs in only about 5% of the cells, IJPs being recorded in the remainder (Furness, 1969*a*). It seems likely that cholinergic nerves innervate most muscle cells but that when transmural stimulating electrodes are used the IJP dominates the response.

However, transmural stimulation is an artificial situation, and it is interesting that when descending inhibition was initiated in guinea pig ileum with a pressure balloon no IJPs were recorded in muscle cells of the longitudinal coat, only in the circular coat (Hirst and McKirdy, 1974).

The EJP appeared more frequently than the IJP in muscle cells of the guinea pig stomach when cholinergic and purinergic nerves were stimulated together via the vagus nerves (Beani *et al.*, 1971). Some cells in the guinea pig stomach, possibly in pacemaker regions, receive only vagal inhibitory innervation; other cells are innervated solely by cholinergic excitatory nerves (Beani *et al.*, 1971). In the avian gizzard, transmural stimulation frequently evoked an EJP followed by an IJP in the same cell (Bennett, 1970). Cells were encountered which responded to stimulation of the vagus nerve with an EJP and to perivascular nerve stimulation with an IJP; other cells showed the opposite responses. EJPs evoked in the same cell by both vagal and perivascular stimulation summed with each other. Some cells responded with IJPs to both vagal and perivascular stimulation.

5. PHYSIOLOGICAL ROLES OF PURINERGIC NERVES

The roles of inhibitory purinergic nerves in gastrointestinal function are beginning to be understood and related to the role of adrenergic inhibitory nerves (see Burnstock and Costa, 1973; Abrahamsson, 1973; Furness and Costa, 1973; Hirst and McKirdy, 1974) (Fig. 4). In general, purinergic nerves are involved in inhibitory reflexes which facilitate passage of material through the alimentary canal by opening sphincters, increasing stomach size, and expanding the intestine in front of an advancing bolus. Thus, as Furness and Costa (1973) described it so vividly, the purinergic neurons compose "the efferent link in a cascade of descending reflexes extending from the esophagus to the anal sphincter." It has also been suggested that intrinsic inhibitory neurons exert a continuous tonic suppression of gut motility, so that stimulation of the gut which leads to increased activity may be due to suppression of inhibitory nerve activity rather than to activation of excitatory nerves (Biber and Fara, 1973). In contrast, adrenergic nerves are concerned largely with modulating reflex activity in the gastrointestinal tract at both neuronal and muscle levels (see Burnstock and Costa, 1973; Furness and Costa, 1974). Adrenergic nerves are involved in the intestinointestinal reflex (Pearcy and Liere, 1926), the enterogastric reflex (Semba, 1954), and reflex inhibition of gastric motility elicited from the gastric antrum (see Abrahamsson, 1973). In view of the findings concerning the role of purinergic nerves in gastrointestinal function, a number of pathological conditions of the alimentary tract should be reexamined (see Christensen, 1971; Pfaffman and McFarlane, 1973).

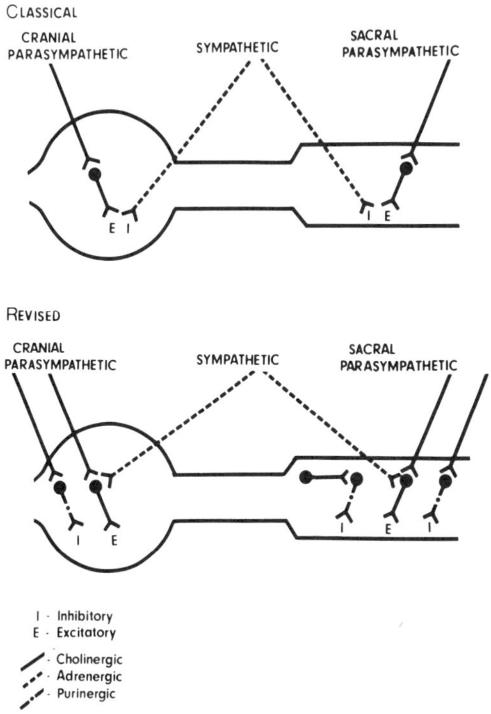

FIG. 4. Diagrammatic representation of the major components in the innervation of the gastrointestinal tract, incorporating the results of recent studies of the distribution of both adrenergic and purinergic nerves. The following qualifications to this simplified picture are necessary: (1) Early workers recognized the existence of some inhibitory fibers in the vagal outflow to the stomach, but they were usually assumed to be of sympathetic origin, so, for the sake of simplicity, they have not been included in the diagram representing the classical situation. (2) Some adrenergic nerves are known to directly innervate the circular muscle coat of parts of the intestine of most vertebrates and of the stomach of some species. (3) The noncholinergic, nonadrenergic *excitatory* innervation of regions of the gut (particularly in lower vertebrates) have not been included. Modified from Burnstock (1972).

The role of purinergic nerves that have been considered to supply organs other than the gut is far more speculative. Nevertheless, some of the ideas put forward have been included since they may stimulate further studies.

5.1. Reflex Relaxation of the Esophagogastric Junction

Relaxation at the junction of the esophagus and stomach occurs in advance of a bolus in the esophagus (Code and Schlegel, 1968; Dimarino and Cohen, 1974). This probably involves purinergic nerves in a similar reflex pathway as that concerned in "receptive relaxation" of the stomach (see below).

5.2. "Receptive Relaxation" of the Stomach

Vagal fibers with their cell bodies in the brain stem have been shown to form excitatory synapses with purinergic neurons in the stomach of several mammalian species (see Section 2.1). When a food bolus passes into the pharynx and upper esophagus, reflex "receptive relaxation" of the stomach (Cannon and Lieb, 1911) occurs, which is mediated by purinergic fibers via afferent and efferent reflex pathways in the vagus nerve (Abrahamsson and Jansson, 1969; Jansson, 1969; Ohga *et al.*, 1970; Abrahamsson, 1973). The vagal gastrogastric reflex mechanism (Barclay, 1936; Abrahamsson, 1971), whereby stimulation of gastric mechanoreceptors leads to relaxation of the stomach wall, also appears to be mediated by purinergic nerves (Abrahamsson and Jansson, 1973).

5.3. "Descending Inhibition" of Peristalsis

Relaxation of intestinal muscle in front of an aborally moving bolus during the process of peristalsis was first described at the end of the last century (Mall, 1896; Bayliss and Starling, 1899). This reflex descending inhibition involves intrinsic nervous pathways, since they are not interrupted by section of the sympathetic or parasympathetic extrinsic nerves. It is likely that purinergic neurons in the intestinal wall mediate these inhibitory reflexes, and various models of their arrangement in the wall of the intestine have been proposed (Furness and Costa, 1973; Burnstock and Costa, 1973; Hirst and McKirdy, 1974) (Figs. 5 and 6). In these models, the main axons of purinergic neurons extend in an anal direction for about 1.5 cm before supplying the circular muscle coat with branching varicose terminal fibers for a further 0.5 cm (Hirst and McKirdy, 1974). Experiments with ganglion blockers suggest that they are controlled by intramural cholinergic interneurons. During peristalsis, contraction occurs behind the bolus as it moves toward the anus (see Kosterlitz, 1968; Crema, 1970). The "rebound contractions" following the inhibitory response of smooth muscle to purinergic nerves (see Section 4.1) are likely to facilitate this phase. It has been proposed that adrenergic nerves may antagonize descending inhibition in intestine by presynaptic inhibition of cholinergic terminals on purinergic neurons (Hirst and McKirdy, personal communication).

5.4. Reflex Relaxation of the Internal Anal Sphincter

Reflex inhibition of the internal anal sphincter in response to rectal distension is likely to be mediated by purinergic nerves since it is unaffected

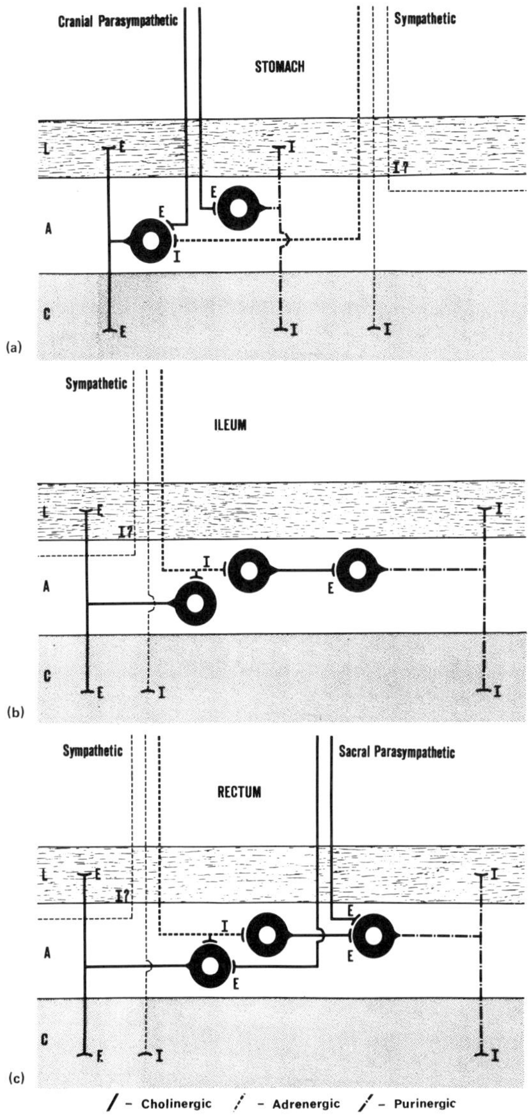

FIG. 5. Diagrammatic representation of the main arrangement of nerve components in the wall of mammalian (a) stomach, (b) ileum, and (c) rectum. Note that the adrenergic nerves are concerned largely with extrinsic modulation of gut motility at both neuronal and muscle levels and are not concerned with normal propulsive function, while the purinergic nerves are concerned with normal propulsive function, including "receptive relaxation" of the stomach, "descending inhibition" in peristalsis, and reflex relaxation of the anal sphincter. Note also that the figure does not include the small number of postganglionic, nonadrenergic fibers to the stomach (in the vagus nerves) and to the rectum (in the pelvic nerves). from Burnstock and Costa (1973).

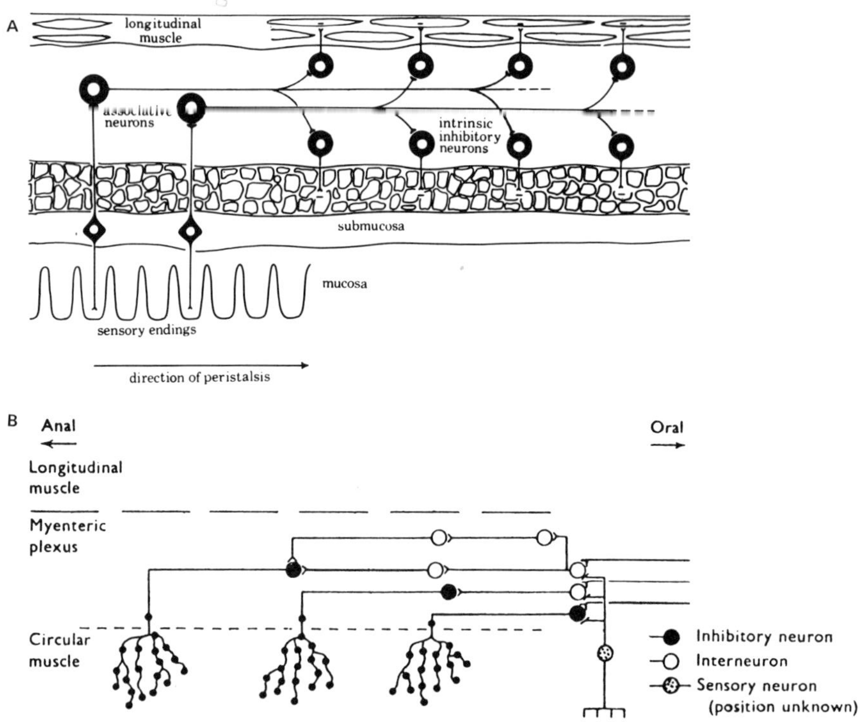

FIG. 6. (A) Diagrammatic representation of the arrangement of the neurons involved in the descending inhibitory reflex in the intestine. Neurons with sensory endings in the mucosa form excitatory connections with associative neurons whose processes run aborally in Auerbach's plexus. Impulses passing down the axons of associative neurons are transmitted to inhibitory cells whose processes innervate both the longitudinal and circular muscle coats. From Furness and Costa (1973). (B) Schematic representation of the descending inhibitory pathway. Afferent processes of the sensory neuron (cell body, stippled circle) are stimulated by distension; efferent processes impinge on the cell body of an interneuron (open circle) or may impinge directly on the cell body of an inhibitory neuron (large filled circle). Inhibitory fibers run in an anal direction; inhibitory transmitter is assumed to be released from varicosities (small filled circles). Note that the direction of the anus is opposite in this model from that depicted in A and in Fig. 5. From Hirst and McKirdy (1974).

by adrenergic and cholinergic receptor blocking agents and both ACh and NE contract the sphincter (Garrett and Howard, 1972; Costa and Furness, 1973). In Hirschsprung's disease, where the rectum is aganglionic, this reflex does not occur (Howard and Nixon, 1968; Ehrenpreis, 1971; see also Webster, 1974).

5.5. Vomiting and Nausea

The involvement of purinergic nerves in the vomiting response has recently been examined (Abrahamsson and Thorén, 1972, 1973;

Abrahamsson *et al.*, 1973). They showed that reflex relaxation of the cat stomach which accompanies or precedes the vomiting response elicited by mechanical or chemical stimulation of ventricle receptors, by stimulation of cardiac afferent fibers or by the centrally acting emetic drug apomorphine (see Lumsden and Holden, 1969) was mediated by the vagal purinergic nerve pathway. Apomorphine acts on the chemoreceptor trigger zone in area postrema from which the vomiting center, located deeper in the medulla, is then activated (Wang and Borison, 1952).

5.6. Bronchodilatation, Asphyxia, Asthma

As discussed earlier (see Section 2.1), purinergic nerves have been implicated in bronchodilatation of the vertebrate lung. Low doses of ATP dilate the bronchioles of adults (Bennett and Drury, 1931; Bianchi *et al.*, 1963; Hauge, 1966). ATP has been used effectively to combat asphyxia in the newborn, although it has been assumed that it acts primarily as a vasodilator (Lobanov, 1961; Znamenáček and Přibylová, 1966; Hanikova *et al.*, 1973). Release of amines from mast cells in the lung can lead to asthmatic spasm, and it is of interest in this respect that of all the putative neurotransmitters tested only ATP degranulates isolated mast cells (Kiernan, 1972*a*).

5.7. Coughing

Noncholinergic, nonadrenergic nerves, which have comparable properties to those of purinergic nerves in the gastrointestinal tract, have been shown to supply the trachea (see Section 2.2). It has been suggested that these nerves may be of importance in control of muscle tone during the cough (Coburn and Tomita, 1973), since they are found in greater abundance in the compressible (thoracic) segment of the trachea, which is considered to be involved in the cough mechanism (Coburn, 1972).

5.8. Inflammation of the Skin

Release of histamine from mast cells in response to ATP released from nerves during "axonal reflexes" has been proposed as the basis of vasodilatation of skin vessels (Kiernan, 1972*b*). Release of histamine and increase in vascular permeability leading to acute inflammation induced by ATP have been demonstrated (Ichikawa *et al.*, 1972), and there are several reports that ATP is the most potent of suspected neurotransmitter substances to release histamine from mast cells (Bloom *et al.*, 1970; Kiernan, 1972*a*; Johansen and Chakravarty, 1972).

5.9. Activities in the CNS

It is clearly premature to think in terms of the role of purinergic nerves in CNS function; however, some interesting observations on the actions of adenyl compounds on CNS activities are reported which may provoke further investigation. Adenine nucleotides have been implicated in depressive illness (Hansen, 1972; Abdulla and McFarlane, 1972; Moyes, 1973). Whole blood ATP and/or adenosine is significantly elevated in patients diagnosed as schizophrenic or in psychotic and neurotic depression (Hansen, 1972). In the hypothesis proposed for the mechanism of depression by Abdulla and McFarlane (1972), the effect of adenine nucleotides on prostaglandin biosynthesis is implicated.

Inherited disorder of purine metabolism in the brain has been related to psychomotor retardation, athetosis, and self-mutilation (Lesch–Nyhan syndrome) (Rosenbloom *et al.*, 1967; Seegmiller *et al.*, 1967; Berman *et al.*, 1969). Adenine therapy has been used for Lesch–Nyhan syndrome (Schulman *et al.*, 1971).

Premature arousal of squirrels from periods of hibernation is evoked by adenosine and adenine nucleotides, but not by other purine nucleotides, and it has been suggested that this effect is due to their action on neurons in the CNS (Twente and Giorgio, 1970).

6. EVIDENCE THAT ATP IS THE PURINERGIC NERVE TRANSMITTER

Several criteria need to be satisfied before a substance can be established as a neurotransmitter: (1) the substance and the enzymes necessary for its formation must be present in the neuron; (2) the substance must be released from the terminal axon when the nerve is activated; (3) the effect of the transmitter released on nerve stimulation must be mimicked by the exogenous application of the substance to the effector; (4) a mechanism for inactivation of the substance must be present, whether it involves enzyme action or uptake or both; (5) drugs which reduce or potentiate nerve-mediated responses should similarly affect the responses to the exogenously applied substance. Application of these criteria appears to establish ATP as the transmitter substance released by purinergic nerves. The evidence has been considered in detail elsewhere (Burnstock, 1972) and will be summarized in this section, with more recent results incorporated. A variety of substances other than ATP have been explored as the possible transmitter released from nonadrenergic, noncholinergic inhibitory nerves in the gut, including catecholamines, 5-HT, cyclic AMP, histamine, prostaglandins, various amino acids such as alanine, arginine, histidine, glycine, glutamic acid, and γ-aminobutyric acid, and the polypeptides bradykinin and substance P. However, these substances were rejected as contenders by most workers on the grounds that they were either inactive or did not mimic the nerve-mediated responses, that specific blocking drugs for these substances did not affect the nerve-mediated response, or that their action was by stimulation of nerves and not by direct action on smooth muscle.

6.1. Formation and Storage of ATP

Both ATP and the enzyme systems which synthesize ATP occur ubiquitously in cells, so that it is not contentious that purinergic nerves are also able to produce and store ATP. The important question, however, is whether ATP is stored in nerve terminals in such a way that it can be released during nerve stimulation. Tritium-labeled adenosine is taken up by preparations of stomach and intestine and rapidly converted largely to [^{3}H]ATP (Su *et al.*, 1971). Analysis of the radioactivity in serial frozen sections shows that most of the labeled ATP is stored in nerves (see Burnstock, 1972). Stimulation of enteric nerves in the guinea-pig taenia coli after [^{3}H]adenosine loading results in release of tritium (Su *et al.*, 1971; Kuchii *et al.*, 1973; Rutherford, personal communication). Some release of tritium from adrenergic nerves has been demonstrated, but this is prevented, as is release of NE, by guanethidine. Release of tritium is markedly reduced by tetrodotoxin and is not correlated with changes in muscle tone *per se*, either spontaneous or drug induced. Kuchii *et al.* (1973) reported that release of tritium from the [^{3}H]adenosine-loaded taenia coli was resistant to tetrodotoxin, but under their experimental conditions it seems likely that most of the labeled compound was being released from a nonnervous pool.

Isolation of LOV from purinergic nerves by differential centrifugation will be necessary before vesicle-bound storage of ATP in these nerves can be established. Electron microscopic–autoradiographic experiments to see if [^{3}H]ATP is localized in LOV should also be carried out.

6.2. Release of ATP

Stimulation of purinergic fibers in the vagus nerves to the stomach increases the venous efflux of adenosine and inosine in both guinea pigs and toads. These are likely to be the breakdown products of adenine nucleotides since ATP introduced into the same perfusing system is quickly broken down into comparable proportions of adenosine and inosine (Burnstock *et al.*, 1970; Satchell and Burnstock, 1971).

Direct support for release of ATP from purinergic nerves to the gut comes from the recent demonstration of an eight- to twentyfold increase in

ATP (determined with the highly sensitive luciferin–luciferase firefly assay technique) in the superfusate of guinea pig taenia coli following stimulation of the intramural nerves in the presence of guanethidine (Paddle and Burnstock, 1975). Relaxations of the same magnitude produced by stimulation of the periarterial sympathetic (adrenergic) nerves produced only about a two- to fivefold increase in ATP release, which was blocked by guanethidine (Fig. 7).

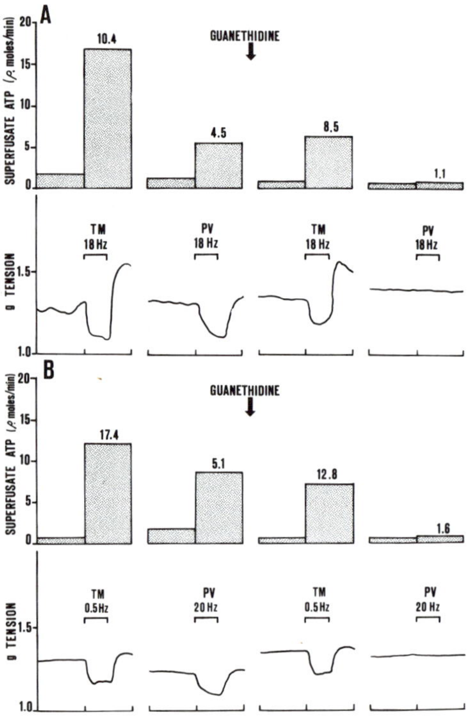

FIG. 7. A comparison of the ATP released determined with the luciferin–luciferase firefly method from guinea pig taenia coli during perivascular (adrenergic) nerve stimulation (PV) and transmural stimulation of intramural nerves (TM). Hyoscine (0.5 μg/ml) was present throughout. Releases during equiamplitude responses are compared. This is achieved in (A) by stimulation of both perivascular nerves and intramural nerves for an equal number of pulses (duration 0.5 ms) at 18 Hz for 30-s periods and in (B) by stimulation (pulse duration 0.5 ms) of perivascular nerves at 20 Hz (600 pulses) and intramural nerves at 0.5 Hz (15 pulses) for 30-s periods. Maximal responses to stimulation of purinergic nerves occur at 5 Hz, while responses to adrenergic nerve stimulation are maximal above 30 Hz. From Burnstock *et al.* (1966). Histograms compare the amounts of ATP (in picomoles) in the superfusate in-60 s periods both before and after stimulation. The numbers represent the percentage increase in ATP release $\times 100$. Note that under both conditions (A and B) of stimulation (1) more ATP is released in response to transmural than to perivascular stimulation and (2) whereas responses to perivascular stimulation and ATP release are blocked by guanethidine (2.4 μg/ml) for 30 min the responses to transmural stimulation are only partially reduced. Courtesy of Paddle and Burnstock (unpublished results).

At least four possibilities that the purine nucleotides or nucleosides released on nerve stimulation are not neurotransmitter substances but appear for other reasons should be considered:

1. Is the ATP being released from nerve membranes during propagation of an action potential? If so, this is not a significant contribution, since the amount of nucleosides collected during stimulation of purinergic nerves is at least a thousandfold greater than that reported to be collected from axons during impulse propagation (Abood *et al.*, 1962; Kuperman *et al.*, 1964; Satchell and Burnstock, 1971).
2. Are the nucleosides coming from muscle? A significant contribution from muscle is unlikely since stimulation of Auerbach's plexus from turkey gizzard (which contains many purinergic inhibitory nerves) dissected free of the underlying muscle still resulted in a substantial efflux of purine nucleotides, in this case mostly AMP. Tetrodotoxin block of most of the label released into the superfusate during transmural stimulation of guinea pig taenia coli incubated in [^{3}H]adenosine (10^{-7}M) also argues against this possibility (Rutherford, personal communication).
3. Is the ATP being released as a result of antidromic stimulation of sensory nerves? This was suggested by Holton (1959) to explain the release of ATP during stimulation of the great auricular nerve. However, this is an unlikely explanation of the release of nucleosides from stomach preparations since the fibers in the vagal trunk mediating gastric inhibition are preganglionic and therefore efferent and no effects on motility attributable to antidromic stimulation of vagal sensory fibers have been observed. This was directly supported by an experiment carried out by B. Cragg, who showed that the purinergic inhibitory response to stimulation of the vagal nerves supplying the rabbit stomach was abolished after surgical degeneration of the efferent, but not afferent, component.
4. Does the ATP released merely accompany the "real" (but unidentified) transmitter substance from purinergic inhibitory nerves? ATP is released together with catecholamine from adrenal medullary vesicles and whole glands (Douglas, 1968; Stevens *et al.*, 1972), and it seems likely that some ATP is released together with NE from adrenergic nerves (Geffen and Livett, 1971; Su *et al.*, 1971; Smith and Winkler, 1972; Paddle and Burnstock, 1974*b*). ATP has also been located together with Ach in a ratio of 1:11 in synaptic vesicles of cholinergic nerves supplying the electric organ of torpedine rays (Whittaker *et al.*, 1972; Bohan *et al.*, 1973). However, whether it is released together with ACh, as has been suggested by Silinsky and Hubbard (1973) for phrenic nerves supplying the rat diaphragm, or whether the fall in vesicular ATP that closely parallels the fall in ACh

is due to hydrolysis of ATP (Zimmerman and Whittaker, 1974) is still not resolved.

6.3. Direct Actions of Purine Nucleotides and Nucleosides on Smooth Muscle

The high sensitivity of smooth muscle to adenine nucleotides was recognized long before ATP was postulated as a neurotransmitter. The form and time course of the response to exogenously applied ATP closely mimic those of the response to purinergic nerve stimulation. Typically the relaxation produced by ATP and nerve stimulation rapidly reaches a maximum, which quickly declines; this is in contrast to the inhibitory responses to NE and sympathetic nerve stimulation, which reach a maximum more slowly and are retained for a longer time. As discussed earlier, electrophysiological studies by Tomita and Watanabe (1973) have shown that while NE and sympathetic nerve stimulation increase the conductance of the smooth muscle membrane to both K^+ and Cl^- the transmitter released from purinergic nerves and ATP both produce a specific increase in K^+ conductance only.

Of the purine compounds, ATP and ADP are the strongest contenders for the transmitter substance in view of their high potency; AMP, cyclic AMP, and adenosine are some ten- to a hundredfold less potent, while inosine and adenine are pharmacologically inactive. ATP is the most likely transmitter, since [^{3}H]adenosine taken up into the taenia coli is rapidly converted and stored largely as [^{3}H]ATP, with only traces of [^{3}H]ADP detectable. ATP does not act indirectly by stimulating purinergic nerves since its action is unaffected by tetrodotoxin.

Boyd (1973) has pointed out that the separation of 4–6 Å between the charged centers in the ATP molecule is similar to the separation of those in the established neurotransmitters, NE and ACh, as well as in 5-HT, γ-aminobutyric acid, and glycine. This similarity in molecular conformation, while not constituting proof of similarity of action, was taken as support for the hypothesis that nucleotides may serve as nerve transmitter substances.

6.4. Inactivation of ATP

By analogy with other neuroeffector systems, if purinergic nerves release ATP, the action of ATP is likely to be terminated by uptake into the nerves and/or by breakdown of ATP by enzymes into compounds with greatly reduced potency. At cholinergic junctions, choline is taken up by the nerves after degradation of released ACh by acetylcholinesterase (Potter, 1970), while at adrenergic junctions there are uptake and reutilization of nerve-released NE (Iversen, 1967; Blakeley *et al.*, 1969).

Mg^{2+}-activated ATPase, 5′-nucleotidase, and adenosine deaminase, enzymes capable of breaking ATP down into pharmacologically inactive compounds, are known to be present in the gut wall, although their precise localization remains to be determined (see Section 3.2).

Double tracer experiments have shown that adenosine, but not ATP, ADP, AMP, or inosine, is taken up by the nerves. This suggests that, by analogy with the inactivation mechanism known for cholinergic nerves, the ATP released from purinergic nerves is rapidly broken down by ATPase and 5′-nucleotidase to adenosine, which is then taken up by the nerves to be resynthesized into ATP and reestablished in physiological stores. Any adenosine which is not taken up would then be broken down by adenosine deaminase to inosine, which is pharmacologically inactive and can diffuse into the circulation. Some support for this suggestion comes from the observation that the overflow of tritium-labeled compounds from taenia coli incubated in [^{3}H]adenosine on stimulation of the nerves at 5 Hz (which produces maximal inhibitory responses) is low, whereas there is a higher overflow with stimulation at 30 Hz. Further, dipyridamole, which is an adenosine uptake inhibitor, potentiates the responses to both purinergic nerve stimulation (particularly at low frequency) and exogenously applied ATP (Satchell *et al.*, 1972).

6.5. Antagonism and Potentiation of Responses to Nerve Stimulation and ATP

There have been a few studies on drugs which affect responses to purine nucleotides that have helped in the search for compounds that block or potentiate purinergic nerve transmission. Several drugs provide evidence which is consistent with the purinergic hypothesis. High concentrations of quinidine (Burnstock *et al.*, 1970) and imidazoline compounds, such as phentolamine (Rikimara *et al.*, 1971*b*; Tomita and Watanabe, 1973), antazoline, and tolazoline (Satchell *et al.*, 1973), produce parallel reduction of the responses of the intestine to purinergic nerve stimulation and ATP, but have less effect on the inhibitory response to other compounds such as amyl nitrite (see also Section 7.2). However, it is unlikely that these drugs are causing specific blockade of purinergic transmission since they are known to have a wide range of pharmacological actions (Nickerson, 1970). It was recently reported that relatively low concentrations of 2-2′-pyridylisatogen (Patterson and Wibberley, 1965) produced specific blockade of the action of ATP on guinea pig taenia coli (Hooper *et al.*, 1974). This drug reduces responses of the preparation to purinergic nerve stimulation and ATP more than responses to perivascular sympathetic nerve stimulation or NE (Satchell, personal communication).

Further support for the purinergic hypothesis comes from experiments on tachyphylaxis to ATP in the rabbit. When tachyphylaxis to repeated doses of ATP is produced in the ileum, there is a consistent depression of the inhibitory responses to purinergic nerve stimulation, but not to adrenergic nerve stimulation (Burnstock *et al.*, 1970). Weston (1973*a,b*) has recently contested this result. However, it is puzzling that in his hands nonadrenergic inhibitory responses continue to increase even at 32 Hz, unlike the findings of other workers, who report optimal responses to nonadrenergic inhibitory nerve stimulation at about 5 Hz. The experiments carried out by Burnstock *et al.*, (1970) were confined to the longitudinal muscle coat of the intestine, which is sparsely innervated by purinergic nerves (Hirst and McKirdy, 1974), while in the experiments of Weston (1973*a*) on the guinea pig ileum the responses of both the longitudinal and circular coat (which is densely innervated by purinergic nerves) during the peristaltic reflex were used as the measure of nonadrenergic inhibitory nerve activity. However, desensitization to ATP was demonstrated only in the longitudinal coat. Higher concentrations of transmitter reaching receptor sites in the circular muscle coat, where close (200 Å) neuromuscular junctions are present, may overcome the desensitizing action of ATP, in contrast to the more diffuse action of exogenously applied ATP or ATP reaching longitudinal muscle from distant purinergic nerves.

Low concentrations of dipyridamole, a drug most commonly used as a coronary vasodilator, potentiate the responses of the guinea pig taenia coli to both purinergic nerve stimulation and ATP, while not altering (or even reducing) the inhibitory response to sympathetic nerve stimulation and NE (Satchell *et al.*, 1972). This drug has been shown to inhibit the uptake of adenosine into the heart (Kolassa *et al.*, 1971; Liu and Feinberg, 1973; Hopkins, 1973*b*) as well as into taenia coli (Satchell *et al.*, 1972). When, following the classical approach of Loewi, two strips of taenia coli in the presence of hyoscine and guanethidine were arranged in series so that the perfusate of one preparation flowed over the second, a short-lasting relaxation of the lower preparation was observed following stimulation of the donor preparation at 30 Hz, but rarely at 5 Hz. However, after addition of dipyridamole the recipient preparation produced prolonged relaxation following stimulation of the donor preparation at both 5 and 30 Hz (Burnstock, 1972).

7. PHARMACOLOGY OF ADENYL COMPOUNDS AND PURINERGIC TRANSMISSION

In this section, drugs which antagonize the action of adenyl compounds and those which potentiate their action on a variety of preparations will be considered, although these drugs consist of a remarkable collection of largely unrelated compounds. Reports of the actions of these drugs on the responses of smooth muscle to stimulation of purinergic nerves will be included, wherever they have been examined, although experiments with blockers or potentiators of a substance such as ATP, which is widely involved in a number of vital cellular processes including muscle contraction, must be interpreted with great care.

7.1. Inhibitory and Excitatory Action of Adenyl Compounds

While the predominant response of mammalian gut to ATP is relaxation, excitatory responses of two kinds are sometimes revealed (see Burnstock, 1972). One kind consists of contractions after washout of ATP, and is probably equivalent to the phenomenon of "rebound excitation" that follows purinergic inhibitory responses rather than a direct response to ATP. The second type of excitatory action occurs while the nucleotide is still present in the organ bath and is probably a direct excitatory effect of ATP. Occasionally a brief contraction precedes relaxation; in some preparations, especially those in which the tone is commonly low (e.g., guinea pig ileum and rabbit stomach), contractions tend to occur only when high concentrations of ATP are applied. Similar dual effects of ATP have also been reported on other gut segments. For example, adenyl compounds have been reported to contract or relax amphibian stomach and guinea pig ileum. The possibility that these effects are related to the presence of excitatory receptors for purinergic nerves should be considered.

If the extrinsic or intramural autonomic nerves supplying a large variety of isolated smooth muscle preparations are stimulated in the presence of atropine and adrenergic neuron blocking agents, nerve responses are often revealed which may be inhibitory or excitatory or a mixture of both. In most preparations so far examined, these responses are mimicked by the direct action of ATP (Ambache and Zar, 1970; Burnstock *et al.*, 1970, 1972*a,b*; Sneddon *et al.*, 1973): if the nerve-mediated response is relaxation (as it is in most mammalian gut segments), then ATP causes a mimicking relaxation; if the nerve-mediated response is contraction (as is the case in the intestine of lower vertebrates or in the urinary bladder), then ATP also causes contraction; if the nerve-mediated response is biphasic (usually relaxation followed by contraction), then ATP produces an identical biphasic response. In those preparations which are supplied by both nonadrenergic inhibitory and noncholinergic excitatory nerves (e.g., guinea pig ileum, toad stomach), the responses to transmural stimulation and applied ATP do not always agree, but this may be explicable in terms of the geometry of electrode placement in relation to the two types of nerve fibers. This situation may be comparable to adrenergic excitatory and inhibitory control of adjacent regions of the gastrointestinal tract (see Furness and Burnstock, 1975).

These observations raise the possibility that receptors mediating either relaxation or contraction may exist for ATP released from purinergic nerves. This would not be surprising, since comparable dual effects are already established for the action of both cholinergic and adrenergic nerves on autonomic effectors. Receptors for catecholamines have been separated into two types, α and β, which are distinguished by the relative potencies of epinephrine, NE, and isoprenaline (Ahlquist, 1948). These receptors may mediate excitation or inhibition, depending on the tissue, and in many tissues mediate antagonistic responses (Triggle, 1965; Ahlquist, 1966). The possibility has been examined that two types of ATP receptors can be distinguished by the criteria developed for adrenoceptors. Thus the potencies of different members of the adenine nucleotide series (ATP, ADP, AMP, and adenosine) were studied on a variety of tissues, including guinea pig taenia coli and bladder and lizard and toad ileum (Smythe, 1971; Burnstock *et al.*, 1972*a,b*; Sneddon *et al.*, 1973). In these preparations, regardless of whether the response was inhibitory or excitatory, ATP was usually the most potent, the order being ATP $\geqslant$ ADP $>$ AMP $\geqslant$ adenosine. Studies of the relative potencies of nucleotides and nucleosides on other tissues have generally given the same result (see Burnstock, 1972). Thus the different actions of adenine nucleotides in causing contraction or relaxation of smooth muscle do not appear to reflect different receptor types which are distinguishable on the basis of relative potencies as is the case for adrenoceptors. However, in view of the evidence for rapid breakdown of ATP and ADP (Hopkins, 1973*a*; Paddle and Burnstock, 1974*a*) and for the uptake of adenosine, but not adenine nucleotides or inosine, into purinergic nerves, the true order of potency may be obscured in isolated organ experiments (Satchell and Burnstock, 1974).

The possibility of distinguishing different muscle receptors for adenyl compounds on the basis of the differential action of blocking agents has also been explored. In a careful study of the effect of adenyl compounds and their antagonists on the isolated uterus of guinea pigs, kittens, rats, and rabbits, Arulappu (1967) concluded that two different receptors were involved: one receptor (related to the contractile action of adenosine) was blocked by the phenothiazines and the dibenzazepines; another receptor (related to the relaxing action of adenosine) was blocked by quinidine. Quinidine has been shown to block the excitatory action of ATP on the gut of lower vertebrates, as well as the inhibitory action of ATP on mammalian gut preparations (Burnstock *et al.*, 1970; Sneddon *et al.*, 1973). In the bladder, the contraction produced by ATP or by noncholinergic, nonadrenergic nerves was blocked by quinidine, but the inhibitory action of adenosine was not (Burnstock *et al.*, 1972*b*). There is some recent evidence to indicate that whereas adenosine acts on a smooth muscle receptor system involving adenyl cyclase and leads to the production of cyclic AMP (see also Section 2.6), ATP does not (Rutherford, personal communication).

The structure–activity relationships of a number of analogues of adenine nucleotides and nucleosides in vascular and intestinal smooth muscle and in cardiac muscle have been described. Activity is increased by attaching a ribose group to the purine nucleus, although the ribose residue itself is not active (Sydow and Ahlquist, 1954). The presence of an amino group on the purine ring is necessary for the activity of these compounds (Bennett and Drury, 1931; Sydow and Ahlquist, 1954), since inosine, the deaminated metabolite of adenosine, has little pharmacological action on smooth muscle. The position of the amino group on the ring also affects activity; 2-aminopurine riboside produces a positive chronotropic effect on the heart, while 6-aminopurine riboside (adenosine) gives the opposite effect (James, 1965). A phosphate group attached to the D-ribose is not essential for the negative chronotropic effect of adenosine, but its position nevertheless modifies the nature of the effect. In the urinary bladder, adenyl compounds containing a pyrophosphate bond produce excitation only. However, sodium pyrophosphate alone has no effect on the bladder, indicating that both a purine compound and a pyrophosphate group are necessary for excitatory activity (Burnstock *et al.*, 1972*b*). In contrast, adenosine (but not inosine or guanosine) causes inhibition of the bladder. Compounds with an extended chain of phosphate groupings or compounds in which methylene substitution confers resistance of the phosphate chain to enzymatic cleavage are more potent than ATP in causing relaxation of smooth muscle of pulmonary vessels and intestine (Gaddum and Holtz, 1933; Gough *et al.*, 1973; Satchell and Maguire, 1974). Compounds with more than one phosphate grouping cause a rapid relaxation of the taenia coli, except for the α,β-methylene substituted nucleotides, which take at least 40% longer to reach maximum. Substitution in the 2-position of the purine nucleus by chloro or methylthio groups markedly increases the relative activity of the diphosphates and triphosphates. It has been suggested (Satchell and Maguire, 1974) that the activity of ATP is rapidly terminated due to cleavage of its phosphate moiety and rapid removal of its adenosine metabolite by further degradation or by uptake into the tissue.

Some studies have been carried out on the vasodilator effects of analogues of adenosine and AMP (Angus *et al.*, 1971; Einstein *et al.*, 1972). Alkylthio and alkylamino substitutions reduce the dilator activity of adenosine. 2-Methylthio- and 2-methylaminoadenosines are less potent than the corresponding ethyl analogues. A further increase in length of the alkylthio side-chain enhances dilator activity, but branching of the propyl chain reduces this effect. The duration of coronary dilator activity is increased by these compounds to 5–15 times that of adenosine. Conversion of the adenosine analogues to their monophosphorylated derivatives generally reduces their dilator activity to about one-third.

The relaxant effects of a series of adenosine analogues were compared on isolated intestinal and aortic smooth muscle of the guinea pig (Leslie *et al.*,

1973). Blood pressure–lowering effects of these compounds were also compared in the guinea pig and dog. Analogues with a modified purine ring system (1-methyladenosine and toyocamycin) were more effective in relaxing intestinal smooth muscle than vascular smooth muscle. Substituents that decreased the basicity of the N_1-position or interfered with hydrogen bonding in the 6-position decreased activity in both vascular and intestinal smooth muscle. Deoxyadenosine, which lacks an oxygen in the 2-position of the ribose portion of the molecule, was ineffective in intestinal smooth muscle but still relaxed vascular smooth muscle. It was concluded that intestinal smooth muscle interacts significantly with the 2-position of the ribose portion of the adenosine molecule whereas vascular smooth muscle requires the adenyl moiety in the molecule for maximal activity.

The possibility that some of the purine analogues discussed might cause the release of ATP from purinergic nerve storage sites cannot be discounted.

7.2. Drugs That Antagonize the Action of Adenyl Compounds

7.2.1. *Mepacrine, Quinine, and Quinidine*

Antimalarial drugs, in particular quinine and mepacrine, inhibit the action of adenosine and ATP on the guinea pig heart (Wayne *et al.*, 1949; Green and Stoner, 1950; Raventos, 1950) and fowl rectal caecum (Madinaveitia and Raventos, 1949). Quinine in concentrations up to 10^{-5} g/ml has no effect on the responses of the guinea pig taenia coli to purinergic nerve stimulation, but neither does it block the direct action of ATP on this tissue (Burnstock *et al.*, 1970).

Antagonism of the actions of adenosine by quinidine (a dextrorotatory stereoisomer of quinine) on the cardiovascular system has been observed by several authors (see Burnstock, 1972). Quinidine has also been shown to antagonize the inhibitory action of adenosine on the isolated guinea pig and kitten uterus (Arulappu, 1967) and of ATP on the rabbit ileum (Bowman and Hall, 1970). Quinidine blocks responses to both ATP and noncholinergic, nonadrenergic nerve stimulation in the gut (Burnstock *et al.*, 1970; Sneddon *et al.*, 1973) and urinary bladder (Burnstock *et al.*, 1972*b*).

7.2.2. *2-Substituted Imidazolines*

High concentrations of phentolamine block the responses of the guinea pig taenia coli to both exogenously applied ATP (Rikimaru *et al.*, 1971*b*) and purinergic nerve stimulation (Satchell *et al.*, 1973; Tomita and Watanabe, 1973). Antazoline, tolazoline, and yohimbine have similar actions (Satchell *et al.*, 1973). It is unlikely that the drugs are causing specific blockade of purinergic transmission, although they are less effective in blocking other smooth muscle relaxants such as amyl nitrate and nitroglycerine.

7.2.3. *Caffeine and Aminophylline*

Caffeine has been reported to block the actions of ATP on the cardiovascular system of a number of mammalian species (Ther *et al.*, 1957; Nichols and Walaszek, 1963; De Gubareff and Sleator, 1965). However, caffeine in concentrations up to 5×10^{-5} g/ml does not affect relaxations of the guinea pig taenia coli in response to either ATP or purinergic nerve stimulation (Burnstock *et al.*, 1970). Higher concentrations of caffeine lower the tone of the preparation and still have no selective blocking action on ATP or nerve stimulation.

Aminophylline has been reported to decrease coronary dilatation produced by intravenous administration of adenosine (Afonso, 1970; Bittar and Pauly, 1971), but not that produced by hypoxia (Afonso *et al.*, 1972). This drug has not yet been tested on purinergic transmission.

7.2.4. *2-2′-Pyridylisatogen*

It has been reported (Hooper *et al.*, 1974) that 2-2′-pyridylisatogen (Patterson and Wibberley, 1965) exerts two actions on the taenia caeci. Concentrations above 2.5 μM gradually relax the smooth muscle over a 30-min contact period; this effect is accompanied by an increase in the frequency of the spontaneous contractions. The second effect, seen after the tone of the smooth muscle has been restored with either histamine or ACh, is a reduction in the submaximal responses to ATP (2–600 μM) after a 15- to 30-min contact of the tissue with 2-2′-pyridylisatogen (2–50 μM). The blockade is specific for ATP and under these conditions cumulative concentration–response curves to ATP are displaced to the right in parallel.

High concentrations of 2-2′-pyridylisatogen (greater than 100 μM for 30 min or longer) cause a general antagonism of ATP, isoprenaline, and NE. These nonspecific effects are not reversed by washing the tissue with McEwen's solution for over 3 h.

7.2.5. *Dinitrophenol and Related Substances*

A variety of drugs known to be uncouplers of oxidative phosphorylation and inhibitors of electron transport (Huijing and Slater, 1961; Webb, 1966) have been tested for their effects on ATP action and, in some cases, purinergic transmission (Hauge *et al.*, 1966; Lunde *et al.*, 1968; Burnstock *et al.*, 1970). In general, they produce nonspecific depression of smooth muscle and do not appear to be a promising group of substances in the search for specific blockers of purinergic transmission.

7.3. Drugs That Potentiate the Action of Adenyl Compounds

7.3.1. Adenosine Uptake Inhibitors

Dipyridamole (Bretschneider *et al.*, 1959) and hexabendine (von Kraup *et al.*, 1966) have been shown to potentiate the effects of adenosine and its derivatives on the guinea pig heart and rabbit and guinea pig intestine, the coronary arteries of dog and cat, cat nictitating membrane, and renal vessels in dogs (see Satchell *et al.*, 1972; Burnstock, 1972; Parratt and Wadsworth, 1972; Satchell and Burnstock, 1974). The mechanism underlying this potentiation has usually been explained in terms of blockade of intracellular uptake of adenosine (Pfleger and Schöndorf, 1969; Kolassa *et al.*, 1970; Liu and Feinberg, 1971, 1973; Hopkins, 1973*b*). Dipyridamole has also been reported to act as an inhibitor of phosphodiesterase (Senft, 1968; Vigdahl *et al.*, 1971) and of adenosine deaminase (Bunag *et al.*, 1964; Stafford, 1966). Papaverine, like dipyridamole, inhibits the uptake of adenosine into red blood cells (von Koss *et al.*, 1962), but produces only slight potentiation of the effect of adenosine on the guinea pig heart *in situ* (Stafford, 1966). Potentiation of lidoflazine (Afonso *et al.*, 1968) could not be explained either by block of adenosine uptake or by inhibition of adenosine deaminase (Hopkins, 1973*b*).

7.3.2. ATPase Inhibitors

Inhibitors of ATPase fall into two main categories: those which act on Na^+/K^+-activated ATPase and those which act on Mg^{2+}-activated ATPase. In general, Na^+/K^+-activated ATPases are considered to be associated with Na and K^+ transport in membranes. On the other hand, the role of Mg^+-activated ATPase is poorly understood.

It is of interest to examine the effect of ATPase inhibitors on relaxations produced by both purinergic nerves and ATP, in view of the likelihood that ATPases are involved in the degradation of ATP released from nerves. If this is the case, ATPase inhibitors would be expected to potentiate both responses. Unfortunately, most of these drugs are potent inhibitors of many cellular activities and depress all activity of smooth muscle preparations in a general way.

Low doses of ouabain, a cardiac glycoside which inhibits Na^+/K^+-activated ATPase (Skou, 1960; Bonting *et al.*, 1962) potentiates the inhibitory effect of ATP on the guinea pig heart (Rand *et al.*, 1955). Ouabain was reported not to affect the inhibition produced by ATP in the guinea pig taenia coli (Axelsson and Holmberg, 1969).

7.3.3. Inhibitors of Adenosine Deaminase

The actions of adenosine and the adenine nucleotides are usually short-lasting. One explanation for this might be that they are readily deaminated in blood and tissues to their corresponding inosine derivatives, which are pharmacologically inactive (Conway and Cooke, 1939), but there may well be other factors involved, such as receptor or uptake mechanisms. By analogy with the role and sites of action of monoamine oxidase and catechol-*O*-methyltransferase in adrenergic transmission (see Iversen, 1967), it would clearly be unwise at this stage to make too many assumptions about the role of adenosine deaminase in purinergic transmission. Investigation of this role will be easier when more reliable adenosine deaminase inhibitors have been found. 8-Azaguanine has been claimed to be an inhibitor of intestinal adenosine deaminase, but little potentiation of adenosine action on heart was detected (Stafford, 1966).

8. SPECULATIONS ON THE EVOLUTION AND DEVELOPMENT OF PURINERGIC NERVES

Purinergic nerves are strongly represented in lower vertebrates (see Burnstock, 1969, 1972). There is purinergic inhibitory nervous control of the stomach in fish (Campbell and Burnstock, 1968; Ito and Kuriyama, 1971), amphibians (Rehm *et al.*, 1970; Satchell and Burnstock, 1971), and birds (Bennett, 1970; Sato *et al.*, 1970), as well as in mammals (Lock and Weber, 1971; see Burnstock, 1972, and Abrahamsson, 1973). The vagal pathway to the stomach in lower vertebrates consists largely, if not entirely, of preganglionic cholinergic nerves forming synapses with purinergic inhibitory neurons in the gut wall. Antagonistic excitatory control of gastric motility is represented by both cholinergic and adrenergic nerve fibers of sympathetic origin. During the course of vertebrate evolution, the purinergic inhibitory pathway in the vagus nerve has been retained (Fig. 8); antagonistic excitatory control of gastric motility in mammals has been taken over by parasympathetic cholinergic neurons in the wall of the gut, while most of the sympathetic adrenergic nerves have come to form terminals about nerve cell bodies in Auerbach's plexus and are concerned with modulating intramural neuron activity (see Burnstock and Costa, 1973). Noncholinergic, nonadrenergic excitatory nerves are a prominent feature in both the small and large intestines of amphibians, reptiles, and birds (Bartlet and Hassan, 1971; Burnstock *et al.*, 1972*a*; Sneddon *et al.*, 1973), and there is some evidence that these may be purinergic nerves (Sneddon *et al.*, 1973). The nerve-mediated contraction is closely mimicked by ATP and blocked by quinidine. The possibility that these nerves release catecholamines, 5-HT, histamine, bradykinin, or prostaglandin E_1 has been excluded. The cell bodies of noncholinergic excitatory neurons do not appear to be in the wall of the small intestine in lower vertebrates; postganglionic fibers reach the gut via sympathetic periarterial nerves. Whether the noncholinergic, nonadrenergic responses to stimulation of periarterial nerves are due to fibers of

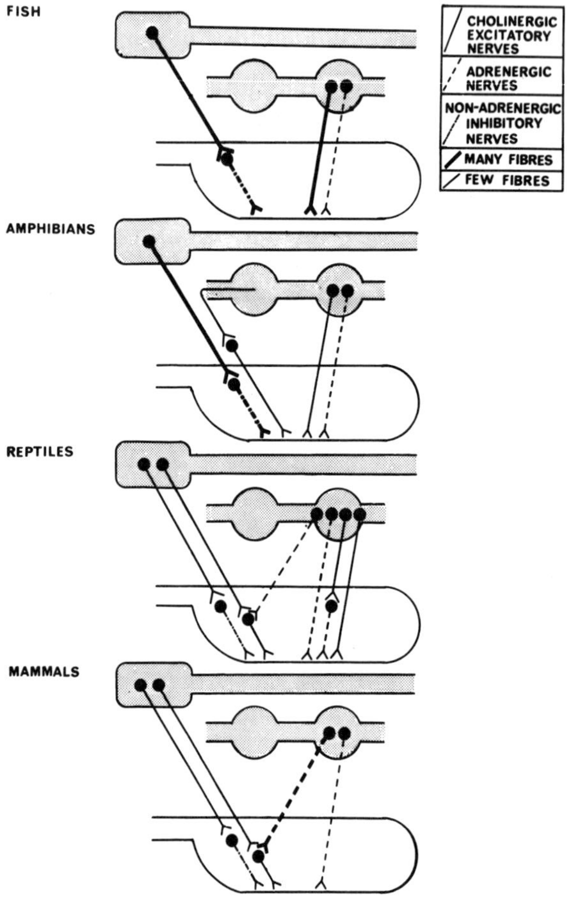

FIG. 8. Diagrammatic representation of the autonomic innervation of the vertebrate stomach. Central nervous system and sympathetic chain are represented by shaded areas. Note that the vagal parasympathetic outflow is purely inhibitory ("purinergic") to the fish and amphibian stomach and is opposed by excitatory cholinergic sympathetic fibers. In reptiles and mammals the cholinergic excitatory nerves have been switched to the parasympathetic outflow, sympathetic fibers becoming adrenergic and inhibitory. Adrenergic modulation of intramural ganglion cell activity is rudimentary in reptiles and strongly developed in mammals. The diagram depicting the innervation of the reptile stomach is largely conjectural. Intramural neurons that are independent of the extrinsic nerve supply are not included in the diagrams. From Burnstock (1969).

sympathetic origin, to parasympathetic fibers invading the sympathetic trunks, to efferent fibers with their cell bodies in the dorsal root ganglia, or possibly to antidromic stimulation of sensory fibers is not yet known (see Campbell and Burnstock, 1968).

There is good evidence for the presence of a prominent purinergic inhibitory nerve supply to the musculature of the lung of amphibians

(Campbell, 1971; Robinson *et al.*, 1971), reptiles (Berger, 1973), and birds (Cook and King, 1970). In mammals there have been reports of bronchodilator responses to vagal stimulation (Widdicombe, 1963); adenosine and AMP dilate the bronchioles (Bennett and Drury, 1931); and, more recently, the presence of nerve profiles with a predominance of LOV has been described in the alveolar ducts and sacs of mouse lung (Hung *et al.*, 1972). The possibility of purinergic innervation of the urinary bladder of fish, amphibians, and reptiles, as well as mammals, has been discussed earlier (see Section 2.4).

This strong representation of purinergic nerves in organs of lower vertebrates opens up the possibility that they may also be present in some invertebrates. Few studies have been carried out to date in this field, but nerve profiles containing a predominance of vesicles which closely resemble LOV have been seen in some invertebrate organs, including body wall muscle of earthworm (Rosenblueth, 1972) and the polychaete *Sabella* (Kryvi, 1971); smooth cardiac muscle of a mollusc (Sathananthan and Burnstock, unpublished results); skeletal muscle of crustacea (Huddart and Bradbury, 1972; Sherman and Fourntner, 1972), insect (Osbourne, 1971), spider (Sherman and Luff, 1971), and mollusc (Barrantes, 1970); muscles in esophagus, vascular walls, and pyloric caecae of starfish (see Pentreath and Cobb, 1972); snail and chiton rectum (Campbell and Burnstock, 1968); and possibly some coelenterate neuromuscular junctions (Westfall, 1973). Despite their close similarity to purinergic nerve profiles in vertebrate gut, some of these profiles seem likely to contain transmitters such as 5-HT, dopamine, and perhaps other as yet unidentified neurohumoral substances. Furthermore, it is not always possible to distinguish profiles of purinergic nerves from processes of "neurosecretory" neurons, although membrane-bound granules in these cells are often larger than LOV (see Bern, 1966; Baumgarten *et al.*, 1972; Miller and Rees, 1973).

While there is no evidence for this proposal, the possibility that a purine nucleotide represents the primitive neurotransmitter developed early in the evolution of nervous communication systems could be considered: that as the needs of animals became more sophisticated and it became a selective advantage to develop differential neurocontrol systems, new enzyme-forming systems were established in neurons, capable of producing other neurotransmitters. In this way, various catecholamines, ACh, GABA, 5-HT, glycine, glutamate, and probably other transmitter substances as yet unidentified may have developed independently as neurotransmitters in different phyla during the course of evolution. Whether the most primitive transmitter in this series of compounds is ATP or not, the question still remains, what is the mechanism whereby new neurotransmitter systems evolve? It seems most unlikely that a new nerve type with a structurally distinct form suddenly appeared during the course of evolution. It is more likely that there was a gradual evolutionary transition from one neurotransmitter to another within homologous neurons. If this is true, then one might begin to look more carefully over a wide range of animals for nerves showing gradations of transmitter mixtures, although this concept challenges the widely accepted view that each nerve releases only one transmitter (Dale, 1935; Rosenblueth, 1950). Burn and Rand (1959, 1965) have proposed that ACh is stored together with NE in sympathetic nerves. ATP is released together with catecholamine from adrenal medullary vesicles and whole glands (Douglas, 1968; Stevens *et al.*, 1972), and it seems likely that some ATP is released together with NE from adrenergic nerves (Geffen and Livett, 1971; Su *et al.*, 1971; Paddle and Burnstock, 1975). ATP has also been located together with ACh in synaptic vesicles of cholinergic nerves supplying the electric organ of torpedine rays (Whittaker *et al.*, 1972; Bohan *et al.*, 1973), and it has been proposed that ATP is released together with ACh from phrenic nerves supplying the rat diaphragm (Silinsky and Hubbard, 1973). The roles of ATP and adenosine in cholinergic transmission are being explored by a number of workers (Smythies *et al.*, 1971; Ginsborg and Hirst, 1972; Kaack, 1972; Takagi and Takayanagi, 1972; Bohan *et al.*, 1973). To quote Whittaker *et al.* (1972), "Although it thus now seems reasonable to conclude that ATP is a constituent of cholinergic vesicles, as of chromaffin granules, rat mast-cell granules and dense-cored synaptic vesicles isolated from adrenergic nerves, the possibilities cannot be entirely excluded at this stage that ATP and acetylcholine are present in separate vesicles . . . ." It is of interest, too, that measurement of the content of ATP and catecholamines in the adrenal medulla of rats and rabbits in the course of pre- and postnatal development revealed that there was a catecholamine:ATP ratio of less than 1 (approximately 1:6 in rats and 1:1.5 in rabbits) in early development (18 days after conception), but that this ratio gradually increased to more than 10:1 in adults (O'Brien *et al.*, 1972). On the basis of these and previous electron microscopic findings (Elfvin, 1967), the authors suggested that the fetal adrenal medulla contains vesicles which store mainly ATP and that in the course of maturation these vesicles take up catecholamines and are transformed into typical chromaffin granules. It has also been proposed that the megakaryocytes—which incidentally contain many granules (Yamada, 1957) that are remarkably similar to LOV seen in purinergic nerves—contain primarily ATP and later accumulate 5-HT after release of the platelets into the circulating blood (Tranzer *et al.*, 1972).

The changes which occur during neuron development appear to be consistent with this hypothesis. Each neuron, being a cell supplied with a complete set of genes, possesses the potential ability for synthesizing the complete enzymatic machinery for a particular transmitter substance. Initially all undifferentiated embryonic nerve cells (or neuroblasts), regardless of the types of transmitter they are destined to contain in their adult form, appear to possess an ACh-synthesizing system (Filogamo and Marchisio, 1971). Whether a maturing neuron emerges at the end of its differentiation as a cholinergic, adrenergic, or purinergic neuron appears to be determined by external factors (possibly "trophic" factors released from nerves or other cells) which trigger the expression of the appropriate genetic mechanism. Studies of cultured mouse neuroblastoma cells (Amano *et al.*, 1972) revealed three types of clones with respect to neurotransmitter synthesis: cholinergic, adrenergic, and clones which do not synthesize ACh or catecholamines, although all clones contain acetylcholinesterase. The authors concluded that "there are relatively few kinds of universal neurotransmitters in the nervous system of both vertebrates and invertebrates" and that "it seems likely that the expression of a gene required for the synthesis of one neurotransmitter may restrict the expression of genes for alternate transmitters . . . simultaneous expression of acetyltransferase and tyrosine hydroxylase genes might inactivate both genes, or might result in a balanced state of mutual inhibition, i.e., a cell with low cholinergic and low adrenergic activities."

9. SUMMARY

1. Purinergic nerves are present throughout the gastrointestinal tract. Their cell bodies are located in Auerbach's plexus and their axons extend for about 1.5 cm in an anal direction before they supply varicose fibers primarily to the circular muscle coat. In the stomach and distal rectum, they are controlled by preganglionic cholinergic fibers of parasympathetic origin. Throughout most of the intestine, they are controlled by intramural cholinergic interneurons. Adrenergic fibers can modify the activity of purinergic neurons by presynaptic inhibition at the cholinergic synapses.

2. The possibility that purinergic nerves are also present in the lung, trachea, retractor penis, uterus, bladder, esophagus, parts of the eye and vascular system, seminal vesicle, and in some regions of the CNS should be considered.

3. The terminal varicosities of purinergic nerves are characterized at the ultrastructural level by a predominance of large opaque vesicles (LOV), which can be distinguished from the large granular vesicles (LGV) found in small numbers in both adrenergic and cholinergic nerves. LOV are larger (800–2000 Å) than LGV (600–1200 Å), have a less prominent halo between the granular core and the vesicle membrane, have a less dense granular matrix, are unaffected by either short-term "loading" or long-term "destruction" by 6-hydroxydopamine, and are unaffected by catecholamine-depleting drugs such as reserpine, metaraminol, and guanethidine.

Redback spider venom destroys LOV in purinergic nerve profiles, and this is associated with loss of inhibitory junction potentials. ATPase has been localized in plasmalemmal vesicles which are often aggregated in the smooth muscle membrane closely apposed to purinergic nerve profiles in the circular smooth muscle coat of the intestine. 5′-Nucleotidase has been localized in the media of many but not all arteries and arterioles and in most visceral smooth muscles, particularly in the longitudinal and outer circular muscle layers of the gut, but not in skeletal muscle or in the cardiac muscle of most species. Adenosine deaminase is found in most tissues with particularly high levels in small intestine.

4. Inhibitory junction potentials (IJPs) have been recorded in single smooth muscle cells in the circular muscle coat and in the longitudinal coat in some regions of the gut in response to stimulation of enteric nerves. IJPs persist in the presence of atropine and adrenergic neuron blocking agents or after degeneration of sympathetic adrenergic nerves, but are abolished when nerve conduction is blocked by tetrodotoxin. Repetitive stimulation of purinergic nerves results in summation of individual IJPs and hyperpolarizations of up to 50 mV; there may be facilitation of the first two or three IJPs in a train. A feature of purinergic transmission is the rapid decay of the response to repetitive nerve stimulation; the amplitude of the response is rarely maintained for more than 20–30 s even at physiological frequences of 5–10 Hz. This is in marked contrast to the inhibitory response of the intestine to adrenergic nerves. The latency of the IJP in response to stimulation of postganglionic purinergic nerves is about 45–80 ms. The time course of IJPs recorded in smooth muscle of the gut has a rise time of 150–250 ms and a total duration of 800–1200 ms. Spontaneous IJPs occur, but mostly only in low-frequency trains.

A characteristic feature of the response to stimulation of purinergic nerves is rebound depolarization associated with spikes and contraction, following the main inhibitory response. Consequently, in low-tone preparations, particularly those with little or no spontaneous spike activity, stimulation of inhibitory purinergic nerves can result in long-latency contraction rather than relaxation. There is evidence that the transmitter released from purinergic nerves acts by producing a specific increase in K^+ conductance, as does exogenously applied ATP (compared to conductance increases to both K^+ and Cl^- in response to sympathetic nerve stimulation and NE). Studies of the interaction of responses of single muscle cells to stimulation of enteric, intrinsic, and extrinsic nerves suggest that most cells in the longitudinal coat receive cholinergic excitatory nerves, while purinergic inhibitory innervation is a prominent feature in the circular coat of the intestine. Purinergic nerves may selectively innervate pacemaker regions in the stomach.

5. The physiological roles of purinergic nerves in the gastrointestinal tract are beginning to be recognized. Purinergic nerves are involved in normal propulsive function, including "receptive relaxation" of the stomach, reflex relaxation of the esophagogastric junction, "descending inhibition" in peristalsis, and reflex relaxation of the internal anal sphincter. (In contrast, adrenergic nerves are concerned largely with extrinsic modulation of gut motility at both neuronal and muscle levels, including intestino-

intestinal and enterogastric reflexes.) Purinergic nerves have also been implicated in the vomiting response. Speculations have been made about the involvement of purinergic nerves which may supply other systems in various normal and pathological conditions, including bronchodilatation, asphyxia, asthma, coughing, inflammation of the skin, hibernation, and depressive illness.

6. Evidence that ATP is the transmitter released from purinergic nerves includes (a) synthesis and storage of ATP in nerves, (b) release of ATP from the nerves when they are stimulated, (c) exogenously applied ATP mimicking the action of nerve-released transmitter, (d) the presence of enzymes which inactivate ATP, and (e) the existence of drugs which produce similar blocking or potentiating effects on the response to exogenously applied ATP and nerve stimulation.

A number of drugs including quinidine and 2-substituted imidazoline compounds have been reported to block the responses both to purinergic nerve stimulation and to exogenously applied ATP, but not to other relaxants. However, high concentrations are required, and they cannot be regarded as specific blockers. 2-2′-Pyridylisatogen has recently been proposed as a specific blocker of ATP acting on smooth muscle and may provide the most promising possibility so far for a specific blocker of purinergic transmission. When tachyphylaxis to repeated administration of ATP is produced, there is consistent depression of the inhibitory responses to stimulation of purinergic nerves, but not to adrenergic nerves. Dipyridamole has been found to produce parallel potentiation of both the responses to purinergic nerve stimulation and to exogenously applied ATP. There is evidence for two kinds of muscle receptors for adenine compounds.

Acknowledgments

Much of the work for this paper was carried out while the author was working in the Department of Zoology, University of Melbourne, and was supported by grants from the Ramaciotti Foundation, the National Heart Foundation, the Australian Research Grants Committee, and the National Health and Medical Research Council. The author is most grateful to his colleagues Bob Cook, Robert Purves, John Furness, Marcello Costa, David Satchell, Angela Rutherford, and Brian Paddle for their helpful criticisms of the manuscript and to Marian Rubio, Gail Liddell, and Jay McKenzie for their willing help in its preparation.

10. REFERENCES

Abdulla, Y. H., and McFarlane, E., 1972, Control of prostaglandin biosynthesis in rat brain homogenates by adenine nucleotides, *Biochem. Pharmacol.* **21**:2841–2847.

Abood, L. G., Koketsu, K., and Miyomoto, S., 1962, Outflux of various phosphates during membrane depolarisation of excitable tissues, *Am. J. Physiol.* **202**:469–474.

Abrahamsson, H., 1971, Vago-vagal gastro-gastric relaxation, *Rend. Romani Gastroenterol.* **3:**114–115.

Abrahamsson, H., 1973, Studies on the inhibitory nervous control of gastric motility, *Acta Physiol. Scand. Suppl.* **390:**1–38.

Abrahamsson, H., and Jansson, G., 1969, Elicitation of reflex vagal relaxation of the stomach from pharynx and esophagus in the cat, *Acta Physiol. Scand.* **77:**172–178.

Abrahamsson, H., and Jansson, G., 1973, Vago-vagal gastro-gastric relaxation in the cat, *Acta Physiol. Scand.* **88:**289–295.

Abrahamsson, H., and Thorén, P., 1972, Reflex relaxation of the stomach elicited from receptors located in the heart: An analysis of the receptors and afferents involved, *Acta Physiol. Scand.* **84:**197–207.

Abrahamsson, H., and Thorén, P., 1973, Vomiting and reflex vagal relaxation of the stomach elicited from heart receptors in the cat, *Acta Physiol. Scand.* **88:**433–439.

Abrahamsson, H., Jansson, G., and Martinson, J., 1973, Vagal relaxation of the stomach induced by apomorphine in the cat, *Acta Physiol. Scand.* **88:**296–302.

Afonso, S., 1970, Inhibition of coronary vasodilating action of dipyridamole and adenosine by aminophylline in the dog, *Circ. Res.* **26:**743–754.

Afonso, S., O'Brien, G. S., and Crumpton, C. W., 1968, Enhancement of coronary vasodilating action of ATP and adenosine by lidoflazine, *Circ. Res.* **22:**43–48.

Afonso, S., Ansfield, T. J., Berndt, T. B., and Rowe, G. G., 1972, Coronary vasodilator responses to hypoxia before and after aminophylline, *J. Physiol.* **221:**589–599.

Ahlquist, R. P., 1948, A study of the adrenotropic receptors, *Am. J. Physiol.* **153:**586–600.

Ahlquist, R. P., 1966, The adrenergic receptor, *J. Pharm. Sci.* **55:**359–367.

Altenähr, E., 1971, Electron microscopic evidence for innervation of chief cells in human parathyroid gland, *Experientia* **27:**1077.

Amano, T., Richelson, E., and Nirenberg, M., 1972, Neurotransmitter synthesis by neuroblastoma clones, *Proc. Natl. Acad. Sci.* **69:**258–263.

Ambache, N., 1957, Properties of irin, a physiological constituent of the rabbit's iris, *J. Physiol.* **135:**114–132.

Ambache, N., and Zar, M., 1970, Non-cholinergic transmission by post-ganglionic motor neurons in the mammalian bladder, *J. Physiol.* **210:**761–783.

Änggård, E., and Samuelsson, B., 1964, Smooth muscle stimulating lipids in sheep iris. The identification of prostaglandin $F_{2\alpha}$, *Biochem. Pharmacol.* **13:**281–283.

Angus, J., Cobbin, L. B., Einstein, R., and Maguire, M. H., 1971, Cardiovascular actions of substituted adenosine analogues, *Brit. J. Pharmacol.* **41:**592–599.

Arulappu, R. G. S., 1967, The actions of nucleic acid derivatives on smooth muscle. Fellowship thesis, Pharmaceutical Society of Victoria, Melbourne.

Axelsson, J., and Holmberg, R., 1969, The effects of extracellularly applied ATP and related compounds on the electrical and mechanical activity of the smooth muscle of taenia coli of the guinea pig, *Acta Physiol. Scand.* **75:**149–156.

Babskiĭ, E. B., and Malkiman, I. I., 1950, Effect of adenosine-triphosphoric acid on the chronaxy of the motor zone of the cerebral cortex, *C. R. Acad. Sci. U.S.S.R.* **74:**1135–1137.

Ballard, D. R., Abboad, F. M., and Mayer, H. E., 1970, Release of a humoral vasodilator substance during neurogenic vasodilatation, *Am. J. Physiol.* **219:**1451–1457.

Barclay, A. E., 1936, *The Digestive Tract: A Radiological Study of Its Anatomy, Physiology and Pathology*, Cambridge University Press, London.

Barrantes, F. J., 1970, The neuromuscular junctions of a pulmonate mollusc. I. Ultrastructural study, *Z. Zellforsch. Mikros. Anat.* **104:**205–212.

Barsoum, G. S., and Gaddum, J. H., 1935, The pharmacological estimation of adenosine and histamine in blood, *J. Physiol.* **85:**1–14.

Bartlet, A. L., 1972, Apparent differences between the affects of hyoscine *in vivo* and *in vitro* on the responses of chicken oesophagus to nerve stimulation, *Brit. J. Pharmacol.* **45:**635–637.

BARTLET A. L., and HASSON, T., 1971, Contraction of chicken rectum to nerve stimulation after blockade of sympathetic and parasympathetic transmission, *Quart. J. Exp. Physiol. Cog–. Med. Sci.* **56:**178–183.

BAUMGARTEN, H. G., HOLSTEIN, A. F., and OWMAN, CH., 1970, Auerbach's plexus of mammals and man: Electron microscopic identification of three different types of neuronal processes in myenteric ganglia of the large intestine from rhesus monkeys, guinea-pigs and man, *Z. Zellforsch. Mikros. Anat.* **106:**376–397.

BAUMGARTEN, H. G., BJÖRKLUND, A., HOLSTEIN, A. F., and NOBIN, A., 1972, Organization and ultrastructural identification of the catecholamine nerve terminals in the neural lobe and pars intermedia of the rat pituitary, *Z. Zellforsch. Mikros. Anat.* **126:**483–517.

BAYLISS, W. M., and STARLING, E. H., 1899, The movement and innervation of the small intestine, *J. Physiol.* **24:**99–143.

BEANI, L., BIANCHI, C., and CREMA, A., 1971, Vagal non-adrenergic inhibition of guinea-pig stomach, *J. Physiol.* **217:**259–279.

BECK, C. S., And OSA, T., 1971, Membrane activity in guinea-pig gastric sling muscle: A nerve-dependent phenomenon, *Am. J. Physiol.* **220:**1397–1403.

BELL, C., 1968, Dual vasoconstrictor and vasodilator innervation of the uterine arterial supply in the guinea-pig, *Circ. Res.* **23:**279–289.

BELL, C., 1969, Transmission from vasoconstrictor and vasodilator nerves to single smooth muscle cells of the guinea-pig uterine artery, *J. Physiol.* **205:**695–708.

BENNETT, A., and STOCKLEY, H. L., 1973, A study of the intrinsic innervation of human isolated gastro-intestinal muscle using electrical stimulation, *J. Physiol.* **233:**34P–35P.

BENNETT, D. W., and DRURY, A. N., 1931, Further observations relating to the physiological activity of adenosine compounds, *J. Physiol.* **72:**288–320.

BENNETT, M. R., 1966*a*, Rebound excitation of the smooth muscle cells of the guinea-pig taenia coli after stimulation of intramural inhibitory nerves, *J. Physiol.* **185:**124–131.

BENNETT, M. R., 1966*b*, Transmission from intramural excitatory nerves to the smooth muscle cells of the guinea-pig taenia coli, *J. Physiol.* **185:**132–147.

BENNETT, M. R., and BURNSTOCK, G., 1968, Electrophysiology of the innervation of intestinal smooth muscle, in: *Handbook of Physiology*, Section 6: Alimentary Canal, IV: Motility, pp. 1709–1732, American Physiological Society, Washington, D.C.

BENNETT, M. R., BURNSTOCK, G., and HOLMAN, M. E., 1963, The effect of potassium and chloride ions on the inhibitory potential recorded in the guinea-pig taenia coli, *J. Physiol.* **169:**33P–34P.

BENNETT, M. R., BURNSTOCK, G., and HOLMAN, M. E., 1966*a*, Transmission from perivascular inhibitory nerves to the smooth muscle of the guinea-pig taenia coli, *J. Physiol.* **182:**527–540.

BENNETT, M., BURNSTOCK, G., and HOLMAN, M. E., 1966*b*, Transmission from intramural inhibitory nerves to the smooth muscle of the guinea-pig taenia coli, *J. Physiol.* **182:**541–558.

BENNETT, T., 1969*a*, The effects of hyoscine and anticholinesterases on cholinergic transmission to the smooth muscle cells of the avian gizzard, *Brit. J. Pharmacol.* **37:**585–594.

BENNETT, T., 1969*b*, Nerve-mediated excitation and inhibition of the smooth muscle cells of the avian gizzard, *J. Physiol.* **204:**669–686.

BENNETT, T., 1970, Interaction of nerve mediated excitation and inhibition of single smooth muscle cells of the avian gizzard, *Comp. Biochem. Physiol.* **32:**669–680.

BERGER, P. J., 1973, Autonomic innervation of the visceral and vascular smooth muscle of the lizard lung, *Comp. Gen. Pharmacol.* **4:**1–10.

BERGSTRÖM, S., CARLSON, L. A., and WEEKS, J. R., 1968, The prostaglandins: A family of biologically active lipids, *Pharmacol. Rev.* **20:**1–48.

BERMAN, P. H., BALIS, M. E., and DANCIS, J., 1969, Congenital hyperuricemia, an inborn error of purine metabolism associated with psychomotor retardation, athetosis, and self-mutilation, *Arch. Neurol.* **20:**44–53.

Bern, H. A., 1966, On the production of hormones by neurones and the role of neurosecretion in neuroendocrine mechanisms, in: Nervous and Hormonal Mechanisms of Integration, *Symp. Soc. Exp. Biol.* **20:**325–344.

Berne, R. M., 1964, Regulation of coronary flow, *Physiol. Rev.* **44:**1–29.

Berne, R. M., Rubio, R., Dobson, J. C., and Cornish, R. R., 1971, Adenosine and adenine nucleotides of possible mediator of cardiac and skeletal muscle blood flow regulation, *Circ. Res.* **28, 29:**115–131 (Suppl. I).

Bianchi, A., de Natale, G., and Giarquinto, S., 1963, The effects of adenosine and its phosphorylated derivatives upon the respiratory apparatus, *Arch. Int. Pharmacodyn. Ther.* **145:**498–517.

Biber, B., and Fara, J., 1973, Intestinal motility increased by tetrodotoxin, lidocaine, and procaine, *Experientia* **29:**551–552.

Biber, B., Lundgren, O., and Svanik, J., 1971, Studies on the intestinal vasodilatation observed after mechanical stimulation of the mucosa of the gut, *Acta Physiol. Scand.* **82:**177–190.

Bittar, N., and Pauly, T. J., 1971, Myocardial reactive hyperemia responses in the dog after aminophylline and lidoflazine, *Am. J. Physiol.* **220:**812–815.

Blakeley, A. G. H., Brown, L., and Geffen, L. B., 1969, Uptake and reuse of sympathetic transmitter in the cat's spleen, *Proc. Roy. Soc. Lond. Ser. B Biol. Sci.* **174:**51–68.

Bloom, F. E., and Aghajanian, G. K., 1968, An electron microscopic analysis of large granular synaptic vesicles of the brain in relation to monoamine content, *J. Pharmacol. Exp. Ther.* **159:**261–273.

Bloom, F. E., Hoffer, B. J., Battenberg, E. R., and Siggins, G. R., 1972, Adenosine 3′5′ monophosphate is localized in cerebellar neurons: Immunofluorescence evidence, *Science* **177:**436–438.

Bloom, G. D., Diamant, B., Hägermark, Ö., and Ritzén, M., 1970, The effects of adenosine-5′-triphosphate (ATP) on structure and amine content of rat peritoneal mast cells, *Exp. Cell. Res.* **62:**61–75.

Blume, A. J., Dalton, C., and Sheppard, H., 1973, Adenosine-mediated elevation of cyclic 3′:5′-adenosine monophosphate concentrations in cultured mouse neuroblastoma cells, *Proc. Natl. Acad. Sci.* **11:**3099–3102.

Bodian, D., 1972, Synaptic diversity and characterization by electron microscopy, in: *Structure and Function of Synapses* (G. D. Pappas and D. F. Purpura, eds.), pp. 45–65, Raven Press, New York.

Bohan, T. P., Boyne, A. F., Guth, P. S., Narayanan, Y., and Williams, T. H., 1973, Electron-dense particle in cholinergic synaptic vesicles, *Nature* **244:**32–34.

Bone, A., 1972, The dogfish neuromuscular junction: Dual innervation of vertebrate striated muscle fibres? *J. Cell Sci.* **10:**657–665.

Bonting, S. L., Carravaggio, L. L., and Hawkins, N. M., 1962, Studies on sodium–potassium-activated adenosinetriphosphatase. IV. Correlation with cation transport sensitive to cardiac glycosides, *Arch. Biochem. Biophys.* **98:**413–419.

Borgers, M., 1971, Cytochemistry and histochemistry of growing collaterals in chronic coronary artery occlusion, in: *The Collateral Circulation of the Heart*, pp. 117–150, W. Schaper, North-Holland, Amsterdam.

Boukma, S. J., Lahti, R. A., and Mathews, J., 1973, Cyclic AMP and phosphodiesterase in synaptic vesicles from mouse brain, *J. Neurochem.* **20:**1387–1392.

Bowman, W. C., and Hall, M. T., 1970, Inhibition of rabbit intestine mediated by α- and β-adreneoreceptors, *Brit. J. Pharmacol.* **38:**399–415.

Boyd, H., 1973, ATP as a nerve transmitter substance, *J. Theor. Biol.* **42:**49–53.

Boyd, I. A., and Martin, A. R., 1956, The end-plate potential in mammalian muscle, *J. Physiol.* **132:**74–91.

Bretschneider, H. J., Frank, A., Bernard, U., Kochsiek, K., and Scheler, F., 1959, Die Wirkung eines Pyrimidopyrimidin-Derivates auf die Sauerstoff-versorgung des Herzmuskels, *Arzneimittel-Forsch.* **9:**49–59.

BRETTSCHNEIDER, H., 1962, Elektronenmikroskopische Untersuchungen über die Innervation der glatten Muskulatur des Darmes, *Z. Mikros.-Anat. Forsch.* **68:**333–360.

BUCHTHAL, F., and KAHLSON, G., 1944, The motor effect of adenosine triphosphate and allied phosphorus compounds on smooth mammalian muscle, *Acta Physiol. Scand.* **8:**325–334.

BUCHTHAL, F., ENGBAEK, L., STEN-KNUDSEN, O., and THOMASEN, E., 1947, Application of adenosinetriphosphate and related compounds to the spinal cord of the cat, *J. Physiol.* **106:**3P–4P.

BÜLBRING, E., and GERSHON, M. D., 1967, 5-Hydroxytryptamine participation in the vagal inhibitory innervation of the stomach, *J. Physiol.* **192:**823–846.

BÜLBRING, E., and TOMITA, T., 1967, Properties of the inhibitory potential of smooth muscle as observed in the response to field stimulation of the guinea-pig taenia coli, *J. Physiol.* **189:**299–316.

BUNAG, R. D., DOUGLAS, C. R., IMAI, S., and BERNE, R. M., 1964, Influence of a pyrimidopyrimidine derivative on deamination of adenosine by blood, *Circ. Res.* **15:**83–88.

BURN, J. H., and RAND, M. J., 1959, Sympathetic postganglionic mechanism, *Nature* **184:**163–165.

BURN, J. H., and RAND, M. J., 1965, Acetylcholine in adrenergic transmission, *Ann. Rev. Pharmacol.* **5:**163–182.

BURNSTOCK, G., 1958, The effects of acetylcholine on membrane potential, spike frequency, conduction velocity and excitability in the taenia coli of the guinea-pig, *J. Physiol.* **143:**165–182.

BURNSTOCK, G., 1969, Evolution of the autonomic innervation of visceral and cardiovascular systems in vertebrates, *Pharmacol. Rev.* **21:**247–324.

BURNSTOCK, G., 1970, Structure of smooth muscle and its innervation, in: *Smooth Muscle* (E. Bülbring, A. F. Brading, A. W. Jones, and T. Tomita, eds.), pp. 1–69, Edward Arnold, London.

BURNSTOCK, G., 1971, Neural nomenclature, *Nature* **229:**282–283.

BURNSTOCK, G., 1972, Purinergic nerves, *Pharmacol. Rev.* **24:**509–581.

BURNSTOCK, G., 1975, Electronmicroscopy: Vesicles, synaptic gaps, pharmacological agents, in: *Methods in Pharmacology*, Vol. III: *Smooth Muscle* (E. E. Daniel and D. M. Paton, eds.), Appleton-Century-Crofts, Edmonton, pp. 113–137.

BURNSTOCK, G., and COSTA, M., 1973, Inhibitory innervation of the gut, *Gastroenterology* **64:**141–144.

BURNSTOCK, G., and HOLMAN, M. E., 1961, The transmission of excitation from autonomic nerve to smooth muscle, *J. Physiol.* **155:**115–133.

BURNSTOCK, G., and IWAYAMA, T., 1971, Fine structural identification of autonomic nerves and their relation to smooth muscle, in: Histochemistry of Nervous Transmission, *Prog. Brain Res.* **34:**389–404.

BURNSTOCK, G., and STRAUB, R. W., 1958, A method for studying the effects of ions and drugs on the resting and action potentials in smooth muscle with external electrodes, *J. Physiol.* **140:**156–167.

BURNSTOCK, G., CAMPBELL, G., BENNETT, M., HOLMAN, M. E., and MERRILLEES, N. C. R., 1963, Inhibition of the smooth muscle of the taenia coli, *Nature* **200:**581–582.

BURNSTOCK, G., CAMPBELL, G., and RAND, M. J., 1966, The inhibitory innervation of the taenia of the guinea-pig caecum, *J. Physiol.* **182:**504–526.

BURNSTOCK, G., CAMPBELL, G., SATCHELL, D. G., and SMYTHE, A., 1970, Evidence that adenosine triphosphate or a related nucleotide is the transmitter substance released by non-adrenergic inhibitory nerves in the gut, *Brit. J. Pharmacol.* **40:**668–688.

BURNSTOCK, G., GANNON, B. J., MALMFORS, T., and ROGERS, D. C., 1971, Changes in the physiology and fine structure of the taenia of the guinea-pig caecum following transplantation into the anterior eye chamber, *J. Physiol.* **219:**139–154.

BURNSTOCK, G., SATCHELL, D. G., and SMYTHE, A., 1972*a*, A comparison of the excitatory and inhibitory effects of non-adrenergic, non-cholinergic nerve stimulation and exogenously applied ATP on a variety of smooth muscle preparations from different vertebrate species, *Brit. J. Pharmacol.* **46:**234–242.

BURNSTOCK, G., DUMSDAY, B., and SMYTHE, A., 1972*b*, Atropine resistant excitation of the urinary bladder: The possibility of transmission via nerves releasing a purine nucleotide, *Brit. J. Pharmacol.* **44:**451–461.

CAMPBELL, G., 1966, Nerve-mediated excitation of the taenia of the guinea-pig caecum, *J. Physiol.* **185:**148–159.

CAMPBELL, G., 1970, Autonomic nervous supply to effector tissues, in: *Smooth Muscle* (E. Bülbring, A. Brading, A. Jones, and T. Tomita, eds.), pp. 451–495, Edward Arnold, London.

CAMPBELL, G., 1971, Autonomic innervation of the lung musculature of a toad (*Bufo marinus*), *Comp. Gen. Pharmacol.* **2:**281–286.

CAMPBELL, G., and BURNSTOCK, G., 1968, The comparative physiology of gastrointestinal motility, in: *Handbook of Physiology*, Section 6: Alimentary Canal, IX: Motility, pp. 2213–2266, American Physiological Society, Washington, D.C.

CANNON, W. B., and LIEB, C. W., 1911, The receptive relaxation of the stomach, *Am. J. Physiol.* **29:**267–273.

CHRISTENSEN, J., 1971, A new neural inhibitor in the gut (editorial), *Gastroenterology* **60:**1130–1131.

COBURN, R. F., 1972, Squeegie of fluid in the compressed canine trachea, *Resp. Physiol.* **16:**33–40.

COBURN, R. F., and TOMITA, T., 1973, Evidence for nonadrenergic inhibitory nerves in guinea-pig trachealis muscle, *Am. J. Physiol.* **224:**1072–1080.

CODE, C. F., and SCHLEGEL, J. F., 1968, Motor action of the esophagus and its sphincters, in: *Handbook of Physiology*, Chap. 90, Section 6: Alimentary Canal, Vol. IV, pp. 1821–1839, American Physiological Society, Washington, D.C.

COLEMAN, R. A., 1973, Evidence for a non-adrenergic inhibitory nervous pathway in guinea-pig trachea, *Brit. J. Pharmacol.* **48:**360P–361P.

COLEMAN, R. A., and LEVY, G. R., 1974, A non-adrenergic inhibitory nervous pathway in guinea-pig trachea, *Brit. J. Pharmacol.* **52:**167–174.

CONWAY, E. J., and COOKE, R., 1939, The deaminases of adenosine and adenylic acid in blood and tissues, *Biochem. J.* **33:**479–492.

COOK, D. B., GILL, G. V., JACKSON, I. M. D., and SMART, G. A., 1974, Inhibition by dexamethasone of adrenocorticotrophin and cortisol release induced by intravenous infusion of ATP and dibutyryl cyclic AMP in piglets, *J. Endocrinol.* **60:**65–73.

COOK, R. D., and KING, A. S., 1970, Observations on the ultrastructure of the smooth muscle and its innervation in the avian lung, *J. Anat.* **106:**273–283.

COSTA, M., and FURNESS, J. B., 1973, The innervation of the internal anal sphincter in the guinea-pig, *Rend. Gastro-enterol.* **5:**47–58.

CREMA, A., 1970, On the polarity of the peristaltic reflex in the colon, in: *Smooth Muscle* (E. Bülbring, A. Brading, A. Jones, and T. Tomita, eds.), pp. 542–548, Edward Arnold, London.

DALE, H. H., 1935, Pharmacology and nerve-endings, *Proc. Roy. Soc. Med.* **28:**319–332.

DARKE, A. C., and SMAJE, L. H., 1973, The effect of chronic duct ligation on the vascular and secretory responses of the cat's submaxillary gland, *J. Physiol.* **228:**361–376.

DE GUBAREFF, T., and SLEATOR, W., 1965, Effects of caffeine on mammalian atrial muscle and its interaction with adenosine and calcium, *J. Pharmacol. Exp. Ther.* **148:**202–214.

DERMIETZEL, R., 1971, Elektronenmikroskopische Untersuchung über die Innervation der Pars pylorica des Mäusemagens, *Z. Mikros.-Anat. Forsch.* **84:**225–256.

DEVINE, C. E, and SIMPSON, F. O., 1968, Localization of tritiated norepinephrine in vascular sympathetic axons of the rat intestine and mesentery by electron microscope radioautography, *J. Cell Biol.* **38:**184–192.

DIAMANT, N. E., 1973, Electrical activity of the cat smooth muscle oesophagus *in vitro*: A study of hyperpolarizing responses occurring with vagal nerve stimulation, intraluminal balloon distension and spontaneous distension and spontaneous contraction of the longitudinal muscle, *Rend. Gastro-enterol.* **5:**26–27.

DIMARINO, A. J., and COHEN, S., 1974, Characteristics of lower esophageal sphincter function in symptomatic diffuse esophageal spasm, *Gastroenterology* **66:**1–6.

DORR, L. D., and BRODY, M. J., 1967, Haemodynamic mechanics of erection in the canine penis, *Am. J. Physiol.* **213:**1526–1531.

DOUGLAS, W. W., 1968, Stimulus–secretion coupling: The concept and clues from chromaffin and other cells, *Brit. J. Pharmacol.* **34:**451–474.

DROLLER, M. J., 1973, Ultrastructure of the platelet release reaction in response to various aggregating agents and their inhibitors, *Lab. Invest.* **29:**595–606.

DUCHON, G., HENDERSON, R., and DANIEL, E. E., 1973, Circular muscle layers in the small intestine, *Rend. Gastro-enterol.* **5:**10.

DUMSDAY, B., 1971, Atropine-resistance of the urinary bladder, *J. Pharm. Pharmacol.* **23:**222–225.

DUNCAN, D., and MORALES, R., 1973*a*, Location of large core synaptic vesicles in the dorsal gray matter of the cat and dog spinal cord, *Am. J. anat.* **136:**123–127.

DUNCAN, D., and MORALES, R., 1973*b*, Location of nerve cells producing the synaptic vesicles situated in the substantia gelatinosa of the spinal cord (1), *Am. J. Anat.* **138:**139–144.

DUTTA, S. P., CHHEDA, G. B. BACZYNSKYJ, L., and MITTELMAN, A., 1973, Characterization of a fluorescent substance derived from N^6-(A^2-isopentenyl)adenosine, *166th Meeting Amer. Chem. Soc. Abs. papers*, MEDI-9.

ECCLES, J. C., and MAGLADERY, J. W., 1937, The excitation and response of smooth muscle, *J. Physiol.* **90:**31–67.

EDVARDSEN, P., 1968, Nervous control of urinary bladder in cats. IV. Effect of autonomic blocking agents on responses to peripheral nerve stimulation, *Acta Physiol. Scand.* **72:**234–247.

EHINGER, B., and FALCK, B., 1971, Autoradiography of some suspected neurotransmitter substances: GABA, Glycine, glutamic acid, histamine, dopamine, and L-DOPA, *Brain Res.* **33:**157–172.

EHRENPREIS, T., 1971, Hirschsprung's disease, *Am. J. Dig. Dis.* **16:**1032–1052.

EINSTEIN, R., ANGUS, J. A., COBBIN, L. B., and MAGUIRE, M. H., 1972, Separation of vasodilator and negative chronotropic actions in analogues of adenosine, *Eur. J. Pharmacol.* **19:**246–250.

ELFVIN, L.-G., 1967, The development of secretory granules in the rat adrenal medulla, *J. Ultrastruct. Res.* **17:**45–62.

EMMELIN, N., and FELDBERG, W., 1948, Systemic effects of adenosine triphosphate, *Brit. J. Pharmacol. Chemother.* **3:**273–284.

FELDBERG, W., and SHERWOOD, S. L., 1954, Injections of drugs into the lateral ventricle of the cat, *J. Physiol.* **123:**148–167.

FILOGAMO, G., and MARCHISIO, P. C., 1971, Acetylcholine system and neural development, in: *Neurosciences Research*, Vol. 4 (S. Ehrenpreis and O. Solnitsky, eds.) pp. 29–64, Academic Press, New York.

FORN, J., and KRISHNA, G., 1971, Effect of norepinephrine, histamine and other drugs on cyclic 3′,5′-AMP formation in brain slices of various animal species, *Pharmacology* **5:**193–204.

FORRESTER, T., 1972, An estimate of adenosine triphosphate release into the venous effluent from exercising human forearm muscle, *J. Physiol.* **224:**611–628.

FORRESTER, T., and HASSAN, M. O., 1973, Appearance of adenosine triphosphate in the perfusate from active frog skeletal muscle, *J. Physiol.* **232:**35P–37P.

FREIMAN, D. G., GOLDMAN, H., and MURRAY, S., 1961, Histochemical studies on hydrolytic enzyme distribution in canine and human muscle and in some human mesenchymal tumors, *Lab. Invest.* **10:**1217–1234

FUMAGALLI, R., BERNAREGGI, V., BERTI, F. and TRABUCCHI, M., 1971, Cyclic AMP formation in human brain: An *in vitro* stimulation by neurotransmitters, *Life Sci.* **10(1):**1111–1115.

FURNESS, J. B., 1969*a*, An electrophysiological study of the innervation of the smooth muscle of the colon, *J. Physiol.* **205:**549–562.

FURNESS, J. B., 1969*b*, The presence of inhibitory fibers in the colon after sympathetic denervation, *Eur. J. Pharmacol.* **6:**349–352.

FURNESS, J. B., 1970, The effect of external potassium ion concentration on autonomic neuro-muscular transmission, *Pflügers Arch.* **317:**310–326.

FURNESS, J. B., 1971, Secondary excitation of intestinal smooth muscle, *Brit. J. Pharmacol.* **41:**213–226.

FURNESS, J. B., and BURNSTOCK, G., 1975, The role of circulating catecholamines in the gastrointestinal tract, in: *Handbook of Physiology*, Section 7: Endocrinology (H. Blaschko and A. D. Smith, eds.), American Physiological Society, Washington, D.C.

FURNESS, J. B., and COSTA, M., 1973, The nervous release and the action of substances which affect intestinal muscle through neither adrenoceptors nor cholinoceptors, in: Recent Developments in Vertebrate Smooth Muscle Physiology, *Phil. Trans. Roy. Soc. London Ser. B Biol. Sci.* **265:**123–133.

FURNESS, J. B., and COSTA, M., 1974, The adrenergic innervation of the gastrointestinal tract, *Ergebn. Physiol.* **69:**1–52.

GAÁL, K., FORGÁCS, I., and SALLAY, P., 1972, Effect of intrarenally infused ATP on renal function, *Acta Physiol. Acad. Sci. Hung.* **41:**213–219.

GABELLA, G., 1970, Electron microscopic observations on the innervation of the intestinal inner muscle layer, *Experientia* **26:**44–46.

GABELLA, G., 1971, Synapses of adrenergic fibers, *Experientia* **27:**280–281.

GABELLA, G., 1972, Innervation of the intestinal muscular coat, *J. Neurocytol.* **1:**341–362.

GADDUM, J. H., and HOLTZ, P., 1933, The localization of the action of drugs on the pulmonary vessels of dogs and cats, *J. Physiol.* **77:**139–158.

GALINDO, A., KRNJEVIĆ, K., and SCHWARTZ, S., 1967, Micro-iontophoretic studies on neurones in the cuneate nucleus, *J. Physiol.* **192:**359–377.

GARRETT, J. R., and HOWARD, E. R., 1972, Effects of rectal distension on the internal anal sphincter of cats, *J. Physiol.* **222:**85P–86P.

GEFFEN, L. B., and LIVETT, B. G., 1971, Synaptic vesicles in sympathetic neurons, *Physiol. Rev.* **51:**98–157.

GERSHON, M. D., and THOMPSON, E. B., 1973, The maturation of neuromuscular function in a multiply innervated structure: Development of longitudinal smooth muscle of foetal mammalian gut and its cholinergic excitatory, adrenergic inhibitory, and non-adrenergic inhibitory innervation, *J. Physiol.* **234:**257–277.

GESCHWIND, I. I., 1970, Mechanism of action of hypothalamic adenohypophysiotropic factors, in: *Hypophysiotropic Hormones of the Hypothalamus Assay and Chemistry* (J. Meites, ed.), pp. 298–319, Williams and Wilkins, Baltimore.

GILLESPIE, J. S., 1962, The electrical and mechanical responses of intestinal smooth muscle cells to stimulation of their extrinsic parasympathetic nerves, *J. Physiol.* **162:**76–92.

GILLESPIE, J. S., 1968, Electrical activity in the colon, in: *Handbook of Physiology*, Section 6: Alimentary Canal, Vol. IV (C. F. Code, ed.), pp. 2093–2120, American Physiological Society, Washington, D.C.

GINSBORG, B. L., and HIRST, G. D. S., 1972, The effect of adenosine on the release of the transmitter from the phrenic nerve of the cat, *J. Physiol.* **224:**629–645.

GLYNN, I. M., 1957, The ionic permiability of the red cell membrane, *Progr. Biophys.* **8:**241–307.

GOUGH, G. R., MAGUIRE, M. H., and SATCHELL, D. G., 1973, Three new adenosine triphosphate analogs: Synthesis and effects on isolated gut, *J. Med. Chem.* **16:**1188–1190.

GREEN, H. N., and STONER, H. B., 1950, *Biological Actions of the Adenine Nucleotides*, Lewis, London.

HADDY, F. J., and SCOTT, J. B., 1968, Metabolically linked vasoactive chemicals in local regulation of blood flow, *Physiol. Rev.* **48:**688–707.

HANIKOVA, M., ZNAMENACK, K., and KRABEC, Z., 1973, ATP and vasoldilan used in cases of asphyxia of newborn rats, *Z. Kinderheilk.* **114:**305–312.

HANSEN, O., 1972, Blood nucleoside and nucleotide studies in mental disease, *Brit. J. Psychiat.* **121:**341–350.

HASHIMOTO, K., and KOKUBUN, H., 1972, Interaction between adenosine compounds and norepinephrine in dog renal circulation, *Tohoku J. Exp. Med.* **107:**373–380.

HASSAN, T., 1969, A hyoscine-resistant contraction of isolated chicken oesophagus in response to stimulation of parasympathetic nerves, *Brit. J. Pharmacol.* **36:**268–275.

HAUGE, A., 1966, Vasoconstriction in isolated blood perfused rabbits lungs and its inhibition by cresols, *Acta Physiol. Scand.* **66:**226–240.

HAUGE, A., LUNDE, P. K. M., WAALER, B. A., and WALLOE, L., 1966, The inhibitory effect of various phenols upon ATP induced vasoconstrictions in isolated perfused lungs, *Acta Physiol. Scand.* **68:**70 (Suppl. 277).

HEIDENHAIN, R., 1872, Ueber die Wirkung einiger Gifte auf die Nerven der glandula submaxillaris, *Pflügers Arch. Ges. Physiol. Menschen Tiere* **5:**309–318.

HELLER, H., and MCILWAIN, H., 1973, Release of [^{14}C] adenine derivatives from isolated sub-systems of the guinea pig brain: Actions of electrical stimulation and of papaverine, *Brain Res.* **53:**105–116.

HERVONEN, A., 1973, Large Vesicles of adrenergic nerves of rabbit uterus, *Acta Physiol. Scand.* **88:**430–432.

HIBBS, R. G., and ELLISON, J. P., 1973, Ultrastructural study of intracardiac autonomic ganglia of guinea-pig, *Tex. Rep. Biol. Med.* **31:**254–255.

HIDAKA, T., and KURIYAMA, H., 1969, Responses of the smooth muscle cell membrane of the guinea-pig jejunum to the field stimulation, *J. Gen. Physiol.* **53:**471–486.

HILTON, S. M., and LEWIS, G. P., 1957, Functional vasodilatation in the submandibular salivary gland, *Brit. Med. Bull.* **13:**189–196.

HILTON, S. M., JEFFRIES, M. G., and VRBOVA, G., 1970, Functional specialisations of the vascular bed of soleus, *J. Physiol.* **206:**543–562.

HIRST, G. D. S., and MCKIRDY, H. C., 1974, A nervous mechanism for descending inhibition in guinea-pig small intestine, *J. Physiol.* **238:**129–143.

HOFFER, B. J., SIGGINS, G. R., and BLOOM, F. E., 1970, Possible cyclic AMP–mediated adrenergic synapses to rat cerebellar Purkinje cells: Combined structural, physiological, and pharmacological analyses, in: *Role of Cyclic AMP in Cell Function*, (P. Greengard and E. Costa, eds.), pp. 1–386, Raven Press, New York.

HÖKFELT, T., 1967, Electron microscopic studies on brain slices from regions rich in catecholamine nerve terminals, *Acta Physiol. Scand.* **69:**119–120.

HOLMAN, M. E., 1958, Membrane potentials recorded with high-resistance microelectrodes and the effects of changes in ionic environment on the electrical and mechanical activity of the smooth muscle of the taenia coli of the guinea-pig, *J. Physiol.* **141:**464–488.

HOLMAN, M. E., 1970, Junction potentials in smooth muscle, in: *Smooth Muscle* (E. Bülbring, A. Brading, A. Jones, and T. Tomita, eds.), pp. 244–288, Edward Arnold, London.

HOLTON, P., 1959, The liberation of adenosine triphosphate on antidromic stimulation of sensory nerves, *J. Physiol.* **145:**494–504.

HONJIN, R., TAKAHASHI, A., SHIMASAKA, S., and MARUYAMA, H., 1965, Two types of synaptic nerve processes in the ganglia of Auerbach's plexus of mice, as revealed by electron microscopy, *J. Electron Micros.* **14:**43–49.

HOOPER, M., SPEDDING, M., SWEETMAN, A. J., and WEETMAN, D. F., 1974, 2-2′pyridylisatogen tosylate: An antagonist of the inhibitory effects of ATP on smooth muscle, *Brit. J. Pharmacol.* **50:**458P–459P.

HOPKINS, S. V., 1973*a*, The action of ATP in the guinea-pig heart, *Biochem. Pharmacol.* **22:**335–339.

HOPKINS, S. V., 1973*b*, The potentiation of the action of adenosine on the guinea-pig heart, *Biochem. Pharmacol.* **22:**341–348.

HÖSLI, L., and HÖSLI, E., 1972, Autoradiographic localization of the uptake of glycine in cultures of rat medulla oblongata, *Brain Res.* **45:**612–616.

HOWARD, E. R., and NIXON, H. H., 1968, Internal anal sphincter: Observations on development and mechanism of inhibitory responses in premature infants and children with Hirschsprung's disease, *Archs. Dis. Child.* **43:**569–578.

HUANG, M., and DALY, J. W., 1974, Adenosine-elicited accumulation of cyclic-AMP in brain slices potentiation by agents which inhibit uptake of adenosine, *Life Sci.* **14:**489–503.

HUANG, M., SHIMIZU, H., and DALY, J. W., 1972, Accumulation of cyclic adenosine monophosphate in incubated slices of brain tissue. 2. Effects of depolarizing agents, membrane stabilizers, phosphodiesterase inhibitors, and adenosine analogs, *J. Med. Chem.* **15:**462–466.

HUDDART, H., and BRADBURY, S. J., 1972, Fine structure of a neurosecretory axon in a crustacean skeletal muscle, *Experientia* **28:**950–951.

HUGHES, J., and VANE, J. R., 1967, An analysis of the responses of the isolated portal vein of the rabbit to electrical stimulation and to drugs, *Brit. J. Pharmacol. Chemother.* **30:**46–66.

HUGHES, J., and VANE, J. R., 1970, Relaxations of the isolated portal vein of the rabbit induced by nicotine and electrical stimulation, *Brit. J. Pharmacol.* **39:**476–489.

HUIJING, F., and SLATER, E. C., 1961, The use of oligomycin as an inhibitor of oxidative phosphorylation, *J. Biochem.* (*Tokyo*) **49:**493–501.

HULTÉN, L., 1969, Reflex control of colonic motility and blood flow, *Acta Physiol. Scand. Suppl.* **335:**77–93.

HUNG, K. S., HERTWECK, M. S., HARDY, J. D., and LOOSLI, C. G., 1972, Innervation of pulmonary alveoli of the mouse lung: An electron microscopic study, *Am. J. Anat.* **135:**477–496.

ICHIKAWA, A., HAYASHI, H., MINAMI, M., and TOMITA, K., 1972, An acute inflammation induced by inorganic pyrophosphate and adenosine triphosphate, and its inhibition by cyclic 3′,5′-adenosine monophosphate, *Biochem. Pharmacol.* **21:**317–331.

ISHII, S., and NAKAMURA, I., 1972, Electron microscopic study on the large granulated vesicles in enlarged axon of the area postrema, *J. Electron Micros.* **21:**85–88.

ITO, Y., and KURIYAMA, H., 1971, Nervous control of the motility of the alimentary canal of the silver carp, *J. Exp. Biol.* **55:**469–487.

ITO, Y., and KURIYAMA, H., 1973, Membrane properties and inhibitory innervation of the circular muscle cells of guinea-pig caecum. *J. Physiol.* **231:**455–470.

IVERSEN, L. L., 1967, *The Uptake and Storage of Noradrenaline in Sympathetic Nerves,* Cambridge University Press, London.

JAMES, T. N., 1965, The chronotropic action of ATP and related compounds studied by direct perfusion of the sinus node. *J. Pharmacol. Exp. Ther.* **149:**233–247.

JANSSON, G., 1969, Extrinsic nervous control of gastric motility: An experimental study in the cat, *Acta Physiol. Scand. Suppl.* **326:**1–42.

JENKINSON, D. H., and MORTON, I. K. M., 1965, Effects of noradrenaline and isoprenaline on the permeability of depolarized intestinal smooth muscle to inorganic ions, *Nature* **205:**505–506.

JOHANSEN, T., and CHAKRAVARTY, N., 1972, Dependence of histamine release from rat mast cells on adenosine triphosphate, *Naunyn-Schmiedebergs Arch. Pharmacol.* **275:**457–463.

JULÉ, Y., and GONELLA, J., 1972, Modifications de l'activité électrique du côlon terminal de lapin par stimulation des fibres nerveuses pelviennes et sympathiques, *J. Physiol. (Paris)* **64:**599–621.

KAACK, B., 1972, Influence of acetylcholine and adrenaline on ATPase activity, *Comp. Gen. Pharmacol.* **3:**296–298.

KAKIUCHI, S., RALL, T. W., and MCILWAIN, H., 1969, The effect of electrical stimulation upon the accumulation of adenosine 3′,5′-phosphate in isolated cerebral tissue, *J. Neurochem.* **16:**485–491.

KERR, F. W. L., 1970, The fine structure of the subnucleus caudalis of the trigeminal nerve, *Brain Res.* **23:**129–145.

KIERNAN, J. A., 1972*a*, Effects of known and suspected neurotransmitter substances and of some nucleotides on isolated mast cells, *Experientia* **28:**653–655.

KIERNAN, J. A., 1972*b*, The involvement of mast cells in vasodilatation due to axon reflexes in infused skin, *Quart. J. Exp. Physiol.* **57:**311–317.

KODAMA, T., MATSUKADO, Y., and SHIMIZU, H., 1973, The cyclic AMP system of human brain, *Brain Res.* **50:**135–146.

KOLASSA, N., PFLEGER, K., and RUMMEL, W., 1970, Specificity of adenosine uptake into the heart and inhibition by dipyridamole *Eur. J. Pharmacol.* **9:**265–268.

KOLASSA, N., PFLEGER, K., and TRÄM, M., 1971, Species differences in action and elimination of adenosine after dipyridamole and hexobendine, *Eur. J. Pharmacol.* **13:**320–325.

KORNELIUSSEN, H., 1973, Dense-core vesicles in motor nerve terminals: Monoaminergic innervation of slow non-twitch muscle fibers in Atlantic hagfish (*Myxine glutinosa,* L.)? *Z. Zellforsch. Mikros. Anat.* **140:**425–432.

KOSTERLITZ, H. W., 1968, Intrinsic and extrinsic nervous control of motility of the stomach and the intestines, in: *Handbook of Physiology,* Section 6: Alimentary Canal, Vol. IV (C. F. Code, ed.), pp. 2147–2171, American Physiological Society, Washington, D.C.

KRYVI, H., 1971, The structure of the longitudinal muscles of *Sabella penicillum* (Annelida, Polychaeta), with a note on the contraction properties, *Norw. J. Zool.* **19:**149–167.

KUCHI, M., MIYAHARA, J. T., and SHIBATA, S., 1973, [^{3}H]-Adenine nucleotide and [^{3}H]-noradrenaline release evoked by electrical field stimulation, perivascular nerve stimulation and nicotine from the taenia of the guinea-pig caecum, *Brit. J. Pharmacol.* **49:**258–267.

KUPERMAN, A. S., VOLPERT, W. A., and OKAMOTO, M., 1964, Release of adenine nucleotide from nerve axons, *Nature* **204:**1000–1001.

KURIYAMA, H., 1963, Electrophysiological observations on the motor innervation of the smooth muscle cells in the guinea-pig vas deferens, *J. Physiol.* **169:**213–228.

KURIYAMA, H., OSA, T., and TOIDA, N., 1967, Nervous factors influencing the membrane activity of intestinal smooth muscle, *J. Physiol.* **191:**257–270.

KURIYAMA, H., OSA, T., and TASAKI, H., 1970, Electrophysiological studies of the antrum muscle fibres of the guinea-pig stomach, *J. Gen. Physiol.* **55:**48–62.

KURODA, Y., and MCILWAIN, H., 1973, Incorporation and release of adenosine derivatives in guinea pig neocortical tissues and derived synaptosomes, in: *4th Int. Soc. Neurochem. Tokyo Meeting,* p. 331.

LANE, B. P., 1967, Localization of products of ATP hydrolysis in mammalian smooth muscle cells, *J. Cell Biol.* **34:**713–720.

LANGLEY, J. N., and ANDERSON, H. K., 1895, The innervation of the pelvic and adjoining viscera. IV. The internal generative organs, *J. Physiol.* **19:**122–130.

LAUWERYNS, J. M., COKELAERC, M., and THEUNYNCK, P., 1973, Serotonin producing neuroepithelial bodies in rabbit respiratory mucosa, *Science* **180:**410–413.

LESLIE, S. W., BOROWITZ, J. L., and MIYA, T. S., 1973, Adenosine analogs: Structure–activity relationshiops in vascular and intestinal smooth-muscle, *J. Pharm. Sci.* **62:**1449–1452.

LIU, M. S., and FEINBERG, H., 1971, Incorporation of adenosine-8-^{14}C and inosine-8-^{14}C into rabbit heart adenine nucleotides, *Am. J. Physiol.* **220:**1242–1248.

LIU, M. S., and FEINBERG, H., 1973, Effect of persantin on nucleoside metabolism of the perfused rabbit heart, *Biochem. Pharmacol.* **22:**1118–1121.

LOBANOV, G. C., 1961, Gas exchange in premature newborns during secondary asphyxia, *Vop. Okhr. Materin. Dets.* **6:**11–17.

LOCK, A., and WEBER, L. J., 1971, The vagal inhibitory reflex in the rat, *Proc. West Pharmacol. Soc.* **14:**88–90.

LUDUENA, F. P., and GRIGAS, E. O., 19666, Pharmacological study of autonomic innervation of dog retractor penis, *Am. J. Physiol.* **210:**435–445.

LUDUENA, F. P., and GRIGAS, E. O., 1972, Effect of some biological substances on the dog retractor penis *in vitro, Arch. Int. Pharmacodyn.* **196:**269–274.

LUMSDEN, K., and HOLDEN, W. S., 1969, The act of vomiting in man, *Gut* **10:**173–179.

LUND, C. F., and CHRISTENSEN, J., 1969, Electrical stimulation of oesophageal smooth muscle and effects of antagonists, *Am. J. Physiol.* **217:**1369–1374.

LUNDE, P. K. M., WAALER, B. A., and WALLØE, L., 1968, The inhibitory effect of various phenols upon ATP-induced vasoconstriction in isolated perfused rabbit lungs, *Acta Physiol. Scand.* **72:**331–337.

MADINAVEITIA, J., and RAVENTOS, J., 1949, Antimalarial compounds as antagonists of adenosine, *Brit. J. Pharmacol. Chemother.* **4:**81–92.

MALL, F. P., 1896, On the reversal of the intestine, *Johns Hopkins Hosp. Rep.* **1:**37–75.

MALMFORS, T., and OLSON, L., 1970, Growth characteristics of adrenergic nerves in the adult rat, *Acta Physiol. Scand. Suppl.* **348:**9–112.

MALMFORS, T., FURNESS, J. B., CAMPBELL, G. R., and BURNSTOCK, G., 1971, Reinnervation of smooth muscle of the vas deferens transplanted into the anterior chamber of the eye, *J. Neurobiol.* **2:**193–207.

MARLEY, E., and NISTICO, G., 1972, Effects of catecholamines and adenosine derivatives given into the brain of fowls, *Brit. J. Pharmacol.* **46:**619–636.

MARX, J. L., 1972, Cyclic AMP in brain: Role in synaptic transmission, *Science* **178:**1188–1190.

MATSUMURA, S., TAIRA, N., and HASHIMOTO, K., 1968, The pharmacological behaviour of the urinary bladder and its vasculature of the dog, *Tohoku J. Exp. Med.* **96:**247–258.

MEVES, H., 1953, Die Wirkung von Adrenalin und Adrenalinverwandten auf Gefässe und Muskulatur der Froschlunge, *Pflügers Arch. Ges. Physiol.* **258:**200–210.

MILLER, T., and REES, D., 1973, Excitatory transmission in insect neuromuscular systems, *Am. Zoologist* **13:**299–313.

MOIR, T. W., and DOWNS, T. D., 1972, Myocardial reactive hyperemia: comparative effects of adenosine, ATP, ADP, and AMP, *Am. J. Physiol.* **222:**1386–1390.

MOYES, I. C. A., 1973, Cyclic AMP in depressive illness, *J. Int. Med. Res.* **1:**321–324.

MCINTYRE, A. M., 1973, Purinergic autonomic neurones (editorial), *J. Clin. Pharmacol.* **13:**241–243.

MCLENNAN, H., 1970, in: *Synaptic Transmission*, 2nd ed., pp. 132–133, Saunders, Philadelphia.

NAGASAWA, J., and MITO, S., 1967, Electron microscopic observations on the innervation of the smooth muscle, *Tohoku J. Exp. Med.* **91:**277–293.

NAKANISHI, H., and TAKEDA, H., 1972, The possibility that adenosine triphosphate is an excitatory transmitter in guinea-pig seminal vesicle, *Jap. J. Pharmacol.* **22:**269–270.

NAKANISHI, H., and TAKEDA, H., 1973, The possible role of adenosine triphosphate in chemical transmission between the hypogastric nerve ending and seminal vesicle in guinea-pig, *Jap. J. Pharmacol.* **23:**479–490.

NAKATSU, K., and DRUMMOND, G. I., 1972, Adenylate metabolism and adenosine formation in the heart, *Am. J. Physiol.* **223:**1119–1127.

NAKAZATO, Y., and OHGA, A., 1971, Relationships between 5-hydroxytryptamine and vagal relaxation in the dog stomach, *Jap. J. Pharmacol.* **21:**829–832.

NICHOLS, R. E., and WALASZEK, E. S., 1963, Antagonism of the vasodepressor effect of ATP by caffeine, *Fed. Proc.* **22:**308.

NICKERSON, M., 1970, in: *The Pharmacological Basis of Therapeutics* (L. S. Goodman and A. Gilman, eds.), Macmillan, New York.

O'BRIEN, R. A., DA PRADA, M., and PLETSCHER, A., 1972, The ontogenesis of catecholamines and adenosine-5'-triphosphate in the adrenal medulla, *Life Sci.* **11(1):**749–759.

OHASHI, H., 1971, An electrophysiological study of transmission from intramural excitatory nerves to the smooth muscle cells of the chicken oesophagus, *Jap. J. Pharmacol.* **21:**585–596.

OHGA, A., NAKAZATO, Y., and SAITO, K., 1970, Considerations of the efferent nervous mechanism of the vago-vagal reflex relaxation of the stomach in the dog, *Jap. J. Pharmacol.* **20:**116–130.

OHKAWA, H., and PROSSER, C. L., 1972, Electrical activity in myenteric and submucous plexuses of cat intestine, *Am. J. Physiol.* **222:**1412–1419.

OLSSON, R. A., SNOW, J. A., GENTRY, M. K., and FRICK., G. P., 1972, Adenosine uptake by canine heart, *Circ. Res.* **31:**767–778.

ONO, H., INAGAKI, K., and HASHIMOTO, K., 1966, A pharmacological approach to the nature of the autoregulation of the renal blood flow, *Jap. J. Physiol.* **16:**625–634.

OSBORNE, M. P., 1971, Neurosecretory endings associated with striated muscles in three insects (*Schistocerca, Carausius,* and *Phormia*) and a frog (*Rana*), *Z. Zellforsch. Mikros. Anat.* **116:**391–404.

PADDLE, B. M., and BURNSTOCK, G., 1974*a*, Release of ATP from perfused heart during coronary vasodilation, *Blood Vessels* **2:**110–119.

PADDLE, B. M., and BURNSTOCK, G., 1975, Nerve-mediated release of ATP from guinea-pig taenia coli, in preparation.

PARRATT, J. R., and WADSWORTH, R. M., 1972, The effects of dipyridamole on the myocardial vasodilator actions of noradrenaline, isoprenaline and adenosine, *Brit. J. Pharmacol.* **46:**585–593.

PATTERSON, D. A., and WIBBERLEY, D. C., 1965, Isatogens. Part II. 2-2'pyridylisatogen, *J. Chem. Soc.* **1965:**1706–1711.

PEARCY, J. F., and LIERE, E. J. VAN, 1926, Studies on the visceral nervous system. XVII. Reflexes from the colon. 1. Reflexes to the stomach, *Am. J. Physiol.* **78:**64–73.

PENTREATH, V. W., and COBB, J. L. S., 1972, Neurobiology of echinodermata, *Biol. Rev.* **47:**363–392.

PFAFFMAN, M. A., and MCFARLAND, S. A., 1973, The effects of theophylline and cyclic AMP on intestinal smooth muscle contractions, *Eur. J. Pharmacol.* **23:**147–152.

PHILLIS, J. W., KOSTOPOULOS, G. K., and LIMACHER, J. L., 1975, A potent depressant action of adenine derivatives on cerebral cortical neurones, *Europ. J. Pharmacol.* **30:**125–129.

PICK, J., 1970, *The Autonomic Nervous System: Morphological, Comparative, Clinical and Surgical Aspects*, Lippincott, Philadelphia.

POTTER, L. T., 1970, Synthesis, storage and release of (^{14}C) acetylcholine in isolated rat diaphragm muscles, *J. Physiol.* **206:**145–166.

PULL, I., and MCILWAIN, H., 1972*a*, Metabolism of (^{14}C) adenine and derivatives by cerebral tissues, superfused and electrically stimulated, *Biochem. J.* **126:**965–973.

PULL, I., and MCILWAIN, H., 1972*b*, Adenine derivatives as neurohumoral agents in the brain: The quantities liberated on excitation of superperfused cerebral tisues, *Biochem. J.* **130:**975–981.

PULL, I., and MCILWAIN, H., 1973, Output of (C–14) adenine nucleotides and their derivatives from cerebral tissues: Tetrodotoxin resistant and calcium ion requiring components, *Biochem. J.* **136:**893–901.

RALL, T., and SATTIN, A., 1970, The effect of adenosine and adenine nucleotides on the cyclic adenosine 3',5'-phosphate content of guinea pig cerebral cortex slices, *Mol. Pharmacol.* **6:**13–23.

RALSTON, H. J., III, 1968, The fine structure of neurons in the dorsal horn of the cat spinal cord, *J. Comp. Neurol.* **132:**275–301.

RAND, M. J., STAFFORD, A., and THORP, R. H., 1955, The potentiation of the action of adenosine on the guinea-pig heart by ouabain, *J. Pharmacol. Exp. Ther.* **114:**119–125.

RAVENTOS, J., 1950, Oral communication, Pharmacological Society, January 1947, in: *Biological Actions of the Adenine Nucleotides* (H. N. Green and H. B. Stoner), p. 260, Lewis, London.

RAYNER, V., 1970, Observations on the functional internal anal sphincter of the vervet monkey, *J. Physiol.* **213:**27P–28P.

REHM, W. S., WHITE, A. S., SANDERS, S. S., and FEAGIN, F. F., 1970, Adenine compounds on changes in optical density and motility of frog gastric mucosa, *Am. J. Physiol.* **218:**1010–1014.

REIS, J. L., 1937, Über die Activität der 5-Nukleotidase in den tierischen und menschlichen Geweben, *Enzymologia* **2:**183–190.

REIS, J. L., 1951, The specificity of phosphomonoesterases in human tissues, *Biochem. J.* **48:**548–551.

RIKIMARU, A., FUKUSHI, Y., and SUZUKI, T., 1971*a*, Evidence for the presence of nonadrenergic inhibitory nerves in the human taenia coli, *Tohoku J. Exp. Med.* **104:**199–200.

RIKIMARU, A., FUKUSHI, Y., and SUZUKI, T., 1971*b*, Effects of imidazole and phentolamine on the relaxant responses of guinea-pig taenia coli to transmural stimulation and to adenosine triphosphate, *Tohoku J. Exp. Med.* **105:**199–200.

ROBINSON, M., MCLEAN, J. R., and BURNSTOCK, G., 1971, Ultrastructural identification of non-adrenergic inhibitory nerve fibres, *J. Pharmacol. Exp. Ther.* **179:**149–160.

ROGERS, A. W., 1973, *Techniques of Autoradiography*, Elsevier, Amsterdam.

ROGERS, D., and BURNSTOCK, G., 1966, Multiaxonal autonomic junctions in intestinal smooth muscle of the toad, *J. Comp. Neurol.* **126:**625–652.

ROMAN, C., and CAR, A., 1967, Contractions oesophagiennes produites par la stimulation du vague ou du bulbe rachidien, *J. Physiol. (Paris)* **59:**377–398.

ROSENBLOOM, F. M., KELLEY, W. N., MILLER, J., HENDERSON, J. E., and SEEGMILLER, J. E., 1967, Inherited disorder of purine metabolism: Correlation between central nervous system dysfunction and biochemical defects, *J. Am. Med. Assoc.* **202:**175–177.

ROSENBLUETH, A., 1950, *The Transmission of Nerve Impulses at Neuroeffector Junctions and Peripheral Synapses*, Technology Press, New York.

ROSENBLUTH, J., 1972, Myoneural junctions of two ultrastructurally distinct types in earthworm body wall muscle, *J. Cell Biol.* **54:**566–579.

ROSS, G., 1973, Vascular effects of periarterial mesenteric nerve stimulation after adrenergic neurone blockade, *Experientia* **29:**289–290.

ROSTGAARD, J., and BARRNETT, R. J., 1964, Fine structure localisation of nucleoside phosphatases in relation to smooth muscle cells and unmyelinated nerves in the small intestine of the rat, *J. Ultrastruct. Res.* **11:**193–207.

ROTH, L. J., and STUMPF, W. E. (eds.), 1969, *Autoradiography of Diffusable Substances*, Academic Press, New York.

RUBIO, R., BERNE, R. M., and KATORI, M., 1969, Release of adenosine in reactive hyperemia of the dog heart, *Am. J. Physiol.* **216:**56–62.

RUBIO, R., BERNE, R. M., and DOBSON, J. G., 1973, Sites of adenosine production in cardiac and skeletal-muscle, *Am. J. Physiol.* **225:**938–953.

SATCHELL, D. G., and BURNSTOCK, G., 1971, Quantitative studies of the release of purine compounds following stimulation of non-adrenergic inhibitory nerves in the stomach, *Biochem. Pharmacol.* **20:**1694–1697.

SATCHELL, D., and BURNSTOCK, G., 1975, Comparison of the effects of adenine nucleotides and adenosine on the guinea-pig taenia coli on the presence and absence of dipyridamole, *Eur. J. Pharmacol.*, in press.

SATCHELL, D. G., and MAGUIRE, M. H., 1975, Inhibitory effects of adenine nucleotide analogues on the isolated guinea-pig taenia coli, *J. Pharmacol. Exp. Ther.*, in press.

SATCHELL, D. G., LYNCH, A., BOURKE, P. M., and BURNSTOCK, G., 1972, Potentiation of the effects of exogenously applied ATP and purinergic nerve stimulation on the guinea-pig taenia coli by dipyridamole and hexobendine, *Eur. J. Pharmacol.* **19:**343–350.

SATCHELL, D., BURNSTOCK, G., and DANN, P., 1973, Antagonism of the effects of purinergic nerve stimulation and exogenously applied ATP on the guinea-pig taenia coli by 2-substituted imidazolines and related compounds, *Eur. J. Pharmacol.* **23:**264–269.

SATO, H., OHGA, A., and NAKAZATO, Y., 1970, The excitatory and inhibitory innervation of the stomachs of the domestic fowl, *Jap. J. Pharmacol.* **20:**382–397.

SATTIN, A., and RALL, T. W., 1970, The effect of adenosine and adenine nucleotides on the cyclic adenosine 3′,5′phosphate content of guinea pig cerebral cortex slices, *Mol. Pharmacol.* **6:**13–23.

SCHACHTER, M., BARTON, S., and KARPINSKI, E., 1973, Analysis of vasodilatation in the submaxillary gland using potentiators of acetylcholine and kinins, *Experientia* **29:**973–974.

SCHNAAR, R. L., and SPARKS, H. V., 1972, Response of large and small coronary arteries to nitroglycerin, $NaNO_2$, and adenosine, *Am. J. Physiol.* **223:**223–228.

SCHULMAN, J. D., GREENE, M. L., FUJIMOTO, W. Y., and SEEGMILLER, J. E., 1971, Adenine therapy for Lesch–Nyhan syndrome, *Pediat. Res.* **5:**77–82.

SCHULTZ, J., and DALY, J. W., 1973*a*, Cyclic adenosine 3′,5′-monophosphate in guinea pig cerebral cortical slices. I. Formation of cyclic adenosine 3′,5′-monophosphate from endogenous adenosine triphosphate and from radioactive adenosine triphosphate formed during a prior incubation with radioactive adenine, *J. Biol. Chem.* **248:**843–852.

SCHULTZ, J., and DALY, J. W., 1973*b*, Cyclic adenosine 3′,5′-monophosphate in guinea pig cerebral cortical slices. III. Formation, degradation, and reformation of cyclic adenosine 3′,5′-monophosphate during sequential stimulations by biogenic amines and adenosine, *J. Biol. Chem.* **248:**860–866.

SECRIST, J. A., III, Barrio, J. R., Leonard, N. J., and Weber, G., 1972, Fluorescent modification of adenosine-containing coenzymes: Biological activities and spectroscopic properties, *Biochemistry* **11:**3499–3506.

SEEGMILLER, J. E., ROSENBLOOM, F. M., and KELLY, W. N., 1967, Enzyme defect associated with a sex-linked human neurological disorder and excessive purine synthesis, *Science* **155:**1682–1684.

SEMBA, T., 1954, Studies on the entero-gastric reflexes, *Hiroshima J. Med. Sci.* **2:**323–327.

SENFT, G., 1968, Biochemical aspects of the hyperglycemic action of diazoxide, *Ann. N.Y. Acad. Sci.* **150:**242–255.

SHEPHERD, J. T., 1963, in: *Physiology of the Circulation in Human Limbs in Health and Disease*, Saunders, Philadelphia.

SHERMAN, R. G., and FOURTNER, C. R., 1972, Ultrastructural features of synaptic regions in walking leg muscles of the horseshoe crab, *Limulus polyphemus* (L.), *J. Ultrastruct. Res.* **40:**44–54.

SHERMAN, R. G., and LUFF, A. R., 1971, Structural features of the tarsal claw muscles of the spider, *Eurypelma marxi* Simon, *Canad. J. Zool.* **49:**1549–1556.

SHIMIZU, H., 1973, Purinergic nerve mechanism in the brain: Uptake, storage, release, and adenyl cyclase as a receptor, in: *4th Int. Soc. Neurochem. Tokyo Meeting*, pp. 88–89.

SHIMIZU, H., and DALY, J., 1970, Formation of cyclic adenosine 3′,5′-monophosphate from adenosine in brain slices, *Biochim. Biophys. Acta* **222:**465–473.

SHIMIZU, H., and OKAYAMA, H., 1973, An ATP pool associated with adenyl cyclase of brain tissue, *J. Neurochem.* **20:**1279–1284.

SHIMIZU, H., CREVELING, C. R., and DALY, J., 1970, Stimulated formation of adenosine 3′,5′-cyclic phosphate in cerebral cortex: Synergism between electrical activity and biogenic amines, *Proc. Natl. Acad. Sci.* **65:**1033–1040.

SHIMIZU, H., TANAKA, S., SUZUKI, T., and MATSUKADO, Y., 1971, The response of human cerebrum adenyl cyclase to biogenic amines, *J. Neurochem.* **18:**1157–1161.

SHNEOUR, E. A., and HANSEN, I. M., 1971, Inhibition by nucleotides of mouse brain UDP galactose 4-epimerase *in vitro*, *J. Neurochem.* **18:**1345–1349.

SILINSKY, E. M., and HUBBARD, J. I., 1973, Release of ATP from rat motor nerve terminals, *Nature* **243:**404–405.

SKOLNICK, P., HUANG, M., DALY, J., and HOFFER, B., 1973, Accumulation of adenosine 3′,5′-monophosphate in incubated slices from discrete regions of squirrel monkey cerebral cortex: Effect of norepinephrine, serotonin and adenosine, *J. Neurochem.* **21:** 237–240.

SKOU, J. C., 1960, Further investigations on a Mg^{++} and Na^{+}-activated adenosintriphosphatase, possibly related to the active, linked transport of Na^{+} and K^{+} across the nerve membrane, *Biochim. Biophys. Acta* **42:**6–23.

SMALL, R. C., 1972, Transmission from intramural inhibitory neurones to circular smooth muscle of the rabbit caecum and the effects of catecholamines, *Brit. J. Pharmacol.* **45:**149P–150P.

SMITH, A. D., and WINKLER, H., 1972, Fundamental mechanisms in the release of catecholamines, in: *Catecholamines*, (H. Blaschko and E. Muscholl, eds.), pp. 538–617, Springer-Verlag, New York.

SMYTHE, A. E., 1971, Studies on the nature of transmitter substances released by non-adrenergic, non-cholinergic nerves to smooth muscle, M.Sc. thesis, University of Melbourne.

SMYTHIES, J. R., ANTUN, F., YANK, G., and YORKE, C., 1971, Molecular mechanisms of storage of transmitters in synaptic terminals, *Nature* **231:**185–188.

SNEDDON, J. D., SMYTHE, A., SATCHELL, D., and BURNSTOCK, G., 1973, Investigation of the identity of the transmitter substance released by non-adrenergic, non-cholinergic excitatory nerves in the gut of lower vertebrates, *Comp. Gen. Pharmacol* **4:**53–60.

SPEDEN, R. N., 1967, Adrenergic transmission in small arteries, *Nature* **216:**289–290.

STAFFORD, A., 1966, Potentiation of adenosine and the adenine nucleotides by dipyridamole, *Brit. J. Pharmacol. Chemother.* **28:**218–227.

STEIN, H. H., 1973, Ethyl adenosine-5′-carboxylate: A potent vasoactive agent in dog, *J. Med. Chem.* **16:**1306–1308.

STEVENS, P., ROBINSON, R. L., VAN DYKE, K., and STITZEL, R., 1972, Studies of the synthesis and release of adenosine triphosphate-8-^{3}H in the isolated perfused cat adrenal gland, *J. Pharmacol. Exp. Ther.* **181:**463–471.

STOCKLEY, H. L., and BENNETT, A., 1973, The intrinsic innervation of human colonic muscle, *Rend. Gastro-enterol.* **5:**17.

SU, C., 1975, Purinergic nerves in blood vessels, *Fol. Pharm. J.* **71:**1–2.

SU, C., BEVAN, J., and BURNSTOCK, G., 1971, (^{3}H) Adenosine triphosphate: Release during stimulation of enteric nerves, *Science*, **173:**337–339.

SURAN, A. A., 1974, 5′-Nucleotidase and an acid phosphatase of spinal cord. Comparative histochemistry and specificity of the enzyme in mouse and cat spinal cords. Cytologic localisation in mouse substantia gelatinosa, *J. Histochem. Cytochem.* **22:**302–311.

SYDOW, V., and AHLQUIST, R. P., 1954, Cardiovascular actions of some simple nucleic acid derivatives, *J. Am. Pharm. Assoc. Sci. Ed.* **43:**166–170.

TAFURI, W. L., 1964, Ultrastructure of the vesicular component in the intramural nervous system of the guinea-pig's intestines, *Z. Naturforsch.* **19:**622–625.

TAFURI, W. L., and MARIA, T. DE A., 1970, Sôbre o comportamento do componente vesicular neurosecretor no megaesôfago da tripanossomiase cruzu humana, *Rev. Inst. Med. Trop. Sao Paulo* **12:**298–309.

TAKAGI, K., and TAKAYANAGI, I., 1972, Effect of N^{6},2′-*O*-dibutyryl 3′5′-cyclic adenosine monophosphate 3′,5′-cyclic adenosine monophosphate and adenosine triphosphate on acetylcholine output from cholinergic nerves in guinea pig ileum, *Jap. J. Pharmacol.* **22:**33–36.

TAXI, J., and DROZ, B., 1966, Etude de l'incorporation de noradrénaline-^{3}H (NA-^{3}H) et de 5-hydroxytryptophane-^{3}H (5-HTP-^{3}H) dans les fibres nerveuses du canal déférent et de l'intestin, *C. R. Hebd. Seances Acad. Sci. Paris* **263:**1237–1240.

TAXI, J., and DROZ, B., 1967, Localization d'amines biogènes dans le système neurovégétatif périphérique: Étude radioautographique en microscopie électronique après injection de noradrenaline-^{3}H et de 5-hydroxytryptophane-^{3}H, in: *Neurosecretion* (F. Stutinsky, ed.), pp. 191–202, Springer-Verlag, Berlin.

THER, L., MUSCHAWEK, R., and HERGOTT, J., 1957, Antagonismus zwischen Adenosin und Methyl-Xanthinen am Reizleitungssystem des Herzens, *Arch. Pharmakol. Exp. Pathol.* **231:**586–590.

TOMINAGA, S., WATANABE, K., SUZUKI, T., and NAKAMURA, T., 1973, Total amount of adenosine and AMP released from canine skeletal muscle after ischemia and during contractions, *Tohoku J. Exp. Med.* **111:**199–200.

TOMITA, T., 1972, Conductance change during the inhibitory potential in the guinea-pig taenia coli, *J. Physiol.* **225:**693–704.

TOMITA, T., and WATANABE, H., 1973, A comparison of the effects of adenosine triphosphate with noradrenaline and with the inhibitory potential of the guinea-pig taenia coli, *J. Physiol.* **231:**167–177.

TRANZER, J. P., DA PRADA, M., and PLETSCHER, A., 1972, Storage of 5-hydroxytryptamine in megakaryocytes, *J. Cell Biol.* **52:**191–197.

TREISTER, G., and BÁRÁNY, E. H., 1970, Degeneration mydriasis and hyperemia of the iris after superior cervical ganglionectomy in the rabbit, *Invest. Ophthalmol.* **9:**873–887.

TRIGGLE, D. J., 1965, *Chemical Aspects of the Autonomic Nervous System*, Academic Press, London.

TWENTE, J., and GIORGIO, N., 1970, Arousing effects of adenosine and adenine nucleotides in hibernating *Citellus lateralis*, *Comp. Gen. Pharmacol.* **1:**485–491.

UCHIZONO, K., and OHSAWA, K., 1973, Morpho-physiological consideration on synaptic transmission in the amphibian sympathetic ganglion, *Acta Physiol. Pol.* **24:**205–214.

UNSICKER, K., 1971, On the innervation of mammalian endocrine glands (anterior pituitary and parathyroids), *Z. Zellforsch. Mikros. Anat.* **121:**283–291.

UNSICKER, K., 1973*a*, Fine structure and innervation of avian adrenal gland. 3. Non-cholinergic nerve fibers, *Z. Zellforsch. Mikros. Anat.* **145:**557–575.

UNSICKER, K., 1973*b*, Innervation of the testicular interstitial tissue in reptiles, *Z. Zellforsch. Mikros. Anat.* **146:**123–138.

UUSITALO, R., and PALKAMA, A., 1971, Evidence for the nervous control of secretion in the ciliary processes, *Prog. Brain Res.* **34:**513–521.

VIGDAHL, R. L., MONGIN, J., JR., and MARQUIS, N. R., 1971, Platelet aggregation. IV. Platelet phosphodiesterase and its inhibition by vasodilators, *Biochem. Biophys. Res. Commun.* **42:**1088–1094.

VON KOSS, F. W., BEISENHERZ, G., and MAERKISCH, R., 1962, Die Eliminierung von Adenosin aus dem Blut unter dem Einfluss von 2,6-Bis(diäthanolamino)-4,8-dipiperidino-pyrimido(5,4-*d*)prymidin und Papaverin, *Arzneimittel-Forsch.* **12:**1130–1131.

VON KRAUPP, O., WOLNER, E., ADLER-KASTNER, L., CHIRIKDJIAN, J. J., PLOSZCZANSKI, B., and TUISL, E., 1966, Die Wirkung von Hexobendin auf Sauerstoffverbrauch, Energetik und Substratsfoffwechsel des Herzens, *Arzneimittel-Forsch.* **16:**692–696.

VON PFLEGER, K., and SCHÖNDORF, H., 1969, Zur Aufklarung des Wirkungsmechanismus von Dipyridamol, *Arzneimittel-Forsch.* **19:**97–102.

WANG, S. C., and BORISON, H. L., 1952, A new concept of organization of the central emetic mechanism: Recent studies on the sites of action of apomorphine, copper sulfate and cardiac glycosides, *Gastroenterology* **22:**1–12.

WAYNE, E. J., GOODWIN, J. F., and STONER, H. B., 1949, Effect of adenosine triphosphate on electrocardiogram of man and animals, *Brit. Heart J.* **11:**55–67.

WEBB, J. L., 1966, Effects of 2-deoxy-D-glucose on carbohydrate metabolism, in: *Enzyme and Metabolic Inhibitors*, Vol. 2, pp. 386–403, Academic Press, New York.

WEBSTER, W., 1974, A ganglionic megacolon in piebald-lethal mice, *Arch. Pathol.* **97:**111–117.

WEISBRODT, N. W., and CHRISTENSEN, J., 1972, Gradients of contractions in the opossum esophagus, *Gastroenterology* **62:**1159–1166.

WEISSEL, M., RABERGER, G., and KRAUPP, O., 1973, The effects of intraarterial adenosine infusion on substrate levels and blood flow in skeletal muscle of the dog, *Naunyn-Schmiedebergs Arch. Pharmacol.* **277:**239–252.

WESTFALL, J. A., 1973, Ultrastructural evidence for neuromuscular systems in coelenterates, *Am. Zoologist* **13:**237–246.

WESTMAN, J., and BOWSHER, D., 1971, The fine structure of "non-specific" grey matter (laminal V and VII) in the cat spinal cord, *Exp. Brain Res.* **12:**379–388.

WESTON, A. H., 1971, Inhibition of the longitudinal muscle of rabbit duodenum, *Brit. J. Pharmacol.* **43:**428P–429P.

WESTON, A. H., 1973*a*, The effect of desensitization to adenosine triphosphate on the peristaltic reflex in guinea-pig ileum, *Brit. J. Pharmacol.* **7:**606–608.

WESTON, A. H., 1973*b*, Nerve-mediated inhibition of mechanical activity in rabbit duodenum and effects of desensitization to adenosine and several of its derivatives, *Brit. J. Pharmacol.* **48:**302–308.

WHITTAKER, V. P., DOWDALL, M. J., and BOYNE, A. F., 1972, The storage and release of acetylcholine by cholinergic nerve terminals: Recent results with non-mammalian preparations, *Biochem. Soc. Symp.* **36:**49–68.

WIDDICOMBE, J. G., 1963, Regulation of tracheobronchial smooth muscle, *Physiol. Rev.* **43:**1–37.

WIEDMEIER, V. T., RUBIO, R., and BERNE, R. M., 1972, Incorporation and turnover of adenosine-U-^{14}C in perfused guinea pig myocardium, *Am. J. Physiol.* **223:**51–54.

WOLFE, D. E., POTTER, L. T., RICHARDSON, K. C., and AXELROD, J., 1962, Localizing tritiated norepinephrine in sympathetic axons by electron microscopic autoradiography, *Science* **138:**440–444.

WOOD, J. D., 1970, Electrical activity from single neurons in Auerbach's plexus, *Am. J. Physiol.* **219:**159–169.

WOOD, J. D., 1973, Electrical discharge of individual neurons within the enteric nervous system, *Rend. Gastro-enterol.* **5:**25–26.

WOOD, J. D., and MARSH, D. R., 1973, Effects of atropine, tetrodotoxin and lidocaine on rebound excitation of guinea-pig small intestine, *J. Pharmacol. Exp. Ther.* **184:** 590–598.

WOOTON, G. F., THOA, N. B., KOPIN, I. J., and AXELROD, J., 1973, Enhanced release of dopamine β-hydroxylase and norepinephrine from sympathetic nerves by dibutyryl cyclic adenosine 3′,5′-monophosphate and theophylline, *Mol. Pharmacol.* **9:**178–183.

YAMADA, E., 1957, The fine structure of the megakaryocyte in the mouse spleen, *Acta Anat.* **29:**267–290.

YIP, K. F., and TSOU, K. C., 1973, Synthesis of fluorescent adenosine derivatives, *Tetrahedron* **33:**3087–3090.

YOKOYAMA, S., 1966, Aktionpotentiale der Ganglienzelle des Auerbachschen Plexus in Kaninchendunndarm, *Pflügers Arch. Ges. Physiol.* **288:**95–102.

ZIMMERMAN, H., and WHITTAKER, V. P., 1974, Effect of electrical stimulation in the yield and composition of synaptic vesicles from the cholinergic synapses of the electric organ of *Torpedo*: a combined biochemical, electrophysiological and morphological study, *J. Neurochem.* **22:**435–450.

ZNAMENÁCEK, K., and PRIBYLOVÁ, H., 1966, Die ATP zur Vorbeugung des asphyktischen Neugeborenensyndroms, *Z. Kinderheilk.* **96:**365.

4

HYPOTHALAMIC HYPOPHYSIOTROPIC HORMONES

Wylie Vale and Catherine Rivier

1. INTRODUCTION

A large body of experimental evidence supports the key role played by hypothalamic neurosecretory cells in coordinating the activities of the central nervous and endocrine systems. The nonapeptides vasopressin and oxytocin, synthesized in nerve cell bodies of the supraoptic and paraventricular nuclei, travel by axoplasmic flow within tracts terminating in the neurohypophysis, from which they are secreted into the general circulation in response to the appropriate hypothalamic inputs (Sachs *et al.*, 1969). Other hypothalamic hormones, the hypophysiotropic releasing and release inhibiting factors, exert a general influence on the homeostasis of the organism via their effects on the adenohypophysis. The portal vessel chemotransmitter theory states that the hypothalamus, in response to various neural and blood-borne signals, secretes factors or hormones which reach the adenohypophysis via the hypothalamic–hypophyseal portal system (Green and Harris, 1947; Friedgood, 1936). The vessels of the primary capillary plexus of this portal system are found in the median eminence of the hypothalamus; these vessels coalesce into veins which pass down the pituitary stalk to the adenohypophysis, where they disperse into a secondary

---

Wylie Vale and Catherine Rivier ● The Salk Institute, Neuroendocrinology Laboratory, La Jolla, California

capillary plexus supplying the various secretory cell types of the adenohypophysis. The demonstration of hypophysiotropic activities attributed to factors in hypothalamic extracts represented a critical part of the evidence supporting this theory. Several of these hormones have now been purified, characterized, and synthesized with subsequent unequivocal demonstration of the biological activities of the synthetic replicates in a number of laboratories. The bulk of this chapter therefore will be concerned with the well-established hypothalamic hypophysiotropic hormones (HHH) TRF (TSH releasing factor), LRF (LH releasing factor), and somatostatin (somatotropin release inhibiting factor, SRIF). The structures of other substances, MRIH (MSH release inhibiting factor) (which will not be discussed) and GHRH (growth hormone releasing hormone), purified from hypothalamic extracts, have also been reported; however, there is no general agreement on the hypophysiotropic activities of their synthetic replicates. Additionally, we will describe recent studies on hypophysiotropic hormones or activities in crude or partially purified hypothalamic extracts which have yet to be characterized: CRF (corticotropin releasing factor), GRF (growth hormone releasing factor), and PIF (prolactin release inhibiting factor).

This chapter will emphasize the *actions* of the characterized and noncharacterized hypothalamic hypophysiotropic hormones. Part of its object is to familarize the reader with the multiplicity of effects of the HHH as well as some of the potential applications of structural analogues of the characterized HHH to the study of basic physiological and pharmacological problems. Investigations of the regulation and mechanisms of HHH biosynthesis and secretion are not covered (for reviews of these topics, see Reichlin *et al.*, 1972; Blackwell and Guillemin, 1973; McCann and Porter, 1969; Van Loon, 1973; Martin, 1973*b*; Reichlin and Mitnick, 1973).

2. HYPOPHYSIOTROPIC HORMONE ACTION

2.1. Characteristics

This section will deal with the characteristics of action of the hypothalamic hormones which stimulate secretion by the adenohypophysis (hypothalamic hypophysiotropic hormones or HHH). The intravenous injection of TRF or LRF results in rapid increase in the secretion rate of the appropriate pituitary hormones. Figure 1 illustrates the effect of two doses of TRF on plasma TSH concentrations in the rat as a function of time. The dose-related rise of plasma TSH is not only rapid but also transient, resulting from the very short biological half-life of TRF *in vivo*. There is evidence that TRF is rapidly excreted in the urine, based on the recovery of intravenously administered tritiated or biologically active (Grant and Vale, 1973) TRF or of immunologically competent (Montoya *et al.*, 1973) TRF in urine.

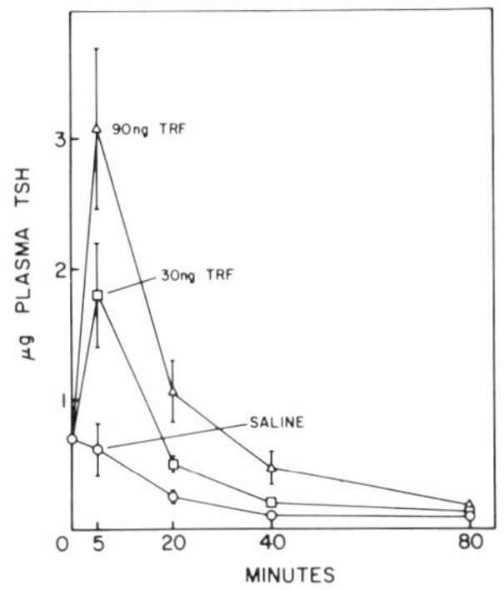

FIG. 1. Effect of two intravenous doses of synthetic TRF on plasma TSH in rats.

Furthermore, in the case of TRF, there is evidence that a plasma enzyme(s) inactivates TRF (Bowers *et al.*, 1966; Vale *et al.*, 1971*b*). It should be noted that endogenous hypothalamic hormones secreted into the portal system are diluted more than 3000-fold by the general circulation after passing through the adenohypophysis; this dilution constitutes an effective means of removing earlier hypothalamic signals, thus allowing a moment-to-moment regulation of hypothalamic inputs to the adenohypophysis.

The hypothalamic hormones act directly at the level of the pituitary, as demonstrated by *in vitro* experiments such as the one shown in Fig. 2, where LRF increases the secretion of LH and FSH from dissociated rat anterior pituitary cells maintained in culture. The high potency of the HHH is revealed in such experiments, with as little as 0.1 nM LRF having some activity; the half-maximal response occurs at 0.5 nM and the plateau response at >3nM, when the secretion rates of LH and FSH are >20 and 12, respectively, times the control rate. The addition of LRF to cultured cells results in a higher rate of secretion that remains constant over the 4-h period

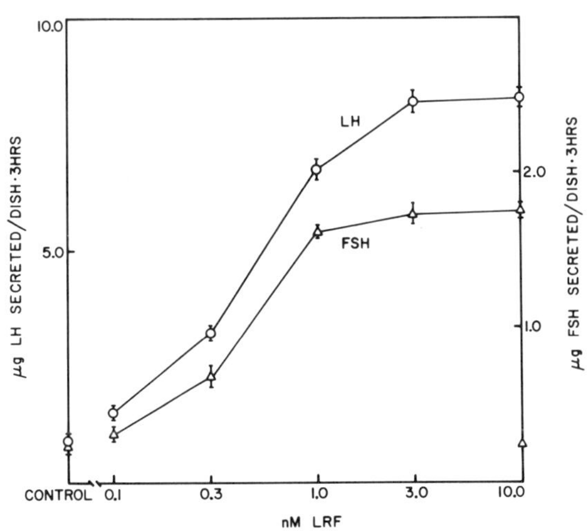

FIG. 2. Effect of synthetic LRF on the secretion of LH and FSH by dissociated pituitary cells in culture.

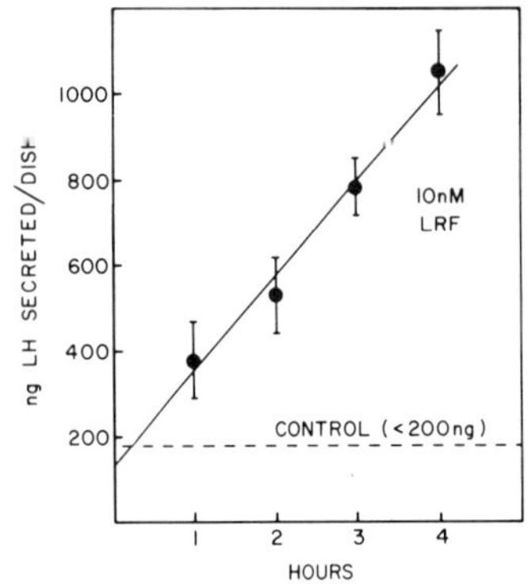

FIG. 3. LRF-stimulated secretion of LH as a function of time.

studied (Fig. 3); this observation indicates that the HHH are capable of influencing pituitary function as long as they are present in the incubation medium.

The initial pituitary response to the HHH involves the release of stored contents. Short-term pretreatment of the pituitary with puromycin or cycloheximide does not decrease the amount of hormones secreted in response to HHH (Vale *et al.*, 1968; Bowers *et al.*, 1968; Redding and Schally, 1969), demonstrating that continuous *de novo* synthesis of the appropriate hormone is not required for the acute response to the HHH.

There is, however, accumulating evidence that the HHH do also influence the rate of synthesis of pituitary hormones. The chronic administration of TRF (Fig. 4a) or LRF (Fig. 4b) to rat pituitary cell cultures leads to increases in TSH or LH concentrations in the medium with concomitant depletions in their pituitary content (Vale *et al.*, 1972*b*; Labrie *et al.*, 1973). The total hormone concentration (cells plus fluids) is increased by the releasing factors. Three-day TRF treatment augments PRL in both the fluids and the cells in the GH_3 GH/PRL-secreting tumor cell line. Hinkle *et al.*, 1973 have recently concluded that the TRF-mediated increase in total culture PRL in the GH_3 cells is best interpreted as an effect of TRF on the synthesis of PRL and not an inhibition of degradation. It has been suggested that the increased synthesis might occur secondarily to the depletion (Fig. 4a,b) of pituitary stores. However, the observation (Gautvik and Tashjian, 1973) that both intracellular and extracellular PRL are increased by TRF (Fig. 4c) would argue against that hypothesis. Of course, the increased rate of secretion might constitute the signal which mediates an increased rate of synthesis.

There have been two basic approaches to the investigation of pituitary secretory mechanisms (for review, see Geschwind, 1969; McCann, 1971; Guillemin *et al.*, 1971; Labrie *et al.*, 1973). One has been to test the effects of various substances or experimental conditions on the rates of secretion of a particular pituitary hormone, which yields information pertinent to specific cell types. The other approach involves the monitoring of a metameter not

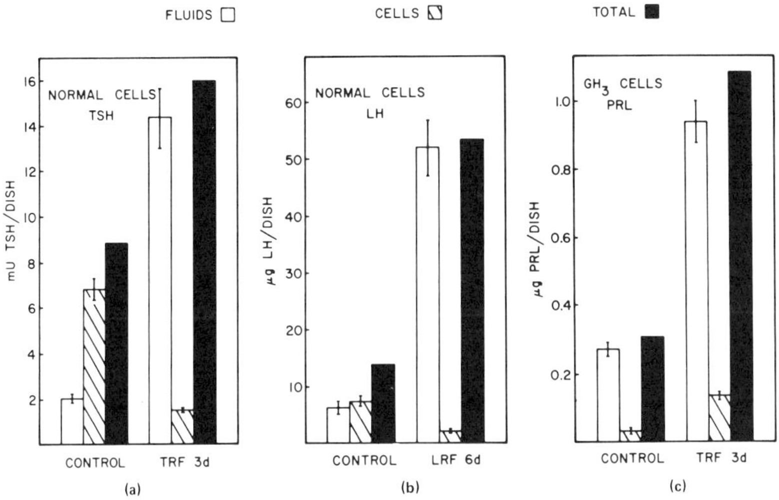

FIG. 4. Effect of TRF or LRF on the distribution (cells or fluids) of TSH (a) or LH (b) in normal pituitary cells and of PRL (c) in cultures on PRL/GH-secreting GH_3 tumor cells.

specific to a pituitary cell type such as adenohypophyseal cyclic AMP metabolism or transmembrane potentials. The results obtained with both approaches can be highlighted as follows:

1. Drugs or conditions known to inhibit energy metabolism (oligomycin, valinomycin, incubation at a low temperature or under anaerobic conditions, etc.) decrease the HHH-stimulated secretion of pituitary hormones (Guillemin *et al.*, 1968; Wilber and Utiger, 1968; Peake, 1973).
2. Elevating the [K^+] of the incubation medium increases the secretion rates of all pituitary hormones (Vale and Guillemin, 1967; Vale *et al.*, 1967*a*; Kraicer *et al.*, 1969; Samli and Geschwind, 1968; Wakabayashi *et al.*, 1969). This result led to the hypothesis that changes in transmembrane potentials or membrane ionic permeability characteristics might precede hormonal secretion.
3. The stimulated secretion of pituitary hormones proceeds as a function of extracellular [Ca^{2+}], suggesting that intracellular calcium might play a role in the secretory mechanism (Vale *et al.*, 1967*b*; Samli and Geschwind, 1968; Watanabe *et al.*, 1968; MacLeod and Fontham, 1970; Jutisz and de la Llosa, 1970). The above observations are consistent with the concept of "stimulus–secretion coupling" proposed by Douglas and his collaborators to explain secretory processes in general (Douglas and Poisner, 1962; Douglas *et al.*, 1967).

4. Cyclic AMP derivatives can stimulate the secretion of GH, ACTH, and PRL (Fleischer and Vale, 1968; MacLeod and Lehmeyer, 1970; Peake, 1973). There are conflicting reports concerning the effects of these derivatives on the release of the glycoprotein hormones TSH, LH, and FSH (Guillemin *et al.*, 1968; Geschwind, 1969; Wilber *et al.*, 1969; Labrie *et al.*, 1973). But agents which increase cyclic AMP levels in many tissues, including the anterior pituitary, such as prostaglandins (de Wied *et al.*, 1969; Bala *et al.*, 1970; MacLeod and Lehmeyer, 1970; Vale *et al.*, 1971*c*; Hedge, 1972) or cyclic nucleotide phosphodiesterase inhibitors (i.e., theophylline, caffeine) (Schofield, 1967; Wilber *et al.*, 1968; Guillemin *et al.*, 1968) stimulate the release of all pituitary hormones and can potentiate the effects of other pituitary hormonal secretagogues (releasing factors, high [K^+]). These results have led to proposals that increased intracellular cyclic AMP concentrations might mediate the actions of the hypothalamic releasing factors. Alternatively, it can be considered, especially in the case of the glycoproteins, that cyclic AMP, while not necessarily the mediator of releasing factor action, might facilitate the secretory process—perhaps by promoting [Ca^{2+}] translocation or by augmenting secretory granule migration (Rasmussen and Tenenhouse, 1968; Grant and Vale, 1973).

The results which correlate changes under various conditions in non-cell-type parameters with modifications in secretory functions of particular cell types present interpretational difficulties. Investigations of the effects of crude or partially purified tissue extracts on such parameters should be considered preliminary. The findings that partially purified hypothalamic extracts increase cyclic AMP levels (Steiner *et al.*, 1969; Zor *et al.*, 1969; Labrie *et al.*, 1973; Peake, 1973), change calcium activities (Peake, 1973), and modify membrane electrophysiological characteristics (Ashworth *et al.*, 1968) only inferentially support the significance of the earlier results relating to secretion mentioned above. Reports (Borgeat *et al.*, 1972, 1974) that pure synthetic hypophysiotropic hormones can modify such parameters as adenohypophyseal cyclic AMP levels are of more consequence and are consistent with a role of adenylate cyclase and cyclic AMP in the mechanism of action of those hypothalamic hormones.

2.2. Mechanisms of Hypophysiotropic Action of Peripheral Hormones

The peripheral hormones feed back to modify the secretion rate of the pituitary hormones. For most pituitary hormones there is some evidence in favor of the feedback occurring at the neural and/or hypophyseal level. The secretion of TSH mediated by TRF can be inhibited by pretreatment with thyroid hormones (Guillemin *et al.*, 1963). Although the interaction between thyroid hormones and TRF is functionally competitive (Vale *et al.*, 1967*c*; Reichlin *et al.*, 1972), thyroid hormones do not exclusively act by competing with TRF for binding to its receptors since the TSH response to high potassium or theophylline is also blocked by thyroxin (Vale and Guillemin, 1967; Wilber and Utiger, 1968). Furthermore, thyroid hormones do not influence the binding of [^{3}H]TRF to pituitary cells (Grant *et al.*, 1972*b*). The thyroid hormone–mediated blockade of TSH secretion can be prevented or reversed by inhibitors of protein synthesis such as puromycin or cycloheximide (Bowers *et al.*, 1968; Vale *et al.*, 1968). Actinomycin D, an inhibitor of DNA-directed RNA synthesis, can prevent but not reverse this blockade (Vale *et al.*, 1968). These results led to the proposal that thyroid hormones induce the synthesis of a stable mRNA coding for the synthesis of a labile protein which blocks TSH secretion by an as yet unknown mechanism. Similar observations have been made for the inhibition of ACTH secretion by glucocorticoids (Arimura *et al.*, 1968).

3. THYROTROPIN RELEASING FACTOR (TRF)

The structure of ovine (Burgus *et al.*, 1970) and porcine (Nair *et al.*, 1970) TRF purified from hypothalamic extracts has been determined to be pGlu-His-Pro-NH_2. There are reports that purified human TRF (Bowers *et al.*, 1970) and radioactive "biosynthesized" (Mitnick and Reichlin, 1971) rat, guinea pig, and frog TRF have mobilities similar to that of pGlu-His-Pro-NH_2 (in several chromatographic systems). Additionally, pGlu-His-Pro-NH_2 has been detected by highly specific radioimmunoassays in brain tissues or urine of various mammals: humans (Montoya *et al.*, 1973); rats and hamsters, birds, reptiles, amphibians, fish, and the lamprey, a cyclostome (Jackson and Reichlin, 1974). It appears that pGlu-His-Pro-NH_2 is phylogenetically widely distributed and represents an ancient molecule whose function is by no means restricted to the regulation of TSH secretion (see below).

TRF was isolated on the basis of its ability to stimulate the secretion of thyrotropin (TSH) and hence was called thyrotropin releasing factor. TRF is effective to release TSH *in vivo* when administered by various routes, intravenously, subcutaneously, sublingually, and orally (for a more detailed review, see Guillemin *et al.*, 1971). In the mouse, $\geqslant$ 1 ng is active; in humans, 50–100 μg, intravenously, elevates TSH levels (Gual *et al.*, 1972; Fleischer and Guillemin, 1972). *In vitro*, the minimal effective dose is about 10^{-10} M; half-maximal response is observed at about 2 nM (corresponding to the apparent dissociation constant) and the plateau response occurs at 30 nM (Vale *et al.*, 1972*b*).

3.1. Effect of TRF on Secretion of Other Pituitary Hormones

TRF exhibits specificity of action since it has no effect on the secretion of ACTH or even of LH and FSH, two glycoproteins with structures closely related to that of TSH. Tashjian *et al.* (1971) found that synthetic TRF could stimulate the secretion of prolactin (PRL) and inhibit the secretion of growth hormone (GH) by cloned GH/PRL-secreting tumor cells. The effect of TRF on PRL has been observed in several mammalian species, including humans, where its administration causes large increases in plasma PRL levels (Jacobs *et al.*, 1971; Convey *et al.*, 1973; Bowers *et al.*, 1973*a*; Fell *et al.*, 1973; Kelly *et al.*, 1973). In the normal rat, however, there is little effect of TRF on PRL secretion (Lu *et al.*, 1972; Vale *et al.*, 1973*d*), whereas the estrogen–progesterone pretreated rat does exhibit a PRL response to TRF (Rivier and Vale, 1974). *In vitro*, pituitary glands in short-term incubation or cells in culture from normal donor rats have no consistent PRL response to TRF, but the PRL secretion rate of thyroidectomized or estrogen–progesterone pretreated rats' pituitaries can be stimulated by TRF (Vale *et al.*, 1973*d*). The effects of the peripheral hormones on the prolactin secreting cell can serve as an excellent example of the permissive action of hormones and of the complexity of the integrative responses of endocrine cells.

The question of whether there is a PRF (PRL releasing factor) in the hypothalamus that is not TRF cannot be conclusively resolved with crude or partially purified hypothalamic extracts. However, the amounts of PRL releasing and TSH releasing activities present in such extracts have been compared *in vivo*, and suggest that there is adequate TSH releasing activity to account for the PRL releasing activities in extracts of rat, pig, and sheep hypothalamus (Rivier and Vale, 1974). Several investigators have claimed separation of PRF and TRF after gel filtration of crude hypothalamus extracts (Valverde-R *et al.*, 1972; Dular *et al.*, 1974). The alternate explanation of their findings is that SRIF, which has been shown to inhibit the TRF-induced release of TSH but not of PRL, was present in the PRF zone that they interpreted as being free of TRF.

A possible physiological role of TRF in the regulation of PRL secretion is somewhat questionable in view of the number of situations (i.e., stress, perphenazine administration) in which the secretion of TSH and PRL can be dissociated; of course, the involvement of specific inhibiting factors (PIF, or a TSH release inhibiting factor such as somatostatin; see Section 8) might provide a mechanism for dissociation of secretion of the two hormones in the presence of a common stimulator (TRF).

While the effect on PRL secretion by the GH_3 and GH_1 tumor cells (Tashjian *et al.*, 1971) has been generally confirmed in untransformed pituitary cells, the TRF-mediated inhibition of GH secretion has been observed only in those tumoral cell lines. In fact, TRF has been found to stimulate GH secretion in several experimental and clinical circumstances, including perfused rat pituitary glands (Carlson and Mariz, 1973) and cell cultures of pituitaries from thyroidectomized rats (Vale *et al.*, unpublished results) and human subjects (Gual *et al.*, 1972) with acromegaly or renal insufficiency (Irie and Tsushima, 1972).

3.2. Psychotropic Actions of TRF

There is accumulating evidence that the hypothalamic hormones can exert an extrahypophyseal effect on the central nervous system. Plotnikoff *et al.* (1972) reported that TRF could potentiate the behavioral effects of L-dopa in the L-dopa–paragyline test used to screen substances for antidepressant action when carried out in normal hypophysectomized or thyroidectomized mice. TRF has been reported by Prange *et al.* (1972) to possess transient antidepressant activity in subjects with unipolar depression; an observation confirmed by some (Kastin *et al.*, 1972; Van der Vis-Melson and Wiener, 1972), but not all (Takahashi *et al.*, 1973) investigators. Segal and Mandell (1974) reported that intraventricular infusion of TRF can increase spontaneous motor activity in freely moving rats. A possible mechanism of these proposed behavioral effects was provided by Keller *et al.* (1974), who reported that TRF probably caused an increase in norepinephrine turnover in the rat brain. In keeping with the suggested psychotropic effects of TRF are the findings of its widespread distribution throughout the brain (Oliver *et al.*, 1973; Jackson and Reichlin, 1974; Winokur and Utiger, 1974).

3.3. TRF Binding Studies

The binding of TRF to pituitary receptor sites has been studied by Grant *et al.* (1972*b*) and Labrie *et al.* (1972) using synthetic [^{3}H]Pro-TRF. Specific binding of [^{3}H]Pro-TRF to mouse thyrotropic and rat somatotropic/prolactotropic tumor or normal bovine pituitary membrane preparations and intact pituitary cells (rat, sheep) has been found to be similar. The binding is saturable with respect to [^{3}H]Pro-TRF, and unlabeled TRF competes stoichiometrically. The apparent overall dissociation constant to pituitary receptors is approximately 20–40 nM (Grant *et al.*, 1972*b*, 1973*a*; Labrie *et al.*, 1972). The greater than tenfold difference between the apparent dissociation constants determined from *in vitro* secretion experiments (Vale *et al.*, 1972*b*) and the binding studies is perhaps best explained by their being a receptor excess (Vale *et al.*, 1973*e*). According to this "spare receptor" concept (Rudinger *et al.*, 1972), only a small percentage of the receptors need be occupied in order to result in a maximum secretory response, thus resulting in TRF's secretory stimulation curve being shifted to the left of its binding curve. Analysis of the binding data of [^{3}H]TRF as well as competition data with TRF analogues shows that the binding process is complex and that pituitary cells possess receptors with two closely related affinity constants.

Due to the presence of two classes of TRF binding sites, the overall dissociation does not follow simple first-order kinetics. The dissociation rate of the [^{3}H]TRF–receptor complex at 0 °C by a 25-fold dilution of the reaction mixture into ice-cold buffer reaches 50% in approximately 3 min. The dissociation rate in the presence of excess nonradioactive TRF is more rapid, a 50% dissociation rate being reached in less than 1 min. The unusual kinetics of TRF binding to its receptors, its dissociation from the receptor, and the slightly different slopes in the competition curves can also be interpreted to suggest the phenomenon of "negative" cooperativity of TRF for its receptor analogous to that proposed for insulin (DeMeyts *et al.*, 1973).

3.4. TRF Structure–Function Relationship Studies

A large number of structural analogues of TRF have been synthesized and tested for activities in several biological systems (Vale *et al.*, 1973*e*). A number of factors can determine the resultant biological activity of a given analogue, such as its volume of distribution, access to the appropriate "target" cells, rate of metabolism, affinity for its receptors, and ability (intrinsic activity) to bring about a response as a result of this binding. By examining these analogues *in vivo* and *in vitro* (using the pituitary cell culture method) and in competitive binding assays, it is possible to determine the factors involved in their altered activity.

The *in vivo* TSH releasing potency of selected TRF analogues is shown in Fig. 5 and Table 1. The relative TRF potencies of these analogues determined *in vivo* correlate well with their ability to compete with TRF for binding to pituitary cells (Grant *et al.*, 1973*a*), indicating that the limiting

TABLE 1
Compared Potencies of TRF Analogues on PRL and TSH Release in EP Rats

Peptide	Potencies (%) relative to TRF (= 100)	
	PRL	TSH
Ac-Gly-His-Pro-NH_2	0.3	0.15
pGlu-Met-Pro-NH_2	0.69	0.60
pGlu-His-azetidine	2.0	1.4
pGlu-His-Pro-Ala-NH_2	0.45	0.43
pGlu-His-Pro-Gly-NH_2	50	40

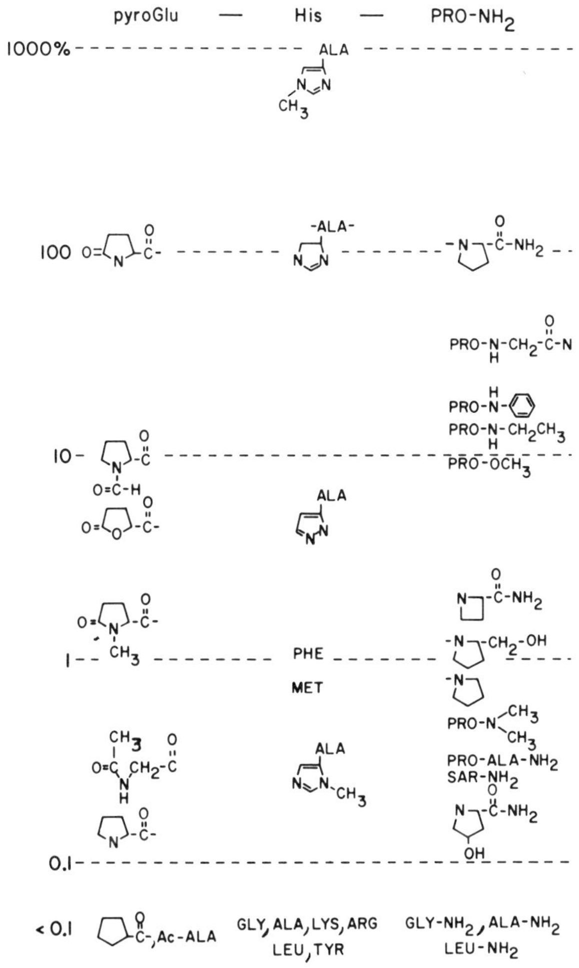

FIG. 5. TSH releasing potency relative to TRF of structural analogues of TRF. Horizontal placement of the displayed structure shows the position in TRF of the modification. Vertical placement is a function of the relative potency of the resultant analogue.

factor involved in their biological activities is their relative affinities for the TRF receptor. These close correlations also provide support for the physiological relevance of the phenomena observed in the TRF binding studies. Additionally, brief trypsin treatment reversibly decreases the cell's abilities to bind labeled TRF and to respond biologically to TRF by TSH secretion, and a TRF analogue linked to dextrans ($>10^6$ daltons) possesses biological activity (see below).

The tripeptide pGlu-His-Pro-NH_2 has been shown to be highly conservative in that alterations to any part of the molecule have marked effects on the biological activity of the modified peptide.

The effect of a given modification of TRF on its relative affinity could reflect the direct involvement of particular moieties in the TRF receptor interaction or might result secondarily from an altered conformation relative to that of TRF. Evidence has been presented for the existence of preferred conformations of TRF. In one model, pGlu-His-Pro-NH_2 was suggested to exist in a "hairpin turn" conformation stabilized by two intramolecular hydrogen bonds (Grant *et al.*, 1972*a*; Blagdon *et al.*, 1973); alternative proposals have also been reported (Fermandjian *et al.*, 1972; Burgess *et al.*, 1973). A valid three-dimensional model of TRF might allow an appreciation of the boundaries of the receptor envelope which recognizes this molecule and thus improve our ability to predict the biological activity of TRF structural analogues. However, the conformation of TRF established in solution may not be relevant to its conformation in the lipoprotein receptor environment.

The importance of the conformation of a TRF analogue to its ability to be recognized by the receptor is illustrated by the low potency of the D-series optical enantiomers of TRF (Wilber and Flouret, 1971).

The vertical placement of each structure under the first column in Fig. 5 represents the biological activity of an analogue with that moiety in place of pyroglutamyl in TRF. As will be seen with each amino acid in TRF, most modifications drastically reduce the biological potency. The importance of the pGlu ring is indicated by the low potency of [Ac-Ala^1]TRF with similar functional groups but lacking the five-membered ring. A possible role of the lactam amide is suggested by the potency of [*N*-methyl-$pGlu^1$]TRF and [γ-hydroxyglutaryl $lactone^1$]TRF. The low activity of [Pro^1]TRF could indicate a requirement for the lactam carbonyl; it could also be a result of the charge carried by the secondary amine at physiological pH as [*N*-formyl-Pro^1]TRF (Monahan *et al.*, unpublished results) is much more potent. In summary, with respect to pGlu, these data and others not presented suggest that the lactam function, and perhaps the degree of nucleophilicity of the 1 position, is of importance to the biological activity.

The specific biological activities of the TRF analogues in which histidine has been replaced by other amino acids are shown in Fig. 5. Substitutions of another basic amino acid, arginine, lysine, or ornithine, yield compounds with little activity. The pK of the histidine residue in TRF is approximately 6.25 (Grant *et al.*, 1972*b*); therefore, most of the TRF molecules are not charged at physiological pH. The three basic amino acids, arginine, lysine, and ornithine, have a positive charge under these conditions, which might explain their low activity. The activity of [Met^2]TRF might be due to the fact that methionine is a residue with a good nucleophil and is fairly close to histidine in size.

Maintenance of the peptide backbone alone with no side chain, as is the case with [Gly^2]TRF or with only alkyl side chains ([Ala^2]TRF, [Leu^2]TRF), yields compounds with very little activity. Sievertsson *et al.* (1972) have reported that [Phe^2]TRF has 10% of the potency of TRF, but since we

(Monahan and Vale, unpublished results) have found [Phe^2]TRF to be only 1% active the role of aromaticity *per se* in the second position should not be overemphasized. Even though all analogues with more than 1% potency are also aromatic, the shape of the ring and position of the imidazole nitrogens are also critical.

The relative importance of the steric and aromatic properties as opposed to the acid–base characteristics of the imidazole ring can be inferred from the observation by Hofmann and Bowers (1970) that substitution of the pyrazole-3-alanine for histidine yields a substance with a 5% TRF potency. The pK of the aromatic pyrazole ring is low (approximately 2–3). If the acid–base characteristics of the 2-position in TRF were critical, it seems that the biological potency would have been affected to a greater extent. The size and the aromaticity in the 2-position therefore appear to be important factors in the recognition of TRF by the receptor.

One of the most striking observations is that methylation of the τ-position of histidine in TRF (Rivier *et al.*, 1972) enhances its biological potency around eightfold (Vale *et al.*, 1971*a*). This is in contrast to the effect of methylation of the π-position, which drastically reduced biological potency. The decreased activity of [$^{\pi}MeHis^2$]TRF could be due to a steric effect that either prevents access to the nitrogen atom which might be a site of interaction with the receptor or, alternately, prevents the molecule from adopting a conformation favorable for TRF activity. The enhanced activity of [$^{\tau}MeHis^2$]TRF might be the result of an inductive effect of the methyl group on the electronic properties of the position which could be a requisite part of the interaction of TRF with the receptor. The effect of a methyl on the τ-position might equally well favor an intramolecular interaction that allows TRF to assume a more preferred conformation (Grant and Vale, 1972).

The third column shows the activities of proline–amide substituted TRF analogues. In some of this series, the amide function is maintained while proline is modified. As the proline ring is reduced to a four-membered ring compound such as azetidine, the biological potency is reduced sixtyfold. Maintenance of the tertiary amide, as in sarcosine amide, still retains some slight activity. Substitution by other hydrophobic groups, such as leucine, or removal of the side chain completely, as in Gly-NH_2, results in a very low biological activity. It is likely that substitution of hydroxyproline sterically restricts the interaction with the receptor. These data suggest that the tertiary amide and the rigid proline ring are required for high activity.

A dipeptide, pGlu-His-OMe, with no hypophysiotropic TRF activity appears to be recognized by the plasma enzyme(s) which inactivates TRF. This dipeptide was found (Vale *et al.*, 1971*b*) to competitively inhibit the inactivation of TRF by plasma.

Substitution of the *C*-terminal amide by the methyl ester reduces the potency to 10% of that of TRF, indicating that neither the amide nor a hydrogen bond that it is proposed to participate in (Blagdon *et al.*, 1973) is obligatory for substantial biological activity. The potency of the free acid of TRF is reduced (<0.1%) probably due to the charge. This is supported by the observation that the prolinol-substituted derivative is considerably more active than the free acid, and the complete removal of the carboxamide moiety, producing the pyrrolidine derivative, still leaves 0.3% of the potency of TRF. Most of the secondary amides have considerable biological activity even when the addition includes a benzene ring, as is the case for the anilide substitution. The most active compound of this series is the tetrapeptide pGlu-His-Pro-Gly-NH_2, which has a potency 35% that of TRF. Another tetrapeptide, pGlu-His-Pro-Ala-NH_2, has a much lower activity, perhaps because the methyl group in optically active alanine sterically interferes with interactions involving the carboxamide. The activity of this latter tetrapeptide is, in fact, similar to that of two of the tertiary amides shown below, and of pGlu-His-Pyr, which lacks the carboxamide residue altogether. It appears that the requirements at the *C*-terminal amide for biological activity are not as stringent as for other parts of the molecule. Accordingly, it is to this portion of TRF that high molecular weight polymers may be tethered (Ling and Vale, in preparation) with the maintenance of biological activity.

Several TRF analogues have been investigated for their effects on the secretion of PRL and TSH *in vivo* in the estrogen–progesterone pretreated rat (Rivier and Vale, 1974) (Fig. 6) and on the secretion of PRL and GH by GH_3 tumor cells in culture (Hinkle *et al.*, 1973). The analogues tested, involving modifications to each part of TRF, have similar potencies when calculated on the basis of their ability to stimulate TSH and PRL or inhibit GH secretion. Furthermore, the kinetics and specificity of TRF binding by mouse TSH (Vale *et al.*, 1973*e*) and rat PRL/GH (Hinkle *et al.*, 1973; Vale *et al.*, 1973*e*) secreting tumor cells are comparable. The above data suggest that the TRF receptors involved in the secretion of these pituitary hormones are closely related.

In contrast, Prange *et al.* (personal communication) have found that the behavioral activities of a series of TRF analogues do not correlate well with their relative hypophysiotropic potencies. It is possible that differences in the pharmacokinetics of the psychotropic compared to hypophysiotropic bioassays, such as penetration through the blood–brain barrier or susceptibility to brain inactivation, are responsible for this lack of correlation. However, Burt and Snyder (in preparation) have observed that the abilities of TRF analogues to compete with [^{3}H]TRF for binding to high-affinity binding sites in membrane preparations of brain tissue also do not correlate well with the hypophysiotropic potencies of these analogues. The possibility exists, therefore, that the receptors involved in the psychotropic actions of TRF exhibit significant differences in their structural preferences. Such differences might well be profitably exploited, allowing the therapeutic administration of a TRF analogue with psychotropic activity without modifying the endocrine status of the patient or *vice versa*.

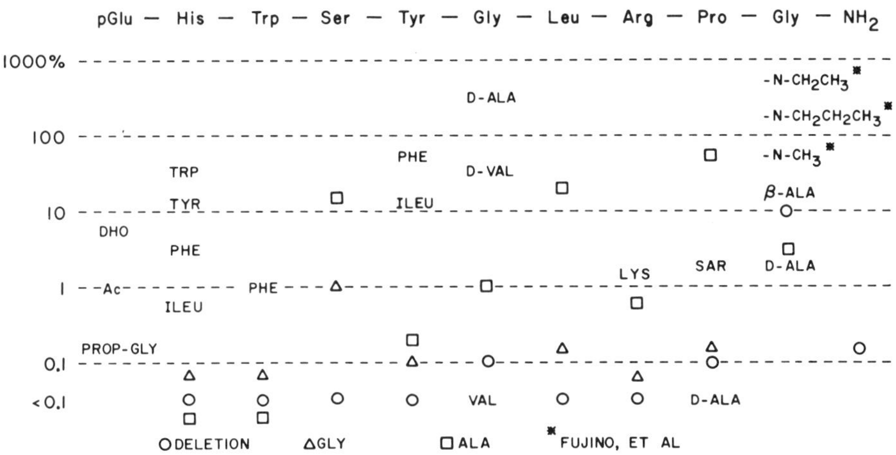

FIG. 6. LH releasing potency relative to LRF of structural analogues of LRF. Horizontal placement of the displayed structure shows the position in TRF of the modification. Vertical placement is a function of the relative potency of the resultant analogue.

4. LUTEINIZING HORMONE RELEASING FACTOR (LRF)

The primary structure of porcine (Matsuo *et al.*, 1971) and subsequently ovine (Burgus *et al.*, 1972) LRF was determined to be the decapeptide pGlu-His-Trp-Ser-Tyr-Gly-Leu-Arg-Pro-Gly-NH_2. LRF was purified on the basis of its ability to stimulate LH secretion; its synthetic replicate has been shown to modify not only the secretion of LH but that of FSH as well. In most biological situations, the maximum LH response (percent increase over control) to LRF is much greater than the maximum FSH response, although other factors (age, sex, steroid pretreatment, etc.) can dramatically affect the relative responses of the two gonadotropins. For example, cultured pituitary cells from normal adult male donors have only a slight increase in FSH secretion rate due to LRF, whereas cultured pituitary cells from immature female rats present a considerable FSH response to LRF (Fig. 2). There are several clinical and experimental circumstances where secretion of the two hormones can be dissociated (Cargille *et al.*, 1969; Goebelsmann *et al.*, 1969; Stevens, 1969; Rubin *et al.*, 1971; Gay and Sheth, 1972). Several possibilities have been raised: that there exists a separate FSH releasing factor (FRF), either devoid of LH releasing activity (McCann *et al.*, 1960; Dhariwal *et al.*, 1965; Schally *et al.*, 1968) or possessing greater FSH releasing intrinsic activity than does LRF. In our hands, no crude extract or partially purified fraction of hypothalamic origin showed greater intrinsic activity than LRF to stimulate FSH secretion. There were reports that a porcine hypothalamic preparation does possess such an FRF, but no further purification or characterization has appeared (Bowers *et al.*, 1973*b*).

Another possibility is that the LRF decapeptide is the sole hypothalamic stimulator of LH and FSH secretion and that neural or gonadal factors, such as steroids, have differential effects on the secretion of LH or FSH. This view is supported by histoimmunological evidence that LH and FSH frequently appear in the same cell and therefore might be secreted by a common cell type. The conditions modifying the ratio of LH to FSH secretion are in general chronic and possibly involve modification of gene transcription of a common gonadotroph population, resulting in differential synthesis and hence differential secretion of LH and FSH in response to the secretory stimulus.

The LRF receptors involved in LH and FSH secretion appear to be similar, as over 100 LRF analogues with agonist or antagonist properties have been found to have identical LH and FSH modifying potencies (Schally *et al.*, 1973*a*; Vale *et al.*, 1973*e*).

The best evidence for a critical role of LRF in the physiology of FSH as well as LH secretion comes from the effects of passive immunization of animals with anti-LRF sera. Koch *et al.* (1973) have reported that the administration of anti-LRF sera to rabbits prevents the reflex ovulatory surge of both LH and FSH and inhibits the rise in the serum gonadotropins in response to castration. Arimura *et al.* (1973) have also observed inhibition of both LH and FSH levels in animals with circulating LRF antibodies.

4.1. LRF Structure–Function Studies

The efforts of a number of laboratories have resulted in the synthesis and testing of hundreds of LRF analogues. Table 2 and Fig. 6 shows the LH and FSH releasing potency of selected analogues tested *in vivo* and *in vitro* for agonistic activities and *in vitro* for antagonistic activities. The biological activities of two series (Rivier *et al.*, 1973*a*, 1974) of LRF analogues shortened from the *C* or *N* terminus are shown in Table 2. With the exception of the two nonapeptides, des-Gly^{10}-LRF (11%) and [Ac^{1}]-LRF (1%), all of these series of shortened LRF analogues less than 0.1% LRF potency. One analogue, Ac-Trp-Ser-Tyr-Gly-Leu-Arg-Pro-Gly-NH_2, is a weak antagonist (see below). An additional series of peptides shortened from the *N* terminus with the *N* terminus unblocked are completely inactive (Rivier *et al.*, unpublished results). It is unlikely, therefore, that the LRF decapeptide is a prohormone in view of the inactivity of the potential fragments of LRF.

The biological activity of a series of nonapeptides in which a single amino acid has been deleted is low (Fig. 6). The activities of the analogues in which one amino acid has been successively replaced by glycine or alanine are generally greater than the activities of the corresponding peptides of the nonapeptide series, indicating that the conservation of the peptide backbone is necessary for high affinity for the LRF receptor. Since the Ala-substituted

TABLE 2
Biological Activity of LRF Analogues

Chain-shortened analogues	Percent LRF potency
pGlu-His-Trp-Ser-Tyr-Gly-Leu-Arg-Pro-Gly-NH_2	100
pGlu-His-Trp-Ser-Tyr-Gly-Leu-Arg-Pro-Gly-OH	0.2
pGlu-His-Trp-Ser-Tyr-Gly-Leu-Arg-Pro-NH_2	11.0
pGlu-His-Trp-Ser-Tyr-Gly-Leu-Arg-NH_2	<0.01
pGlu-His-Trp-Ser-Tyr-Gly-Leu-NH_2	<0.01
pGlu-His-Trp-Ser-Tyr-Gly-NH_2	<0.01
pGlu-His-Trp-Ser-Tyr-NH_2	<0.01
pGlu-His-Trp-Ser-NH_2	<0.01
pGlu-His-Trp-NH_2	<0.01
Des-His^2-LRF	<0.01
pGlu-His-Trp-Ser-Tyr-Gly-Leu-Arg-Pro-Gly-NH_2	100
Ac-His-Trp-Ser-Tyr-Gly-Leu-Arg-Pro-Gly-NH_2	0.2
Ac-Trp-Ser-Tyr-Gly-Leu-Arg-Pro-Gly-NH_2	<0.01
Ac-Ser-Tyr-Gly-Leu-Arg-Pro-Gly-NH_2	<0.01
Ac-Tyr-Gly-Leu-Arg-Pro-Gly-NH_2	<0.01
Ac-Gly-Leu-Arg-Pro-Gly-NH_2	<0.01
Ac-Leu-Arg-Pro-Gly-NH_2	<0.01
Ac-Arg-Pro-Gly-NH_2	<0.01
Ac-Pro-Gly-NH_2	<0.01

peptides are usually more active than the Gly-substituted peptides, the conformation of the backbone would also appear to be important. At no position in LRF does L-alanine substitution result in full activity, indicating the significance of various functional groups to the activity of LRF.

Substitution of L-Ala for Gly in the 6-position in LRF considerably decreases its potency. However, the potency of [D-Ala^6]LRF is 450% that of LRF (Monahan *et al.*, 1973*a*). These data can be interpreted as resulting from a restriction in the conformational degrees of freedom of LRF when D- or L-alanine replaces glycine. In [D-Ala^6]LRF, this restriction might lead to the stabilization of conformations which have a higher affinity for the LRF receptor. Consistently the D-amino acid substituted LRF analogues at the 6-position have more activity than the corresponding L-amino acid substituted peptides: [D-Val^6]LRF = 32%; [L-Val^6]LRF < 0.1%; [D-Lys^6]LRF= 400%; [L-Lys^6]LRF < 0.1% (Monahan *et al.*, 1973). The [D-Lys^6]LRF was synthesized specifically to provide an LRF analogue which could be coupled to other molecules and retain high potency. The coupling of [D-Lys^6]LRF to dextran T2000 has been accomplished (Ling *et al.*, in preparation) and found (Vale *et al.*, in preparation) to have high LRF potency *in vivo* and *in vitro*. The observation that an LRF analogue linked to a $>10^6$ dalton polymer at the 6 position has high biological activity is consistent with our suggestion (Grant and Vale, 1972) that the LRF molecule is "hinged" at the 6-position, allowing the *N* and *C* terminals to present the face that interacts with the LRF receptor. Fujino *et al.* (1972) have reported that alkylated amides of des-Gly-amide^{10}LRF have high LRF activity, with des-Gly-amide^{10}[Pro-*N*-ethylamide^{9}] possessing 3–5 times more activity than LRF. In addition to being more potent than LRF *in vivo* (Fujino *et al.*, 1973; Arnold *et al.*, 1974) and *in vitro* (Vale *et al.*, in preparation), this analogue has prolonged biological activity *in vivo* (Rippel *et al.*, 1973).

Most of the abovementioned LRF analogues give parallel responses to LRF with similar amounts of LH and FSH secreted at plateau doses *in vitro*, suggesting that the limiting factor in their biological activities is affinity for the LRF receptor. In contrast, several peptides with modifications to the 2(His)- or 3(Trp)-position in LRF have altered dose–response curves with lower response maxima. For example, [Gly^{2}]LRF (Fig. 7) at highest doses releases approximately 30% of the LRF released by plateau concentrations of LRF, and hence possesses lower intrinsic activity than does LRF and is considered to be a partial agonist. The intrinsic activity of the histidine-deleted nonapeptide, des-His^{2}-LRF, is lower still, releasing no LH at any dose in this *in vitro* test (Monahan *et al.*, 1972; Vale *et al.*, 1972*c*). *In vivo*, des-His^{2}-LRF does have slight LH releasing activity, although considerably less than does LRF. The difference between the intrinsic activity of des-His^{2}-LRF in the two-assay system is not without precedence; the expression by an analogue of antagonistic or partial agonistic properties as a function of the conditions of bioassay has been observed with several analogues of vasopressin and oxytocin (Rudinger *et al.*, 1972). [Ileu^{2}]LRF has full (measurable) intrinsic activity, although its affinity is still quite low, indicating that the requirements for intrinsic activity can be satisfied by a bulky hydrophobic amino acid; however, there are more stringent requirements for high affinity for the LH receptor, with the aromatic amino acid substitutions yielding higher potency.

As was anticipated from its lower intrinsic activity, [Gly^{2}]LRF was shown to be an antagonist of LRF (Vale *et al.*, 1973*e*). Des-His^{2}-LRF, with very low intrinsic activity, does have affinity for the LRF receptor as evidenced by its

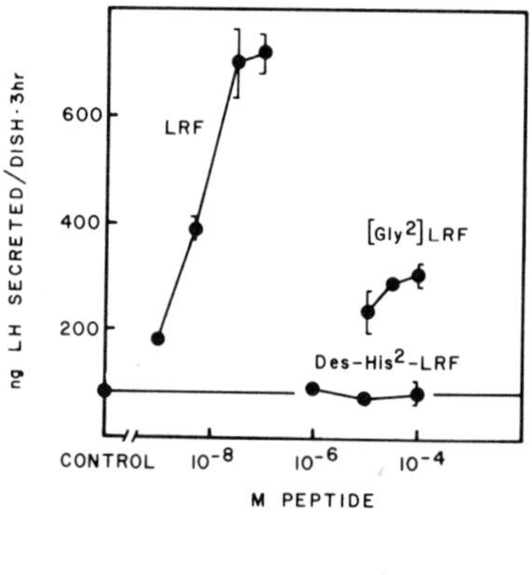

FIG. 7. Effect of LRF, des-His^{2}-LRF and [Gly^{2}]LRF on secretion of LH by pituitary cell cultures.

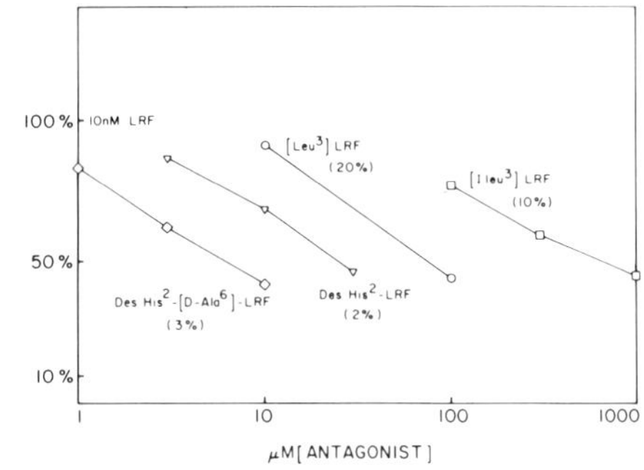

FIG. 8. Inhibition of the LRF-mediated secretion of FSH by LRF analogues *in vitro*.

inhibition of the release of LH due to LRF, indicating that the histidine moiety, while required for the process coupling receptor binding to stimulation of secretion, is not required for recognition.

Des-His^2-LRF behaves as a competitive antagonist, with its effect being overcome by increasing the concentration of LRF. Des-His^2-LRF inhibits neither release of LH and FSH due to high [K^+] nor the release of TSH due to TRF, showing its specificity for the LRF-mediated gonadotropin secretory process. Furthermore, des-His^2-LRF and its derivatives, i.e., des-His^2-des-Gly^{10}[Pro-*N*-ethylamide^9]LRF (Coy *et al.*, 1973) and des-His^2[D-Ala^6]LRF (Amoss *et al.*, 1974), have been found to block the LRF induced secretion of LH and FSH *in vivo.*

Incorporating the D-Ala^6 modification into des-His^2-LRF increases its antagonist potency around threefold (Fig. 8). A similar approach has been reported for the des-Gly^{10}-Pro-ethylamide modification (Coy *et al.*, 1973; Fujino *et al.*, 1974). While we find that this modification increases the potency of agonists (des-Gly^{10}·[D-Ala^6, Pro-*N*-ethylamide] = 13 × LRF), we see no increase in the potency of antagonists (des-His^2, Gly^{10}-[Pro-*N*-ethylamide^9] = des-His^2-LRF). These analogues are still rather weak inhibitors. A 700-fold molar excess of des-His^2[D-Ala^6]LRF is required *in vitro* to inhibit the LH secretory rate by 50% (Vale *et al.*, in preparation). The antagonists involving changes to the Trp^3 in LRF are less potent still (Fig. 8).

4.2. LRF Binding Studies

Studies of the binding of high specific activity [^{3}H-Pro^9]LRF to normal rat cells indicates the presence of two populations of binding sites: a high-affinity class with a K_d of 2 nM and appropriate specificity (based on the lack of competability of various biologically inactive analogues) and a lower-affinity class which is less specific (Grant *et al.*, 1973*b*; Spona, 1973). In fact, it was possible to investigate the high-affinity sites by saturating the nonspecific low-affinity sites with des-Arg^8-LRF, an analogue with no agonist or antagonist activity. As is the case with TRF, the apparent K_d of the LRF receptor interaction of approximately 0.4 nM is lower than the K_d of high-affinity LRF binding sites (Grant *et al.*, 1973*b*).

4.3. Behavioral Effects of LRF

Moss and McCann (1973) have reported that ovariectomized rats treated with low doses of estrogen displayed mating behavior when given subcutaneous injections of LRF and not LH, FSH, or TRF, suggesting a direct CNS effect of LRF on this behavior. Pfaff (1973) has found similar effects of LRF in hypophysectomized rats, providing additional evidence that these psychotropic effects of LRF are not mediated by the hypophysis.

5. CORTICOTROPIN RELEASING FACTOR (CRF)

The first evidence of a hypothalamic factor influencing ACTH secretion was found by Guillemin and Rosenberg (1955), who showed that addition of a crude hypothalamic extract to long-term cultures of pituitary cells that had ceased producing ACTH cells would reinitiate their ACTH secretion, and by Saffran and Schally (1955), who reported that the addition of catecholamines to coincubates of hypothalamic and pituitary fragments increased the secretion of ACTH by the pituitaries. Purification of CRF (corticotropin releasing factor) (Guillemin *et al.*, 1962; Schally *et al.*, 1962) of neurohypophyseal origin led to the isolation of two peptides, α- and β-CRF. Because of the instability of these compounds as well as their scarcity, it was not possible to determine their complete structure, but the amino acid composition showed α-CRF to be closely related to α-MSH and β-CRF to vasopressin. The close similarity between β-CRF and vasopressin on the one hand and the ability of vasopressin to stimulate ACTH secretion on the other hand led to the hypothesis that vasopressin might be CRF itself (McCann and Fruit, 1957). However, this view was abandoned since physiological situations occur with dissociated secretion of ACTH and vasopressin, for example, in rats suffering from diabetes insipidus. Also, antidiuretic amounts of VP can be released physiologically without causing simultaneous release of ACTH in normal animals (for review, see Ganong, 1963). Additional evidence was provided by *in vitro* experiments showing that the dose–response curve and the maximal secretion rate of ACTH following exposure to vasopressin and crude hypothalamic extract were significantly different (Portanova and Sayers, 1973; Rivier and Vale, unpublished observation). Furthermore, addition of vasopressin to a hypothalamic extract inhibits the secretion of ACTH caused by the extract alone, an observation which led Portanova and Sayers (1973) to propose that neurohypophyseal polypeptides are partial agonists of ACTH secretion. Lymangrover and Brodish (1973/1974) recently proposed the existence of an extrahypothalamic CRF which they called "tissue-CRF." These investigators proposed that tissue-CRF might represent an extra source of CRF released in conditions when hypothalamic CRF is secreted in inadequate amounts and would provide an explanation for several puzzling physiological studies which showed that debrained animals possess a "stress" response (Egdahl, 1960).

More recently, Chan *et al.* (1969) submitted acetic acid extracts of rat median eminences to gel filtration and ion exchange chromatography. The ACTH-releasing activity was found in a retarded fraction after Sephadex G25, but was lost during further purification steps. Pepsin and thioglycolate treatment led to only partial inactivation; several substances might be responsible for CRF activity in this preparation with differential sensitivity to pepsin and thioglycolate treatment, or the degradation products of a single CRF might be active, or a single CRF might be protected in crude extracts.

Our own findings indicate the presence in sheep hypothalami of a compound devoid of vasopressin activity and intrinsic ACTH activities and capable of stimulating the *in vitro* secretion of radioimmunoassayable ACTH.

6. PROLACTIN RELEASE INHIBITING FACTOR (PIF)

Evidence that the hypothalamus tonically inhibits prolactin secretion has been provided both *in vivo* and *in vitro* by results showing that pituitaries transplanted away from the sella turcica or maintained in culture (Everett, 1956; Chen *et al.*, 1970; Pasteels, 1961*a*) have elevated PRL secretion rates and that hypothalamic lesions result in increased plasma PRL levels (Bishop *et al.*, 1972).

Extraction and purification of PIF (PRL release inhibiting factor) activity from the hypothalamus have been reported (Pasteels, 1961*a,b*; Talwalker *et al.*, 1963; Dhariwal *et al.*, 1968; Valverde-R *et al.*, 1972; Dular *et al.*, 1974; Schally *et al.*, 1974; Bowers *et al.*, 1973*c*). Interpretation of these activities is, however, complicated by the ability of other substances to inhibit PRL secretion at the pituitary level.

Infusion of dopamine into the third ventricle inhibits PRL secretion and results in higher bioassayable concentrations of PIF in hypothalamohypophyseal portal blood (Kamberi *et al.*, 1971). There appears to be some possibility (Takahara *et al.*, 1974) that the PIF bioassay used by Kamberi *et al.* (1971) was responding to dopamine itself (having reached the portal blood from the third ventricle); however, Kamberi *et al.* reported that dopamine was ineffective in their assay. The differential lability of catecholamines in various perfusion media might explain the discrepancy between these reports. Quijada *et al.* (1973/1974) have obtained additional evidence from *in vitro* experiments, using incubates of hypothalamus and pituitary, that dopamine might stimulate the secretion of PIF by the hypothalamus. The effect of dopamine on pituitary itself in this study was eliminated pharmacologically (see below).

There is little question that catecholamines can *directly* inhibit the secretion of PRL by pituitary glands incubated *in vitro* (MacLeod, 1969; Birge *et al.*, 1970) or cells maintained in culture. Catecholamines are found in high concentrations in the hypothalamus (Dahlstrom, 1971) and have been detected in purified extracts associated with PIF activity (Schally *et al.*, 1974). Furthermore, agents such as perphenazine (Ben-David *et al.*, 1970) and haloperidol (Table 3), which elevate plasma PRL levels *in vivo*, can reverse the catecholamine inhibition of PRL secretion *in vitro* (MacLeod and Leymeyer, 1973) (Fig. 9). There would appear to be PIF activity in hypothalamic (Vale *et al.*, 1974*a*; Quijada *et al.*, 1973/1974) and extrahypothalamic (Vale *et al.*, 1974*a*) brain extracts that is not due to catecholamines as perphenazine or haloperidol does not block the *in vitro* inhibition of PRL secretion due to these extracts.

We have recently observed that cholinergic agonists such as carbachol can also inhibit PRL secretion *in vitro*. Either atropine or higher doses of D-tubocurarine will block the PRL release inhibition (Table 4) due to carbachol and not influence the brain extracts' inhibition of PRL secretion.

Somatostatin, which inhibits GH and TSH secretion in most biological assays (see Section 8), under some circumstances inhibits the secretion of PRL as well (Fig. 15). Since the partially purified PIF described by Bowers *et al.* (1973*c*) inhibited both GH and TSH, the possibility that somatostatin might participate in those activities must be considered. It would appear

TABLE 3

Effect of Catecholamines on in Vivo PRL Secretion in Steroid-Primed Male Rats

Treatment	*N*	ng PRL/ml plasma	SE	*P*
Experiment 1				
Control	5	39.4	3.7	
Perphenazine 40 μg	5	59.6	4.1	<0.01
Dopamine 100 μg	5	25.9	3.2	<0.01
Perphenazine + dopamine	5	51.2	3.9	<0.05
Experiment 2				
Control	5	55.0	4.2	
Dopamine 100 μg	5	36.1	4.8	<0.05
Dibenzyline (2.5 mg, −24 h)	5	59.1	4.7	—
Haloperidol 100 μg	5	104.4	5.2	<0.01
Propranolol 100 μg	5	46.6	4.9	—
Dibenzyline + dopamine	5	48.7	4.9	—
Haloperidol + dopamine	5	99.1	5.0	<0.01
Propranolol + dopamine	5	33.3	4.8	<0.01

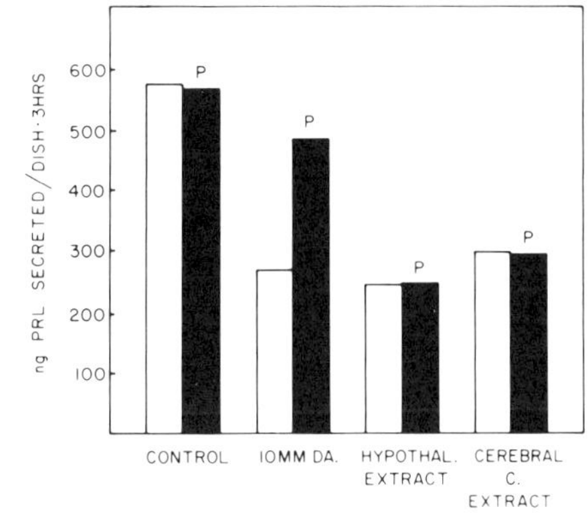

FIG. 9. Effect of perphenazine on inhibition *in vitro* of PRL secretion by dopamine (DA), hypothalamic extract and cerebral cortical extract.

that not all PRL release inhibiting activity in our brain extracts is due to somatostatin as it gives a flatter slope with lower response maxima than do hypothalamic extracts.

In summary, a variety of substances, neurotransmitters (dopamine, norepinephrine), cholinergic agonists, hypothalamic peptide hormones (somatostatin, TRF), and peripheral hormones (estrogens, thyroid hormones) can modify PRL secretion by the anterior pituitary. The existence of such a vast array of effectors for a single cell type (implying the presence of multiple functional receptors), while providing an exciting model system for the study of the interactions of the various classes of hormones, certainly complicates the task of those searching for additional substances modifying PRL secretion. All of the data considered, it would appear that an additional hormone(s) that is neither dopamine, acetylcholine, nor somatostatin exists

TABLE 4

Effect of Cholinergic Agents and Brain Extracts on PRL Secretion in Vitro

Treatment	Percent control
Atropine (ATR) 100 μM	108
Tubocurarine (TUB) 100 μM	100
Carbachol (CAR) 1 μM	60
Carbachol (CAR) 10 μM	43
CAR 10 μM + ATR 1 μM	100
CAR 10 μM + TUB 1 μM	81
CAR 10 μM + TUB 10 μM	92
CAR 10 μM + TUB 100 μM	100
Brain extract (Br Extr)	47
Br Extr + TUB 100 μM	42
Br Extr + ATR 100 μM	46

in brain extracts and is capable of inhibiting PRL secretion; the physiological role of this PIF, and, indeed, of all of the other hormones influencing PRL secretion, remains at issue.

7. GROWTH HORMONE RELEASING FACTOR (GRF)

Physiological and clinical evidence supported the involvement of the central nervous system in the regulation of growth hormone secretion (Bala *et al.*, 1970; Frohman and Bernardis, 1970). Several laboratories have reported the demonstration with various hormone bioassay procedures of releasing factor activity in hypothalamic extracts. A decapeptide isolated from porcine hypothalami, termed "GH-RH" on the basis of its ability to increase the levels of bioassayable GH, was identified to be Val-His-Leu-Ser-Ala-Glu-Glu-Lys-Glu-Ala (Schally *et al.*, 1971). Synthetic GH-RH was found to be ineffective in modifying the secretion rate of immunoactive GH *in vitro* and *in vivo* in several species including man. Furthermore, Verber *et al.* (1971) called attention to the structural similarity between this decapeptide and the amino-terminal sequence of the β-chain of porcine hemoglobin. The physiological significance, if any, of this GH-RH is questionable.

Subsequently, other investigators have found that crude and partially purified hypothalamic extracts can stimulate the secretion of radioimmunoassayable GH (Malacara and Reichlin, 1971; Wilber *et al.*, 1971). This GH-releasing factor remains to be characterized.

8. SOMATOSTATIN–SOMATOTROPIN RELEASE INHIBITING FACTOR (SRIF)

Krulich *et al.* (1972) had reported that the hypothalamus contains a substance that could inhibit the secretion of immunoassayable GH *in vitro*. On the basis of the migration of activities to stimulate or inhibit radioimmunoassayable GH release following ultrafiltration and Sephadex G15 chromatography, it was suggested that SRIF (having a molecular weight of 2000–4000 daltons) was larger than GRF.

In the search for hypophysiotropic substances in ovine hypothalamic extracts that could modify the secretion of radioimmunoassayable GH by monolayer cultures of dissociated anterior pituitary cells (Vale *et al.*, 1972*b*), it was routinely observed that an acid–ethanol–chloroform extract was highly active to inhibit GH release at concentrations as low as 0.0015 fragment per milliliter of culture medium. This extract of almost 0.5 million ovine hypothalamic fragments was submitted to countercurrent distribution

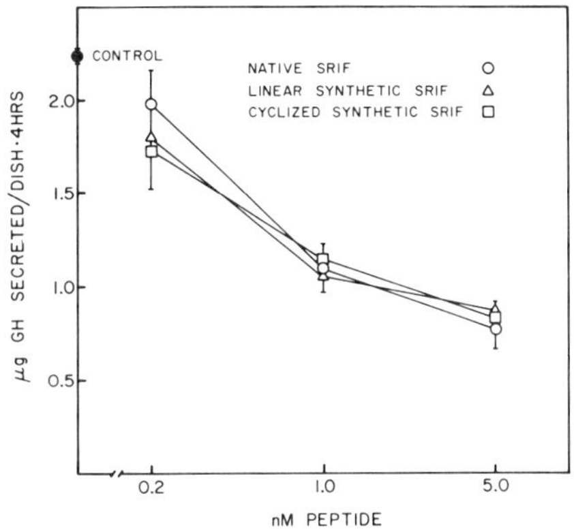

FIG. 10. Effect of native or synthetic somatostatin or (linear) dihydrosomatostatin on the secretion of GH by pituitary cell cultures.

in two systems, cation exchange chromatography and gel filtration and partition chromatography, yielding 8.5 mg purified somatostatin (Brazeau *et al.*, 1974*c*; Burgus *et al.*, 1973*b*). The primary structure was established by submitting the carboxymethylated peptide, the carboxymethylated tryptic digest, and the chymotryptic digest of the peptide to Edman degradation (Burgus *et al.*, 1973*a*). Degradation products were analyzed by amino acid analysis as well as in some cases by determination of the *N* termini by dansylation and determination of phenylthiohydantions by mass spectrometry. The establishment of the 5–9 pentapeptide fragment was carried out simultaneously by mass spectrometry (Ling *et al.*, 1973).

The sequence of native (cyclic) somatostatin was determined to be H-Ala-Gly-*Cys-Lys-Asn-Phe-Phe-Trp-Lys-Thr-Phe-Thr-Ser-Cys*-OH (Brazeau *et al.*, 1973; Burgus *et al.*, 1973*a*; Vale *et al.*, 1972*a*), and synthetic replicates were prepared (Rivier *et al.*, 1973*b*) by Merrifield solid phase procedures. The *in vitro* biological activity (Fig 10) of native somatostatin was not distinguishable from the activities of either synthetic dihydrosomatostatin (in which the cysteine residues are reduced prior to the bioassay) or cyclic synthetic somatostatin containing a disulfide bridge (Vale *et al.*, 1973*c*). It is possible that other intramolecular associations maintain somatostatin in a conformation favorable to receptor interaction regardless of whether the disulfide bond is formed (i.e., reduced and oxidized somatostatin might have similar conformations). The biological activity of two analogues of somatostatin which cannot form a disulfide bond ([$Ala^{3,14}$]somatostatin = 0.2%; [SM3-$Cys^{3,14}$]somatostatin = 1%) (Vale *et al.*, 1973*c*) would suggest that only a small portion of these analogues exists in a favorable form for receptor recognition, and hence the disulfide bond would be important to activity. Since these analogues differ from somatostatin in respects other than being able to cyclize, alternative explanations cannot be ruled out. The most compelling hypothesis is that cyclized somatostatin is the most potent form of somatostatin and that dihydrosomatostatin is rapidly oxidized under the conditions of the bioassays.

Both forms of somatostatin are equally active *in vitro* at ≤1 nM in most experiments, indicating that somatostatin has a potency similar to that of the other characterized hypophysiotropic hormones, TRF and LRF (Vale *et al.*, 1927*b*).

Also, as with TRF and LRF, studies with synthetic somatostatin analogues indicate strict structural requirements at some parts of somatostatin for high potency. For example, [Ala^8]somatostatin (alanine replacing tryptophan) < 1%, [$Cys\text{-}NH_2$]somatostatin < 1%. On the other hand, des-Ala^1-Gly^2-somatostatin = 50% and [Tyr^{11}]somatostatin = 50–100% (synthesized in order to obtain iodinateable molecules) indicate that the structural requirements for receptor recognition are not absolute.

As reported by Schally *et al.* (1973*b*), α-MSH, which bears little apparent resemblance to somatostatin, does possess some SRIF activity *in vitro* (Vale *et al.* 1973*c*), although the potency is extremely low (less than 1/10,000 that of somatostatin). Because of its low potency, the response to doses up to 100 μM was too low to allow comparison of response maxima and slopes with somatostatin. Since no such comparison was reported by Schally *et al.* (1973*b*) either, it is not known if somatostatin and α-MSH inhibit secretion *in vitro* through similar mechanisms. The possibilities that α-MSH plays a physiological role to inhibit the secretion of GH are limited in view of its low potency and reported (Schally *et al.*, 1973*b*) inactivity in the intact rat. In fact, it should be noted here that α-MSH has been reported to be a potent *stimulator* of GH secretion in man *in vivo* (Zahnd *et al.*, 1972).

The cultured pituitary cells secrete GH at a constant rate of GH following medium change; treatment with somatostatin results in a constant but lower secretion rate of GH, indicating that somatostatin is active as long as it is present in the medium (Vale *et al.*, 1972*a*). From a practical standpoint, it means that the amounts of GH in fluids sampled at one time reflect effects on secretion rates.

The secretion rate of GH can be stimulated by various means, including derivatives of cyclic AMP, theophylline, and prostaglandins, which led several investigators to propose that an increase in intracellular cyclic AMP (Schofield, 1967; MacLeod and Leymeyer, 1970) levels mediates an increase in GH secretion. Somatostatin inhibits the GH secretion stimulated by all of these agents (Vale *et al.*, 1972*a*, 1973*c*), as the amount of inhibition by somatostatin cannot be completely explained by a lowering of the baseline release. Since somatostatin blocks the response to exogenously applied cyclic AMP derivatives (Vale *et al.*, 1972*a*) (Fig. 11), it is unlikely that somatostatin acts *exclusively* through an inhibition of cyclic AMP synthesis, although it would be possible for somatostatin to inhibit the formation as well as the expression of cyclic AMP. Borgeat *et al.* (1974) have in fact reported that somatostatin does indeed inhibit the increase in cyclic AMP due to theophylline and prostaglandins.

The secretion of GH following the administration of a fraction of ovine hypothalamic extracts containing GRF activity is also suppressible by

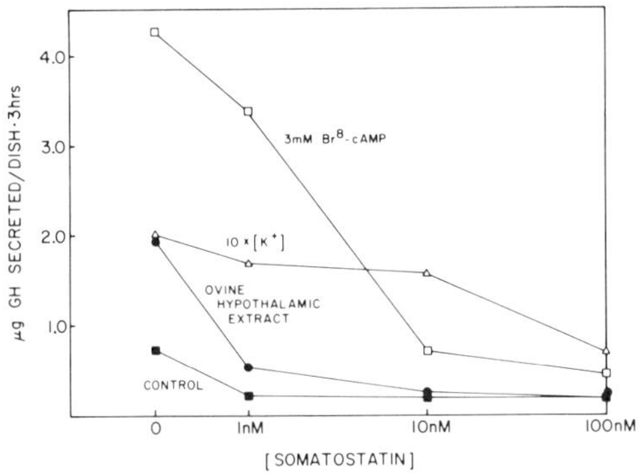

FIG. 11. Somatostatin inhibition of GH secretion stimulated by ^{8}Br cyclic AMP, $10 \times [K^+]$, or ovine hypothalamic extract.

somatostatin (Fig. 11); this is in contrast to the relative insensitivity of the high $[K^+]$-mediated secretion of GH. This may provide evidence that the mechanism of secretion stimulated by high potassium differs from that mediated by GRF factor or cyclic AMP. Observations of the pharmacological interaction of high $[K^+]$ and TRF or LRF are consistent with such a difference (Samli and Geschwind, 1968; Guillemin *et al.*, 1968).

The actions of certain peripheral hormones exerting their negative feedback effects on the secretion of particular pituitary hormones have been shown (Bowers *et al.*, 1968; Vale *et al.*, 1968) to be blocked by inhibitors of DNA-directed RNA synthesis (actinomycin D) or protein synthesis (cycloheximide, puromycin). Considering the proposed mode of action of these hormonal inhibitors (see Section 1) of pituitary hormone secretion, the effect of cycloheximide on the inhibition of GH by somatostatin was studied. A concentration of cycloheximide that inhibits 98% of the incorporation of [^{3}H]leucine into TCA-precipitable materials by the pituitary cells in culture has little effect on the spontaneous secretion of GH in short-term (3-h) experiments and furthermore does not prevent the action of somatostatin (Vale *et al.*, 1973*c*). Hence somatostatin does not require uninterrupted protein synthesis for its action and can be contrasted with thyroxin in this regard. Also, these data indicate that most of the radioimmunoassayable GH secreted by the cells was synthesized prior to the 3-h incubation period and that somatostatin can inhibit the secretion of previously synthesized GH. This conclusion is supported by experiments on the effect of somatostatin on the secretion of biolabeled GH and PRL (Vale *et al.*, 1972*a*). Cultured cells were preincubated with [^{14}C]leucine for 12 h, washed, incubated without label for 2 h, washed again, and then incubated with ^{3}H for 12 h. ^{14}C-Labeled and ^{3}H-labeled GH and PRL were separated by immunoprecipitation with specific antisera and anti-γ-globulin. The results indicated that somatostatin inhibits the secretion of both previously synthesized (^{14}C-labeled) and acutely synthesized (^{3}H-labeled) GH with no effect on the secretion of previously or acutely synthesized PRL by those normal cells.

Because somatostatin was purified exclusively on the basis of an *in vitro* assay, it was critical to test it in the intact rat under a number of experimental situations. Surgical stress decreases GH secretion in the rat (Schalch and Reichlin, 1968); it is therefore difficult to observe further inhibition of GH in normal anesthetized rats because the GH levels are already low. An approach taken in one series of experiments was to test the effect of somatostatin on the release of GH stimulated by pentobarbital (Brazeau *et al.*, 1974*d*), shown by Howard and Martin (1971) to release GH in the rat. Rats under ether anesthesia were intravenously injected with pentobarbital and various amounts of somatostatin were administered subcutaneously. We observed a dose-related inhibition of GH secretion by somatostatin, with as little as 2 μg inhibiting the response to pentobarbital.

Another approach (Brazeau *et al.*, 1974*a*) was to condition the animals to the experimental procedures used for several days prior to the assay. Takahashi *et al.* (1971) reported that such "gentling" prevents the usual fall in plasma GH levels observed in response to handling. In a time study, somatostatin given subcutaneously to previously gentled rats either 10 or 20 min prior to decapitation inhibited GH levels while having no effect when administered 40 min prior to decapitation. Since somatostatin produces continuous suppression of the GH secretion rate *in vitro* for at least 3 h, that experiment suggests that somatostatin is rapidly cleared from its pituitary site of action. We have observed that somatostatin, as is the case for TRF, is partially inactivated by incubation in rat serum; obviously, additional mechanisms such as excretion by the kidney are operative in the removal of somatostatin. If 15 min prior to blood sampling is chosen as a reasonable time for injection, multiple doses of somatostatin yield a dose–response curve (Brazeau *et al.*, 1974*a*) with as little as 0.4 μg somatostatin blocking GH secretion in the gentled rat.

The hypothalamic releasing factors TRF and LRF are active *in vivo* in the rat at much lower doses (<10 ng) than is somatostatin, while the three hormones are all active in the same range *in vitro* (<1 nM). The releasing factors need act only briefly to have a measurable effect, whereas an inhibitor need be present in an effective concentration for a longer period of time; hence the higher doses are probably required to extend the period of action of the inhibitor. Because of its short period of action, studies on the chronic effects of somatostatin will require longer-acting preparations.

The suspending of somatostatin with protamine D zinc has provided one means of achieving a long-acting inhibitor of GH secretion: 300 μg somatostatin–protamine–zinc was found to lower plasma GH in gentled rats for up to 10 h (Brazeau *et al.*, 1974*a*). This and other long-acting preparations offer promise for future physiological and clinical studies.

In summary, these early *in vivo* experiments indicated that the activity of somatostatin was not an artifact of the *in vitro* cell culture system.

Subsequently, somatostatin was found to inhibit GH secretion under various circumstances: by administration of L-dopa, arginine, morphine, or insulin; during hypoglycemia; by injection of norepinephrine into the ventromedial nucleus; by electrical stimulation of the amygdala or hypothalamus; or during sleep—in rats (Martin, 1973*a*), dogs (Lovinger *et al.*, 1973), baboons (Gale *et al.*, 1973), and humans (Hall *et al.*, 1973; Prange *et al.*, 1973; Siler *et al.*, 1973; Yen *et al.*, 1973). In the original description (Brazeau *et al.*, 1973) of the biological activity of somatostatin, we had reported that somatostatin inhibited the secretion of GH by cultured pituitary cells obtained from a human subject with acromegaly. This was the first evidence that somatostatin would be effective in humans and furthermore might be of therapeutic significance in the management of acromegaly. However, in view of the present concepts of the role of cAMP in the regulation of cell function and multiplication and the reported inhibition of pituitary cAMP levels by somatostatin, it is certainly possible that somatostatin, while inhibiting the secretory functions of some pituitary adenomas, might actually stimulate the growth of such tumors. Somatostatin might prove efficacious in the management of tumors dependent on GH, PRL, or TSH (see below). Because of the high intrinsic PRL activity of human GH, the inhibition of GH (by somatostatin) as well as PRL secretion (by ergot derivatives or a PIF) may be indicated in some mammary cancers. The therapeutic value of somatostatin in the treatment of diabetes is also under experimental consideration (Hall *et al.*, 1973; Lundbaeck *et al.*, 1973; Gerich, 1974; Yen *et al.*, 1973) in view of the possible role of GH in the development of diabetic microangiopathies (Luft *et al.*, 1955; Lundbaeck *et al.*, 1970).

Perhaps the most surprising aspect of the biological activities of somatostatin has been its effects on the secretion of hormones other than GH—thyrotropin, prolactin, glucagon, and insulin. The first indication of these multiple effects was the observation that somatostatin inhibits secretion of thyrotropin (Vale *et al.*, 1973*b,c*) in response to various stimuli. Somatostatin decreases the secretion of TSH in the cells exposed to high potassium while having no effect on the spontaneous secretion of TSH, showing that the effect on TSH secretion is independent of the stimulus used (the release of TSH due to theophylline is also blocked by somatostatin, Vale *et al.*, 1972*a*). Somatostatin exhibits some specificity of action as it blocks the release of TSH due to TRF and has no effect on the release of LH by LRF (Vale *et al.*, 1973*c*).

Somatostatin also inhibits (as a function of the dose administered) the secretion of TSH due to TRF *in vivo* (Vale *et al.*, 1973*c*) (Fig. 12) in the estrogen–progesterone primed (EP) rat (Rivier and Vale, 1974), but doe not inhibit the secretion of PRL due to TRF in the same animals whose TSH secretion is lowered, thus providing more evidence that the effect of

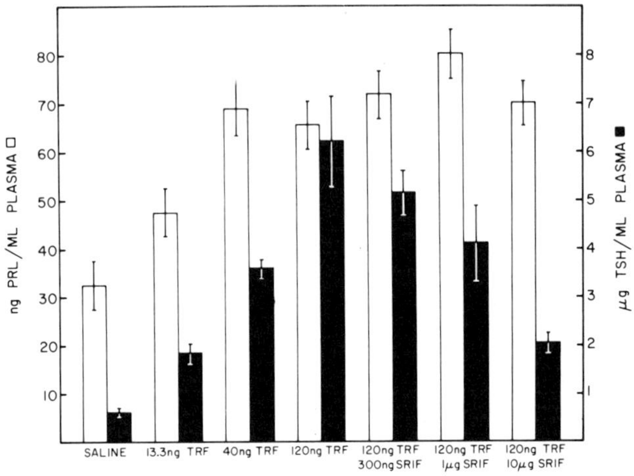

FIG. 12. Effect of somatostatin (SRIF) on the secretion of TSH and PRL mediated by TRF in the estrogen–progesterone pretreated rat.

somatostatin is not mediated by competition for binding to cellular TRF receptors. A dose-related response to TRF can be obtained *in vivo* in the presence of somatostatin. Somatostatin administered intravenously simultaneously with TRF inhibits the rise in plasma TSH levels sampled 5 min later (Fig. 13). If somatostatin is administered intravenously 5 min prior to TRF injection, it has no effect on plasma TSH levels sampled 5 min after TRF administration (Vale *et al.*, 1973*c*; Fig. 21). Therefore, as is the case for its action on GH, the somatostatin effect on TSH is rapid in onset and of short duration.

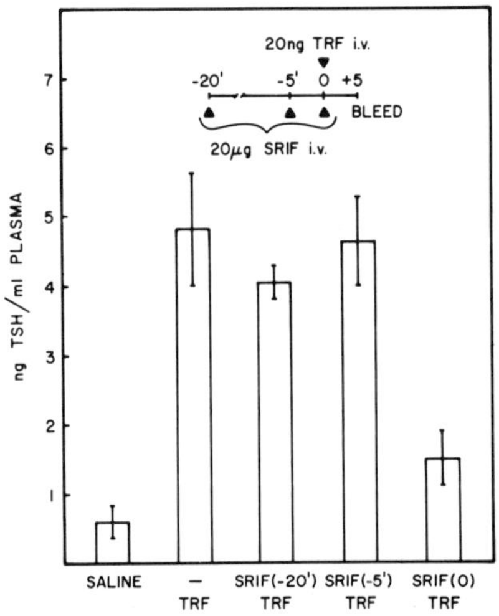

FIG. 13. Effect of time of pretreatment with somatostatin (SRIF) on the inhibition of TSH secretion mediated by TRF.

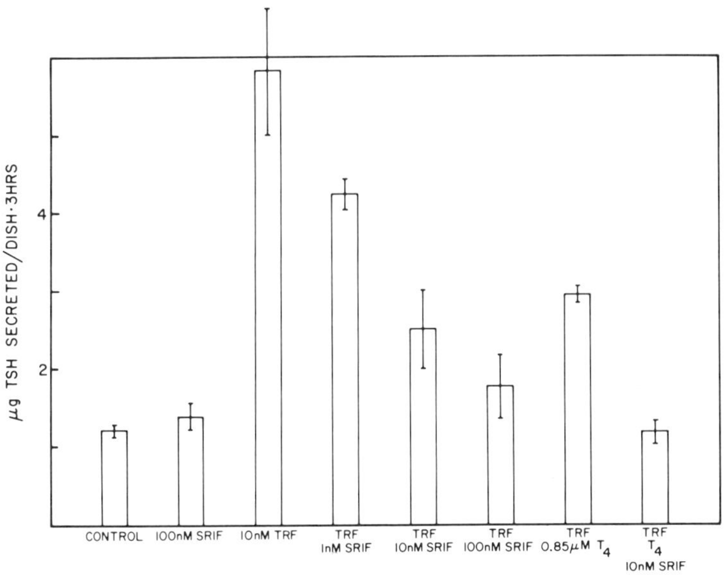

FIG. 14. Interaction of somatostatin (SRIF), TRF, and thyroxin (T_4) on the secretion of TSH by pituitary cell cultures.

The effect of somatostatin on TSH secretion *in vitro* is dose related, with as little as 1 nM somatostatin partially inhibiting the response to 10 nM TRF (Fig. 14). However, the noncompetitive nature of this inhibition has been demonstrated in other *in vitro* experiments in which up to 10 μM TRF cannot completely overcome the block due to 10 nM somatostatin.

Thyroid hormones have long been known to act at the pituitary level to inhibit the secretion of thyrotropin due to TRF and other substances (Section 1). Unlike somatostatin, thyroid hormones have a long latent period but a prolonged period of action and can be blocked by inhibitors of protein synthesis. In spite of these marked differences, somatostatin and thyroid hormones exhibit pharmacological summation *in vitro* (Fig. 14) and *in vivo* (Vale *et al.*, 1973*c*, 1974*b*) on the inhibition of TRF-stimulated TSH release, suggesting perhaps a common step at some point in their respective mechanisms of action. Thus the experimental evidence raises the possibility that the secretion of TSH is under acute positive control by TRF and negative control chronically by thyroid hormones and acutely by somatostatin, with all three elements modulating TSH secretion in a concentration and time-dependent manner.

Although somatostatin does not inhibit the secretion of PRL stimulated by TRF *in vivo*, we usually observe an inhibition of PRL secretion by somatostatin *in vitro* (Fig. 15). This effect is seen often with pituitary cells from normal or estrogen–progesterone treated rats and invariably with

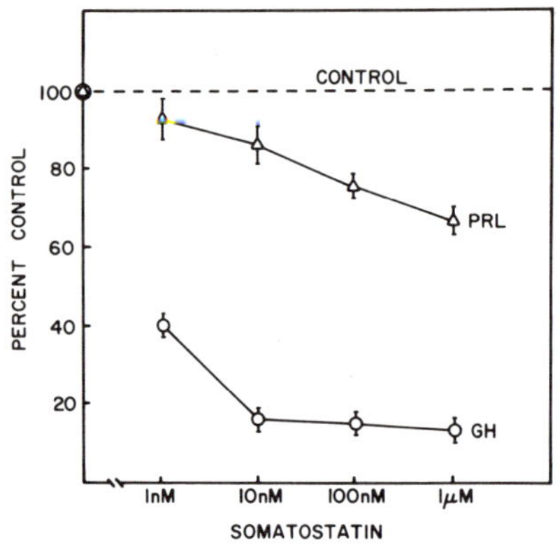

FIG. 15. Effect of somatostatin on the secretion of GH and PRL by cultured pituitary cells from gonadectomized rats.

pituitary cells from castrated donor rats (Vale *et al.*, 1973*c*). As described in Section 2.2, the ability of the rat anterior pituitary to secrete PRL in response to TRF is modified by the presence or absence of peripheral hormones. It would therefore appear that the secretion of PRL can be influenced by a number of factors whose interrelations are not fully defined at the moment (see also Section 6).

The *in vitro* influence of somatostatin on the secretion rate of PRL is considerably less than on the secretion of GH. Since this effect on PRL has not been seen *in vivo* in the rat, its significance is open to question, but we had anticipated that one might be rewarded by looking closely at the effects of somatostatin on the secretion of PRL in other species and under various pathological conditions. Indeed, somatostatin has been found (Vale *et al.*, 1973*c*) to lower plasma PRL levels in some acromegalic patients but not in normal subjects, an observation reminiscent of the effects of TRF (Irie and Tsushina, 1972) and LRF (Rubin *et al.*, 1973) on the secretion of GH in acromegalics. It would appear that there is a nonexclusive distribution of hypothalamic hormone receptors among the several pituitary cell types and that a variety of pathological and experimental circumstances (including the levels of peripheral hormones) influence the functionality of those receptors.

Gale and his colleagues (1973; Koerker *et al.*, 1974) have found that the infusion of somatostatin not only lowered GH levels but also produced a hypoglycemia which was preceded by a dramatic fall in glucagon and insulin concentrations in the unanesthetized baboon. There is evidence from *in vitro* (Leffert *et al.*, in preparation) and perfusion (Gerich and Forsham, 1974) studies that this inhibitory effect can be exerted directly on the endocrine cells of pancreas. The pancreatotropic effects on somatostatin have also been observed in clinical studies (Siler *et al.*, 1973; Mortimer *et al.*, 1974) and have added to its potential clinical significance. Both GH (see above) and glucagon (Unger, 1972) are secreted inappropriately in many juvenile diabetics. Since somatostatin lowers both GH and glucagon, it might be of considerable therapeutic benefit to the juvenile diabetic.

As is the case for TRF and LRF, somatostatin appears to possess psychotropic activity. During the early clinical trials, some of the subjects receiving somatostatin mentioned feelings of mild tranquilization. Monkeys given much higher doses on a weight basis became calm and, although awake, relatively insensitive to environmental stimuli. Segal and Mandell (1974) have reported that intraventricular infusions of somatostatin suppressed the spontaneous motor activity of freely moving rats. Consistently, Prange *et al.* (1973) have found that somatostatin can extend the period of anesthesia following pentobarbital administration. It is interesting that somatostatin, which inhibits one of the hypophysiotropic actions of TRF, would appear to have opposing effects on gross behavior. Further, it can be speculated that somatostatin might be beneficial in some types of (excited) mental disorders. Since depressed subjects often exhibit blunted thyrotropin responses to TRF (Prange *et al.*, 1972; Takahashi *et al.*, 1973) and decreased GH secretion due to various stimuli (Sachar *et al.*, 1971), it is tempting to suggest that inappropriate somatostatin secretion might play a role in some of the behavioral manifestations of depression.

We have found (Vale *et al.*, 1974*a*) that somatostatin-like activity is distributed throughout the brain. Although the highest concentrations appear in the hypothalamus, because of differences in regional weights the cerebral cortex contains more than 10 times more somatostatin-like activity. Therefore, as is the case for TRF, there is evidence for somatostatin presence in and actions on the central nervous system.

All of the characterized hypothalamic hormones have been found to have multiple actions—TRF releases TSH, PRL, and in some conditions GH; LRF stimulates the secretion of LH and FSH; both TRF and LRF have reported psychotropic effects. Somatostatin inhibits the secretion of the pancreatic hormones glucagon and insulin in addition to suppressing the release of GH, TSH, and possibly PRL. Whether these multiple activities represent important mechanisms for the synchronization of endocrine events remains to be determined.

Acknowledgments

Research carried out in the Laboratories of Neuroendocrinology, of which the authors are members, is supported by AID (Contract No. csd-2785), NIH (AM 16707-01), the Rockefeller Foundation, the Ford Foundation, and the Edna McConnell Clark Foundation.

9. REFERENCES

AMOSS, M. S., MONAHAN, M., RIVIER, J., and GUILLEMIN, R., 1974, Inhibition of LRF induced LH release *In Vivo* by LRF analogues, *Endocrinology* **93:**A78.

ARIMURA, A., BOWERS, C. Y., and SCHALLY, A. V., 1968, Suppression by dexamethasome of the action of hypothalamic CRF: Its elimination by actinomycin D or cycloheximide, *Fed. Proc.* **27:**5(abst.).

ARIMURA, A., DEBELJUH, L., and SCHALLY, A. V., 1972, Stimulation of FSH release *in vivo* by prolonged infusion of synthetic LH-RH *Endocrinology* **91:**529–532.

ARIMURA, A., SATO, H., KUMASAKA, T., WOROBEC, R. B., DEBELJUH, L., DUNN, J., and SCHALLY, A. V., 1973, Production of antiserum to LH-releasing hormone (LH-RH) associated with gonadoal atrophy in rabbits: Development of radioimmunoassays for LH-RH, *Endocrinology* **93:**1092–1103.

ARNOLD, W., FLOURET, G., MORGAN, R., RIPPEL, R., and WHITE, W., 1974, Synthesis and biological activity of some analogs of the gonadotropin releasing hormone, *J. Med. Chem.* **17:**314–319.

ASHWORTH, R., WAKABAYASHI, K., MCGOVERN, W., DHARIWAL, A. P. S., and MCCANN, S. M., 1968, The possible relationship between membrane depolarization and the action of the hypothalamic releasing factors on the pituitary cell, *Proc. 24th Int. Cong. Physiol. Sci.* **2:**19 (abst.).

BALA, R. M., BURGUS, R., FERGUSON, K. A., GUILLEMIN, R., KUDO, C., OLIVER, G. C., RODGER, N. W., and BECK, J. C., 1970, Control of growth hormone secretion, in: *The Hypothalamus* (L. Martini, M. Motta, and E. Fraschini, eds.), pp. 401–448, Academic Press, New York.

BEN-DAVID, M., DANON, A., and SULMAN, F. G., 1970, Acute changes in blood and pituitary prolactin after a single injection of perphenazine, *Neuroendocrinology* **7:**193–201.

BIRGE, C. A., JACOBS, L. S., HAMMER, C. T., and DAUGHADAY, W. H., 1970, Catecholamine inhibition of prolactin secretion by isolated rat adenohypophyses, *Endocrinology* **86:**120–130.

BISHOP, W., FAWCETT, C. P., KRULICH, L., and MCCANN, S. M., 1972, Acute and chronic effects of hypothalamic lesions on the release of FSH, LH and prolactin in intact and castrated rats, *Endocrinology* **91:**643–656.

BLACKWELL, R., and GUILLEMIN, R., 1973, Hypothalamic control of adenohypophysial secretions, *Ann. Rev. Physiol.* **35:**357–390.

BLAGDON, D. E., RIVIER, J., and GOODMAN, M., 1973, Proposed tertiary structure for the hypothalamic thyrotropin releasing factor, *Proc. Natl. Acad. Sci.* **70:**1166–1168.

BORGEAT, P., CHAVANCY, G., DUPONT, A., LABRIE, F., ARIMURA, A., and SCHALLY, A. V., 1972, Stimulation of adenosine 3′,5′-cyclic monophosphate accumulation in anterior pituitary gland *in vitro* by luteinizing hormone–releasing hormone, *Proc. Natl. Acad. Sci.* **69:**2677–2681.

BORGEAT, P., LABRIE, F., DROUIN, J., and BELANGER, A., 1974, Inhibition of adenosine 3′,5′-monophosphate accumulation in anterior pituitary gland *in vitro* by growth hormone–release inhibiting hormone, *Biochem. Biophys. Res. Commun.* **56:**1052–1059.

BOWERS, C. Y., REDDING, T., and HAWLEY, W. D., 1966, The effect of thyrotropin releasing factor (TRF) in animals and man, *Proc. 48th Meet. Endocrine Soc. (Chicago)*, p. 43 (abst.).

BOWERS, C. Y., LEE, K. L., and SCHALLY, A. V., 1968, Effect of actinomycin D on hormones that control the release of thyrotropin from the anterior pituitary glands of mice, *Endocrinology* **82:**303–310.

BOWERS, C. Y., SCHALLY, A. V., WEIL, A., REYNOLD, G. A., and FOLKERS, K., 1970, Chemical and biological identity of thyrotropin releasing hormones (TRH) of bovine and human origin, *Proc. Int. Thyroid Conf. (Vienna)* **2:**1019–1040.

BOWERS, C. Y., FRIESEN, H. G., and FOLKERS, K., 1973*a*, Further evidence that TRF is also a physiological regulator of PRL secretion in man, *Biochem. Biophys. Res. Commun.* **51:**512–521.

BOWERS, C. Y., CURRIE, B. L., JOHANSSON, K. N. G., and FOLKERS, K., 1973*b*, Biological evidence that separate hypothalamic hormones release the follicle stimulating and luteinizing hormone, *Biochem. Biophys. Res. Commun.* **50:**20–26.

BOWERS, C. Y., CURRIE, B. L., JOHANSSON, K. N. G., and FOLKERS, K., 1973*c*, Influence of estradiol, triiodothyronine and partially purified porcine prolactin inhibiting factor (PP-PIF) on the TRF induced release of TSH and PRL, *Proc. 55th Meet. Endocrine Soc. (Chicago)*, p. 141 (abst.).

BRAZEAU, P., VALE, W., BURGUS, R., LING, N., BUTCHER, M., RIVIER, J., and GUILLEMIN, R., 1973, A hypothalamic polypeptide that inhibits the secretion of pituitary growth hormone, *Science* **179:**77–79.

BRAZEAU, P., RIVIER, J., VALE, W., and GUILLEMIN, R., 1974*a*, Inhibition of growth hormone secretion in the rat by synthetic somatostatin, *Endocrinology* **94:**184.

BRAZEAU, P., VALE, W., RIVIER, J., and GUILLEMIN, R., 1974*b*, Biological potency of synthetic somatostatin in the oxidized and reduced form on the inhibition of secretion of growth hormone, *Life Sci.* **15:**2, 351–357.

BRAZEAU, P., VALE, W., GUILLEMIN, R., and BURGUS, R., 1974*c*, Isolation of somatostatin (a somatotropin release inhibiting factor) of ovine hypothalamic origin, *Canad. J. Biochem.* **52:**1067–1072.

BRAZEAU, P., RIVIER, J., VALE, W., and GUILLEMIN, R., 1974*d*, Further biological studies with somatostatin and various analogs, *Proc. Endocrine Soc. (Atlanta)*.

BURGESS, A. W., MOMANY, F. A., and SCHERAGA, H. A., 1973, Conformational analysis of thyrotropin releasing factor, *Proc. Natl. Acad. Sci.* **70:**1456–1460.

BURGUS, R., DUNN, T. F., DESIDERIO, D., WARD, D. N., VALE, W., and GUILLEMIN, R., 1970, Characterization of the hypothalamic hypophysiotropic TSH-releasing factor (TRF) of ovine origin, *Nature* **226:**321–325.

BURGUS, R., BUTCHER, M., AMOSS, M., LING, N., MONAHAN, M., RIVIER, J., FELLOWS, R., BLACKWELL, R., VALE, W., and GUILLEMIN, R., 1972, Primary structure of the hypothalamic luteinizing hormone–releasing factor (LRF) of ovine origin, *Proc. Natl. Acad. Sci.* **69:**278–282.

BURGUS, R., LING, N., BUTCHER, M., and GUILLEMIN, R., 1973*a*, Primary structure of somatostatin, a hypothalamic peptide that inhibits the secretion of pituitary growth hormone, *Proc. Natl. Acad. Sci.* **70:**684–688.

BURGUS, R., BRAZEAU, P., and VALE, W., 1973*b*, Isolation and determination of the primary structure of somatostatin (a somatotropin release inhibiting factor) of ovine hypothalamic origin, *Proc. Natl. Pit. Agency hGH Symp. (Baltimore)*, Oct. 9–12.

CARGILLE, C. M., ROSS, G. T., and YOSHINI, T., 1969, Daily variations in plasma follicle stimulating hormone luteinizing hormone and progesterone in the normal menstrual cycle, *J. Clin. Endocrinol.* **29:**12–19.

CARLSON, H., and MARIZ, I., 1973, TRH: A releasing factor for GH in perifused rat pituitaries, *Endocrinology* **93:**A–141.

CHAN, L. T., SCHAAL, S. M., and SAFFRAN, M., 1969, Properties of the corticotropin-releasing factor of the rat median eminence, *Endocrinology* **85:**644–651.

CHEN, C. L., AMENOMOFI, Y., LU, K. H., VOOGT, J. L., and MEITES, J., 1970, Serum prolactin levels in rats with pituitary transplants or hypothalamic lesions, *Neuroendocrinology* **6:**220–227.

CONVEY, E. M., TUCKER, H. A., SMITH, V. G., and ZOLMAN, J., 1973, Bovine prolactin, growth hormone, thyroxine and corticoid response to thyrotropin-releasing hormone, *Endocrinology* **92:**471–476.

COY, D. H., VILCHEZ-MARTINEZ, J. A., COY, E. J., ARIMURA, A., and SCHALLY, A. V., 1973, A peptide inhibitor of luteinizing-hormon-releasing hormone (LH-RH), *J. Clin. Endocrinol. Metab.* **37:**331–333.

COY, D. H., COY, E. J., SCHALLY, A. V., VILCHEZ-MARTINEZ, J. A., HIROTSU, Y., and ARIMURA, A., 1974, Synthesis and biological properties of [D-Ala-6, Des-Gly-NH_2-10]-LH-RH ethyl-amide, a peptide which greatly enhances LH- and FSH-releasing activity, *Biochem. Biophys. Res. Commun.* **57:**335–360.

DAHLSTROM, A., 1971, Regional distribution of brain catecholamines and serotonin, *Neurosci. Res. Prog. Bull.* **9:**197–205.

DEMEYTS, P., ROTH, J., NEVILLE, D. M., GAVIN, J. R., and LESMIAH, M. A., 1973, Insulin interactions with its receptor: Experimental evidence for negative cooperativity, *Biochem. Biophys. Res. Commun.* **55:**154–161.

DE WIED, D., MILLER, A., VERSTEEG, D. H. G., and MULDER, A. H., 1969, Release of ACTH by substances of central nervous system origin, *Endocrinology* **85:**561–569.

DHARIWAL, A. P. S., NALLER, R., BATT, M., and MCCANN, S. M., 1965, Separation of follicle-stimulating hormone–releasing factor from luteinizing hormone–releasing factor, *Endocrinology* **76:**290–294.

DHARIWAL, A. P. S., GROSVENOR, C. E., ANTUNES-RODRIGUES, J., and MCCANN, S. M., 1968, Studies on the purification of ovine prolactin-inhibiting factor, *Endocrinology* **82:**1236–1241.

DOUGLAS, W. W., and POISNER, A. M., 1962, Importance of calcium for acetylcholine in evoking adrenal medullary secretion, *Nature* **196:**379–380.

DOUGLAS, W. W., KANNO, T., and SAMPSON, S. R., 1967, Influence of the ionic environment on the membrane potential of adrenal chromaffine cells and on the depolarizing effect of acetylcholine, *J. Physiol.* **191:**107–121.

DULAR, R., LAZELLA, F., VIVIAN, S., and EDDIE, L., 1974, Purification of prolactin-releasing and inhibiting factors from beef, *Endocrinology* **94:**563–567.

EGDAHL, R. H., 1960, The effect of brain removal, decortication and midbrain transection on adrenal cortical function in dogs, *Acta Endocrinol.* **35**(Suppl. 51):49–50.

EVERETT, J. W., 1956, Functional corporalutea maintained for months by autografts of rat hypophysis, *Endocrinology* **58:**786–796.

FELL, L. R., FINDLAY, J. K., CUMMING, I. A., and GODING, J. R., 1973, Effect of synthetic TRF on prolactin release in the sheep, *Endocrinology* **93:**487–491.

FERMANDJIAN, S., PRADELLES, P., and FROMAGEOT, P., 1972, Proton NMR studies on thyrotropin releasing factor, *FEBS Letters* **28:**156–160.

FLEISCHER, N., and GUILLEMIN, R., 1972, Clinical applications of hypothalamic releasing factors, in: *Advances in Internal Medicine* (G. H. Stollerman and M. Siperstein, eds.), pp. 303–323, Year Book Medical Publishers, Chicago.

FLEISCHER, N., and VALE, W., 1968, Vasopressin induced ACTH release *in vitro* inhibition by glucocorticoids and possible mediation by cyclic AMP, *Clin. Res.* **161:**266.

FRIEDGOOD, H. B., 1936 (personal communication to J. Porter), see PORTER, J. C., GOLDMAN, B. D., and WILBER, J. F., 1970, Hypophysiotropic hormones in portal vessel blood, in: *Hypophysiotropic Hormones of the Hypothalamus: Assay and Chemistry* (J. Meites, ed.), pp. 282–297, Williams and Wilkins Co., Baltimore.

FROHMAN, L. A., and BERNARDIS, L. L., 1970, Growth hormone secretion in the rat: Metabolic clearance and secretion rates, *Endocrinology* **86:**305–312.

FUJINO, M. S., KOBAYASHI, S., OBAYASHI, M., SHINAGAWA, S., FUKUDA, T., KITALA, C., NAKAYAMA, R., IAMAZAKI, I., WHITE, W., and RIPPEL, R., 1972, Structure–activity relationship in the *C*-terminal part of luteinizing hormone releasing hormone (LH-RH), *Biochem. Biophys. Res. Commun.* **49:**863–869.

FUJINO, M. S., SHINAGAWA, S., OBAYASHI, M., KOBAYASHI, S., FUKUDA, T., YAMAZAKI, I., and NAKAYAMA, R., 1973, Further studies on the structure-activity relationship in the *C*-terminal part of luteinizing hormone-releasing hormone, *J. Med. Chem.* **16:**1144–1147.

FUJINO, M., YAMAZAKI, I., KOBAYASHI, S., FUKUDA, T., SHINAGAWA, S., NAYAMA, R., WHITE, F. W., and RIPPEL, R. H., 1974, Some analogs of luteinizing hormone releasing hormone (LH-RH) having intense ovulation-inducing activity, *Biochem. Biophys. Res. Commun.* **57:**1248–1256.

GALE, C., *et al.*, 1973, Paper presented at *Natl. Pit. Agency hGH Symp. (Baltimore)*, Oct. 9–12.

GANONG, W. F., 1963, The central nervous system and the synthesis and release of adrenocorticotropic hormone, in: *Advances in Neuroendocrinology* (A. V. Nalbandov, ed.), pp. 92–149, University of Illinois Press, Urbana.

GAUTVIK, F. M., and TASHJIAN, A. H., 1973, Effects of cations and colchicine on the release of prolactin and growth hormone by functional pituitary tumor cells in culture, *Endocrinology* **93:**793–799.

GAY, V. L., and SHETH, N. A., 1972, Evidence for a periodic release of LH in castrated male and female rats, *Endocrinology* **90:**158–162.

GAY, V. L., MIDGLEY, A. R., and NISWENDER, G. D., 1970, Patterns of gonadotropin secretion associated with ovulation, *Fed. Proc.* **29:**1880–1887.

GERICH, E. J., LORENZI, M., SCHNEIDER, V., KWAN, C. W., KARAM, J. H., GUILLEMIN, R., and FORSHAM, P. H., 1974, Inhibition of pancreatic glucagon responses to arginine by somatostatin in normal man and in insulin-dependent diabetics, *Diabetes* **23:**876–880.

GESCHWIND, I. I., 1969, Mechanism of action of releasing factors, in: *Frontiers in Neuroendocrinology* (W. F. Ganong and L. Martini, eds.), pp. 389–431, Oxford University Press, New York.

GOEBELSMANN, U., MIDGLEY, A. R., and JAPTE, R. B., 1969, Regulation of human gonadotropin. VII. Daily individual urinary estrogens pregnanediol and serum luteinizing and follicle stimulating hormones during the menstrual cycle, *J. Clin. Endocrinol.* **29:**1222–1230.

GRANT, G., and VALE, W., 1972, Speculations on structural relationships between the hypothalamic releasing factors of pituitary hormones, *Nature New Biol.* **237:**182–183.

GRANT, G., and VALE, W., 1973, Hypothalamic control of anterior pituitary hormone secretion—Characterized hypothalamic hypophysiotropic peptides, in: *Current Topics in Experimental Endocrinology*, Vol. II (V. H. T. James, ed.), Academic Press, New York.

GRANT, G., LING, N., RIVIER, J., and VALE, W., 1972*a*, Orientation restrictions of the peptide hormone, thyrotropin releasing factor, due to intramolecular hydrogen bonding, *Biochemistry* **11:**3070–3073.

GRANT, G., VALE, W., and GUILLEMIN, R., 1972*b*, Interaction of thyrotropin releasing factor with membrane receptors of pituitary cells, *Biochem. Biophys. Res. Commun.* **46:**28–36.

GRANT, G., VALE, W., and GUILLEMIN, R., 1973*a*, Characteristics of the pituitary receptor for thyrotropin releasing factor, *Endocrinology* **92:**1629.

GRANT, G., VALE, W., and RIVIER, J., 1973*b*, Pituitary binding sites for [^{3}H]-labelled luteinizing hormone releasing factor (LRF), *Biochem. Biophys. Res. Commun.* **50:**771–778.

GREEN, J. D., and HARRIS, G. W., 1947, The neurovascular link between the neurohypophysis and adenohypophysis, *J. Endocrinol.* **5:**136–146.

GUAL, C., KASTIN, A. J., and SCHALLY, A. V., 1972, Clinical experience with hypothalamic releasing hormones. Part I. Thyrotropin releasing hormone, in: *Recent Progress in Hormone Research* (E. B. Astwood, ed.), pp. 173–200, Academic Press, New York.

GUILLEMIN, R., and ROSENBERG, B., 1955, Humoral hypothalamic control of anterior pituitary: A study with combined tissue cultures, *Endocrinology* **57:**599–607.

GUILLEMIN, R., SCHALLY, A. V., LIPSCOMB, H. S., ANDERSEN, R. N., and LONG, J. M., 1962, On the presence in hog hypothalamus of β-corticotropin releasing factor, α- and β-melanocyte stimulating hormones, adrenocorticotropin, lysine-vasopressin and oxytocin, *Endocrinology* **70:**471–477.

GUILLEMIN, R., YAMAZAKI, E., GARD, D. A., JUTISA, M., and SAKIZ, E., 1963, *In vitro* secretion of thyrotropin (TSH): Stimulation by a hypothalamic peptide (TRF), *Endocrinology* **73:**564–572.

GUILLEMIN, R., BURGUS, R., and VALE, W., 1968, TRF-releasing factor: an RF model study. *Proc. 2nd Int. Cong. Endocrinol.*, series No. 184, 577, Excerpta Medica, Amsterdam.

GUILLEMIN, R., BURGUS, R., and VALE, W., 1971, The hypothalamic hypophysiotropic thyrotropin releasing factor (TRF), *Vitam. Horm. (N.Y.)* **29:**1–39.

GUILLEMIN, R., AMOSS, M., BLACKWELL, R., BURGUS, R., GRANT, G., LING, N., MONAHAN, M., RIVIER, J., and VALE, W., 1972, Polypeptides antagonists of the hypothalamic luteinizing hormone releasing factors, *Gynecol. Invest.* **2:**2–12.

HALL, R., SCHALLY, A. V., EVERED, D., KASTIN, A. J., MORTIMER, C. H., TUNBRIDGE, W. M. G., BESSER, G. M., COY, D. H., GOLDIE, D. J., MCNEILLY, A. S., PHENEKOS, C., and WEIGHTMAN, D., 1973, Action of growth hormone release inhibitory hormone in healthy men and in acromegaly, *Lancet* **2:**581–584.

HEDGE, A., 1972, The effects of prostaglandins on ACTH secretion, *Endocrinology* **91:**925–933.

HINKLE, P. M., WOROCH, E. L., and TASHJIAN, A. H., 1973, Activity of analogs of thyrotropin releasing hormone (THR) on prolactin synthesis and binding to TRF receptors in pituitary cells in culture, *Proc. 53rd Meet. Endocrine Soc. (Chicago)*, p. 140 (abst.).

HOFMANN, K., and BOWERS, C. Y., 1970, Polypeptides. XLVII. Effect of the pyrazole–imidazole replacement on the biological activity of thyrotropin releasing hormone, *J. Med. Chem.* **13:**1099–1101.

HOWARD, H., and MARTIN, J. M., 1971, A stimulatory test for growth hormone release in the rat, *Endocrinology* **88:**497–499.

IRIE, M., and TSUSHIMA, T., 1972, Increase of serum growth hormone concentration following thyrotropin-releasing hormone injection in patients with acromegaly or gigantism, *J. Clin. Endocrinol. Metab.* **35:**97–100.

JACKSON, I., and REICHLIN, S., 1974, Thyrotropin releasing hormone (TRH): Distribution in hypothalamic and extrahypothalamic brain tissues of mammalian and submammalian chordates, *Endocrinology* **95:**854–862.

JACOBS, L. S., SNYDER, P. J., WILBER, J. F., UTIGER, R. D., and DAUGHADAY, W. H., 1971, Increased serum prolactin after administration of synthetic thyrotropin-releasing hormone (TRF) in man, *J. Clin. Endocrinol.* **33:**996–998.

JUTISZ, M., and DE LA LLOSA, M. P., 1970, Requirements of Ca^{++} and Mg^{++} ions for the *in vitro* release of follicle-stimulating hormone from rat pituitary glands and its subsequent biosynthesis, *Endocrinology* **86:**761–768.

KAMBERI, I. A., MICAL, R. S., and PORTER, J. C., 1971, Effect of anterior pituitary perfusion and intraventricular injection of catecholamines on prolactin release, *Endocrinology* **88:**1012–1020.

KASTIN, A. J., EHRENSING, R. H., SCHALCH, D. S., and ANDERSON, M. S., 1972, Improvement in neural depression with decreased thyrotropin response after administration of thyrotropin-releasing hormone, *Lancet* **2:**740–742.

KELLER, H. H., BARTHOLINI, G., and PLETSCHER, A., 1974, Enhancement of cerebral norepinephrine turnover by thyrotropin-releasing hormone, *Nature* **248:**528–529.

KELLY, P. A., BEDIRIAN, K. N., BAKER, R. D., and FRIESEN, H. G., 1973, Effect of synthetic TRH on serum prolactin, TSH and milk production in the cow, *Endocrinology* **92:**1289–1293.

KOCH, Y., CHOBSIENG, P., ZOR, U., FRIDKIN, M., and LINDNER, H. R., 1973, Suppression of gonadotropin secretion and prevention of ovulation in the rat by antiserum to synthetic gonadotropin-releasing hormone, *Biochem. Biophys. Res. Commun.* **55:**623–629.

KOERKER, D., RUCH, W., CHIDECKEL, E., PALMER, J., GOODNER, C., ENSINCK, J., and GALE, C., 1974, Somatostatin: Hypothalamic inhibitor of the endocrine pancreas, *Science* **184:**482–484.

KRAICER, J. J., MILLIGAN, V., GOSBEE, J. L., CONRAD, R. G., and BRANSON, C. M., 1969, *In vitro* release of ACTH: Effects of potassium, calcium and corticosterone, *Endocrinology* **85:**1144–1153.

KRULICH, L., ILLNER, P., FAWCETT, C. P., QUIJADA, M., and MCCANN, S. M., 1972, Dual hypothalamic regulation of growth hormone secretion, in: *Growth and Growth Hormone* (A. Pecile and E. E. Muller, eds.), pp. 306–316, Excerpta Medica, Amsterdam.

LABRIE, F., BORDEN, N., POIRIER, G., and DELEAN, A., 1972, Binding of TRF to plasma membranes of bovine anterior pituitary gland, *Proc. Natl. Acad. Sci.* **69:**283–287.

LABRIE, F., PELLETIER, G., LEMAY, A., BORGEDT, P., BARDEN, N., DUPONT, A., SAVARY, M., CÔTE, and BOUCHER, R., 1973, Control of protein synthesis in anterior pituitary gland, in: *Karolinska Symposium on Research Methods in Reproductive Endocrinology* (E. Diczfalusy, ed.), pp. 301–340, Karolinska Institutet, Stockholm.

LING, N., BURGUS, R., RIVIER, J., VALE, W., and BRAZEAU, P., 1973, The use of mass spectrometry in deducing the sequence of somatostatin—a hypothalamic polypeptide that inhibits the secretion of growth hormone, *Biochem. Biophys. Res. Commun.* **50:**127–133.

LOVINGER, R., CONNORS, M., BORYZEHA, A., KAPLAN, S. L., and GRUMBACH, M. M., 1973, Suppression of L-dopa induced rise in plasma growth hormone by somatotropin release inhibiting factor (SRIF) in the dog, *Proc. 55th Meet. Endocrine Soc. (Chicago)*, p. 82 (abst.).

LU, K. H., SHAAR, C. J., KORTRIGUI, K. H., and MEITES, J., 1972, Effects of synthetic TRF on *in vitro* and *in vivo* prolactin release in the rat, *Endocrinology* **91:**1540–1545.

LUFT, R., OLIVECRONA, H., and SJOGREN, B., 1955, Hypophysectomy in man: Experiences in severe diabetes mellitis, *J. Clin. Endocrinol. Metab.* **15:**391–408.

LUNDBAECK, F., JENSEN, V. A., STEEN OLSEN, T., ØRSKOV, H., JUEL CHRISTENSEN, N., JOHANSEN, K., PRANGE HANSEN, A., and ØSTERBY, R., 1970, Diabetes, diabetic angiopathy, and growth hormone, *Lancet* **2:**131–133.

LUNDBAECK, K., CHRISTENSEN, S. E., and PRANGE HANSEN, A., 1973, Growth hormone in acromegaly, *Lancet* **2:**913.

LYMANGROVER, J. R., and BRODISH, A., 1973/1974, Physiological regulation of tissue-CRF, *Neuroendocrinology* **13:**234–245.

MACLEOD, R. M., 1969, Influence of norepinephrine and catecholamine-depleting agents on the synthesis and release of prolactin and growth hormone, *Endocrinology* **85:**916–923.

MACLEOD, R. M., and FONTHAM, E. H., 1970, Influence of ionic environment on the *in vitro* synthesis and release of pituitary hormones, *Endocrinology* **86:**863–869.

MACLEOD, R. M., and LEHMEYER, J. E., 1970, Release of pituitary growth hormone by prostaglandins and dibutyryl adenosine cyclic 3′,5′-mono-phosphate in the absence of protein synthesis, *Proc. Natl. Acad. Sci.* **67:**1172–1179.

MACLEOD, R. M., and LEHMEYER, J. E., 1973, Pituitary gland alpha-adrenergic receptors and their function in prolactin secretion, *Proc. 55th Meet. Endocrine Soc. (Chicago)*, p. 50 (abst.).

MACLEOD, R. M., FONTHAM, G. H., and LEYMEYER, J. E., 1970, Prolactin and growth hormone production as influenced by catacholamines and agents that affect brain catacholamines, *Neuroendocrinology* **6:**283–294.

MALACARA, J. M., and REICHLIN, S., 1971, Elevation of radioimmunoassayable plasma growth hormone in rat induced by porcine hypothalamic extract, *Fed. Proc.* **30:**198 (abst.).

MARTIN, J., 1973*a*, Hypothalamic and extrahypothalamic mechanisms for control of gGH secretion, *Proc. Natl. Pit. Agency hGH Symp. (Baltimore)*, Oct. 9–12.

MARTIN, J., 1973*b*, Neural regulation of growth hormone secretion, *New Engl. J. Med.* **288:**1384–1393.

MATSUO, H., BABA, Y., NAIR, R. M. G., ARIMURA, A., and SCHALLY, A. V., 1971, Structure of the porcine LH- and FSH-releasing hormone. I. Proposed amino acid sequence, *Biochem. Biophys. Res. Commun.* **43:**1374–1339.

MCCANN, S. M., 1971, Mechanism of action of hypothalamic-hypophysial stimulating and inhibiting hormone, in: *Frontiers in Neuroendocrinology* (W. F. Ganong and L. Martini, eds.), pp. 209–235, Oxford University Press, New York.

MCCANN, S. M., and FRUIT, A. J., 1957, Effect of synthetic vasopressin on release of adrenocorticotropin in rats with hypothalamic lesions, *Proc. Soc. Exp. Biol. Med.* **96:**566–567.

MCCANN, S. M., and PORTER, J. E., 1969, Hypothalamic pituitary stimulating and inhibiting hormones, *Physiol. Rev.* **49:**240–284.

McCann, S. M., Taleishik, S., and Friedman, H. M., 1960, LH-releasing activity in hypothalamic extracts, *Proc. Soc. Exp. Biol. Med.* **104:**432–434.

Mitnick, M., and Reichlin, S., 1971, Thyrotropin-releasing hormone: Biosynthesis by rat hypothalamic fragments *in vitro*, *Science* **172:**1241–1243.

Monahan, M. W., Rivier, J., Vale, W., Guillemin, R., and Burgus, R., 1972, [Gly[2]]LRF and des-His[2]-LRF: The synthesis, purification and characterization of two LRF analogues antagonistic to LRF, *Biochem. Biophys. Res. Commun.* **47:**551–556.

Monahan, M., Amoss, M., Anderson, H., and Vale, W., 1973, Synthetic analogs of the hypothalamic luteinizing hormone releasing factor with increased agonist or antagonist properties, *Biochemistry* **12:**4616.

Montoya, E., Seibel, M. J., and Wilber, J., 1973, Studies of thyrotropin releasing hormone (TRH) in the rat by means of radioimmunoassay: Normal values and response to cold exposure, *Endocrinology* **92:**A138.

Mortimer, C. H., Carr, D., Lind, T., Bloom, S. R., Mallinson, C. N., Schally, A. V., Tunbridge, W. M. G., Yeomans, L., Coy, D. Y., Kastin, A., Besser, G. M., and Hall, R., 1974, Effects of growth hormone release–inhibiting hormones on circulating glucagon, insulin and growth hormone in normal, diabetic, acromegalic, and hypopituitary patients, *Lancet* **2:**697–701

Moss, R. L., and McCann, S. M., 1973, Induction of mating behavior in rats by luteinizing hormone–releasing factor, *Science* **181:**177–179.

Nair, R. M. G., Barrett, J. F., Bowers, C. Y., and Schally, A. V., 1970, Structure of porcine thyrotropin releasing hormone, *Biochemistry* **9:**1103–1106.

Oliver, C. R., Estray, L., Mical, R. S., and Porter, J. C., 1973, *Proc. 49th Meet. Am. Thyroid Assoc.*, p. T4 (abst.). Title not available to us.

Pasteels, J.-L., 1961*a*, Sécrétion de prolactine par l'hypophyse en culture de tissue, *C. R. Acad. Sci. Paris Ser. D* **253:**2140–2142.

Pasteels, J.-L., 1961*b*, Premiers résultats de culture combinée *in vitro* d'hypophyse et d'hypothalamus, dans le but d'en apprécier la sécrétion de prolactine, *C. R. Acad. Sci. Paris Ser. D* **253:**3074–3075.

Peake, G. T., 1973, The role of cyclic nucleotides in the secretion of pituitary growth hormone, in: *Frontiers in Neuroendocrinology* (W. F. Ganong and L. Martini, eds.), pp. 173–208, Oxford University Press, New York.

Pfaff, D. W., 1973, Luteinizing hormone–releasing factor potentiates lordosis behavior in hypophysectomized ovariectomized female rats, *Science* **182:**1148–1149.

Plotnikoff, M. P., Prange, A. J., Breese, G. R., Anderson, M. S., and Wilson, I. C., 1972, Thyrotropin releasing hormone: Enhancement of dopa activity by a hypothalamic hormone, *Science* **178:**417–418.

Portanova, R., and Sayers, G., 1973, Isolated pituitary cells: CRF-like activity of neurohypophysial and related polypeptides, *Proc. Soc. Exp. Biol. Med.* **143:**661–666.

Prange, A. J., Jr., Wilson, I. C., Lara, P. P., Alltrop, L. B., and Breese, G. R., 1972, Effects of thyrotropin-releasing hormone in depression, *Lancet* **2:**999–1002.

Prange, H., Ørskov, A. H., Seyer-Hansen, K., and Lundbaeck, K., 1973, Some actions of growth hormone release inhibiting factor, *Brit. Med. J.* **3:**523–524.

Quijada, M., Illner, P., Krulick, L., and McCann, S. M., 1973/1974, The effect of catecholamines on hormone release from anterior pituitary and ventral hypothalami incubated *in vitro*, *Neuroendocrinology* **13:**151–163.

Rasmussen, H., and Tenenhouse, A., 1968, Cyclic adenosine monophophate, Ca^{++} and membranes, *Proc. Natl. Acad. Sci.* **59:**1364–1370.

Redding, T. W., and Schally, A. V., 1969, Studies on the inactivation of thyrotropin-releasing hormone (TRH), *Proc. Soc. Exp. Biol. Med.* **131:**415–420.

Reichlin, S., and Mitnick, M., 1973, Biosynthesis of hypothalamic hypophysiotropic factors, in: *Frontiers in Neuroendocrinology* (W. F. Ganong and L. Martini, eds.), pp. 61–88, Oxford University Press, New York.

REICHLIN, S., MARTIN, J. B., MITNICK, M., BOSHANS, R. L., GRIMM, Y., BOLLINGER, L., GORDON, J., and MALACARA, J., 1972, The hypothalamus in pituitary–thyroid regulation, in: *Recent Progress in Hormone Research* (E. B. Astwood, ed.), pp. 229–286, Academic Press, New York.

RIPPEL, R. H., JOHNSON, E. S., WHITE, W. F., FUJINO, M., YAMAZAKI, I., and NAKAYAMA, R., 1973, Ovulating and LH-releasing activity of a highly potent analog of synthetic gonadotropin-releasing hormone, *Endocrinology* **93:**1449–1452.

RIVIER, C., and VALE, W., 1974, *In vivo* stimulation of prolactin secretion in the rat by thyrotropin releasing factor, related peptides and hypothalamic extracts, *Endocrinology* **95:**978–983.

RIVIER, J., VALE, W., MONAHAN, M., LING, N., and BURGUS, R., 1972, Synthetic TRF (thyrotropin releasing factor) analogs. III: Effect of replacement or modification of histidine residue on biological activity, *J. Med. Chem.* **15:**479–482.

RIVIER, J., VALE, W., BURGUS, R., LING, N., AMOSS, M., BLACKWELL, R., and GUILLEMIN, R., 1973*a*, Synthetic luteinizing hormone releasing factor analogs: Series of short-chain amide LRF homologs converging to the amino terminus, *J. Med. Chem.* **16:**545–549.

RIVIER, J., BRAZEAU, P., VALE, W., LING, N., BURGUS, R., GILON, C., YARDLEY, H., and GUILLEMIN, R., 1973*b*, Synthèse totale par phase solide d'un tétradécapeptide ayant les propriétés chimiques et biologiques de la somatostatine, *C. R. Acad. Sci. Paris* **276:**2737.

RIVIER, J., AMOSS, M., RIVIER, C., and VALE, W., 1974, Synthetic luteinizing hormone releasing factor: Short chain analogs, *J. Med. Chem.* **17:**230–233.

RUBIN, A. L., LEVIN, S. R., BERNSTEIN, R. I., TYRRELL, J., NOACCO, C., and FORSHAM, P., 1973, Stimulation of growth hormone by luteinizing hormone–releasing hormone in active acromegaly, *J. Clin. Endocrinol. Metab.* **37:**160–162.

RUBIN, R. P., KALES, A., ADLER, R., FAGAN, T., and ODELL, W., 1971, Gonadotropin secretion during sleep in normal adult men, *Science* **175:**196–198.

RUDINGER, J., PLIŠKA, V., and KREJČI, I., 1972, Oxytocin analogs in the analysis of some phases of hormone action, in: *Recent Progress in Hormone Research*, Vol. 28 (E. B. Astwood, ed.), pp. 131–172, Academic Press, New York and London.

SACHAR, E. J., FINKELSTEIN, J., and HELLMAN, L., 1971, Growth hormone responses in depressive illness. I. Response to insulin tolerance test, *Arch. Gen. Psychiat.* **25:**263–269.

SACHS, H., FAWCETT, P., TAKABATAKE, Y., and PORTANOVA, R., 1969, Biosynthesis and release of vasopressin and neurophysin, in: *Recent Progress in Hormone Research* (E. B. Astwood, ed.), pp. 447–491, Academic Press, New York.

SAFFRAN, M., and SCHALLY, A. V., 1955, The release of corticotropin by anterior pituitary tissue *in vitro, Canad. J. Biochem. Physiol.* **33:**408–415.

SAMLI, M. H., and GESCHWIND, I. I., 1968, Some effects of energy-transfer inhibitors and of Ca^{++}-free and of K^{+}-enhanced media on the release of luteinizing hormone from the rat pituitary gland *in vitro, Endocrinology* **82:**225–231.

SCHALCH, and REICHLIN, 1968, Stress and growth hormone release, in: *Growth Hormone* (A. Pecile and E. E. Muller, eds.), Excerpta Medica Foundation, Amsterdam, pp. 211–225.

SCHALLY, A. V., LIPSCOMBE, H. S., and GUILLEMIN, R., 1962, Isolation and amino acid sequence of α-corticotropin releasing factor (α_2-CRF) from hog pituitary glands, *Endocrinology* **71:**164–173.

SCHALLY, A. V., ARIMURA, A., BOWERS, C. Y., KASTIN, A. J., SAWANS, S., and READING, T. W., 1968, Hypothalamic neurohormones regulating anterior pituitary function, in: *Recent Progress in Hormone Research* (E. B. Astwood, ed.), pp. 497–588, Academic Press, New York.

SCHALLY, A. V., BABA, Y., NAIR, R. M. G., and BENNETT, C. D., 1971, The amino acid sequence of a peptide with growth hormone–releasing activity isolated from porcine hypothalamus, *J. Biol. Chem.* **246:**6647–6650.

SCHALLY, A. V., REDDING, T. V., MATSUO, H., and ARIMURA, A., 1972, Stimulation of FSH and LH release *in vitro* by natural and synthetic LH and FSH releasing hormone, *Endocrinology* **90:**1561–1568.

SCHALLY, A. V., ARIMURA, A., and KASTIN, A. J., 1973*a*, Hypothalamic regulatory hormones, *Science* **179:**341–349.

SCHALLY, A. V., ARIMURA, A., KASTIN, A. J., UEHARA, T., COY, D. H., COY, E. J., and TAKAHARA, J., 1973*b*, Inhibition of the release of growth hormone *in vitro* by α-melanocyte stimulating hormone, *Biochem. Biophys. Res. Commun.* **52:**1314–1319.

SCHALLY, A. V., ARIMURA, A., TAKAHARA, J., REDDING, T. W., and DUPONT, A., 1974, Inhibition of prolactin release *in vitro* and *in vivo* by catecholamines, *Fed. Proc.*, abst. 190.

SCHOFIELD, J. C., 1967, Role of cyclic 3′,5′-AMP in the release of GH *in vitro, Nature* **215:**1382–1383.

SEGAL, D. S., and MANDELL, A. J., 1974, Differential behavioral effects of hypothalamic polypeptides, in: *The Thyroid Axis, Drugs and Behavior* (A. J. Prange, ed.), Raven Press, New York.

SIEVERTSSON, H., CHANG, J. F., FOLKERS, K., and BOWERS, C. Y., 1972, Synthesis of di- and tri-peptides and assay *in vivo* for activity in the thyrotropin releasing hormone and luteinizing releasing hormone systems, *J. Med. Chem.* **15:**3–11.

SILER, T. M., VANDENBERG, G., and YEN, S. S. C., 1973, Inhibition of growth hormone release in humans by somatostatin, *J. Clin. Endocrinol. Metab.* **37:**632–634.

SPONA. J., 1973, LH-RH stimulated gonadotropin release mediated by two distinct pituitary receptors, *FEBS Letters* **35:**59–62.

STEINER, A. L., PEAKE, G. T., UTIGER, R. D., KARL, I. E., and KIPNER, D. M., 1969, Hypothalamic stimulation of growth hormone and thyrotropin release *in vitro* and pituitary 3′,5′-adenosine cyclic monophosphate, *Endocrinology* **86:**1354–1360.

STEVENS, V. C., 1969, Comparison of FSH and LH patterns in plasma urine and urinary extracts during the menstrual cycle, *J. Clin. Endocrinol. Metab.* **29:**904–910.

TAKAHARA, J., ARIMURA, A., and SCHALLY, A. V., 1974, Effect of catecholamines infused into a hypophysial portal vessel on serum prolactin levels in the rat, *Fed. Proc.*, abst. 191.

TAKAHASHI, K., DAUGHADAY, W. H., and KIPNIR, D. M., 1971, Regulation of immunoreactive growth hormone secretion in male rats, *Endocrinology* **88:**909–917.

TAKAHASHI, S., KONDO, H., YOSHIMURA, M., and OCHI, Y., 1973, Antidepressant effect of thyrotropin-releasing hormone (TRH) and the plasma thyrotropin levels in depression, *Folia Psychiat. Neurol. Jap.* **27:**305–314.

TALWALKER, P. K., RATNER, A., and MEITES, J., 1963, *In vitro* inhibition of pituitary prolactin synthesis and release by hypothalamic extract, *Am. J. Physiol.* **205:**213–218.

TASHJIAN, A. H., BAROWSKY, N. J., and JENSEN, D. K., 1971, Thyrotropin releasing hormone: Direct evidence for stimulation of prolactin by pituitary cells in culture, *Biochem. Biophys. Res. Commun.* **43:**516–523.

UNGER, R. H., 1972, Pancreatic alpha-cell function in diabetes mellitus, in: *Glucagon* (P. J. Lefebvre and R. H. Unger, eds.), pp. 245–258, Pergamon Press, New York.

VALE, W., and GUILLEMIN, R., 1967, Potassium induced stimulation of thyrotropin release *in vitro*: Requirement for presence of calcium and inhibition by thyroxine, *Experientia* **23:**855–857.

VALE, W., AMOSS, M., BURGUS, R., and GUILLEMIN, R., 1967*a*, On the mode of action of hypothalamic releasing factors in their stimulating release of pituitary hormones, *Int. Symp. Pharmacol. Horm. Polypep. (Milan)*, Sept. 14–16, p. 58 (abst.).

VALE, W., BURGUS, R., and GUILLEMIN, R., 1967*b*, Presence of calcium ions as a requisite for the *in vitro* stimulation of TSH release by hypothalamic TRF, *Experientia* **23:**853–855.

VALE, W., BURGUS, R., and GUILLEMIN, R., 1967*c*, Competition between thyroxine and TRF at the pituitary level in the release of TSH, *Proc. Soc. Exp. Biol. Med.* **125:**210–213.

VALE, W., BURGUS, R., and GUILLEMIN, R., 1968, On the mechanism of action of TRF: Effects of cycloheximide and actinomycin on the release of TSH stimulated *in vitro* by TRF and its inhibition by thyroxine, *Neuroendocrinology* **3:**34–46.

VALE, W., RIVIER, J., and BURGUS, R., 1971*a*, Synthetic TRF (thyrotropin releasing factor) analogues. II. pGlu-N^{3im}Me-His-Pro-NH_2: A synthetic analogue with specific activity greater than that of TRF, *Endocrinology* **89:**1485–1488.

VALE, W., BURGUS, R., DUNN, T. F., and GUILLEMIN, R., 1971*b*, *In vitro* plasma inactivation of thyrotropin releasing factor (TRF) and related peptides: Its inhibition by various means and by the synthetic dipeptide PCA-His-OMe, *Hormones* **2:**193–203.

VALE, W., RIVIER, C., and GUILLEMIN, R., 1971*c*, A "prostaglandin receptor" in the mechanisms involved in the secretion of anterior pituitary hormones, *Fed. Proc.* **30:**363.

VALE, W., BRAZEAU, P., GRANT, G., NUSSEY, A., BURGUS, R., RIVIER, J., LING, N., and GUILLEMIN, R., 1972*a*, Premières observations sue le mode d'action de la somatostatine un facteur hypothalamique qui inhibe la sécrétion de l'hormone de croissance, *C. R. Acad. Sci. Paris* **275:**2913.

VALE, W., GRANT, G., AMOSS, M., BLACKWELL, R., and GUILLEMIN, R., 1972*b*, Culture of enzymatically dispersed anterior pituitary cells: Functional validation of a method, *Endocrinology* **91:**562–572.

VALE, W., GRANT, G., RIVIER, J., MONAHAN, M., AMOSS, M., BLACKWELL, R., BURGUS, R., and GUILLEMIN, R., 1972*c*, Synthetic polypeptide antagonists of the hypothalamic luteinizing hormone releasing factor, *Science* **176:**933–934.

VALE, W., BRAZEAU, P., RIVIER, C., RIVIER, J., GRANT, G., BURGUS, R., and GUILLEMIN, R., 1973*a*, Inhibitory hypophysiotropic activities of hypothalamic somatostatin, *Fed. Proc.* **32:**211.

VALE, W., BRAZEAU, P., RIVIER, C., RIVIER, J., GRANT, G., BURGUS, R., and GUILLEMIN, R., 1973*b*, Biological activities of somatostatin, *Proc. 55th Meet. Endocrine Society (Chicago)*, p. 118 (abst.).

VALE, W., BRAZEAU, P., RIVIER, C., RIVIER, J., and GUILLEMIN, R., 1973*c*, Biological studies with somatostatin, *Proc. Natl. Pit. Agency hGH Synp. (Baltimore)*, Oct. 9–12.

VALE, W., BLACKWELL, R., GRANT, G., and GUILLEMIN, R., 1973*d*, TRF and thyroid hormones on prolactin secretion by rat anterior pituitary cells *in vitro*, *Endocrinology* **93:**26–33.

VALE, W., GRANT, G., and GUILLEMIN, R., 1973*e*, Chemistry of the hypothalamic releasing factors—Studies on structure–function relationships, in: *Frontiers in Neuroendocrinology* (W. F. Ganong and L. Martini, eds.), pp. 375–414, Oxford University Press, New York.

VALE, W., RIVIER, C., PALKOVITIS, M., SAAVEDRNA, J. M., and BROWNSTEIN, M., 1974*a*, Ubiquitous brain distribution of inhibitors of adenohypophysial secretion, *Proc. Endocrine Soc. (Atlanta)*, p. 128 (abst. 146).

VALE, W., RIVIER, C., BRAZEAU, P., and GUILLEMIN, R., 1974*b*, Effects of somatostatin on the secretion of thyrotropin and prolactin, *Endocrinology* **95:**968–977.

VALVERDE-R, C., CHIEFFO, V., and REICHLIN, S., 1972, Prolactin-releasing factor in porcine and rat hypothalamic tissue, *Endocrinology* **91:**982–993.

VAN DER VIS-MELSON, M. J. E., and WIENER, J. D., 1972, Improvement in neural depression with decreased thyrotropin response after administration of thyrotropin releasing hormone, *Lancet* **2:**1415.

VAN LOON, G. R. 1973, Brain catecholamines and ACTH secretion, in: *Frontiers in Neuroendocrinology* (W. F. Ganong and L. Martini, eds.), pp. 209–248, Oxford University Press, New York.

VERBER, D. F., BENNETT, C. D., MICKOWSKI, J. D., GAL, G., DENKEWATLER, R. G., and HIRSCHMANN, R., 1971, Synthesis of a proposed growth hormone releasing factor, *Biochem. Biophys. Res. Commun.* **45:**235–239.

WAKABAYASHI, K., KAMBERI, I. A., and MCCANN, S. M., 1969, *In vitro* response of the rat pituitary to gonadotropin-releasing factors and to ions, *Endocrinology* **85:**1046–1056.

WATANBE, S., DHARIWAL, A. P. S., and MCCANN, S. M., 1968, Effect of inhibitors of protein synthesis on the FSH-releasing action of hypothalamic extracts *in vitro*, *Endocrinology* **82:**674–684.

WILBER, J., and FLOURET, G., 1971, Thyrotropin releasing hormone (TRH) analogues: Stimulation of thyrotropin (TSH) secretion *in vitro*, *Proc. 53rd Meet. Endocrine Soc. (San Francisco)*, p. 90 (abst.).

WILBER, J. F., and UTIGER, R. D., 1968, *In vitro* studies on the mechanisms of action of TRF, *Proc. Soc. Exp. Biol. Med.* **127:**488–490.

WILBER, J. F., PEAKE, G. T., PARKER, M. I., UTIGER, R. D., and DAUGHADAY, W. H., 1968, Theophylline and epinephrine effects upon the secretion of GH and TSH *in vitro, Clin. Res.* **16:**277 (abst.).

WILBER, J. F., PEAKE, G. T., and UTIGER, R. D., 1969, Thyrotropin release *in vitro*: Stimulation of 3′,5′-adenosine monophosphate, *Endocrinology* **84:**758–760.

WILBER, J., NAGEL, T., and WHITE, W. F., 1971, Hypothalamic growth hormone–releasing activity (GRA): Characterization by the *in vitro* rat pituitary and radioimmunoassay, *Endocrinology* **89:**1419–1424.

WINOKUR, A., and UTIGER, R. D., 1974, Regional distribution of thyrotropin releasing hormone in rat brain, *Science* **185:**265–267.

YEN, S. S. C., SILER, T., DEVANE, G., RIVIER, J., VALE, W., BRAZEAU, P., and GUILLEMIN, R., 1973, Biological effects of somatostatin in normal and acromegalic subjects, *Natl. Pit. Agency hGH Symp. (Baltimore).*

ZHAND, G. R., NADEAN, A., and VON MUHLENDAHL, K. E., 1972, Growth hormone, insulin release and acromegaly, *Israeli J. Med. Sci.* **8:**874.

ZOR, T. F., SCHNEIDER, H., MCCANN, S. M., LOWER, I., BLOOM, G., BORLAND, B., and FIELD, J. B., 1969, Stimulation of anterior pituitary adenyl cyclase activity and adenosine 3′,5′-cyclic phosphate by hypothalamic extract and prostaglandin E_1, *Proc. Natl. Acad. Sci.* **63:**918–925.

5

BINDING, METABOLISM, AND ACTION OF STEROID HORMONES IN THE CENTRAL NERVOUS SYSTEM

Richard E. Zigmond

> We may now believe that in the interstitial tissues of the gonads special chemical substances are produced which, taken up in the blood stream, permit the charge of definite parts of the central nervous system with sexual tension.
>
> —SIGMUND FREUD, *Three Contributions to the Theory of Sex*, 1905.

1. INTRODUCTION

Evidence that steroid hormones can act directly on the central nervous system comes largely from implantation studies. The work of Harris *et al.* (1958), Lisk (1967), Davidson (1969), and others established that many of the effects on behavior and on gonadotropin secretion produced by peripheral injections of estrogens and androgens could also be produced by

Richard E. Zigmond ● M.R.C. Neurochemical Pharmacology Unit, Medical School, Cambridge, England. Alfred P. Sloan Foundation Research Fellow

direct implantation of these compounds in certain areas of the brain. Effective sites were clustered in the preoptic area and hypothalamus. Implants in many other regions of the brain had no detectable effects (for review, see McEwen *et al.*, 1972*b*).

In an experiment designed to measure the extent of diffusion from such implants, Michael (1962) placed [^{14}C]diethylstilbestrol di-*n*-butyrate, a synthetic estrogen (Fig. 1), into the hypothalamus of a female cat and measured the spread of the compound autoradiographically. While examining the autoradiographs, he found that certain cell bodies in the vicinity of the implant seemed to concentrate the labeled estrogen. Subsequent experiments with peripheral injections of [^{3}H]hexesterol (another synthetic estrogen) (Fig. 1) suggested that this ability to concentrate estrogens was limited to cells in certain parts of the brain (Glascock and Michael, 1962; Michael, 1964, 1965*a,b*). Heavily labeled cells were found only in the lateral septum and the medial hypothalamus. To ascertain whether significant metabolism of the tritiated compound had occurred, the labeled material was extracted from the brain and chromatographed. The material was found to be "hexesterol or a simple conjugate" (Glascock and Michael, 1962). The concentration of hexesterol in different regions was examined by scintillation counting. At various times from 2 to 24 h after a subcutaneous injection, the preoptic area and hypothalamus retained more [^{3}H]hexesterol than did the cerebral cortex or the blood. As a result of these experiments,

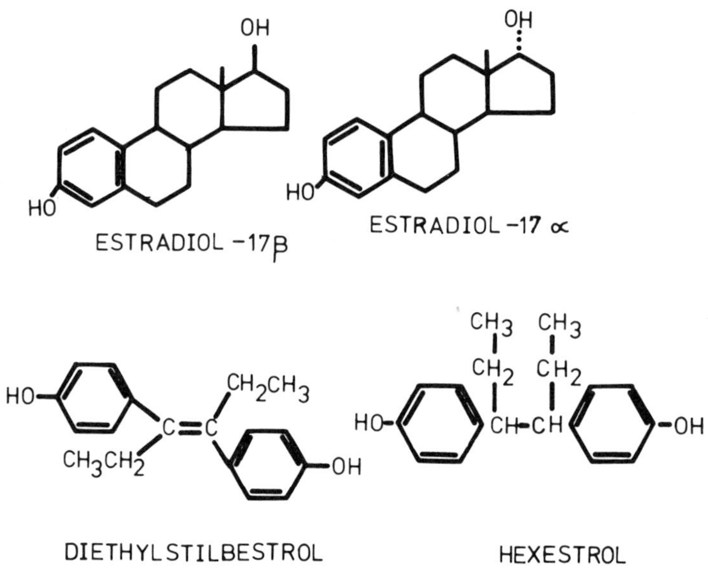

FIG. 1. Chemical structure of estradiol-17β, its stereoisomer, estradiol-17α, and two synthetic nonsteroidal estrogens, diethylstilbestrol and hexestrol.

Michael (1962) proposed that certain cells in particular parts of the central nervous system have a selective affinity for estrogens.

During the past 12 years, a great deal of biochemical and histochemical work has been devoted to studying the interaction of steroid hormones with the nervous system. The purpose of this chapter is to review our knowledge of the binding and metabolism of estrogens, androgens, glucocorticoids, and progestins in the central nervous system and to relate these data to the behavioral and physiological effects of the hormones.

2. ESTROGENS

2.1. Determination of the Estradiol Concentration in Dissected Brain Regions

2.1.1. Methodological Considerations

The low endogenous level of estradiol in the brain and the absence of a histochemical technique for its detection have prevented the direct study of the distribution of this hormone in the undisturbed animal. Our knowledge of the distribution of estrogens in the brain (and in other tissues) depends almost entirely on the administration of radioactive estrogens and the localization of these molecules in different parts of the brain by scintillation counting of dissected regions or by autoradiography. In most experiments, about 0·1–0·2 μg [^{3}H]estradiol is injected intraperitoneally or intravenously per 100 g body weight in an attempt to achieve a "physiological" level of estradiol in the plasma. However, it is virtually impossible to mimic normal plasma levels of a hormone by a single injection, particularly in a saline–ethanol vehicle as is usually used. After such an injection, plasma hormone levels reach their peak fairly rapidly and then decline exponentially. Thus if the plasma levels are approximately physiological shortly after the injection they will be below the physiological range 1 or 2 h later, when most measurements of the distribution of the hormone are made (Pfaff and Keiner, 1973). An alternative approach adopted by Lemaire *et al.* (1974) in their study of [^{3}H]corticosterone is to continuously infuse the compound intravenously at a rate which maintains a normal circulatory level of the hormone.

One limitation in the study of the distribution of any substance in dissected brain regions is the anatomical resolution which is achieved. In most studies, it is impossible to be sure exactly which cell groups are included in a particular dissection. For instance, when one author refers to a median eminence sample does this include the cell bodies of the arcuate and perhaps the ventral part of the ventromedial nucleus or does it only include the axons, nerve terminals, and nonneuronal cells of the median eminence?

Similarly, does an anterior hypothalamus sample also contain cells of the preoptic area? These anatomical problems are shared to some extent by all the studies described in this section and point to the importance of using both biochemical and histological (e.g., autoradiographic) techniques. Due to these considerations, the anatomical designations used here refer to regions of the brain (e.g., preoptic region) rather than to specific nuclei (e.g., medial preoptic nucleus).

2.1.2. Regional Distribution of [^{3}H]Estradiol in the Ovariectomized Rat

In most studies on the localization of estrogens in the brain since those of Michael (1964) on diethylstilbestrol in cats, [^{3}H]estradiol has been injected into ovariectomized rats. After peripheral administration of the labeled hormone, a higher retention of tritium was found in the hypothalamus, preoptic area, amygdala, septum, and midbrain than in the cerebral cortex (Attramadal, 1964; Eisenfeld and Axelrod, 1965; Kato and Villee, 1967*a*). Kato and Villee (1967*a*) showed that, within the hypothalamus, the median eminence and the anterior hypothalamus retained more radioactivity than other regions. Greater than 85% of the tritium extracted from the hypothalamus and preoptic area co-chromatographed with authentic estradiol (Eisenfeld and Axelrod, 1965; Kato and Villee, 1967*a*). A more definite identification of this material as unmetabolized [^{3}H]estradiol was achieved by recrystallization to constant specific activity (Kato and Villee, 1967*a*). A small amount of [^{3}H]estrone was also found. Slightly more of this metabolite was found in regions of low estrogen retention (e.g., posterior hypothalamus and cerebral cortex) than in regions of high retention (e.g., anterior hypothalamus and median eminence) (Kato and Villee, 1967*a*; Luttge and Whalen, 1970*a*; Wade and Feder, 1972*b*).

In an attempt to correlate the sites of [^{3}H]estradiol binding more precisely with estrogen-sensitive sites found in implantation studies, McGuire and Lisk (1969) determined the content of radioactivity in frontal sections of the brain. They found higher retention of radioactivity in sections through the preoptic and arcuate nuclei than in those through the mammillary bodies or through other areas of the brain. However, since they used complete frontal sections the site of retention within the section remains unclear. Dissection of individual cell groups in the hypothalamus has been attempted in a study of steroid hormone localization only in the case of glucocorticoids (Eik-Nes and Brizee, 1965).

Differences in the retention of estradiol by different regions of the brain could result from a number of factors. Three possibilities are (1) unequal blood flow; (2) a difference in the chemical composition of different regions such as their lipid content, resulting in differences in their ability to retain steroids and other lipophilic molecules; or (3) a difference in the content of specific binding sites for estradiol. Eisenfeld (1967) observed that the initial uptake of labeled hormone after an injection of [^{3}H]estradiol was similar in the hypothalamus and cortex and that regional differences appeared only at longer time intervals, suggesting that differences in blood flow were not important.

Competition studies with unlabeled steroids made the second explanation unlikely. If the differences in hormone retention between areas were due to a difference in their "partition coefficient" for the steroid, one would expect to see competition effects first in areas of low hormone uptake (e.g., cerebral cortex) rather than in areas of high hormone uptake (e.g., hypothalamus). However, concurrent injections of unlabeled estradiol, estrone or estriol decreased the amount of [^{3}H]estradiol retained in the hypothalamus but not in the cerebral cortex (Eisenfeld and Axelrod, 1965, 1966). In a study of nine brain areas, McEwen and Pfaff (1970) found that areas which retained the most [^{3}H]estradiol showed the largest decrement in retention when animals were pretreated with unlabeled hormone (Fig. 2). The largest and most consistent effects of pretreatment were seen in the hypothalamus, preoptic area, septum, and amygdala.

Eisenfeld (1967) found that his kinetic data fitted a model in which estradiol could be present in an area in one of two compartments—a "free" pool in rapid equilibrium with plasma and a "bound" pool. The free pool was assumed to be the same size in both the hypothalamus and cerebral cortex, while a measurable number of bound molecules seemed to be present only in the hypothalamus.

The idea that saturable binding sites for estradiol are concentrated in certain regions of the brain is supported by the "dose–response" curves of Kato and Villee (1967*b*). By injecting different amounts of estradiol into rats, these authors showed that the retention of estradiol by the anterior hypothalamus was almost completely saturated at a dose of about 3 μg/100 g, while in the cerebral cortex the retention was proportional to the dose injected. The middle hypothalamus and the posterior hypothalamus showed partial saturation. These results and those of other workers (Wade and Feder, 1972*a,b*; Lemaire *et al.*, 1974) (see Fig. 22) indicate that the amount of "nonsaturable" binding may also differ between brain areas, thus suggesting a necessary modification of the model proposed by Eisenfeld (1967).

How specific are the binding sites for estradiol? As has already been mentioned, estrone and estriol inhibit estradiol retention in the hypothalamus when injected concurrently. However, unlabeled testosterone, progesterone, and hydrocortisone have no effect even when injected in milligram doses (Eisenfeld and Axelrod, 1966). Other compounds which can inhibit estradiol retention include norethynodrel, a 17α-ethynyl norprogestin present in certain oral contraceptives; diethylstilbestrol, a potent synthetic estrogen; and U-11,100A, Mer-25, and CI-628, all three synthetic compounds with antiestrogenic properties (Eisenfeld, 1972; Rotsztejn,

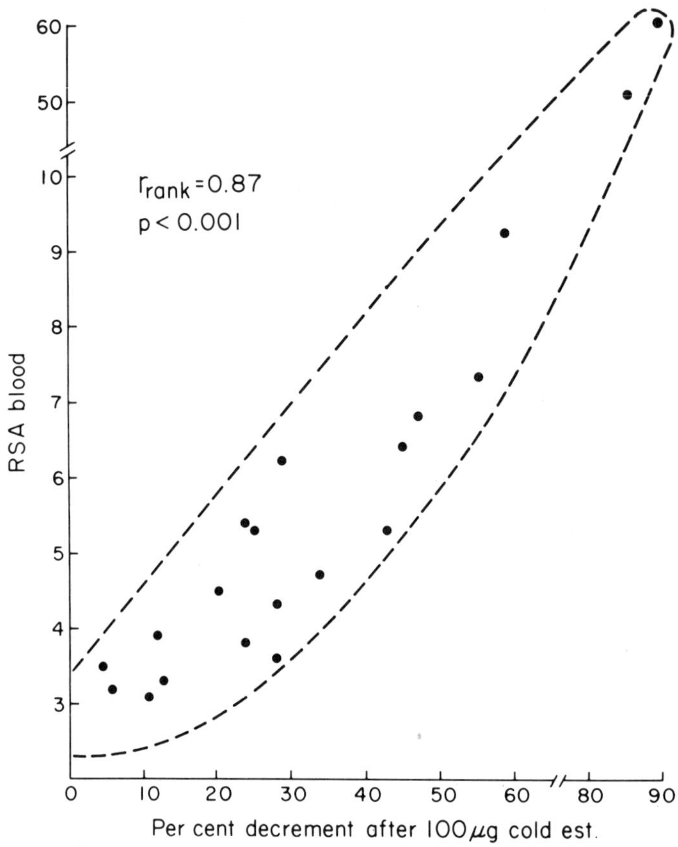

FIG. 2. Correlation between the amount of estradiol retained in different brain regions and the saturability of this retention. Male and female rats were injected with [^{3}H]estradiol with or without a prior injection of unlabeled hormone and the amount of radioactivity retained in various parts of the brain and in the pituitary gland was determined. The extent of uptake in animals given no pretreatment is expressed as the concentration of radioactivity in a brain region relative to the concentration in the blood (RSA blood). Each point represents the mean of several determinations for a given tissue sample. Points toward the upper right include the pituitary gland, preoptic area, and hypothalamus, while points toward the lower left include the cortex and cerebellum. From Pfaff (1971), reprinted with permission of the Regents of the University of California.

1973) (Table 1). However, the most dramatic evidence of stereoselectivity was the finding that pretreatment with estradiol-17β but not estradiol-17α decreased the retention of [^{3}H]estradiol-17β (Kato and Villee, 1967*b*). Since most of the compounds which inhibit estradiol retention had no effect on the plasma concentration of [^{3}H]estradiol or on its retention by the cerebral

TABLE 1
Effect of Various Compounds on the Retention of [^{3}H]Estradiol in the Hypothalamus[a]

Effective inhibitors	Compounds with no effect
Estriol (25 μg)[b]	Testosterone (1 mg)
Estrone (25 μg)	Progesterone (1 mg)
Diethylstilbestrol (25 μg)	Hydrocortisone (1 mg)
Dimethylstilbestrol (100 μg)	Chlormadinone (1 mg)
Norethynodrel (200 μg)	Medroxyprogesterone (1 mg)
Norethindrone (800 μg)	
U-11,100A (1 mg)	
Clomiphene (5 mg)	

[a]Data from review by Eisenfeld (1972). Animals were intravenously injected with these compounds 30 seconds before administration of 0.1 μg/100 g[^{3}H]estradiol. One hour later, the hypothalamus was removed and the total number of counts/min extractable in toluene–isoamyl alcohol was determined. For experimental details, see original articles (Eisenfeld and Axelrod, 1965, 1966, 1967).
[b]All drug doses are given per 100 g body weight.

cortex, they probably competed directly with estradiol at the level of the hypothalamus.

Although concurrent injections of testosterone do not decrease estradiol retention, pretreatment with testosterone is effective. McEwen and Pfaff (1970) found that a prior injection of testosterone decreased estradiol retention in the preoptic area and hypothalamus, although at low doses (10 μg) testosterone was less effective than estradiol. Perhaps prior injection of testosterone leads to a formation of a metabolite (e.g., estradiol? see Section 3.3.) which competes for estradiol binding.

Once bound, [^{3}H]estradiol is not displaced by subsequent injections of unlabeled estradiol or norethynodrel (Eisenfeld and Axelrod, 1965; Kato and Villee, 1967*b*). Although Saucier *et al.* (1970) reported a decrease in hypothalamic estradiol retention when norethynodrel is given after [^{3}H]estradiol, plasma [^{3}H]estradiol was also reduced, leaving the tissue-to-plasma ratio unchanged.

2.2. Determination of the Cellular Localization of [^{3}H]Estradiol by Autoradiography

While experiments using scintillation counting techniques demonstrated that regions of the brain differed in their ability to retain [^{3}H]estradiol, autoradiographic studies have provided a detailed cellular description of the distribution of the labeled hormone. As already indicated, early autoradiographic experiments established two important facts: first, that following injections of labeled estrogens ([^{3}H]hexestrol or [^{3}H]diethylstilbestrol) grains could be found concentrated over cell bodies in the brain, and, second, that these labeled cell bodies were found only in certain parts of the nervous system (Attramadal, 1964; Michael, 1964, 1965*a,b*). Recent studies have provided detailed descriptions of the distribution of such "estradiol-concentrating cells" throughout the brain. The results agree well with the biochemical experiments reported in the previous section in that the highest retention is found in the preoptic area, hypothalamus, amygdala, and septum. However, in addition, these autoradiographic studies have established that only specific cell groups within these regions are heavily labeled.

2.2.1. Methodological Considerations

a. Preparation of the Autoradiographs. Discussions of the methodological problems involved in the autoradiographic localization of steroids have dealt primarily with the probability of translocating the radioactive compound during the preparation of tissue sections (for extensive discussion of this subject, see Stumpf and Roth, 1966; Roth and Stumpf, 1969; Stumpf, 1970*b*; Rogers, 1973). It has been found that the conventional techniques of fixing, dehydrating, embedding, and dipping sections often result in the extraction of diffusible substances, such as steroids, from the tissue and may result in translocation within the tissue (Stumpf and Roth, 1966). Thus such techniques can be used safely only if conditions are chosen which eliminate or minimize these problems (Rogers, 1973). Most recent work has employed methods in which unfixed, unembedded, frozen sections are cut. The most commonly used techniques are the freeze-dry and the thaw-mount methods. Both seem to give good resolution of the cellular distribution of tritiated steroids, with some evidence indicating that the freeze-dry method preserves the true subcellular distribution better (Stumpf and Roth, 1966; Stumpf, 1970*b*). In the freeze-dry method developed by Stumpf and Roth (1965, 1966, 1967), frozen sections are dried under vacuum at low temperatures (below −60 °C). In the thaw-mount method, the frozen sections are air-dried on slides at room temperature (Stumpf and Roth, 1966). Appleton (1964) introduced a variant of the latter method in which frozen sections were placed on cold slides (−5 to −10 °C) to avoid thawing. In all these methods, as a precaution against translocation due to contact between the section and the liquid emulsion, slides are precoated with emulsion and allowed to dry before the tissue sections are placed on them. The results on the localization of cells which concentrate estradiol in the rat and mouse brain determined using these three techniques are quite comparable and as pointed out below the discrepancies which exist are probably not due to translocation artifacts.

b. Analysis of the Autoradiographs—Criteria for an "Estrogen-Concentrating Cell." In most studies, after the autoradiographs are developed the sections are stained with a "cell-body stain" (e.g., cresyl violet) and the distribution of silver grains is examined under the light microscope.* The data are usually presented in the form of neuroanatomical drawings showing the positions of "estradiol-concentrating cells." Before discussing these results, however, it is important to consider the evidence that these cells actually concentrate estradiol. In other words, what criteria are used to decide whether or not a cell is labeled? What is the evidence that the labeled material is [^{3}H]estradiol? And should these cells be considered "estradiol-concentrating cells" or, more generally "steroid-concentrating cells"?

In many published reports showing the anatomical distribution of labeled cells, the criterion used by the experimenter is not given. The problem of criteria is particularly important in areas of the brain where few, scattered, weakly labeled cells are found, such as, for instance, in the cerebral cortex (Stumpf, 1970*a*; Pfaff and Keiner, 1973). Do these cells bind estradiol or do they represent the chance accumulation of unbound hormone which one expects over a certain number of cells? Introducing a fixed criterion (e.g., a labeled cell must have at least 5 times the number of grains over it as is found over a comparable area of neuropil; see Pfaff and Keiner, 1973; Zigmond *et al.*, 1973) may help to reduce experimenter bias, but the problem of false positives and also false negatives is still present, as discussed by England *et al.* (1973). However, the solution proposed by these authors to solve this problem is based on the assumption that the grain densities over labeled cells fit a Poisson distribution (England *et al.*, 1973), and existing evidence suggests that this assumption does not hold for steroid-concentrating cells in the brain (e.g., see Fig. 13 and Stumpf and Sar, 1973). The number of estradiol binding sites or the affinity of these sites for the hormone may vary in different cells and this heterogeneity complicates the analysis. At present, then, the analysis of autoradiographs prepared from animals injected with [^{3}H]estradiol depends on the reliable appearance of cells in particular anatomical locations showing a concentration of radioactivity above that in the surrounding neuropil. The significance of occasional labeled cells such as those found in parts of the cerebral cortex remains questionable.

Since biochemical studies indicate that greater than 85% of the tritium in the brain after an injection of [^{3}H]estradiol is still in the form of the unmetabolized hormone, it can be assumed that most of the reduced silver grains represent labeled estradiol. However, since a small amount of [^{3}H]estrone is also present, the possibility exists that a small number of cells might concentrate estrone or some other metabolite of estradiol. The possibility that different cells may concentrate different metabolites of a hormone seems quite likely in the case of androgens (see Section 3.9).

* It should be noted that this method essentially precludes the discovery of axons, dendrites, or nerve endings, which are heavily labeled. Detection of such structures probably must await the development of an electron microscopic method for doing autoradiography with labeled steroids.

Having shown that cells in a certain area of the brain retain estradiol, it remains to be determined whether this retention process is specific for estrogenic hormones. One method for investigating this problem is to see which steroids inhibit estradiol retention (see Section 2.1). Another is to compare the distribution of [^{3}H]estradiol with that of other labeled steroids. Anderson and Greenwald (1969) found that the number of labeled cells in the preoptic area and basal hypothalamus after an injection of [^{3}H]estradiol was greatly reduced by pretreatment with 2 μg of unlabeled estradiol but was not affected by 2.5 mg of cortisone acetate. Progesterone (2.5 mg) had an intermediate effect (Table 2). Comparison of the distribution of tritiated estradiol, testosterone, progesterone, and corticosterone reveals important differences in the retention of these four steroids. However some cells seem able to concentrate more than one hormone. For example, the high percentage of cells in the medial preoptic area which are labeled after an injection of [^{3}H]estradiol and [^{3}H]testosterone (more than 50%) suggests that some of the cells in this area can concentrate both hormones (Sar and Stumpf, 1973*a*). Nevertheless, these cells may still have separate binding sites for the two hormones.

Finally, it is important to know to what extent the distribution of estradiol-concentrating cells varies depending on conditions of the experiment such as hormone dose, interval between injection and sacrifice, or length of exposure of the autoradiographs. Although little information is available on these points, it should be noted that labeled cells were not detected in the hippocampus in early experiments but were later found when the dose of hormone administered was increased or the exposure period lengthened (Stumpf, 1970*a*). Furthermore, the number of labeled cells found in the preoptic area and basal hypothalamus depended on the length of the interval between hormone injection and sacrifice (Anderson and Greenwald, 1969) (Table 3).

TABLE 2

Effect of Pretreatment with Unlabeled Steroids on the Retention of [^{3}H]Estradiol[a]

Hormone treatment	Number of labeled cells (expressed as % vehicle control)	
	Preoptic area	Ventromedial and arcuate nuclei
None	100	100
2.0 μg estradiol-17β	17	4
2.5 mg progesterone	51	36
2.5 mg cortisone acetate	102	104

[a]One hour before injection of [^{3}H]estradiol (about 2 μg), ovariectomized rats were pretreated with unlabeled estradiol (2 μg), progesterone (2.5 mg), cortisone acetate (2.5 mg), or vehicle alone. Two hours after injection of the labeled hormone, the animals were killed and autoradiograms were prepared by the thaw-mount method. Data from Anderson and Greenwald (1969).

TABLE 3

Effect of Time of Sacrifice on the Number of Labeled Cells Found in the Brain[a]

Interval between injection and sacrifice (h)	Number of labeled cells ± SEM	
	Preoptic area	Ventromedial and arcuate nuclei
2	342 ± 17 (100%)	461 ± 47 (100%)
4	238 ± 43 (70%)	264 ± 31 (57%)
6	147 ± 24 (43%)	125 ± 30 (27%)
8	5 ± 2 (1%)	8 ± 2 (2%)

[a]Ovariectomized rats were injected subcutaneously with about 2 μg of [^{3}H]estradiol. Two, four, six, and eight hours later, the animals were killed and autoradiograms were prepared by the thaw-mount method. The number of labeled cells is expressed in parentheses as a percentage of the "2-h" group. Data are from Anderson and Greenwald (1969).

2.2.2. *Distribution of Labeled Cells After [^{3}H]Estradiol Administration*

The autoradiographic results presented here are a compilation of the work of Stumpf (1968*a*, 1970*a*, 1971, 1972), Anderson and Greenwald (1969), and Pfaff and Keiner (1972, 1973) on the rat and that of Warembourg (1970*a,b*, 1971) on the mouse. An attempt has been made to list the nuclei which contain labeled cells under anatomical headings which roughly correspond to the dissected regions used in biochemical studies (Section 2.1).

a. Preoptic Area. Many labeled cells are found in the medial preoptic area, in the suprachiasmatic portion of the preoptic area, and in the ventral

TABLE 4

Distribution of Estradiol-Concentrating Cells in the Ovariectomized Female Mouse[a]

Brain region	Percentage of labeled cells	Average number of grains per labeled cell[b]
Bed nucleus of the stria terminalis	95	120
Medial preoptic area		
Anterior part	52	100
Middle part	32	100
Amygdaloid complex	44	50
Arcuate nucleus	30	90
Nucleus triangularis septi	22	35
Subfornical organ	18	38

[a]Ovariectomized female mice were injected with 0.2–0.7 μg [^{3}H]estradiol subcutaneously. One and one-half to two hours later, the animals were killed and the brain was processed for autoradiography by the Appleton (1964) technique. The data are from Warembourg (1970*b*).
[b]The background level of radioactivity was 6 grains over a comparable area.

part of the bed nucleus of the stria terminalis (below the anterior commissure, Table 4, Fig. 3A). Rostral to the preoptic area, labeled cells are also found in the islands of Calleja and in the diagonal band of Broca.

b. Anterior Hypothalamus. The anterior hypothalamic area represents the region of greatest disagreement among different laboratories. Tuohimaa (1971) and Pfaff and Keiner (1973) have found many labeled cells in the medial portion of this area (see Fig. 2H in Pfaff and Keiner, 1973), while Stumpf (1968*a*, 1970*a*) and Warembourg (1970) did not. Stumpf (1968*a*, 1970*a*), Anderson and Greenwald (1969) and Pfaff and Keiner (1973) all found labeled cells in the periventricular nucleus at the level of the anterior hypothalamus.

c. Middle Hypothalamus. Heavily labeled cells are found in the periventricular nucleus, the arcuate nucleus, and the ventrolateral portion of the ventromedial nucleus (Fig. 3B).

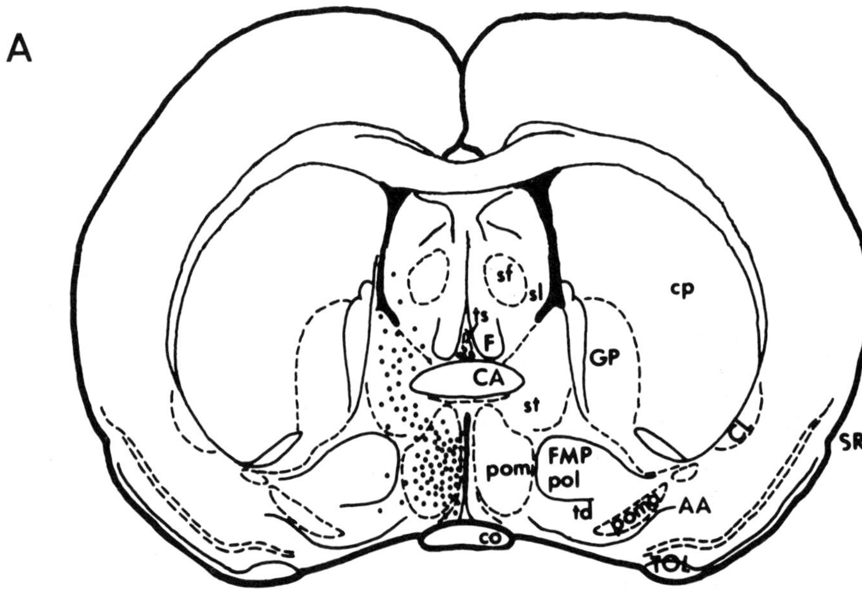

FIG. 3A,B. Distribution of labeled cells in two frontal sections of the rat brain 1 h after an injection of [^{3}H]estradiol. Abbreviations: AA, anterior amygdaloid area; abl, basal amygdaloid nucleus, lateral part; abm, basal amygdaloid nucleus, medial part; ac, central amygdaloid nucleus; aco, cortical amygdaloid nucleus; ala, lateral amygdaloid nucleus, anterior part; alp, lateral amygdaloid nucleus, posterior part; am, medial amygdaloid nucleus; CA, anterior commissure; CAI, internal capsule; CAIR, internal capsule, retrolenticular part; CI, claustrum; co, optic chiasm; cp, caudate putamen; F, fornix; FH, fimbria hippocampi; FMP, medial forebrain bundle; FMT, mammillothalamic tract; g, nucleus gelatinosus; GP, globus pallidus; hdd, dorsomedial hypothalamic nucleus, dorsal part; hdv, dorsomedial hypothalamic nucleus,

d. Posterior Hypothalamus. Heavily labeled cells are found in the arcuate nucleus and the ventral premammillary nucleus.

e. Septum. Labeled cells are found in the lateral septum, the nucleus triangularis septi, the subfornical organ, and the dorsal portion of the bed nucleus of the stria terminalis (Fig. 3A).

f. Amygdala. The most heavily labeled cells in the amygdala are in the medial and cortical nuclei (Fig. 3B). The central nucleus and the medial part of the basal nucleus also contain labeled cells. A few labeled cells are present in the entorhinal cortex.

g. Hippocampus. Some labeled cells are present in the hippocampus, particularly in the ventral area.

h. Midbrain. Labeled cells can be found in the central gray.

Several of the areas mentioned above were found not to contain labeled cells by Anderson and Greenwald (1969), namely, the nucleus triangularis

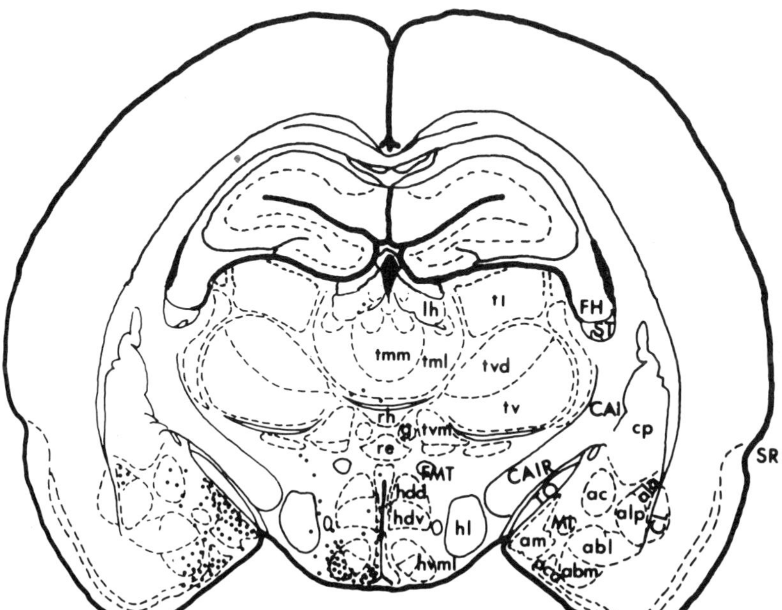

ventral part; hl, lateral hypothalamic nucleus; hvml, ventromedial hypothalamic nucleus, lateral part; lh, lateral habenular nucleus; MI, massa intercalata; pol, lateral preoptic nucleus; pom, medial preoptic nucleus; poma, magnocellular preoptic nucleus; re, nucleus reuniens; rh, rhomboid nucleus; sf, septofimbrial nucleus; sl, lateral septal nucleus; SR, rhinal sulcus; st, stria terminalis; td, nucleus of the diagonal tract of Broca; tl, lateral thalamic nucleus; tml, medial thalamic nucleus, lateral part; tmm, medial thalamic nucleus, medial part; TO, optic tract; TOL, lateral olfactory tract; ts, nucleus triangularis septi; tv, ventral thalamic nucleus; tvd, ventral thalamic nucleus, dorsal part; tvm, ventral thalamic nucleus, magnocellular part. Modified from Stumpf (1970*a*).

septi, the subfornical organ, the hippocampus, and all areas of the amygdala other than a portion of the medial amygdaloid nucleus. The reason for the discrepancy between their findings and those of Stumpf, Warembourg, and Pfaff and Keiner and also the reason for the different results found concerning the anterior hypothalamic area are unclear. However, these differences seem unlikely to be due to translocation artifacts since results using different techniques have proved quite comparable in most parts of the brain. For instance, all the studies show that only a portion of the ventromedial nucleus (i.e., the ventrolateral part) is heavily labeled. The differences seem more likely to be due to such factors as dose of hormone used and length of exposure period. As mentioned previously, for instance, the weakly labeled cells of the hippocampus are discernible only after long exposure periods (Stumpf, 1970*a*).

In addition to these cells in the brain, labeled cells have been found in the spinal cord, particularly in laminae I and II and in lamina X in the lumbar region (Pfaff, 1971; Keefer *et al.*, 1973).

2.3. Subcellular Distribution of Estradiol

2.3.1. Nuclear Binding

The data discussed thus far demonstrate that cells in particular parts of the brain retain estradiol by a mechanism which is highly stereoselective and is saturated by low doses of the hormone. Experiments using cell fractionation techniques have elucidated the subcellular distribution of the retained hormone.

Zigmond and McEwen (1970) injected ovariectomized rats with [^{3}H]estradiol; 2 h later they dissected out different brain areas, homogenized the tissue, and subjected the homogenates to a series of differential centrifugations. In a pooled brain sample containing areas of the brain thought to contain estradiol binding sites (i.e., septum, preoptic area, hypothalamus, olfactory bulbs, and amygdala; abbreviated SPHOA), the highest concentration of radioactivity was found in a purified nuclear pellet (Table 5). The concentration of radioactivity in this fraction was 12 times higher than the concentration in the whole homogenate. Most of the tritium (more than 85%) co-chromatographed with unlabeled estradiol in a thin-layer chromatographic system (Table 6). In the hippocampus the nuclear fraction also contained more radioactivity than the whole homogenate, but in the cerebral cortex there was no significant difference between the two (Tables 5 and 7). About 75% of the radioactivityextraced from nuclei prepared from the hippocampus and cerebral cortex had the same chromatographic mobility as estradiol (Table 6). The higher percentage of metabolites in this sample than in the SPHOA together with the results of

TABLE 5

Concentration of Tritium in Subcellular Fractions of Brain Tissue After an Intraperitoneal Injection of [^{3}H]Estradiol[a]

	SPHOA		Hippocampus		Cortex	
	Concentration[b]	Concentration ratio[c]	Concentration	Concentration ratio	Concentration	Concentration ratio
Whole homogenate	138	1.0	78	1.0	88	1.0
1. High-speed supernatant	243	1.8	332	4.3	460	5.2
2. High-speed pellet	70	0.5	46	0.7	71	0.8
3. Nuclear supernatant	154	1.1	69	0.9	98	1.1
4. Nuclear pellet	1745	12.6	309	4.0	135	1.5

[a]Two hours after an intraperitoneal injection of 0.1 mCi (about 0.6 μg) of [^{3}H]estradiol, animals were sacrificed and three brain samples were taken: SPHOA (a pooled sample including septum, preoptic area, hypothalamus, olfactory bulbs, and amygdala), hippocampus, and cerebral cortex. Subcellular fractions were prepared by differential centrifugation (for further details, see Zigmond and McEwen, 1970).

[b]Radioactive steroid concentration is expressed as counts/min/mg of protein.

[c]Ratio of concentration of radioactivity in a particular fraction to that in the whole homogenate.

TABLE 6

Thin-Layer Chromatography of Labeled Material Extractable into Dichloromethane[a]

		Brain (percentage of total extract)	
		SPHOA	Hippocampus and cortex
Whole homogenate	Estradiol	81	82
	Estrone	14	12
	Estriol	1	0
	Others	4	7
Nuclear pellet	Estradiol	87	76
	Estrone	5	8
	Estriol	2	5
	Others	7	13
		Blood (percentage of total extract)	
	Estradiol	59	
	Estrone	12	
	Estriol	5	
	Others	23	

[a]Two animals were injected 2 h before sacrifice with 0.1 mCi (0.57 μg) of [^{3}H]estradiol and two brain samples were taken from each: a pooled sample designated SPHOA (containing the septum, preoptic area, hypothalamus, olfactory bulbs, and amygdala) and a sample consisting of hippocampus and cerebral cortex. Dichloromethane extracts of the whole homogenate and of a purified nuclear pellet were run on silica gel plates using benzene–ethanol (9:1, v/v) as a solvent. Authentic estradiol, estrone, and estriol were run as standards. The data, expressed as the percentage of the extracted tritium which ran with the same R_f value as each standard, are the average of two runs. Blood samples from both animals were pooled and processed together.

Kato and Villee (1967*a*), Luttge and Whalen (1970*a*), and Wade and Wade and Feder (1972*b*) suggests that there is a regional difference in the extent of estradiol metabolism and/or that estradiol metabolites produced peripherally or centrally are retained to a different extent in different parts of the brain.

The high-speed supernatant or "cytosol" fraction was the only other subcellular fraction which showed a higher concentration of radioactivity than the whole homogenate. The mechanism of the retention of estradiol in this fraction is discussed in detail in the next section. It should be noted here, however, that hormone found in this fraction could be either free or bound to a soluble molecule.

Pretreatment of animals with unlabeled estradiol (1 mg) 30 min before the injection of [^{3}H]estradiol (0.6 μg) abolished the nuclear retention of the radioactive hormone in all three brain samples (Table 7). The concentration of estradiol was also decreased in the whole homogenates, but to a lesser extent. These findings suggest that all the estradiol in the nuclear fraction may be bound in the sense used by Eisenfeld (1967), while much of the estradiol in the whole homogenate may be free (see Section 2.1). It is

TABLE 7

Retention of [^{3}H]Estradiol by Whole Homogenates and Nuclear Pellets and the Effect of Pretreatment with Unlabeled Estradiol[a]

Brain region	Pretreatment	*N*	Whole homogenate (WH) (counts/min/mg)	Nuclear pellet (NP) (counts/min/mg)	Concentration ratio (NP/WH)	Percent total counts/min in homogenate recovered in nuclear pellet
SPHOA	None	5	216 ± 115	1311 ± 249	7.5 ± 2.2	13.3 ± 3.4
	Estradiol	2	76 ± 10	3 ± 2	0.1 ± 0.0	0.1 ± 0.0
Hippocampus	None	6	177 ± 60	211 ± 59	1.9 ± 0.6	2.9 ± 0.5
	Estradiol	4	57 ± 5	4 ± 2	0.1 ± 0.0	0.3 ± 0.2
Cortex	None	6	181 ± 65	112 ± 17	0.8 ± 0.2	1.2 ± 0.3
	Estradiol	4	73 ± 16	5 ± 1	0.1 ± 0.0	0.1 ± 0.0

[a]Nuclear pellets were isolated from animals given an intraperitoneal injection of 0.1 mCi (about 0.6 μg) of [^{3}H]estradiol with and without a prior injection (at −30 min) of 1 mg of unlabeled estradiol. Concentrations are expressed as counts/min of tritium per milligram of protein. *N* equals the number of replicates for each condition. Data from Žigmond and McEwen (1970).

interesting that although cortical nuclei did not concentrate estradiol they did show saturable retention of the hormone.

One methodological difficulty in cell fractionation experiments is the possibility of redistribution of compounds during homogenization and centrifugation. In order to see whether [^{3}H]estradiol was adsorbing to cell nuclei during the fractionation procedure, labeled hormone was added to homogenates prepared from uninjected animals. The percentage of radioactivity recovered in the nuclear pellets of the three brain samples (SPHOA, hippocampus, and cerebral cortex) was only 0.1%. The percentage of radioactivity recovered in each of these fractions after an intraperitoneal injection of [^{3}H]estradiol was significantly higher (1.2–13.3%).

Another critical feature of cell fractionation experiments is the purity of the fractions studied. The method used by Zigmond and McEwen (1970) to isolate brain cell nuclei was a modification of the procedure described by Løvtrup-Rein and McEwen (1966). Light and electron microscopic examination of a number of nuclear pellets prepared by this method indicated that they contained highly purified cell nuclei with little cytoplasmic debris (Zigmond and McEwen, 1970; McEwen and Zigmond, 1972). Furthermore, biochemical measurements of cytochrome oxidase, a mitochondrial marker enzyme, suggested that there was little mitochondrial contamination of the nuclear pellet (McEwen and Zigmond, 1972).

Measurements of DNA content indicated that the nuclear pellet contains 35% of the nuclei present in the initial homogenate (Zigmond and McEwen, 1970). Examination of the size distribution of cell nuclei in the nuclear pellet and in the whole homogenate showed that at least by this criterion the nuclear pellet isolated by this method is a representative sample of the cell nuclei present in the brain (Løvtrup-Rein and McEwen, 1966). It should be remembered that both neuronal and glial nuclei are present in the pellet.

A more precise regional study of the nuclear retention of estradiol revealed that nuclei from the preoptic–hypothalamic and amygdaloid regions showed the greatest retention of the hormone (Fig. 4). After correction for the nuclear yield, it was estimated that 44% and 31% of the labeled hormone in the whole homogenate was retained by cell nuclei in the two brain areas. Because it showed the highest percentage of nuclear retention, the preoptic–hypothalamic sample was used in further studies on the time course and chemical specificity of estradiol binding.

The disappearance of radioactivity from the whole homogenate of the preoptic–hypothalamic sample was only slightly slower than the disappearance from the blood. A similar result had been reported previously by Jensen (1966) and prompted him to suggest that the hypothalamus might not be a target organ for steroid hormones. However, examination of the time course of disappearance of radioactivity from the nuclear pellet isolated from this brain area indicates a clear-cut retention of the hormone for at least 4 h after an intraperitoneal injection (Fig. 5). This means that the percentage of counts in the hypothalamus retained in cell nuclei increases with time (Fig. 5).

Concurrent injections of 10 μg of unlabeled estradiol-17β and 0.6 μg of [^{3}H]estradiol-17β decreased the nuclear retention of [^{3}H]estradiol by about 90%. Similar treatment with unlabeled estradiol-17α or testosterone had no significant effect (Fig. 6). Even at a dose of 1 mg, testosterone had no effect on the nuclear retention of estradiol, indicating the stereoselectivity of the retention process. On the other hand, 50 μg of diethystilbestrol significantly decreased the nuclear retention both in the preoptic–hypothalamic area and in the amygdala (Fig. 7). In other words, potent estrogens (i.e., estradiol-17β and diethylstilbestrol) inhibit [^{3}H]estradiol retention while compounds with weak estrogenic activity (i.e., estradiol-17α and testosterone) have little effect.

Chader and Villee (1970, 1971) studied the subcellular localization of estradiol after incubating brain tissue *in vitro* with a low concentration of [^{3}H]estradiol (10^{-10} M). Radioactivity was more concentrated in the nuclear fraction prepared from hypothalamic tissue than in the mitochondrial, microsomal, or supernatant fraction. After a 60-min incubation, all the

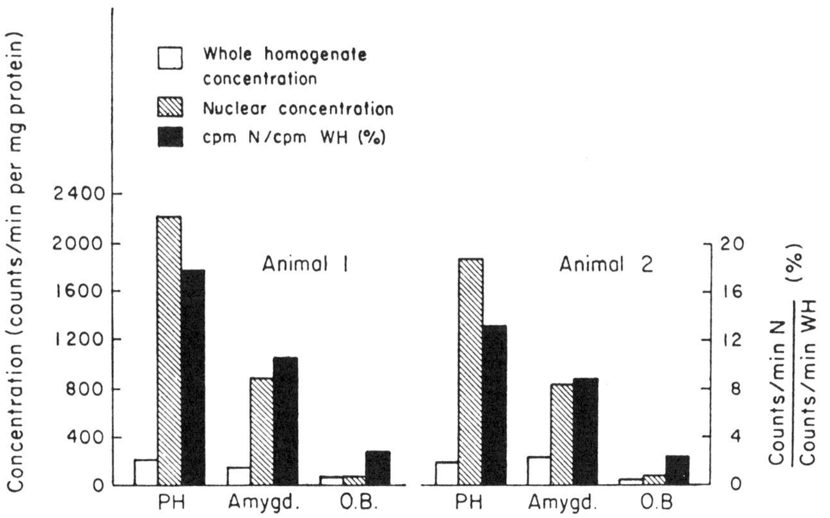

FIG. 4. Regional differences in estradiol retention in the brain. Ovariectomized rats were injected with [^{3}H]estradiol and 2 h later the concentration of labeled hormone was measured in the whole homogenate and in a purified nuclear fraction from three brain areas: PH, preoptic–hypothalamic area; Amygd., amygdala plus overlying cortex; O.B., olfactory bulbs. The amount of radioactivity recovered in the nuclear pellet is expressed both in counts/min/mg protein (left ordinate) and as a percentage of the total counts in the whole homogenate (right ordinate). From Zigmond and McEwen (1970).

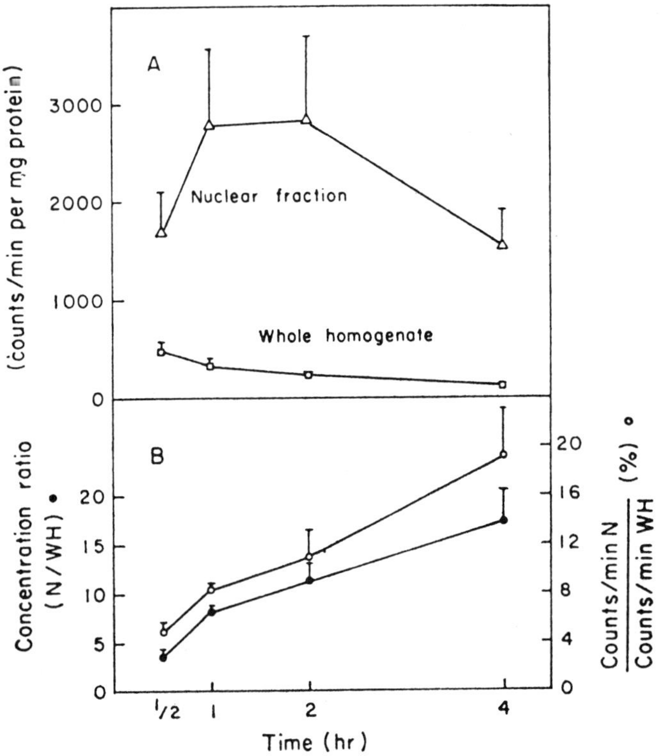

FIG. 5. Time course of estradiol retention in the whole homogenate and nuclear fraction from the preoptic–hypothalamic area after a peripheral injection of [^{3}H]estradiol. A: Concentration of radioactivity (counts/min/mg protein). B: Ratios of the concentration of radioactivity in the nuclear fraction (N) to that in the whole homogenate (WH) (●, left ordinate), and the percentage of the total radioactivity in the whole homogenate recovered in the nuclear fraction (○, right ordinate). Each point represents the means ± SEM for six animals. From Zigmond and McEwen (1970).

radioactivity extracted from the hypothalamus was unmetabolized [^{3}H]estradiol. Thus the small amounts of [^{3}H]estrone and other metabolites found in the hypothalamus after *in vivo* administration of [^{3}H]estradiol may be formed peripherally.

After *in vitro* labeling, Chader and Villee (1970) dialyzed their four fractions for 24 h at 4 °C against a large volume of buffer. The nuclear fraction was the only fraction which retained a large percentage (76%) of the hormone it had contained prior to dialysis, suggesting that estradiol is bound to macromolecules within this fraction. Further support for this idea comes from the demonstration by sucrose gradient centrifugation of a bound peak

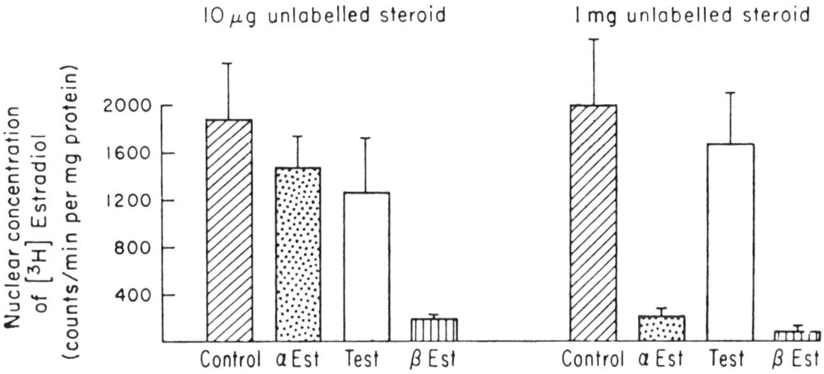

FIG. 6. Effect of concurrent injections of three unlabeled steroids on the retention of [^{3}H]estradiol by cell nuclei from the preoptic–hypothalamic area. Animals were injected with about 0.6 μg of [^{3}H]estradiol together with estradiol-17α (α Est), testosterone (Test), or estradiol-17β (β Est) at two doses, 10 μg or 1 mg. Controls received the vehicle, 95% ethanol, together with the radioactive steroid. From Zigmond and McEwen (1970).

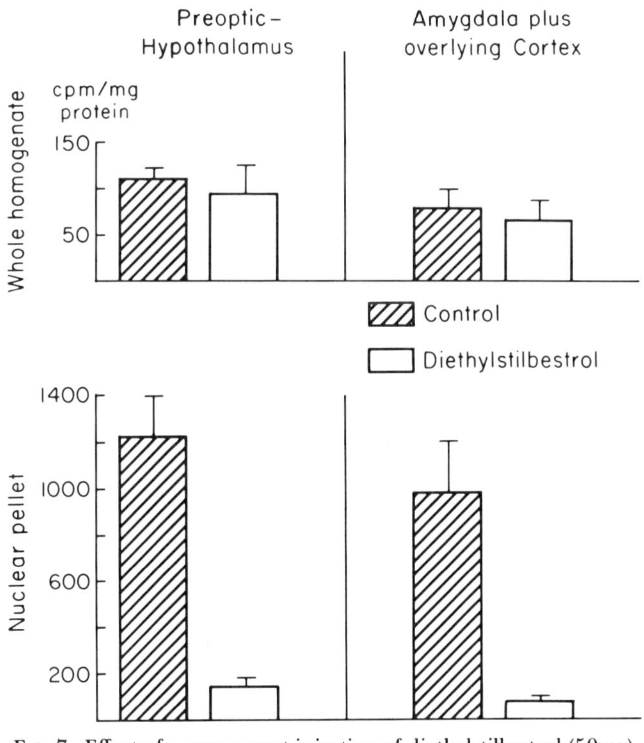

FIG. 7. Effect of a concurrent injection of diethylstilbestrol (50 μg) on the retention of [^{3}H]estradiol by cell nuclei in the preoptic–hypothalamic area and the amygdaloid region. Control animals received the vehicle together with the radioactive steroid. From Zigmond (1971).

of estradiol in 0.4 M KCl extracts of hypothalamic nuclei (Mowles *et al.*, 1971).

Clark *et al.* (1972) estimated that the dissociation constant of estradiol and its hypothalamic nuclear binding site was 1×10^{-9} M and that the binding capacity of hypothalamic nuclei was 0.1–0.5 pmol estradiol per gram of tissue. These figures were derived from experiments in which hypothalamic tissue was incubated with [^{3}H]estradiol with and without a hundred-fold excess of unlabeled diethylstilbestrol. The amount of specifically bound estradiol in a crude nuclear pellet was assumed to be the difference between the amount of estradiol bound in the absence and in the presence of diethylstilbestrol.

More recently, Anderson *et al.* (1973) have estimated these same parameters using a [^{3}H]estradiol exchange assay. In this method, animals are injected with unlabeled estradiol, a nuclear fraction is isolated, and the fraction is incubated with labeled hormone. Under the conditions of the incubation, the estradiol bound in the nuclei exchanges completely with the tritiated estradiol in the medium, thus providing a measure of the number of nuclear binding sites. The dissociation constant for the binding of estradiol in hypothalamic nuclei measured by this technique was $0.39 \pm 0.19 \times 10^{-9}$ M and the binding capacity of the nuclei was 0.47 pmol per gram of tissue. The binding capacity of isolated nuclei was about half maximal after *in vivo* administration of 0.5 μg estradiol.

When examing estradiol binding in various parts of the hypothalamus, Anderson *et al.* (1973) found nuclear binding sites only in the "basal hypothalamus–median eminence region." However, their data suggest that this area can account for only about half of the total estradiol bound per hypothalamus. Furthermore, results using other techniques, in particular autoradiography, clearly indicate that cell nuclei in other parts of the hypothalamus concentrate estradiol (e.g., see Stumpf, 1968*a*).

In the uterus, estradiol seems to be transported into the nucleus by a process which requires some component(s) from the cytoplasm (Jensen and De Sombre, 1973). A similar process may occur in the brain. When isolated hypothalamic nuclei are incubated with [^{3}H]estradiol, the radioactivity which is retained is lost upon dialysis. However, if a supernatant fraction ("cytosol") is added to the incubation and the nuclei are subsequently isolated, the hormone is found to be tightly bound to the nuclear fraction (Chader and Villee, 1970).

2.3.2. *Cytosol Binding*

The first observations on the molecular basis of estradiol binding in the central nervous system were reported by Kahwanago *et al.* (1969, 1970) and by Eisenfeld (1969, 1970). These authors demonstrated that estradiol at low concentrations (10^{-8}–10^{-9} M) bound *in vitro* to macromolecules present in a "high-speed supernatant" fraction (approximately 100,000*g*) prepared from the hypothalamus. Kahwanago *et al.* (1969, 1970) studied the bovine hypothalamus and separated free from bound hormone by sucrose gradient centrifugation. Eisenfeld (1969, 1970) studied the rat hypothalamus by polyacrylamide gel filtration (Table 8). Estradiol binding to macromolecules in the rat hypothalamus and amygdala has also been demonstrated by equilibrium dialysis (Zigmond, 1971).

The binding of estradiol to hypothalamic macromolecules was inhibited by chymotrypsin and papain (proteolytic agents) and by *p*-chloromercuriphenylsulfonic acid (a sulfhydryl-group blocking agent) but not by ribonuclease or deoxyribonuclease (Eisenfeld, 1970; Kahwanago *et al.*, 1970). These results suggest that the binding macromolecules are proteins or at least that a protein component is essential for the binding to occur. The stereoselectivity of the binding was demonstrated by the observations that unlabeled estradiol or clomiphene inhibited [^{3}H]estradiol binding while unlabeled progesterone and testosterone had no effect (Eisenfeld, 1970; Kahwanago *et al.*, 1970). Furthermore, no evidence for macromolecular binding of [^{3}H]progesterone or [^{3}H]testosterone was found under comparable conditions (Kahwanago *et al.*, 1970).

In the rat, the hypothalamus and the amygdala bound more estradiol per unit weight than did the cerebral cortex (Eisenfeld, 1970; Zigmond, 1971). In the cow, a regional difference within the hypothalamus was found, the median eminence area being significantly higher than the rest of the hypothalamus (Kahwanago *et al.*, 1970).

Estradiol binding to soluble macromolecules has also been demonstrated in the brain after an *in vivo* injection (Zigmond, 1971). High-speed supernatant fractions were prepared 10 min after an intracarotid injection

TABLE 8

Macromolecular Binding of Estradiol in Vitro in Cytosol Fractions[a]

	Dpm bound/mg protein + SEM
Hypothalamus	1,520 ± 160
Cerebral cortex	320 ± 40
Cerebellum	250 ± 40
Plasma	55 ± 20
Heart	200 ± 40
Anterior pituitary	10,500 ± 2,200
Uterus	17,800 ± 3,700

[a]Cytosol fractions were prepared from various tissues and incubated with [^{3}H]estradiol (2×10^{-9} M) for 1 h at 4 °C. Bound and free steroid were separated by polyacrylamide gel filtration. Data from Eisenfeld (1970).

and free and bound hormone were separated by gel filtration. More bound estradiol was found in a sample containing septum, preoptic area, hypothalamus, and amygdala than in a sample of cerebral cortex (Fig. 8). The amount of bound [^{3}H]estradiol was reduced by concurrent injections of unlabeled estradiol (10 μg).

2.4. Developmental Changes in the Estradiol Binding System

2.4.1. Changes in Estradiol Binding in the Female with Age

While rats retain more [^{3}H]estradiol in the central nervous system during the first 2 wk of life than at later times, most evidence suggests that the early retention is not saturable and shows no regional differentiation. The high retention of estradiol seems to reflect the extremely high blood levels present after hormone administration in young animals rather than a well-developed binding system (Wooley *et al.*, 1969; Presl *et al.*, 1970; Kato *et al.*, 1971*a*). The brains of these animals do not concentrate estradiol from the blood, as shown by the brain/plasma ratios of radioactivity per unit weight, which are well below 1 in neonates but range from 2 to 10 in adults (Wooley *et al.*, 1969; McEwen and Pfaff, 1970). The first *in vivo* evidence of regional differentiation of the retention mechanism—as judged by tissue/cortex ratios of radioactivity—was found at 12–15 days for the median eminence and at 20–25 days for the anterior hypothalamus (Presl *et al.*, 1970; Kato *et al.*, 1971*a*). These results are in apparent conflict with the report of Kulin and Reiter (1972) that the highest hypothalamus/cortex ratio after an *in vitro* incubation occurred in fetal and neonatal animals and that the ratio decreased with age. Another difference between estradiol retention in neonates and adults is the inability of low doses of unlabeled steroids to saturate the retention in neonates (Kato *et al.*, 1971*a*).

Sucrose gradient studies indicate a gradual development of the adult cytosol receptor from day 6 to day 33 (Kato *et al.*, 1971*b*; Plapinger and McEwen, 1973) (Fig. 9). On the other hand, there is a sharp rise in nuclear retention between day 20 and day 26 (Plapinger and McEwen, 1973). No evidence is available as to what limits nuclear retention before this time.

In contrast to these findings using biochemical techniques, Sheridan *et al.* (1973) found labeled cells autoradiographically in neonatal rats as early as day 2. The distribution of these cells was very similar to the distribution of estradiol-concentrating cells seen in the adult. As noted below, a similar discrepancy between results from biochemical and autoradiographic studies exists concerning [^{3}H]testosterone retention in the adult rat. Although the explanation for these discrepancies is not certain, they may result from a disruption of hormone binding during homogenization and centrifugation.

Less is known about changes in estradiol binding with age after puberty. Peng and Peng (1973) reported decreased hormone retention in the

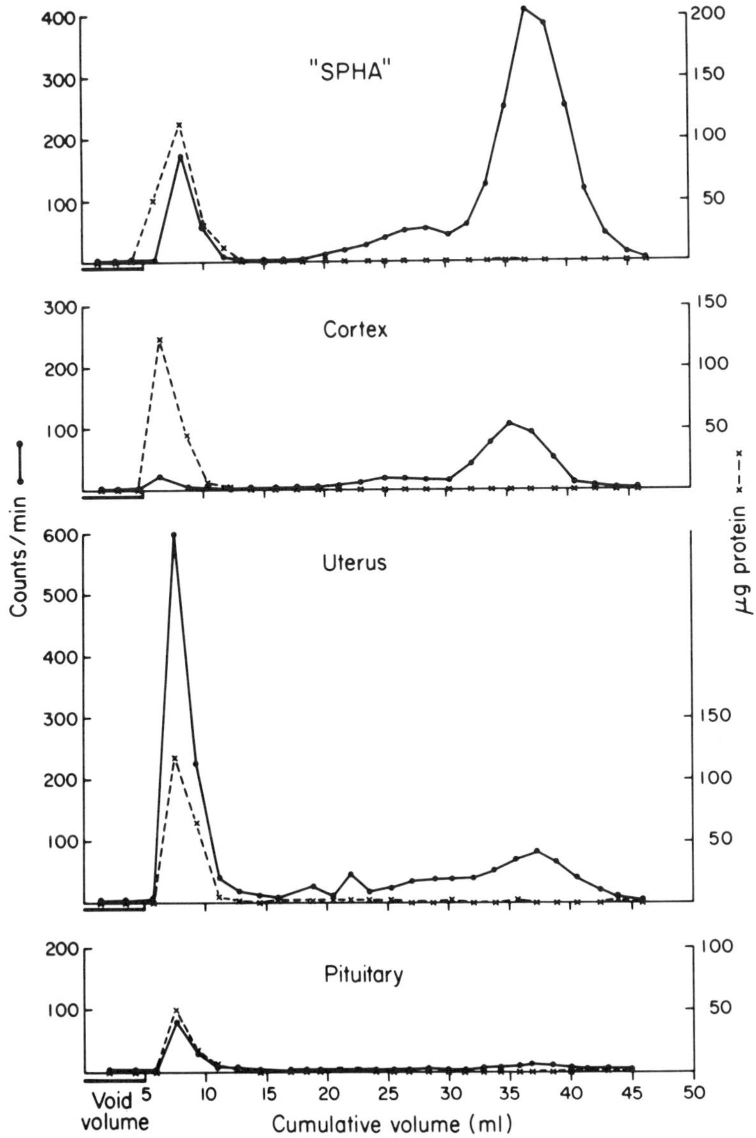

FIG. 8. *In vivo* cytosol binding of estradiol. Ovariectomized rats were injected intravenously with 0.1 mCi (0.6 μg) of [^{3}H]estradiol and 10 min later the animals were killed. Four samples were taken: SPHA (includes septum, preoptic area, hypothalamus, and amygdala), cerebral cortex, uterus, and pituitary gland. High-speed supernatant fractions were prepared and layered on Bio-Gel 10 columns. The void volume was determined with blue dextran 2000. The solid line represents the amount of radioactivity eluted in successive fractions in counts/min. The dashed line shows the elution pattern for protein. From Zigmond (1971).

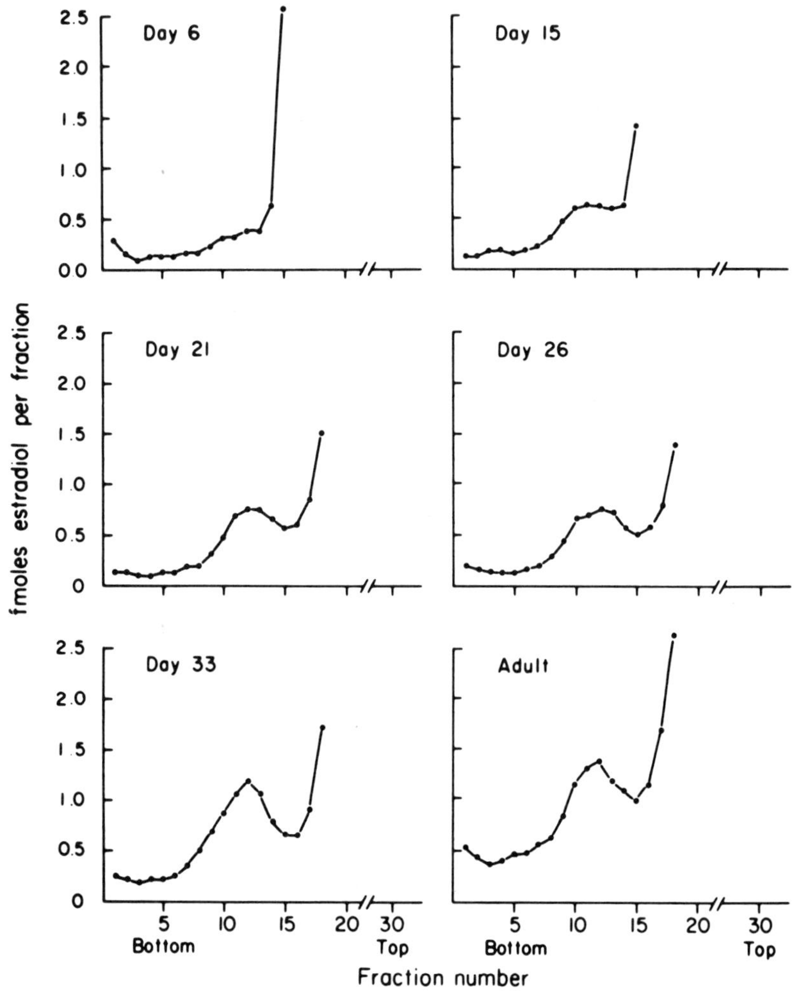

FIG. 9. Ontogeny of "adult-like" cytosol binding of estradiol. Cytosol fractions were prepared from a brain sample including the preoptic–hypothalamic area, the amygdala, and the midbrain and were incubated with [^{3}H]estradiol (1×10^{-9} M) for 2 h at 4 °C. After this incubation, the fractions were layered on a linear sucrose gradient and centrifuged for 1 h at 127,000 × *g*. The points represent the amount of labeled hormone recovered from successive gradient fractions. From Plapinger and McEwen (1973), reprinted by permission of J. B. Lippincott Company, Philadelphia.

anterior hypothalamus, uterus, and anterior pituitary *in vitro* and *in vivo* in 2-yr-old female rats compared to 5-month-old animals. No change was found in the posterior hypothalamus and cerebral cortex, areas of the brain which contain few specific binding sites for estradiol.

Although young rats show little estradiol binding in the brain of the type seen in adults, there are macromolecules in these animals which bind estradiol (Plapinger *et al.*, 1973). The neonatal binding macromolecules differ from the adult variety in their (1) sedimentation coefficient, (2) lack of regional localization, (3) extremely high binding capacity (200 times higher than in the adult), and (4) specificity of binding (they do not bind diethylstilbestrol). The concentration of these macromolecules was highest in fetal animals and decreased progressively with age until they were undetectable 22 days after birth. A similar binding macromolecule has been described in fetal and neonatal rat plasma (Raynaud *et al.*, 1971; Nunez *et al.*, 1971). However, the brain binding macromolecule does not seem to be an artifact due to plasma contamination. It has been proposed that these binding systems may protect the fetal and neonatal rat from the potentially masculinizing effect of maternal estrogens (McEwen *et al.*, 1974*b*).

2.4.2. Effects of Early Hormone Manipulation and Normal Sexual Differentiation on Estradiol Binding

Sexual differentiation of the central nervous system in the rat depends to a large extent on the presence or absence of circulating androgens during the first week of life (for review, see Pfaff *et al.*, 1974). Thus several aspects of brain function (e.g., control of reproductive behavior and control of pituitary gonadotrophin secretion) can be "masculinized" by an injection of testosterone propionate into the developing female or by putting an implant of the androgen into the hypothalamus (Nadler, 1973). As adults, these animals appear to be less sensitive to androgens (Petrusz and Nagy, 1967; Barraclough and Haller, 1970; Edwards and Thompson, 1970; Gerall and Kenney, 1970; Pfaff and Zigmond, 1971; Whalen *et al.*, 1971). Flerko and coworkers found that neonatal androgenization also results in the decreased ability of a number of target tissues to retain [^{3}H]estradiol (Flerko and Mess, 1968; Flerko *et al.*, 1969). When androgenized and control rats were injected with [^{3}H]estradiol (about 0.5 μg) as adults, less radioactive hormone was retained 2 h later in the anterior hypothalamus (35% less), "middle" hypothalamus (30%), anterior pituitary (28%), and uterus (37%). No difference was found in estradiol retention in the two groups in the posterior hypothalamus or parietal cortex, areas of the brain which contain many fewer specific binding sites.

Subsequent studies have confirmed the finding of decreased estradiol retention in the hypothalamus of the androgenized female (McEwen and Pfaff, 1970; Flerko *et al.*, 1971; Tuohimaa and Johansson, 1971; Maurer and Wooley, 1971). Using an autoradiographic technique, Anderson and Greenwald (1969) found fewer labeled cells in the preoptic area (a decrease of 54%) and in the ventromedial and arcuate nuclei (50%) of androgenized rats. Vertes and King (1971) showed that estradiol retention in the crude nuclear pellet and cytosol fraction prepared from the hypothalamus was also decreased by this early hormone treatment.

The effect of neonatal androgen injections on estradiol binding sites may only occur in certain estrogen target tissues. Thus in spite of the early report by Flerko *et al.* (1969) of decreased estradiol retention in the pituitary, most subsequent studies have found no effect in this tissue (Anderson and Greenwald, 1969; McEwen and Pfaff, 1970; Flerko *et al.*, 1971; Tuohimaa and Johansson, 1971; Maurer and Wooley, 1971).

Masculinization can be prevented in normal male rats by castrating neonates during the first few days of life or by injecting them daily with cyproterone acetate, a compound with antiandrogenic activity (see Pfaff *et al.*, 1974). Although no difference was found in estradiol retention between neonatal castrates and sham-operated rats (McEwen and Pfaff, 1970), less retention was found in the "rostral middle hypothalamus" of cyproterone-treated males than in controls (Tuohimaa and Niemi, 1972*b*).

Although it is generally assumed that these neonatal hormone manipulations mimic normal developmental processes, it is not at all clear whether there is a normal male–female difference in estradiol retention. Stumpf (1968*a*) reported that the anatomical distribution of estradiol-concentrating cells was similar in male and female rats, and several other authors found no quantitative difference in the amount of hormone retained (Eisenfeld and Axelrod, 1966; Green *et al.*, 1969; Anderson *et al.*, 1973). On the other hand, Pfaff (1968), McEwen and Pfaff (1970), Tuohimaa (1971), and Clark *et al.* (1972) found less retention in adult males than in adult females.

2.5. Changes in Estradiol Binding During the Estrus Cycle

Because of the possibility that estradiol binding sites in intact animals might be saturated by endogenous estrogens, most experiments on estradiol retention are performed on ovariectomized animals. However, to test directly the extent to which these sites are saturated under physiological conditions, several workers have injected normal cycling rats with [^{3}H]estradiol and attempted to correlate the uptake of labeled hormone with the circulating levels of endogenous hormone. About 50% less [^{3}H]estradiol was retained by hypothalamus (particularly the anterior hypothalamus) during proestrus than during diestrus (McGuire and Lisk, 1968; Kato *et al.*, 1969; Luttge, 1972*a*). In the cerebral cortex, on the other hand, no changes were seen during the cycle. Somewhat surprisingly, however, no changes were found in the median eminence sample, either (Kato *et al.*, 1969), an area shown to have limited-capacity binding sites for estradiol (Kato and Villee, 1967*b*). Kato *et al.* (1969) reported that if the anterior hypothalamus is incubated *in vitro* with labeled estradiol (10^{-7} M) tissue from proestrous animals takes up less hormone than tissue from diestrous animals. These results are consistent with the interpretation that endogenous estradiol, which is higher at proestrus than at diestrus (Fig. 10), is partially saturating

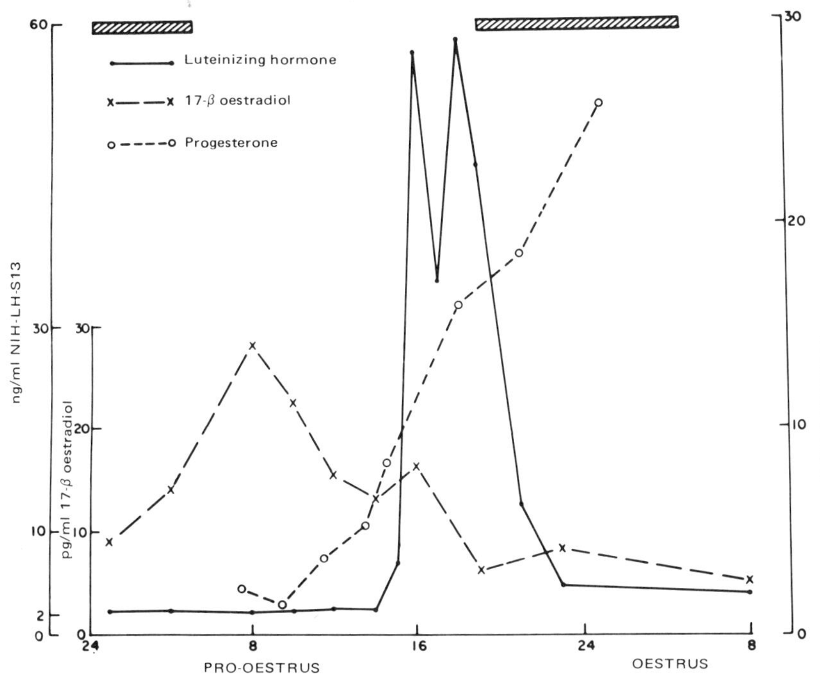

FIG. 10. Plasma concentrations of estradiol, progesterone, and luteinizing hormone on the day of proestrus in the rat. Shaded bar indicates time when the lights were off. From Brown-Grant (1971), reprinted with permission of the Regents of the University of California.

the binding sites in the hypothalamus and that the endogenous steroid is not readily displaced under the conditions of incubation. It should be remembered, however, that this interpretation is based on the assumptions that fluctuations in other hormones during the estrus cycle are unimportant and that the number of estrogen binding sites and their affinity for the hormone remain constant throughout the cycle.

2.6. Behavioral and Physiological Effects of Estrogen Agonists and Antagonists

Of the naturally occurring estrogens, estradiol-17β seems to be the most potent in stimulating mating behavior in ovariectomized rats (Beyer *et al.*, 1971*b*; Meyerson, 1972). Estrone, estriol, estrone sulfate, and estradiol-17α (in decreasing order of potency) have less stimulatory ability. On the other hand, the synthetic estrogen, hexestrol, is very effective in the rat and diethylstilbestrol is even slightly more potent than estradiol-17β in the cat

(Michael, 1966; Meyerson, 1972). These results, together with the competition experiments discussed above, suggest that there is a relationship between the potency of a compound to stimulate lordosis behavior and its ability to bind to "estrophilic" macromolecules in the brain.

The study of estrogen action has been aided by the synthesis of a number of compounds with antiestrogenic activity. The drugs listed in Table 9 and Fig. 11 have been shown to inhibit a number of peripheral effects of estradiol, including the uterotrophic response and may act by inhibiting estradiol binding in target cells (see references, Table 9). These compounds can also antagonize certain of the effects of estradiol on the central nervous system.

Mer-25, CI-628, and *cis*-clomiphene can block the effects of estradiol on female mating behavior. For instance, when Mer-25 was injected either 2 h before or 2 or 8 h after estradiol benzoate, the percentage of female rats exhibiting lordosis when tested with males and the ratio of lordoses to mounts was significantly reduced (Meyerson and Lindstrom, 1968; Komisaruk and Beyer, 1972). Mer-25 injections 24 h after or, surprisingly, at the same time as estrogen administration had no effect (Meyerson and Lindstrom, 1968). An injection of Mer-25 into an intact, 5-day cyclic rat, 24 h before the normal onset of receptivity, inhibited mating as judged by the absence of vaginal plugs and the absence of sperm in the vagina (Shirley *et al.*, 1968).

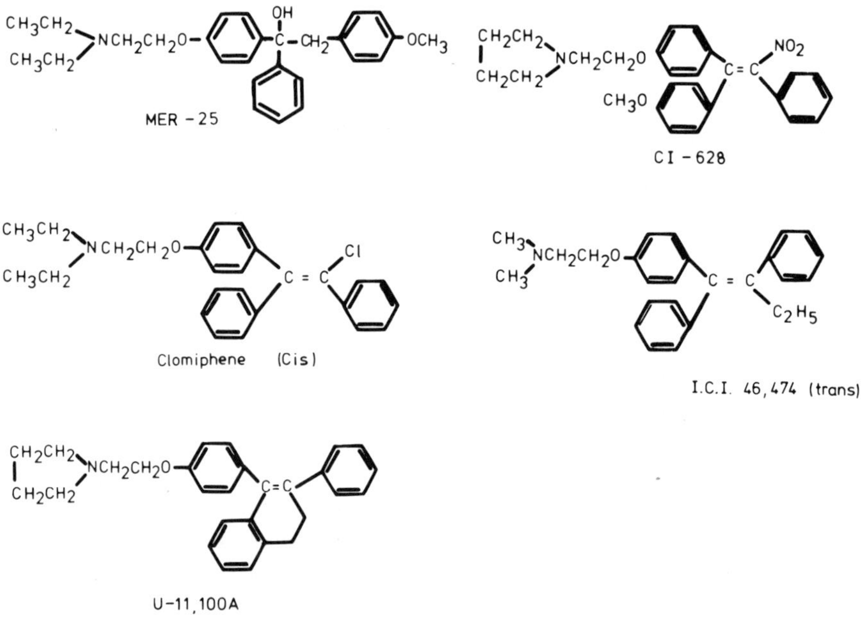

FIG. 11. Chemical structures of five compounds shown to have antiestrogenic activity.

TABLE 9

References on the Effects of Several Antiestrogens on Estrogen Action and Binding

Drug	Antiestrogenic effects on peripheral tissues	Effects on estradiol binding in uterus	Effects on estradiol binding in brain
Mer-25	Lerner *et al.* (1958)	Jensen (1966)	—
CI-628 (formerly CN-55,945-27)	Callantine *et al.* (1966)	Callantine (1967)	Whalen and Gorzalka (1973)
I.C.I. 46,474	Harper and Walpole (1967)	Quoted in Labhsetwar (1970*c*)	—
Clomiphene	Holtkamp *et al.* (1960)	Roy *et al.* (1964), Wyss *et al.* (1968)	Eisenfeld and Axelrod (1967) Kato *et al.* (1968) Maurer and Wooley (1971)
U-11,100A	Duncan *et al.* (1963)	Jensen (1966)	Eisenfeld and Axelrod (1967)

CI-628 antagonized the effects of estrogen treatment on mating behavior if given to ovariectomized rats at the time of estrogen treatment or 4 or 6 h later, but like Mer 25 it was ineffective if given 24 h later (Arai and Gorski, 1968; Whalen and Gorzalka, 1973). Clomiphene exists in both a *cis* and *trans* form and the two isomers have very different effects on lordosis behavior. Pretreatment of rats for 4 days with *cis*-clomiphene (1 mg) inhibits the stimulation of lordosis behavior by estradiol benzoate (Ross *et al.*, 1973*a*). *trans*-Clomiphene facilitates lordosis behavior and can act synergistically with low doses of estradiol (Ross *et al.*, 1973*a,b*).

Mer-25, *cis*-clomiphene, and I.C.I. 46,474 can also inhibit ovulation if administered to cycling rats the day before proestrus (Shirley *et al.*, 1968; Labhsetwar, 1970*a,b,c*). *trans*-Clomiphene and I.C.I. 47,699 (the *cis*-isomer of I.C.I. 46,474) are ineffective. The blockade of ovulation caused by *cis*-clomiphene and I.C.I. 46,474 can be overcome by injections of LH, a median eminence extract containing LH releasing factor, or a large dose of estradiol benzoate. These findings suggest that the drugs act by antagonizing the effects of estradiol in the central nervous system rather than at the level of the pituitary or ovary. More direct evidence for a central site of action of I.C.I. 46,474 was provided by implantation studies (Bainbridge and Labhsetwar, 1971; Billard and McDonald, 1973). Implants of the drug in the arcuate nucleus–median eminence region on the day before proestrus were effective in blocking ovulation. More anteriorally placed implants in the preoptic–anterior hypothalamic area were less effective.

While it is often assumed that these antiestrogenic drugs exert their effects in the central nervous system by blocking estradiol binding, direct evidence for this idea is not available on Mer-25 and I.C.I. 46,474, and the data on clomiphene and CI-628 are inconclusive. While clomiphene has been shown to inhibit the binding of estradiol in the hypothalamus (Eisenfeld and Axelrod, 1967; Kato *et al.*, 1968; Kahwanago *et al.*, 1970; Mauer and Wooley, 1971), the doses required to produce a significant decrease *in vivo* are larger than those used in the behavioral and endocrinological studies quoted above (Kato *et al.*, 1968). Rotsztejn (1973) found an inhibition of estradiol retention in the anterior hypothalamus when rats were pretreated with CI-628; however, again the dose used (about 30 mg/kg intravenously) was in excess of that required to inhibit the behavioral effects of estradiol (2mg/kg by gavage) (Arai and Gorski, 1968). Further studies using lower doses of these drugs are required.

One of the puzzling features of the studies on Mer-25 and CI-628 is the finding that these drugs can antagonize the effects of estradiol on lordosis behavior even if injected several hours after the hormone (Meyerson and Lindstrom, 1968; Whalen and Gorzalka, 1973). If the mechanism of action of these drugs does depend on an antagonism of estradiol binding, this would suggest that (1) Mer-25 and CI-628 can displace bound hormone and that (2) estradiol is bound in the central nervous system for several hours after an injection. In regard to the first point, Callantine *et al.* (1968) reported that CI-628 can displace bound estradiol in the uterus. However, although Whalen and Gorzalka (1973) replicated this effect in the uterus, they could find no evidence for displacement of bound estradiol in the brain. It is difficult to estimate the duration of estradiol binding in the behavioral studies referred to above as the dose and method of hormone injection (usually microgram quantities of estradiol benzoate injected subcutaneously in oil) differ markedly from those used in binding studies (usually a few tenths of a microgram of [^{3}H]estradiol injected intraperitoneally or intravenously in saline–ethanol). However, if one compares the binding study of Anderson *et al.* (1973) with the behavioral study of Whalen and Gorzalka (1973), two experiments in which the estrogen injections were *roughly* similar, it appears that CI-628 is still effective at a time in which there is little estrogen remaining in the brain. Clearly we still have a lot to learn about the mechanism of action of these "antiestrogens" in the brain.

2.7. Sites of Estrogen Action

As was mentioned in Section 1, estrous behavior can be restored in ovariectomized animals by direct hypothalamic implantation of an estrogen into the preoptic–hypothalamic area. The most effective sites within this region vary from species to species. In the rat, the medial preoptic–anterior hypothalamic area seems to be the best site (Lisk, 1962), while in the rabbit the ventromedial–premammillary region is best (Palka and Sawyer, 1966*a*). In the cat, effective sites can be found in both the anterior and posterior hypothalamus (Michael, 1964).

Implants of estradiol in the arcuate–median eminence region in the rat and rabbit inhibit pituitary gonadotropin secretion (Davidson, 1969). Implants of the hormone directly into the anterior pituitary are less effective. These experiments are generally interpreted to indicate that the medial basal hypothalamus is the site of the inhibitory feedback action of estrogens. Bogdanove (1963), however, has pointed out a paradox in these experiments. Since the median eminence is connected to the anterior pituitary gland by a system of portal blood vessels, it is conceivable that the most efficient way to deliver estradiol to anterior pituitary cells is to implant the hormone in the basal hypothalamus. Proof that hormone reaches the pituitary gland after implantation in the median eminence region was provided by Palka *et al.* (1966). While the problems caused by the "implantation paradox" still remain to be resolved experimentally, most authors accept that estradiol is probably acting both in the arcuate–median eminence region and in the anterior pituitary (Davidson, 1969). Feedback sites for the hormone may also exist in the preoptic–anterior hypothalamic area and in the amygdala (Davidson, 1969; Sawyer, 1972).

2.8. Temporal Aspects of Estrogen Action

While ovariectomy leads to the disappearance of the lordosis response in the rat, the ovaries need not be present at the exact time of mating. In the intact rat the ovary secretes little estrogen during the period of behavioral receptivity. In rats with 4-day cycles, the level of plasma estradiol begins to rise during diestrus, reaches a maximum on the morning of proestrus, and decreases the same afternoon (Schwartz, 1969; Brown-Grant, 1971) (Fig. 10). Behavioral receptivity begins in the afternoon of proestrus and continues into the evening (Schwartz, 1969; Nequin and Schwartz, 1971; Brown-Grant, personal communication). If animals are ovariectomized at 8 A.M. on proestrus, mating still occurs in the afternoon. However, if they are ovariectomized earlier that morning or on the previous afternoon mating is prevented (Schwartz and Talley, 1965; Nequin and Schwartz, 1971).

Ovarian estrogens, then, seem to have a triggering effect on female mating behavior. The length of the interval between an injection of estradiol in an ovariectomized rat or cat and the first appearance of lordosis behavior can be influenced by the dose of hormone, the method of administration, and the amount of behavioral testing the animal receives (Michael, 1964; Chambers and Howe, 1968; Green *et al.*, 1970). However, there seems to be a minimal latency, which has been estimated to be 16 h in the rat (Green *et al.*, 1970), 1–2 days in the rabbit (Palka and Sawyer, 1966*a*), and 2–3 days in the cat (Michael, 1964; Peretz, 1968). Thus the first signs of behavioral receptivity after a single injection of estradiol occur at a time at which both plasma and brain concentrations of the hormone would be extremely low (Jensen and Jacobson, 1962; Michael, 1966; Anderson *et al.*, 1973).

The stimulation of ovulation by estradiol is similarly a delayed phenomenon. Injections of antibodies to estradiol-17β at 5 P.M. on diestrus blocked the LH surge and ovulation, but when the antiserum was injected at 10 A.M. on proestrus ovulation occurred normally that afternoon.

At present we do not know the minimum period estradiol must be present in the brain in order to initiate the sequence of events leading to the onset of lordosis behavior or ovulation. Experiments with Mer-25 and CI-628 suggest that the hormone must be present for at least 8 h to fully stimulate female mating behavior. However, as pointed out above (Section 2.6), more work needs to be done on the exact mechanism by which these compounds inhibit lordosis behavior.

The sequence of biochemical events which intervene between the injection of estradiol and the appearance of mating behavior remains to be elucidated. Is binding to specific macromolecules in the target cells a necessary first step? Does the hormone act by altering RNA and protein synthesis as it does in peripheral target tissues such as the uterus (Hamilton, 1968)? If so, which proteins are involved?

One reason for suggesting that estradiol affects RNA and protein synthesis is the fact that the hormone concentrates in brain cell nuclei. It has been postulated that the hormone–receptor complex alters the transcription of the genome in estrogen target cells (McEwen *et al.*, 1972*b*). It is conceivable, however, that estrogens (and other steroid hormones) influence nuclear events in a more indirect way.

In the last few years, a great deal of evidence has been accumulated suggesting that specific changes in protein synthesis can occur in a neuron as a result of an increase in transsynaptic stimulation (see Chap. 8, Vol. 3). Such biochemical alterations take some time to develop and, for instance, in the case of tyrosine hydroxylase in the superior cervical ganglion changes may not be detected for as long as 24 h after the onset of increased neurophysiological activity (Zigmond *et al.*, 1974). Nevertheless, the increased stimulation need not continue throughout the entire period but is required only for a short time (Zigmond and Mackay, 1974; Zigmond *et al.*, 1974). Thus the increased neural input acts like a trigger to initiate a change in the level of a particular enzyme. Such a time course is reminiscent of the events following estrogen administration. Since changes in neural activity have been recorded following administration of estrogens, androgens, glucocorticoids, and progestins (see, for instance, Sawyer and Gorski, 1971), the possibility arises that steroid hormones could alter protein synthesis in a neuron (or other biochemical parameters) indirectly by temporarily changing the neural input to the cell. To what extent the biochemical changes seen after estrogen administration are caused by such indirect mechanisms or by the more usually envisioned direct mechanism remains to be determined.

3. ANDROGENS

3.1. Regional and Cellular Distribution of Radioactivity After an Injection of [^{3}H]Testosterone in the Castrated Male Rat

After an injection of [^{3}H]testosterone in a castrated male rat, the highest concentration of radioactivity was found in the hypothalamus, preoptic area, septum, amygdala, and brain stem (Roy and Laumas, 1969; McEwen *et al.*, 1970*a*; Stern and Eisenfeld, 1971). This regional pattern was similar to that found after injection of [^{3}H]estradiol in ovariectomized females; however, the differences between brain regions and between the brain and the blood were smaller after [^{3}H]testosterone (McEwen and Pfaff, 1970; McEwen *et al.*, 1970*a*).

The cellular localization of [^{3}H]testosterone and/or its metabolites has been studied autoradiographically. At 30 min and 3 h after testosterone administration, cells in the preoptic area, septum, and olfactory tubercle were more heavily labeled than cells in the sensory-motor cortex (Pfaff,

1968). At 30 min, cells in the amygdala, hippocampus, ventromedial hypothalamus, cingulate gyrus, and cerebellum were also heavily labeled (Pfaff, 1968). Tuohimaa (1971) estimated that within the hypothalamus 30% of the cells in the ventromedial and arcuate nuclei concentrated labeled testosterone and metabolites but that only 1% of the cells in the dorsomedial or lateral hypothalamus did so.

Sar and Stumpf (1972, 1973*a*), using a freeze-dry method, found the highest concentration of labeled cells in the lateral septum, bed nucleus of the stria terminalis, medial preoptic nucleus, periventricular nuclei of the preoptic area and hypothalamus, arcuate nucleus, ventromedial nucleus, ventral premammillary nucleus, hippocampus, dentate gyrus, subiculum, and cortical and medial amygdaloid nuclei. Scattered labeled cells were reported in the diagonal band of Broca, islands of Calleja, nucleus triangularis septi, suprachiasmatic nucleus, anterior hypothalamic area, lateral hypothalamus at the level of the ventromedial nucleus, and medial part of the basal amygdaloid nucleus.

Compared to the distribution of labeled cells after an injection of [^{3}H]estradiol, more labeled cells were found after [^{3}H]testosterone in the lateral septum, hippocampus, dentate gyrus, and subiculum and fewer were found in the arcuate nucleus (Stumpf, 1970*a*; Sar and Stumpf, 1973*a*). Labeled cells were found throughout the ventromedial hypothalamus after [^{3}H]testosterone treatment but only in the ventrolateral portion of the nucleus after [^{3}H]estradiol (Stumpf, 1970*a*; Sar and Stumpf, 1973*a*). Differences in the retention of the two hormones were also found in the anterior pituitary. After an injection of [^{3}H]testosterone only 15% of the cells in the pituitary were labeled (mainly basophils), whereas after [^{3}H]estradiol 60–80% were labeled (Stumpf, 1968*b*; Sar and Stumpf, 1973*b*).

3.2. Testosterone Metabolism in Peripheral Tissues: The Idea of Testosterone as a "Prehormone"

While estradiol and corticosterone are retained by their target cells primarily in an unmetabolized form, significant amounts of testosterone metabolites are retained both in the brain and in peripheral androgen target tissues. For example, 1 min after an intravenous injection of [^{3}H]testosterone only 10% of the radioactivity extracted from the cytoplasmic fraction of the prostate gland was unmetabolized testosterone and 70% was dihydrotestosterone and 3α-androstanediol (Bruchovsky and Wilson, 1968) (Table 10, Figs. 12 and 13). 50% of the radioactivity in the nuclear fraction was dihydrotestosterone and 35% was testosterone (Fig. 13). In the plasma, on the other hand, 75% of the radioactivity was still unmetabolized [^{3}H]testosterone and no [^{3}H]dihydrotestosterone could be detected (Fig. 13).

TABLE 10

Trivial and Systematic Names of Androgens and Antiandrogens

Trivial name	Systematic name
Testosterone	17β-Hydroxy-4-androsten-3-one
Dihydrotestosterone	17β-Hydroxy-5α-androstan-3-one
Androstenedione	4-Androstene-3,17-dione
Androstanedione	5α-Androstane-3,17-dione
3α-Androstanediol (allotetrahydrotestosterone)	3α, 17β-Dihydroxy-5α-androstane
Androsterone	3α-Hydroxy-5α-androstan-17-one
Etiocholanolone	3α-Hydroxy-5β-androstan-17-one
Fluoxymesterone	9α-Fluoro-11β,17β-dihydroxy-17α-methyl-4-androsten-3-one
Cyproterone	1,2α-Methylene-6-chloro-17α-hydroxy-4,6-pregnadiene-3,20-dione

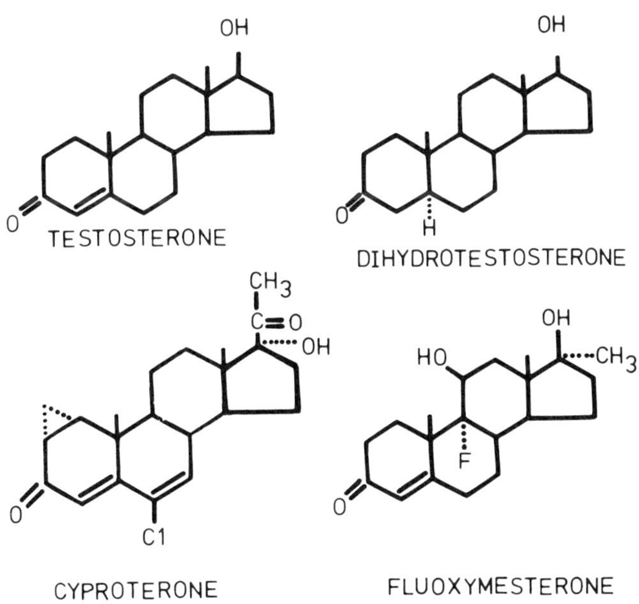

FIG. 12. Chemical structures of testosterone, its 5α-reduced metabolite, dihydrotestosterone, cyproterone (a compound with antiandrogenic activity), and fluoxymesterone (a compound with androgenic activity in certain tissues).

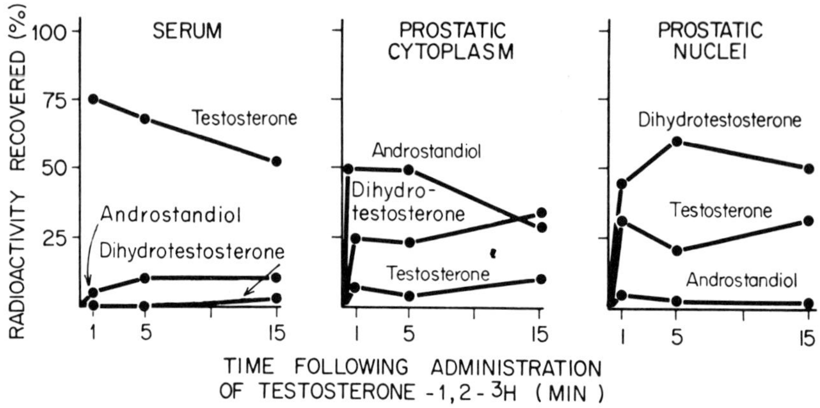

FIG. 13. Appearance of testosterone metabolites in serum, prostatic cytosol, and prostatic nuclei after an intravenous injection of [^{3}H]testosterone. The percentage of the total radioactivity identified as testosterone, dihydrotestosterone, and androstanediol is plotted as a function of time after the injection. From Wilson *et al.* (1969), reprinted with permission of Excerpta Medica Foundation.

The presence of a higher proportion of metabolites in the prostate than in the plasma immediately after an injection of testosterone suggested that the hormone was being metabolized within the prostate itself. This idea is supported by the finding that after prostate tissue is incubated with [^{3}H]testosterone, [^{3}H]dihydrotestosterone is found in the nuclear fraction (Anderson and Liao, 1968). Subcellular fractionation studies on the prostate have demonstrated the presence of an NADPH-dependent Δ^4-3-ketosteroid-5α-reductase (E.C. 1.3.1.99), the enzyme responsible for the conversion of testosterone to dihydrotestosterone, in the microsomal and nuclear fractions (Bruchovsky and Wilson, 1968; Anderson and Liao, 1968). The enzyme responsible for the conversion of dihydrotestosterone to 3α-androstanediol, NADPH:3α-ketosteroid dehydrogenase (E.C. 1.1.1.50), was found in the soluble fraction (Bruchovsky and Wilson, 1968).

Not only is dihydrotestosterone formed and retained by the prostate but it also has a higher affinity for the androgen-binding macromolecules in the cytosol than does testosterone (Mainwaring, 1969) and is more potent in promoting prostate growth (Baulieu *et al.*, 1968; Wilson and Gloyna, 1970). Thus testosterone can be considered a "prehormone" which is taken up and converted to a more active metabolite within a target cell. It is clear, however, that dihydrotestosterone is not the only active androgen even in the prostate. The relative potency of different androgens varies with the tissue and response studied. For instance, comparing dihydrotestosterone and testosterone, the former is more potent in stimulating growth in the rat seminal vesicle and the latter in the capon's comb (Dorfman and Shipley, 1956) (Table 11). In cultures of prostate, dihydrotestosterone is more potent in

TABLE 11

Relative Activities of Testosterone and Some Metabolites in Stimulating Growth in Two Androgen-Dependent Tissues[a]

	Relative activity (%)	
	Immature rat seminal vesicles	Capon's comb
Testosterone	100	100
Dihydrotestosterone	200	75
3α-Androstanediol	33	75
Androstenedione	20	12
Androstanedione	14	12
Androsterone	10	10

[a]The growth-promoting activities of different steroids are expressed as a percentage of the testosterone activity. Data from Dorfman and Shipley (1956).

stimulating cell division, but testosterone is more potent in maintaining epithelial cell height and secretory activity (Baulieu *et al.*, 1968). Although dihydrotestosterone has been found in a number of androgen target tissues in the rat (e.g., seminal vesicle, epididymis, and preputial gland) and in prostate glands of several species, it has not been found in rat skeletal muscle, which is also responsive to androgens, nor in the prostates of rabbits (Wilson and Gloyna, 1970). Skeletal muscle also seems to have little 5α-steroid reductase activity, and androgen-binding macromolecules isolated from this tissue have a higher affinity for testosterone than for

TABLE 12

Endogenous Concentration of Testosterone and 5α-Dihydrotestosterone in Rat Tissues (ng/g)[a]

	Testosterone	5α-Dihydrotestosterone
Plasma	2.5 ± 0.3	N.D.
Hypothalamus	13.7 ± 2.0	2.0 ± 0.4
Parietal cortex	1.3 ± 0.1	N.D.
Seminal vesicle	2.2 ± 0.3	3.0 ± 0.6
Ventral prostate	2.0 ± 0.4	2.8 ± 0.5
Levator ani muscle	7.9 ± 0.5	N.D.
Thigh muscle	2.9 ± 0.5	N.D.
Pituitary gland	60.5 ± 5.5	N.D.

[a]The endogenous concentration of testosterone and 5α-dihydrotestosterone in various tissues was measured by gas-liquid chromatography. N.D., Not detectable. Data from Robel *et al.* (1973).

dihydrotestosterone (Jung and Baulieu, 1972). Measurements of endogenous testosterone and dihydrotestosterone show that the prostate and seminal vesicle contain approximately equal concentrations of the two hormones while skeletal muscle contains no detectable dihydrotestosterone (Robel *et al.*, 1973) (Table 12). Thus it is possible that in skeletal muscle testosterone itself is the active androgen.

In addition to dihydrotestosterone, it is quite likely that other metabolites of testosterone have important physiological effects. For instance, the 5β- rather than the 5α-reduced metabolites seem to be important in stimulating heme biosynthesis (Levere *et al.*, 1967) and erythropoiesis (Gordon *et al.*, 1970).

3.3. Metabolism of Testosterone in the Brain

A number of metabolites of testosterone have been identified in the brain after a peripheral injection of labeled hormone into castrated rats. These include dihydrotestosterone, androstenedione, and 3α-androstanediol (Resko *et al.*, 1967; Appelgren, 1970; Stern and Eisenfeld, 1971; Sholiton *et al.*, 1972; Whalen and Rezek, 1972). [^{3}H]Dihydrotestosterone, but not [^{3}H]testosterone or [^{3}H]androstenedione, was more concentrated in the hypothalamus than in the cerebral cortex (Stern and Eisenfeld, 1971). On the other hand, measurements of the endogenous concentration of testosterone and dihydrotestosterone in intact rats have shown that under these conditions both hormones are more concentrated in the hypothalamus (Robel *et al.*, 1973) (Table 12). The discrepancy in these results may indicate changes in the retention mechanism after castration or the inadequacy of the dose and method of hormone administration used in studies with labeled testosterone. In the castrated guinea pig, both [^{3}H]testosterone and its less polar metabolites (dihydrotestosterone?) were more concentrated in the hypothalamus than in the cerebellum (Resko *et al.*, 1967).

When [^{3}H]testosterone is injected peripherally, it is impossible to determine whether testosterone is metabolized in the brain or whether the metabolites are taken up from the blood. The finding of labeled dihydrotestosterone, 3α-androstanediol, and androstenedione in the brains of hepatectomized rats strengthens the possibility that the metabolites are formed in the brain since the liver is the major peripheral site of steroid metabolism (Sholiton *et al.*, 1972). Furthermore, *in vitro* experiments have established the presence of the enzymes 5α-steroid reductase, 3α-hydroxysteroid dehydrogenase, and 17β-hydroxysteroid dehydrogenase (E.C. 1.1.1.51) in the rat brain. The 5α-steroid reductase was localized in the microsomal (and possibly nuclear) fraction, while the 3α- and 17β-hydroxysteroid dehydrogenases were present in the cytosol fraction (Rommerts and van der Molan, 1971). Rat brain slices or homogenates incubated with testosterone can form dihydrotestosterone, 3α-androstanediol, androstanedione, etiocholanolone, and androsterone, as demonstrated by recrystallization to constant specific activity (Sholiton and Werk, 1969; Jaffe, 1969; Sholiton *et al.*, 1970; Rommerts and van der Molen, 1971; Denef *et al.*, 1973) (Table 10). The predominant metabolite found was dihydrotestosterone (Jaffe, 1969; Rommerts and van der Molen, 1971; Denef *et al.*, 1973). Tissues incubated with androstenedione formed testosterone, 5α-androstanedione, androsterone, and the estrogenic steroid estrone (Rommerts and van der Molen, 1971; Naftolin *et al.*, 1972; Reddy *et al.*, 1974).

Details of androgen metabolism in the brain vary with species, brain region, age, sex, and hormonal condition. In the dog, for instance, in addition to dihydrotestosterone an androstenedione, 5α-androstanedione, was identified after incubation of hypothalamus with tritiated testosterone (Perez-Palacios *et al.*, 1970). In the cow, unlike the rat, testosterone was not metabolized to 3α-androstanediol, etiocholanolone, or androsterone (Sholiton and Werk, 1969; Sholiton *et al.*, 1970).

5α-Steroid reductase activity is unevenly distributed in the rat brain: midbrain, brain stem > hypothalamus, thalamus > cerebellum, cerebral cortex, hippocampus, caudate, preoptic area, amygdala, and pineal (Jaffe, 1969; Rommerts and van der Molen, 1971; Massa *et al.*, 1972; Denef *et al.*, 1973). A similar regional pattern was found for the formation of 3α-androstanediol, but no significant differences were found in androstenedione formation (Jaffe, 1969; Denef *et al.*, 1973). The aromatization of androstenedione to estrone was also found to be higher in the hypothalamus and "limbic" system (i.e., amygdala and hippocampus) than in the cerebral cortex in rats, rabbits, and humans (Naftolin *et al.*, 1971*a,b*; 1972; Reddy *et al.*, 1973, 1974).

Dihydrotestosterone formation in both the rat hypothalamus and cerebral cortex declines with age, being highest during the first week of life (Massa *et al.*, 1971; Weisz and Philpott, 1971). In adulthood, the male hypothalamus has a greater ability to convert testosterone to dihydrotestosterone and androstenedione to estrone than the female (Naftolin *et al.*, 1972; Denef *et al.*, 1973; Reddy *et al.*, 1973; 1974). Both enzymatic activities increase in both sexes after gonadectomy (Denef *et al.*, 1973; Reddy *et al.*, 1973). Although Sholiton *et al.* (1970) reported that homogenates of female brains produced more 3α-androstanediol than homogenates of male brain, no sex difference in the formation of this metabolite was found in tissue slices (Denef *et al.*, 1973).

Evidence from behavioral and endocrinological experiments referred to below suggests that the metabolism of testosterone in the brain may be an important step in a number of androgen-sensitive processes. It has been proposed that conversion of testosterone to dihydrotestosterone may be involved in the inhibitory action of androgens on the secretion of gonadotropins (see Section 3.9). Furthermore, a great deal of interest has arisen in the idea that aromatization of testosterone to an estrogen may be involved in the behavioral and developmental effects of androgens (see Section 3.9). However, the importance of changes in the extent of hormone metabolism with age, sex, or hormonal status cannot be evaluated at present as it is not known whether the metabolism of androgens is ever a rate-limiting step in androgen action.

3.4. Saturability and Stereoselectivity of Androgen Retention

Pretreatment of castrated rats with unlabeled testosterone prior to an injection of labeled hormone and comparisons of androgen retention in intact and castrated animals suggest that saturable androgen-binding sites exist in the preoptic area, septum, and amygdala (McEwen *et al.*, 1970*b*; Stern and Eisenfeld, 1971). With testosterone, as was previously shown with estradiol, brain areas which retain the most labeled hormone show the largest effects of pretreatment with unlabeled hormone (McEwen and Pfaff, 1970; McEwen *et al.*, 1970*b*). However, the percentage reduction in hormone retention found for testosterone (20–30%) was less than that found for estradiol (20–70%) (McEwen and Pfaff, 1970; McEwen *et al.*, 1970*b*).

Cyproterone, a compound with antiandrogenic activity, has been shown to reduce androgen binding in the prostate and seminal vesicle by competitive inhibition (Liao and Fang, 1969; Stern and Eisenfeld, 1969) (Fig. 12). Whalen *et al.* (1969) found no effect of this synthetic steroid on testosterone retention in the brain. However, later studies reported a decreased retention of testosterone in the preoptic area, septum, and amygdala (McEwen *et al.*, 1970*b*; Stern and Eisenfeld, 1971; Sar and Stumpf, 1973*c*) and of dihydrotestosterone in the preoptic–hypothalamic area (Stern and Eisenfeld, 1971).

The specificity of androgen retention was tested by injecting a variety of unlabeled steroids before an injection of [^{3}H]testosterone. Pretreatment with 2.5 mg of progesterone (5 min before an injection of [^{3}H]testosterone) was less effective in reducing the retention of labeled androgens than pretreatment with 60 μg of unlabeled testosterone (Stern and Eisenfeld, 1971). On the other hand, 1 mg of unlabeled estradiol and 1 mg of unlabeled testosterone were equally effective in reducing testosterone retention if given 30 min before the labeled hormone (McEwen *et al.*, 1972*b*). The latter results could be due to the existence of common binding sites for estrogens and androgens or to the metabolism of testosterone to an estrogen and subsequent binding to "estrophilic" marcromolecule (Naftolin *et al.*, 1972).

3.5. Androgen-Binding Macromolecules

Although tissue retention experiments indicate the presence of a small number of androgen-binding sites in the brain, there is little biochemical evidence demonstrating the existence of specific androgen-binding macromolecules. Kahwanago *et al.* (1970), using the same techniques they had used studying estradiol, found no evidence for macromolecular binding of androgens *in vitro* to cytosol fractions from bovine basal hypothalamus. On the other hand, Jouan *et al.* (1971) reported androgen binding to soluble macromolecules in the rat hypothalamus after *in vivo* and *in vitro* administration of labeled testosterone. However, under the conditions of their experiment only a small portion of the binding was saturable by testosterone (12%), dihydrotestosterone (28%), or androstenedione (10%). Furthermore, only 30% of the labeled material extracted from the macromolecular fraction could be accounted for by labeled testosterone, dihydrotestosterone, or androstenedione.

After an *in vivo* injection of [^{3}H]testosterone, no nuclear concentration of radioactivity was found in any of the brain regions studied. Also, there were only small regional differences in the amount of radioactivity retained by the nuclear fraction, although the nuclear pellet from the preoptic–hypothalamic area had the highest concentration of radioactivity (Zigmond and McEwen, 1970; McEwen *et al.*, 1972*b*). Preliminary results using labeled testosterone with a higher specific activity than previously available and castrated–adrenalectomized rats suggest that nuclei from the preoptic–hypothalamic area do contain slightly more androgen-binding sites than nuclei from the cerebral cortex (Zigmond, Gerlach, and McEwen, unpublished observations).

These biochemical results are compatible with the idea that there are fewer androgen- than estrogen-binding sites in the brain and/or that the macromolecular binding of androgens is weaker than that of estrogens and perhaps is disrupted by the biochemical techniques currently in use. Results from autoradiographic studies lead to similar conclusions. For instance, the percentage of labeled cells in the hypothalamus and the density of grains per labeled cell were lower after an injection of [^{3}H]testosterone than after [^{3}H]estradiol (Tuohimaa, 1971). Although nuclear concentration of grains was seen autoradiographically after [^{3}H]testosterone, a higher percentage of the grains were found over the cytoplasm and extracellular space than after [^{3}H]estradiol (Stumpf, 1970*b*; Sar and Stumpf, 1973*a*). It should also be noted that in their study on androgen localization Stumpf and coworkers used a higher dose of labeled hormone and a longer exposure period than in their earlier study on estrogen localization (Stumpf, 1970*b*; Sar and Stumpf, 1973*a*).

3.6. Androgen Retention in Birds

A number of studies have been published on sites of androgen retention in the avian brain. After an injection of labeled testosterone in the castrated

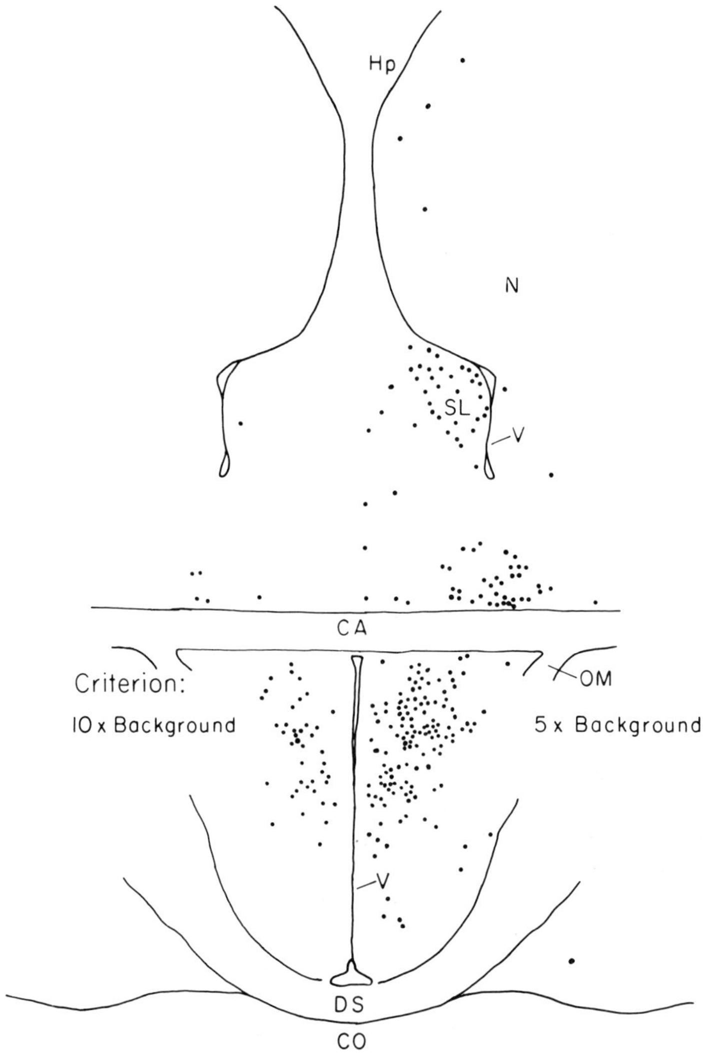

FIG. 14. Distribution of labeled cells in the hypothalamus and septum of the chaffinch 1 h after an injection of [^{3}H]testosterone. On the right-hand side of the figure, each dot represents a cell body over which the density of silver grains was 5 times the density over the surrounding neuropil. On the left-hand side, the criterion for a labeled cell was set at 10 times "background." Abbreviations: CA, anterior commissure; CO, optic chiasm; DS, supraoptic decussation; Hp, hippocampus; N, neostriatum; OM, tractus occipitomesencephalicus; SL, lateral septum; V, ventricle. From Zigmond (unpublished).

ring dove, both testosterone and dihydrotestosterone were more concentrated in the hypothalamus than in the cerebrum or plasma (Stern, 1972). These differences were abolished by pretreatment with unlabeled testosterone, but unlabeled corticosterone had no effect. Subcellular fractionation studies showed an enrichment of radioactivity in nuclei isolated from the hypothalamus (Zigmond *et al.*, 1972*a*). The concentration of radioactivity was 14 times higher in nuclei isolated from this area than in those isolated from the cerebrum.

Androgen-concentrating cells were studied autoradiographically in the chaffinch 1 h after an intramuscular injection (Zigmond *et al.*, 1972*b*, 1973). At this time, essentially all the radioactivity present in brain cell nuclei was identified as testosterone and dihydrotestosterone—the two steroids being present in approximately equal amounts. Labeled cells were found particularly in the medial preoptic area, medial hypothalamus, lateral septum, and the nucleus intercollicularis, an area in the midbrain (Figs. 14, 15 and 16). Grain counting showed that quantitative differences existed among these regions. Thus cells were more heavily labeled in the hypothalamus than in the septum (Fig. 14).

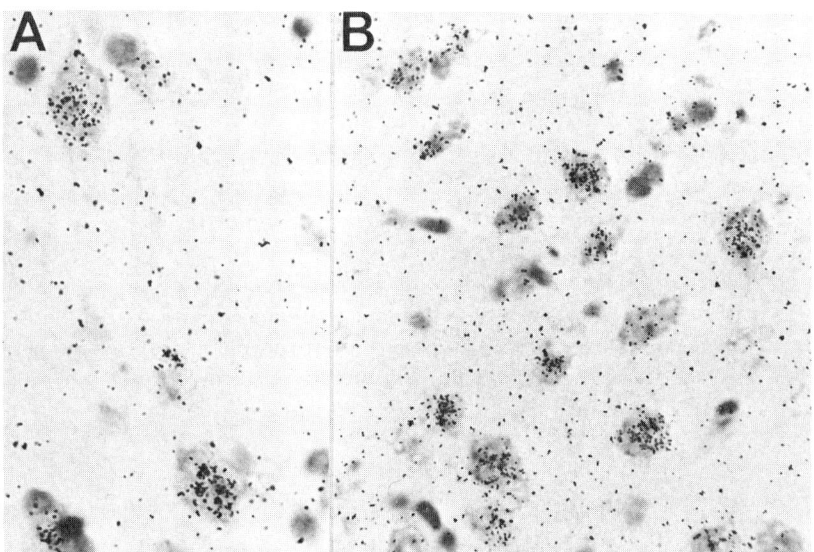

FIG. 15. Autoradiograms of the nucleus intercollicularis from the midbrain of a male chaffinch. Two days after castration, 0.46 μg of [^{3}H]testosterone was injected into the breast muscle. An hour later, the brain was removed and frozen. Unfixed and unembedded sections 6 μm thick were cut at $-19\,^{\circ}$C. Sections from which these photographs were taken were exposed for 96 days and then developed, fixed, and stained with cresyl violet. A: ×690; B: ×525. From Zigmond *et al.* (1973), copyright by the American Association for the Advancement of Science.

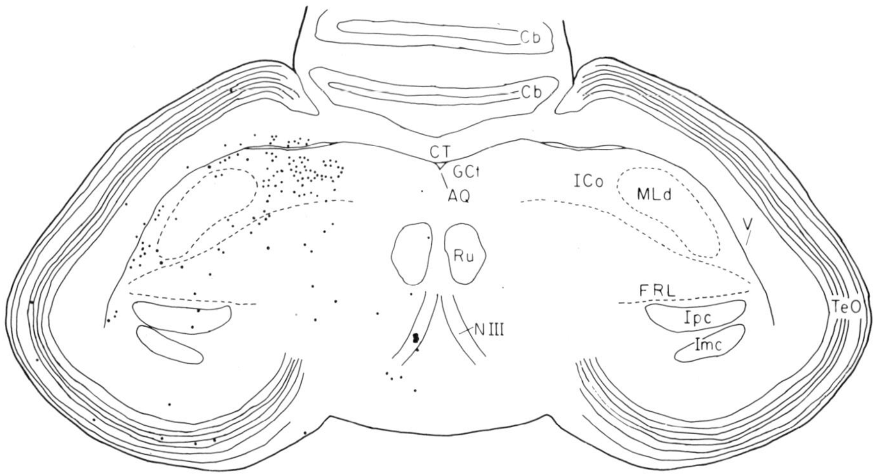

FIG. 16. Distribution of labeled cell bodies in a section through the midbrain of a chaffinch 1 h after an injection of [^{3}H]testosterone. Each dot represents the location of a cell body containing 5 times the density of grains found between cell bodies. Abbreviations: AQ, aqueductus cerebri; Cb, cerebellum; CT, commissura tectalis; FRL, formatio reticularis lateralis mesencephali; GCt, substantia grisea centralis; ICo, nucleus intercollicularis; Imc, nucleus isthmi, pars magnocellularis; Ipc, nucleus isthmi, pars parvocellularis; MLd, nucleus mesencephalicus lateralis, pars dorsalis; NIII, nervus oculomotorius; Ru, nucleus ruber; TeO, tectum opticum; V, ventriculus. From Zigmond *et al.* (1973), copyright by the American Association for the Advancement of Science.

Labeled cells have also been found in the chick brain after injection of [^{3}H]testosterone (Meyer, 1973). The nucleus preopticus paraventricularis magnocellularis had the highest proportion of labeled cells and also the highest mean density of grains per cell. No decrease in the number of grains per cell occurred in this nucleus from 30 min to 3 h after the administration of the radioactive hormone, indicating long-term retention. At this later time, labeled cells were also found in the supraoptic and paraventricular nuclei, the medial preoptic area, the anterior hypothalamus, the medial posterior hypothalamus, and the nucleus rotundus.

3.7. Comparison of Sites of Androgen Binding and Androgen Action in the Adult

Male reproductive behavior in many species is dependent on testicular androgens. In the rat, for instance, castration results in the gradual decreased appearance of the mounting, intromission, and ejaculatory patterns characteristic of the normal male. These changes can be prevented or reversed by peripheral injections of testosterone (Beach, 1948). Copulatory behavior can also be restored by direct implantation of testosterone propionate into the preoptic–anterior hypothalamic area (Davidson, 1966; Lisk, 1967; Johnston and Davidson, 1972). Compared to the implants of estrogen necessary to stimulate sexual behavior in the gonadectomized female rat; larger implants of androgen are required in the male. This difference may be related to a difference in the strength of binding of the two hormones in the brain (see Section 3.5). The preoptic area is also an important site of action of testosterone in promoting reproductive behavior in male chicks, chickens, and ring doves (for review, see Hutchinson, 1975) (Fig. 17). Studies in spinal rats and dogs indicate that, in addition to acting in the brain, testosterone can act on the spinal cord (Hart, 1967, 1968; Hart and Haugen, 1968). As yet, no studies on testosterone retention in the spinal cord have been reported.

Implantation studies suggest that, in addition to these behavioral effects, androgens act in the brain to inhibit the secretion of gonadotropins by the pituitary gland (Davidson, 1969). In the rat, duck, and Japanese quail, implants were most effective in the medial basal hypothalamus (i.e., the arcuate nucleus in rats) (Gogan, 1968; Davidson, 1969). As with comparable experiments implanting estrogens, it is difficult to rule out the possibility that the hormone is leaking into the portal circulation and acting directly on the pituitary gland (see Section 2.7). However, Smith and Davidson (1967) have shown that implants of testosterone in the rat hypothalamus inhibit the secretion of gonadotropins by pituitary glands which have been transplanted to the kidney capsule. Their data strongly suggest that testosterone is acting at the level of the hypothalamus.

These androgen-sensitive sites in the preoptic area and hypothalamus determined by implantation studies correlate well with known sites of androgen binding determined by autoradiography (Fig. 17). One of the strengths of the latter technique is that it can be used relatively easily to map the entire brain. Practically speaking, implantation studies are limited to investigations of circumscribed parts of the nervous system. Since in those areas of the brain where the two techniques have both been used sites of binding and sites of action overlap, it seems reasonable to use maps of androgen-concentrating cells to select areas to be studied with implants.

An example of such an area is the nucleus intercollicularis in songbirds. As shown in Fig. 16, the nucleus contains a large number of androgen-concentrating cells (Zigmond *et al.*, 1973). Other parts of the midbrain such as the adjoining nucleus mesencephalicus lateralis dorsalis contain few if any labeled cells. The results of electrical stimulation studies suggest that the nucleus intercollicularis is involved in the control of vocal behavior in a number of avian species (for references, see Zigmond *et al.*, 1973) (Fig. 18). The nucleus mesencephalicus lateralis dorsalis, on the other hand, has been shown by a number of techniques to be an auditory relay nucleus, comparable to the inferior colliculus in mammals (Fig. 18). Since a number of the vocalizations of birds are dependent on testicular androgens, it is plausible that the nucleus intercollicularis is one of the sites of androgen action in promoting vocal behavior. This hypothesis can be tested directly with androgen implants.

3.8. Androgen Binding and Action During Development

In addition to acting on the adult brain, androgenic hormones affect the development of the nervous system (for review, see Pfaff *et al.*, 1974). The presence or absence of these hormones during the first week of life greatly influences the pattern of sexual behavior and gonadotropin secretion seen in adulthood. Females injected with testosterone during this period show increased male behavior, decreased female behavior, and an acyclic pattern of gonadotropin secretion in adulthood. Males castrated during this period show increased female behavior, decreased male behavior, and (given an

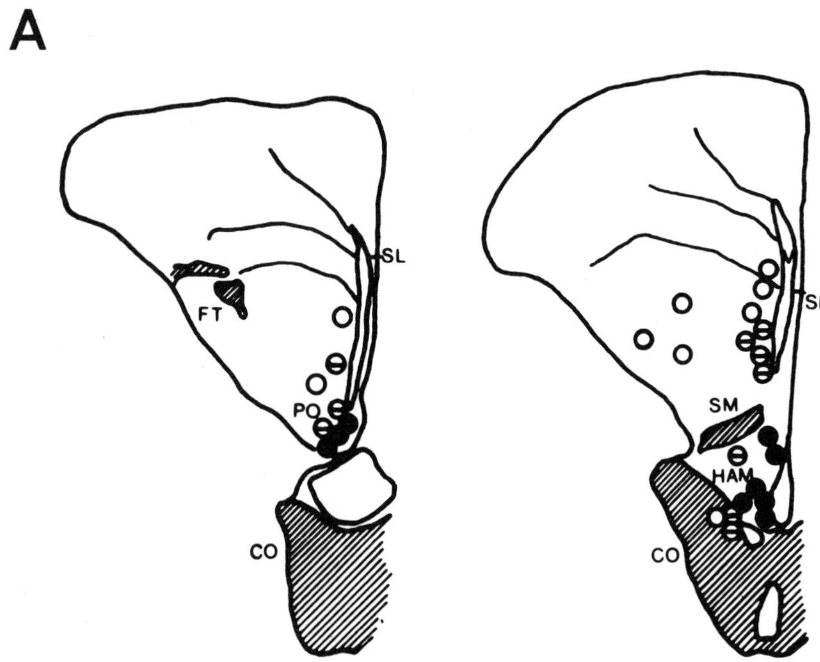

FIG. 17. Comparison of the distribution of androgen-sensitive sites and sites of androgen binding in the avian preoptic area. A: Sites of implants of testosterone propionate in castrated Barbary doves. ●, Sites from which complete courtship behavior was restored including aggressive and nest-oriented behavior; ⊖, sites from which incomplete courtship behavior was elicited lacking in either aggressive or nest-oriented behavior; ○, sites from which no change in courtship

ovarian graft) a cyclical pattern of gonadotropin secretion as adults. Evidence based on implantation studies indicates that at least one important site of testosterone action during this neonatal period is the basal hypothalamus (Nadler, 1973).

As a result of these findings, a great deal of interest has centered on the ability of the hypothalamus to bind testosterone during the first week of life. However, despite a preliminary report indicating that the neonatal hypothalamus could retain [^{3}H]testosterone and/or its metabolites to a greater extent than the neonatal cerebral cortex (Diamond and Dale, 1967), a large number of studies have been unable to replicate this result (Sheratt *et al.*, 1969; Alvarez and Ramirez, 1970; Kincl, 1970; Weisz and Philpott, 1971; Barnea *et al.*, 1972; Tuohimaa and Niemi, 1972*a*; Whitsett *et al.*, 1972; Vertes *et al.*, 1973; Heffner and van Tienhoven, 1973). In these studies, no evidence was found for regional differences in hormone retention, saturable retention in any brain region, or cytosol or nuclear binding.

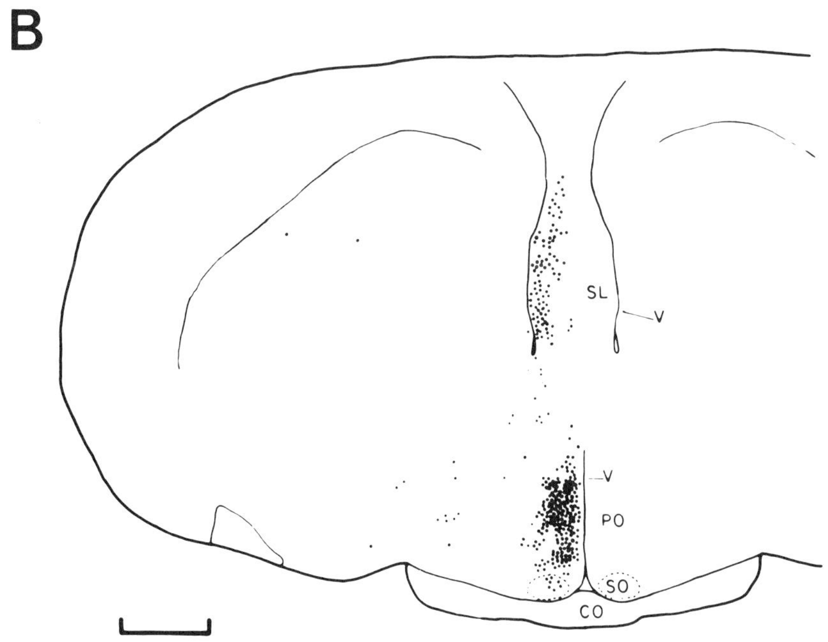

behavior was seen. B: Distribution of labeled cells in the castrated chaffinch 1 h after systemic administration of [^{3}H]testosterone. Abbreviations: CO, optic chiasm; FT, frontothalamic tract; HAM, anterior medial hypothalamic nucleus; PO, medial preoptic area; SL, lateral septal nucleus; SM, septomesencephalic tract; SO, supraoptic nucleus; V, ventricle. Scale represents 1 mm. Data from Hutchison (1970) and Zigmond (unpublished).

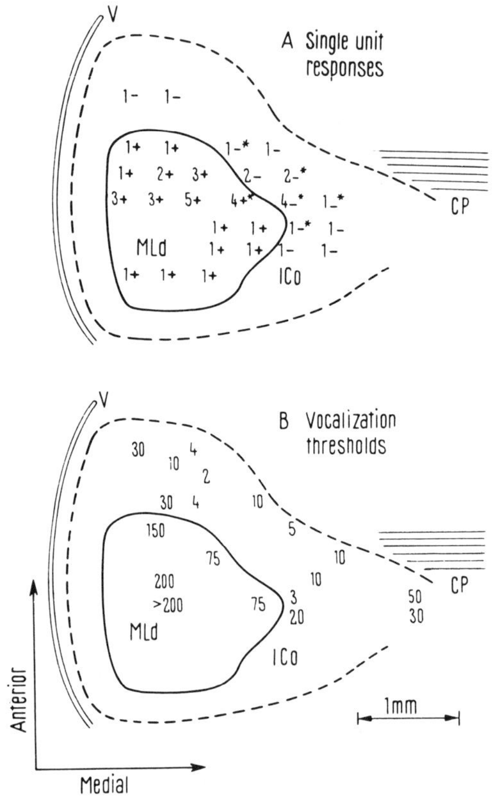

FIG. 18. Sites in the midbrain of the Japanese quail from which neurons respond to auditory stimulation and from which electrical stimulation elicits vocalizations. A: The numbers refer to the number of electrode penetrations made in an area and + or − refers to whether or not units responding to auditory stimulation were found. The region is drawn from a dorsal view. * indicates auditory units in the formatio reticularis lateralis, an area ventral to the section shown. B: The numbers refer to the threshold (μA) for eliciting vocalizations at each site. Abbreviations: CP, posterior commissure; ICo, nucleus intercollicularis; MLd, nucleus mesencephalicus lateralis. From Potash (1970), reprinted with permission.

3.9. Chemical Specificity of Androgen Action: Is There More Than One Type of Androgen Receptor in the Brain?

Following the studies referred to above on androgen metabolism by brain tissue (Section 3.3), a great deal of interest has focused on the ability of various androgens, and in particular dihydrotestosterone, to act in the central nervous system. In the rat, dihydrotestosterone was as effective as testosterone in inhibiting gonadotropin secretion by the pituitary but was only marginally effective in stimulating copulatory behavior whether injected or implanted in the brain (McDonald *et al.*, 1970*b*; McDonald, 1971; Beyer *et al.*, 1971*a*, 1972; Feder, 1971; Whalen and Luttge, 1971*c*; Johnston and Davidson, 1972). These results raise the possibility that hypothalamic receptors mediating androgen effects on behavior and on pituitary secretion differ in their chemical specificities.

The existence of two types of androgen receptors is also suggested by experiments with cyproterone. This compound antagonizes the growth-promoting effects of testosterone in the prostate gland and seminal vesicle and is known to compete with testosterone for macromolecular binding in these tissues (Liao and Fang, 1969; Stern and Eisenfeld, 1971). Cyproterone stimulated gonadotropin secretion when injected into rats or implanted directly into the medial basal hypothalamus, as would be expected if it antagonized the inhibitory feedback effects of gonadal androgens (Bloch and Davidson, 1967; von Berswordt-Wallrabe and Neumann, 1967; Davidson and Bloch, 1969). On the other hand, cyproterone showed no antiandrogenic activity in regard to male sexual behavior in the rat or guinea pig (Zucker, 1966*a*; Beach and Westbrook, 1968*a*; Whalen and Edwards, 1969; Bloch and Davidson, 1971).

Other aspects of male behavior in other species have also been shown to be unaffected by dihydrotestosterone or cyproterone. For instance, intermale fighting in mice and scent marking in gerbils can be restored in castrates by testosterone but not by dihydrotestosterone (Luttge, 1972*b*; Thiessen *et al.*, 1973). Cyproterone does not significantly reduce aggressive behavior or scent marking in intact gerbils, although a tendency in that direction is seen (Sayler, 1970).

Nevertheless, the generalization that androgen feedback receptors are stimulated by dihydrotestosterone and blocked by cyproterone while behavioral receptors are only marginally affected by either compound does not hold for all species. Studies on the guinea pig and rhesus monkey show that in these animals dihydrotestosterone can stimulate male sexual behavior in castrates (Phoenix, 1973; Goy, personal communication). Furthermore, in humans dihydrotestosterone was reported to be ineffective in inhibiting gonadotropin secretion (Sherins and Loriaux, 1973).

3.10. Role of Aromatization in Androgen Action

The effects of testosterone on male reproductive behavior and on sexual differentiation can be closely mimicked by estradiol (Gorski, 1963; Pfaff, 1970*a*; Feder *et al.*, 1974). This apparent nonspecificity also operates in the reverse direction in that testosterone can stimulate female sexual behavior in several species (rats, cats, and rabbits), even though this behavior is usually thought to be under estrogenic control (Ball, 1940; Beach, 1942*a*; Green *et al.*, 1957; Palka and Sawyer, 1966*b*; Pfaff, 1970*a,b*; Whalen and Hardy, 1970; Beyer and Komisaruk, 1971; Pfaff and Zigmond, 1971). Beach (1942*a*) suggested that the effect of testosterone on female sexual behavior may involve the hormone first being metabolized to an estrogen. Recently it has been proposed that the effects of testosterone on male behavior and on development may also involve aromatization (i.e., conversion of testosterone to an estrogenic steroid with an aromatic A ring) (McDonald *et al.*, 1970*b*; McDonald and Doughty, 1972*b*; Ryan *et al.*, 1972; Naftolin *et al.*, 1974).

Evidence supporting this hypothesis comes from three main sources:

1. Brain tissue from adult male and female rats, rabbits, and rhesus monkeys, from neonatal rats, and from human and rat fetuses can convert androstendione to estrone *in vitro* (Naftolin *et al.*, 1971*a,b*, 1972; Ryan *et al.*, 1972; Reddy *et al.*, 1973, 1974). This aromatization activity is primarily localized in the anterior hypothalamus and "limbic system" (i.e., amygdala and hippocampus). The percentage conversion in all cases is quite low (less than 0.2%). Nevertheless, as Ryan *et al.* (1972) have pointed out, estrogens are much more potent than androgens on a per weight basis and since aromatization probably takes place only in a fraction of the cells in any brain area the local concentration of estrogen may be quite high. The formation of estrone and estradiol from androstenedione has been shown to occur *in vivo* in the isolated perfused rhesus monkey brain (Flores *et al.*, 1973).
2. Not all androgens can be converted to estrogens (Ryan, 1960; Gual *et al.*, 1962) (Table 13). By comparing the ability of different androgens to stimulate both mounting and lordosis in ovariectomized rabbits, Beyer *et al.* (1970*a,b*) concluded that only aromatizable androgens increased the frequency of these behaviors. For instance, testosterone, androstenedione, and 19-hydroxyandrostenedione were effective, while dihydrotestosterone and androsterone were not. The latter two compounds have saturated A rings and do not seem to be converted to estrogens (Ryan, 1960; Gual *et al.*, 1962). A similar correlation between effective androgens and androgens which can be aromatized has been found for the stimulation of male behavior in castrated rats and for the masculinization of neonatal female rats

TABLE 13

Relative Substrate Activity of Several Androgens for Steroid Aromatization[a]

	Relative activity (%)
Testosterone	100
Androstenedione	100
19-Hydroxyandrostenedione	113
11β-Hydroxytestosterone	4
Dihydrotestosterone	0
Androstanedione	0

[a]Microsomal fractions prepared from human placenta were incubated with different androgenic steroids and the amount of phenolic estrogens formed was determined. The relative conversion rates are expressed as a percentage of the testosterone rate. Data from Ryan (1960) and Gual *et al.* (1962).

(McDonald *et al.*, 1970*b*; Feder, 1971; McDonald, 1971; Whalen and Luttge, 1971*c*; McDonald and Doughty, 1972*a*). In both instances, testosterone and androstenedione were effective while dihydrotestosterone was ineffective. 5α-Androstanediol—another nonaromatizable androgen—was also ineffective in masculinizing female rats (Gual *et al.*, 1962; Brown-Grant *et al.*, 1971). Beach and Westbrook (1968*b*) reported that fluoxymesterone (Table 10), a synthetic steroid which exhibits androgenic activity in peripheral tissues, did not stimulate male sexual behavior in castrated rats. Based on the criteria proposed by Ryan (1960) and Gual *et al.* (1962), fluoxymesterone should not be aromatized due to its 11β-hydroxyl group (Fig. 12).

3. Certain of the actions of testosterone can be antagonized by Mer-25, a compound shown to have antiestrogenic activity (see Section 2.6) (Fig. 11). Administration of Mer-25 has been shown to prevent the effects of testosterone on lordosis behavior in rats (Meyerson *et al.*, 1971) and rabbits (Beyer and Vidal, 1971) and on sexual differentiation in neonatal female rats (McDonald and Doughty, 1972*b*).

Although the idea of testosterone being a prehormone and estradiol being the active metabolite is intriguing, there are a number of points which need clarification. For instance, although the conversion of androstenedione to estrone has been demonstrated in the rat and rabbit brain, no studies have been reported on the aromatization of testosterone in this species or on the conversion of either androgen to estradiol (Naftolin *et al.*, 1974). On the other hand, most of our knowledge on the hormonal control of behavior and sexual differentiation and on the antagonistic actions of Mer-25 is based on experiments using testosterone and estradiol. Therefore, the case for the aromatization hypothesis would be strengthened by the demonstration that testosterone can be converted by the rat or rabbit brain to estradiol or another potent estrogen whose actions can be antagonized by Mer-25. Also, the distinction between aromatizable and nonaromatizable androgens is based on experiments in which these compounds were incubated with human placental tissue. These findings should be corroborated using brain tissue from rats and rabbits. Besides these general qualifications, there are also aspects of the data concerning each of the phenomena where aromatization has been invoked that require further experimentation.

a. Sexual Differentiation. Gorski (1963) found that while both testosterone and estradiol produced acyclicity when given to neonatal female rats, there were significant differences in the effects of the two hormones. Furthermore, the finding that cyproterone acetate—usually considered an antiandrogen—blocks the masculinizing effects of testosterone has been interpreted as indicating that testosterone (or an androgenic metabolite) is the active compound involved in sexual differentiation (see Pfaff *et al.*, 1974). However, Brown-Grant (1974) has reported his inability to replicate this developmental effect of cyproterone acetate and Naftolin *et al.* (1974) have reported preliminary evidence that in addition to blocking the binding of testosterone in the brain this compound can inhibit aromatization in the rabbit brain. Obviously, caution must be taken in viewing all the actions of cyproterone acetate in the brain as "antiandrogenic" and in assuming that it blocks all the effects of testosterone (see also Section 3.9).

b. Male Sexual Behavior. Exceptions to the generalization that only aromatizable androgens stimulate male sexual behavior have been found. In the castrated rhesus monkey and guinea pig, injections of dihydrotestosterone increase copulatory behavior (Phoenix, 1973; Goy, personal communication). Implants of dihydrotestosterone directly into the preoptic–anterior hypothalamic area produce a weak but significant stimulation of reproductive behavior in castrated rats (Johnston and Davidson, 1972). Furthermore, the effects of testosterone on sexual behavior in the castrated rat are not antagonized by Mer-25, suggesting that aromatization may not be involved (Whalen *et al.*, 1972).

c. Female Sexual Behavior. Although dihydrotestosterone is ineffective in stimulating female sexual behavior in ovariectomized rabbits or Sprague-Dawley rats, it is weakly effective in Wistar rats both after peripheral injection and after hypothalamic implantation (Beyer *et al.*, 1970*a*, 1971*a*; Beyer and Komisaruk, 1971).

Finally, it should be noted that the ability of different androgens and estrogens to stimulate male (or female) sexual behavior may simply reflect the stereo-selectivity of the receptors involved rather than indicate a requirement for aromatization.

4. GLUCOCORTICOIDS

4.1. Anatomical Distribution of Corticosterone Binding Sites in the Rat

In the rat, the principal glucocorticoid secreted by the adrenal gland is corticosterone (Bush, 1953) (Fig. 19). Extensive studies on the retention of this hormone in the rat brain have revealed a phenomenon of stereoselective limited-capacity binding similar to that described above for estradiol (see Section 2). The primary differences in the binding of the two hormones are in the neuroanatomical distribution and chemical specificity of the binding sites. Two hours after an injection of [^{3}H]corticosterone (0.7 μg) into adrenalectomized male rats, a higher concentration of radioactivity was found in the hippocampus and septum than in the hypothalamus, amygdala, cerebral cortex, medulla–pons, or plasma (McEwen *et al.*, 1968, 1969).

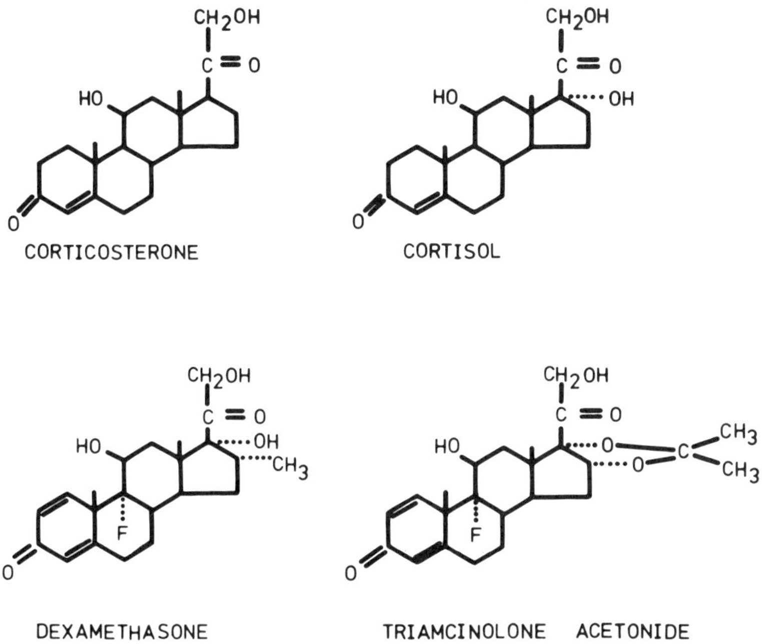

FIG. 19. Chemical structures of two naturally occurring glucocorticoids (corticosterone and cortisol) and two synthetic glucocorticoids (dexamethasone and triamcinolone acetonide).

Seventy to eighty percent of the radioactivity in the hippocampus was unmetabolized [^{3}H]corticosterone, as judged by thin-layer chromatography. Slightly more radioactivity was found in the dorsal than in the ventral hippocampus.

A more precise anatomical description of the distribution of corticosterone in the brain has been achieved using autoradiographic techniques (Gerlach and McEwen, 1972; Stumpf and Sar, 1973; Warembourg, 1973). One hour after a subcutaneous injection of [^{3}H]corticosterone, reduced silver grains were found concentrated over cell bodies in discrete parts of the brain, with the pyramidal cells of the hippocampus being particularly heavily labeled (Fig. 20A). Corticosterone was more concentrated in the pyramidal cells of regions CA_1 and CA_2 than in regions CA_3 and CA_4, but most neurons throughout the hippocampus were clearly labeled. As in the biochemical experiments mentioned above, retention was somewhat higher in the dorsal than in the ventral hippocampus. The granule cells of the dentate gyrus and cells in the subiculum were also labeled (Gerlach and McEwen, 1972; Stumpf and Sar, 1973; Warembourg, 1973). Heavily labeled cells were found in the septum—particularly the hippocampal, dorsal, and lateral septal nuclei—and in the precommissural hippocampus (Fig. 20A).

Less heavily labeled cells were found in the anterior olfactory nucleus (particularly the lateral and dorsal parts), the amygdala (in the medial and cortical nuclei and the medial part of the basal nucleus), and the amygdalocortico transition zone (Fig. 20B). Certain portions of the cerebral cortex also contain cells which concentrated corticosterone, particularly the entorhinal cortex, the indusium griseum, the periamygdaloid cortex, and the pyriform cortex (Warembourg, 1973).

Ependymal cells were not labeled. Interestingly, in comparison to the distribution of cells which concentrate gonadal steroids only a few scattered, weakly labeled cells were found in the bed nucleus of the stria terminalis or in the medial hypothalamus (Warembourg, 1973).

4.2. Saturability and Stereoselectivity of Corticosterone Retention

In contrast to these results in adrenalectomized rats, no difference was found between the concentrations of [^{3}H]corticosterone in the hippocampus

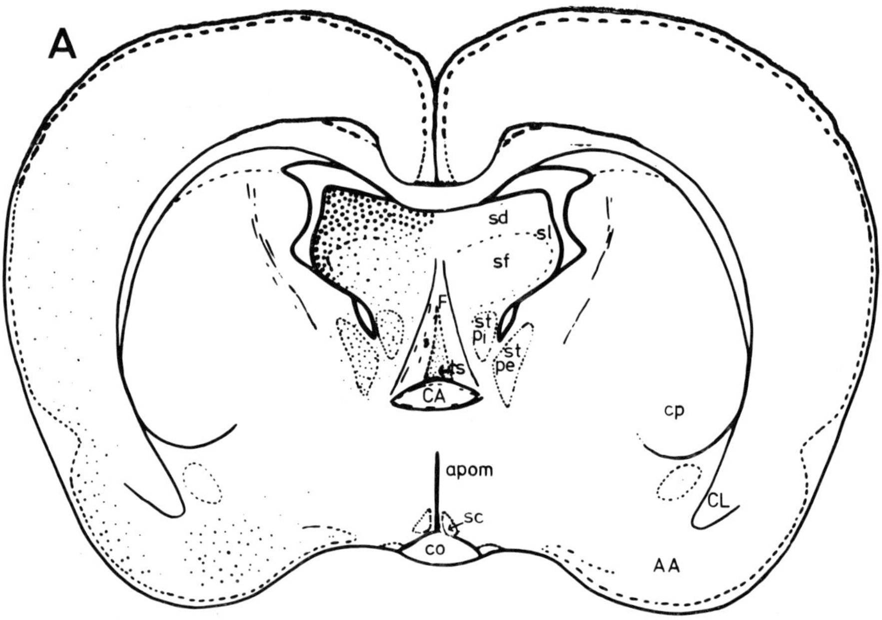

FIG. 20A,B. Two frontal sections showing the distribution of labeled cells after an injection of [^{3}H]corticosterone. Abbreviations: AA, anterior amygdaloid area; ac, central amygdaloid nucleus; aco, cortical amygdaloid nucleus; ar, arcuate nucleus; al, lateral amygdaloid nucleus; am, medial amygdaloid nucleus; apom, medial preoptic nucleus, anterior part; CA, anterior commissure; CA_1, CA_2, parts of Ammon's horn; CL, claustrum; co, optic chiasm; cp, caudate

and cerebral cortex in intact rats, suggesting that circulating corticosterone may saturate the binding sites in the hippocampus and block the retention of exogenously administered hormone (McEwen *et al.*, 1969). This idea was supported by the finding that unlabeled corticosterone (3 mg) injected 30 min prior to a tracer dose of [^{3}H]corticosterone (0.7 μg) reduced the retention of labeled hormone in the hippocampus and abolished the difference in hormone retention between the hippocampus and cerebral cortex (McEwen *et al.*, 1969). (In contrast, the retention of corticosterone by the septum is not saturated in the intact animal and is less influenced by the prior injection of unlabeled hormone.) Dexamethasone (3 mg), a potent synthetic glucocorticoid, was equally effective as corticosterone in decreasing hippocampal retention, while cortisol (hydrocortisone) at the same dose was less effective (Fig. 19). Knizley (1972) confirmed the finding that corticosterone retention in the brain was highest in the hippocampus and septum and found that hippocampal sites were partially saturated by an injection of 20 μg of corticosterone.

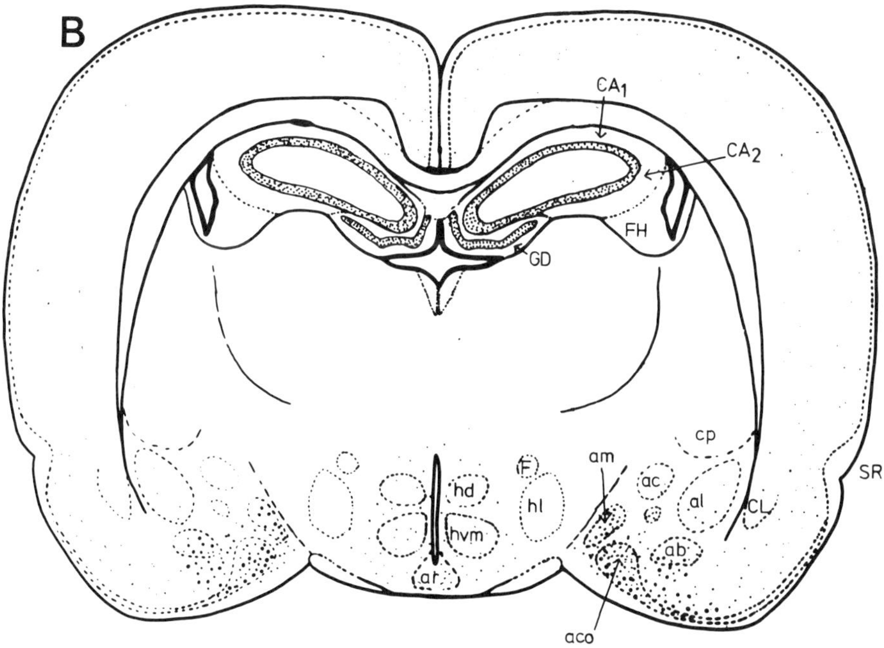

putamen; F, fornix; FH, hippocampal fimbria; GD, dentate gyrus; hd, dorsomedial hypothalamic nucleus; hvm, ventromedial hypothalamic nucleus; sc, suprachiasmatic nucleus; sd, dorsal septal nucleus; sf, septofimbrial nucleus; sl, lateral septal nucleus; SR, rhinal sulcus; stpi, stria terminalis, internal part; stpe, stria terminalis, external part; ts, nucleus trinagularis septi. Modified from Warembourg (1973).

4.3. Subcellular Distribution of Corticosterone

Subcellular fractionation of hippocampus from adrenalectomized rats showed the highest concentration of radioactivity in a purified nuclear pellet (McEwen *et al.*, 1970*c*) (Fig. 21). Thirty-six percent of the radioactivity in the whole homogenate could be accounted for by nuclear binding, and more than 90% of the radioactivity in the nuclear pellet cochromatographed with authentic corticosterone. Retention of corticosterone by cell nuclei in the hippocampus reached a maximum 1 h after an injection and declined to a low level by 4 h (McEwen *et al.*, 1970*c*; McEwen and Wallach, 1973).

Experiments in which animals were pretreated with a number of different steroids demonstrated both the saturability and the stereoselectivity of corticosterone retention by hippocampal cell nuclei. At a dose of

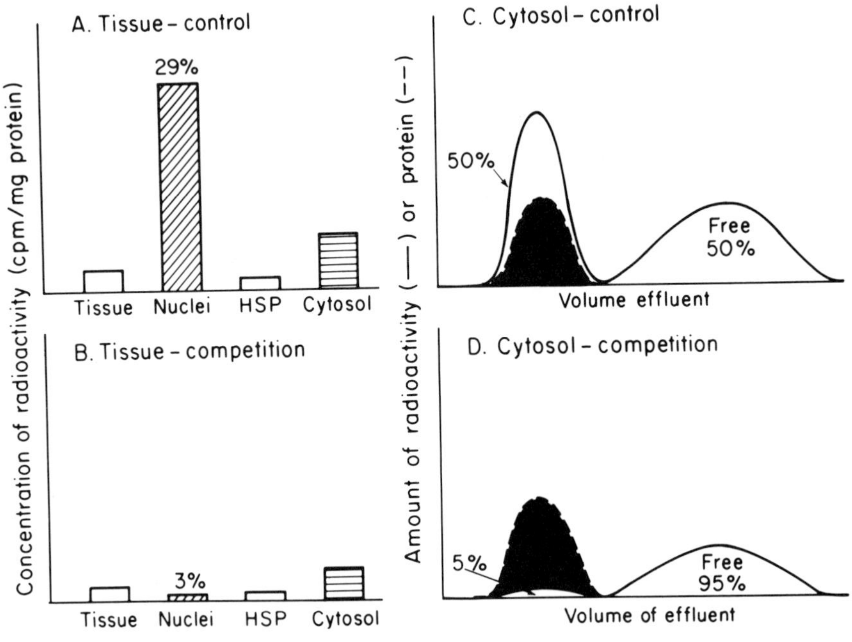

FIG. 21. Distribution of [^{3}H]corticosterone in hippocampus 1 h after a systemic injection to an adrenalectomized rat. The subcellular localization of the labeled hormone is shown in (A) and the effect of a prior injection of unlabeled corticosterone is shown in (B). The gel filtration pattern of labeled cytosol is shown in (C) and the effect of pretreatment with unlabeled hormone on this pattern is shown in (D). In C and D, the dark area represents protein distribution and the clear zone represents radioactivity. "Free" refers to [^{3}H]corticosterone not bound to a macromolecular component, "Tissue" to whole homogenate, "Nuclei" to purified nuclear pellet, "HSP" to high-speed (100,000*g* for 60 min) pellet, "Cytosol" to high-speed supernatant. From McEwen *et al.* (1971), reprinted with permission of the Regents of the University of California.

0.5 mg unlabeled corticosterone but not dexamethasone, cortisol, or desoxycorticosterone inhibited this retention (McEwen *et al.*, 1970*c*) (Fig. 21). Also, less corticosterone was retained by hippocampal nuclei in intact than in adrenalectomized animals, suggesting competition from endogenous glucocorticoids.

Nuclear localization of corticosterone has also been shown autoradiographically, particularly in the labeled neurons of the hippocampus and cortex (Gerlach and McEwen, 1972; Stumpf and Sar, 1973; Warembourg, 1973). Within the nucleus, the nucleolus does not seem to be labeled (McEwen and Pfaff, 1973). Pretreatment with 3 mg of unlabeled corticosterone virtually abolished the nuclear labeling of hippocampal pyramidal cells (McEwen and Pfaff, 1973).

In addition to the nuclear pellet, the high-speed supernatant fraction also contained a high concentration of corticosterone (McEwen *et al.*, 1970*c*). Lemaire *et al.* (1974) studied the distribution of [^{3}H]corticosterone in soluble and particulate fractions prepared from the hippocampus and cortex after intravenous infusion of the hormone into adrenalectomized rats for a period of 45 min. Different doses of the hormone were given and the plasma corticosterone concentrations were measured at the time of sacrifice in order to correlate the extent of binding with the level of the hormone circulating in the blood. Both the supernatant and particulate fractions from the cerebral cortex showed a linear increase in concentration of corticosterone with increasing plasma levels over the range of 4–30 μg/100 ml. However, comparable fractions from the hippocampus showed complete saturation of the binding within this range, indicating that circulating levels of corticosterone comparable to those found in the intact animal can saturate the binding sites in the hippocampus (Fig. 22).

4.4. Corticosterone-Binding Macromolecules in the Nucleus and Cytoplasm *in Vivo*

By use of the technique of gel filtration, corticosterone binding to macromolecules both in the high-speed supernatant (Grosser *et al.*, 1971; McEwen *et al.*, 1971; Stevens *et al.*, 1971) and in the nuclear fraction (McEwen and Plapinger, 1970) was demonstrated after *in vivo* administration of the hormone (Fig. 21). As would be expected, more macromolecular binding was found in the hippocampus and septum than in other brain regions (McEwen *et al.*, 1971; Stevens *et al.*, 1971). Enzymatic digestion studies indicated that the macromolecules involved were protein or at least had a protein component which was essential for the binding. Thus addition of proteolytic enzymes to cytosol or nuclear fractions which were prepared from rats previously injected with [^{3}H]corticosterone released the bound hormone while deoxyribonuclease, ribonuclease, neuraminidase, and alkaline phosphatase left the binding unaffected (McEwen and Plapinger, 1970; McEwen *et al.*, 1972*a*).

Since corticosterone is bound in the blood to the protein transcortin, it was important to determine to what extent protein binding in the brain was due to residual blood. Perfusion of the brain does in fact reduce the amount of cytosol (although not nuclear) binding (McEwen *et al.*, 1972*a*). Nonetheless, the existence of a corticosterone-binding protein distinct from transcortin has been demonstrated by polyacrylamide gel electrophoresis and protamine sulfate precipitation (McEwen *et al.*, 1972*a*). The cytosol-binding protein (although not the serum-binding protein) is precipitated by protamine sulfate, suggesting that it is an acidic protein (see Steggles and King, 1970, for the first use of this method to study steroid-binding proteins).

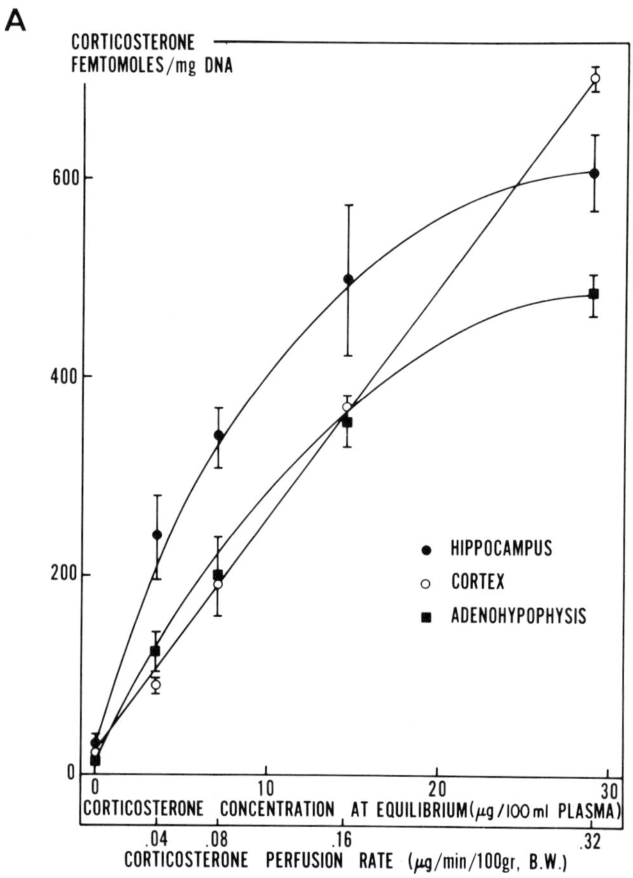

FIG. 22. Binding of [^{3}H]corticosterone to supernatant (A) and particulate (B) fractions following intravenous perfusion of the labeled hormone for 45 min. The perfusion rate and

Cytosol binding of [^{3}H]corticosterone, like nuclear binding, is greatly reduced by pretreatment with a large dose of unlabeled hormone and is higher in adrenalectomized than in intact rats (Grosser *et al.*, 1971; McEwen *et al.*, 1971) (Fig. 21). During the first few hours after adrenalectomy, the increase in cytosol binding of exogenous corticosterone seems inversely related to the disappearance curve for endogenous corticosterone (McEwen *et al.*, 1971). As mentioned in the section on estradiol, changes in hormone binding in different endocrine conditions may be due not only to changes in endogenous hormone levels but also to changes in the number of binding macromolecules. This possibility is strengthened in the case of corticosterone binding by the finding that the ability of the hippocampus to bind corticosterone continues even after all endogenous hormone has disappeared (McEwen *et al.*, 1969, 1973*b*). Binding of corticosterone mac-

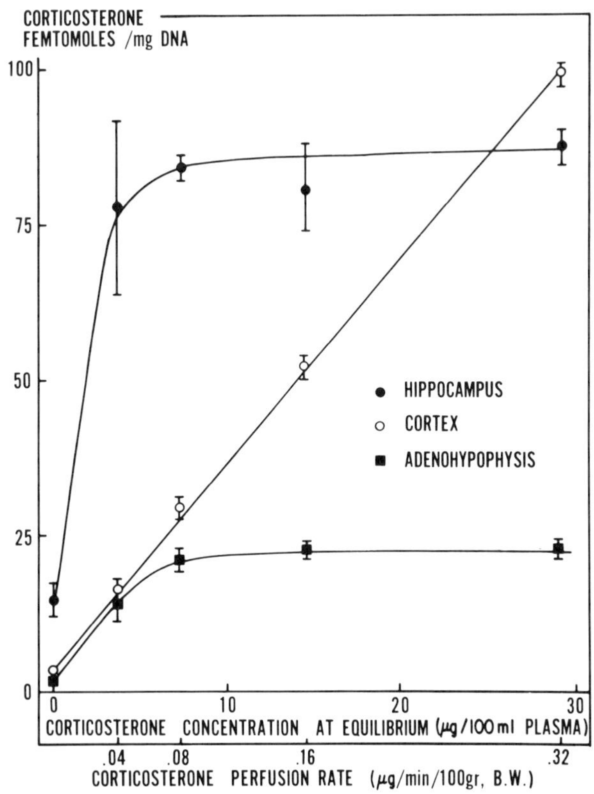

the resulting plasma corticosterone levels measured at the end of the perfusion are given. The data are the means ± SE for four determinations. From Lemaire *et al.* (1974), reprinted with permission.

romolecules in the cytosol shows considerable stereoselectivity. Pretreatment with 3 mg of progesterone, testosterone, or estradiol had no effect, cortisol and cortisone partially inhibited the binding, and 11-dehydrocorticosterone was as effective as unlabeled corticosterone (Grosser *et al.*, 1971).

4.5. Corticosterone Binding *in Vitro*

In vitro methods have been employed to study corticosterone binding in more detail. Incubating cytosol fractions prepared from whole brain with labeled corticosterone and then separating free from bound hormone by gel filtration, Grosser *et al.* (1973) estimated that the dissociation constant of the protein–hormone complex was 2.7×10^{-10} M and that the binding capacity of the fraction was 0.47 pmol of corticosterone per milligram of protein. McEwen and Wallach (1973) estimated the same parameters using a charcoal absorption method for removing free steroid and reported a somewhat higher dissociation constant (2.3×10^{-9} M) and a binding capacity

TABLE 14

Specificity of [^{3}H]Corticosterone Binding to Cytosol Proteins in Vitro[a]

Competing steroid	Percent inhibition
Corticosterone	84
Cortisol	75
Desoxycorticosterone	77
11β-Hydroxyprogesterone	66
Progesterone	66
11-Deoxycortisol	50
Dexamethasone	47
Aldosterone	35
Cortisol-21-acetate	31
11α-Corticosterone	23
Testosterone	13
11-Dehydrocorticosterone	10
17β-Estradiol	4

[a]Cytosol fractions prepared from perfused brains of adrenalectomized rats were incubated for 30 min at 4 °C with 6×10^{-9} M [^{3}H]corticosterone and a 25-fold greater concentration of unlabeled steroids. [^{3}H]Corticosterone binding was assayed by gel filtration on Sephadex G25. Data from Grosser *et al.* (1973).

of 0.58 pmol/mg protein. They also found the binding to be partially inhibited by sulfhydryl-group blocking agents (McEwen and Wallach, 1973).

Grosser *et al.* (1973) tested the ability of a large number of steroids to inhibit the binding of corticosterone *in vitro* (Table 14). The main differences between these *in vitro* data and the *in vivo* data published by the same laboratory (Grosser *et al.*, 1971) are that 11-dehydrocorticosterone was effective in inhibiting corticosterone binding only *in vivo* while progesterone was effective only *in vitro.* The authors suggest that the first discrepancy might be due to the *in vivo* conversion of 11-dehydrocorticosterone to corticosterone (Grosser *et al.*, 1973).

When cytosol fractions were prepared from intact rats at 4-h intervals throughout the day, their ability to bind corticosterone *in vitro* was inversely related to the circulating level of corticosterone at the time of sacrifice (Stevens *et al.*, 1973). This result is consistent with the observation of McEwen *et al.* (1972*a*) that corticosterone bound *in vivo* to soluble proteins is not easily displaced *in vitro.*

Retention of labeled corticosterone by cell nuclei has also been demonstrated *in vitro* in slices of hippocampus. Nuclear retention was maximal at 25 °C, was not affected by inhibitors of respiration or glycolysis, and was not greatly diminished by subsequent addition of unlabeled corticosterone (McEwen and Wallach, 1973).

4.6. Experiments on Other Glucocorticoids and Other Species

4.6.1. Cortisol

While most of our knowledge of glucocorticoid binding in the brain comes from experiments with [^{3}H]corticosterone and adrenalectomized rats, a number of experiments have been reported on the retention of labeled cortisol. Except where indicated, these studies have been performed on animals with intact adrenal glands.

Peterson and Chaikoff (1963) injected different amounts of [^{14}C]cortisol into rats and found a linear relationship between the amounts of radioactivity in brain and plasma. In the dog, 15 min to 24 h after an injection of [^{3}H]cortisol, the concentration of radioactivity was at least 10 times higher in the hypothalamus than in the cerebral cortex or plasma (Eik-Nes and Brizee, 1965). In contrast to this, in the pig the ratio of concentraction of radioactivity in brain to plasma was 0.4 for both hypothalamus and cerebral cortex (Bottoms *et al.*, 1969).

Subcellular fractionation of the cat brain followed by equilibrium dialysis of the fractions indicated that cortisol is bound in a crude nuclear fraction (Fontana *et al.*, 1970). Nuclear and cytosol binding of cortisol has also been demonstrated in the brains of adrenalectomized rats (Grosser *et al.*, 1971; McEwen and Wallach, 1973) and in the chick retina (Chader, 1973).

The rat brain bound half as much cortisol as corticosterone (Grosser *et al.*, 1971; McEwen and Wallach, 1973), although the anatomical distributions of the cells that bind the two glucocorticoids were similar (Stumpf and Sar, 1973). Since corticosterone is the main adrenal steroid in the rat, the possibility remains that cortisol binding might be stronger than corticosterone binding in an animal that had higher circulating levels of cortisol (e.g., hamster, dog, cat, guinea pig). It should be noted, however, that Warembourg (1973) failed to find any cellular retention of [^{3}H]cortisol in the guinea pig brain using an autoradiographic technique which had shown clear-cut retention of [^{3}H]corticosterone in the rat.

4.6.2. Triamcinolone and Dexamethasone

Some evidence suggests that there is more than one type of glucocorticoid binding protein in the brain. Chytil and Toft (1972) showed that the synthetic glucocorticoid triamcinolone acetonide bound *in vitro* to a cytosol macromolecule with a high affinity (dissociation constant about 10^{-9} M) and low capacity (about 0.22 pmol bound per milligram of protein) (Fig. 19). They suggested that this binding macromolecule might be the same as that which binds [^{3}H]corticosterone; however, results from competition experiments suggest a difference in the specificity of the binding. For instance, dexamethasone was as effective as unlabeled corticosterone in reducing [^{3}H]triamcinolone acetonide binding but much less effective in reducing [^{3}H]corticosterone binding (Grosser *et al.*, 1973) (Table 14).

Regional differences in the binding of [^{3}H]dexamethasone and [^{3}H]corticosterone have also been reported. In the hypothalamus, cell nuclei had a higher binding capacity for dexamethasone than for corticosterone, while in the hippocampus the reverse was true (McEwen, 1973*b*; de Kloet *et al.*, 1974). Thus more than one glucocorticoid-binding protein might exist in the brain, differing in chemical specificity and in anatomical distribution. The physiological significance of macromolecules which bind synthetic glucocorticoids remains to be determined.

4.6.3. Glucocorticoid Retention in Other Species

Rhees *et al.* (1972) found labeled cells in the hippocampus and septum of the duck brain after an injection of [^{3}H]corticosterone. Labeled cells were also found in the medial portions of the hyperstriatum dorsale and ventrale and associated with tractus quintofrontalis. The hypothalamus contained only a few labeled cells. In the duck, unlike the rat, a similar distribution of labeled cells was found using either [^{3}H]corticosterone or [^{3}H]progesterone. Binding of [^{3}H]corticosterone in the hippocampus has also been demonstrated in the hamster, mouse, and monkey (McEwen *et al.*, 1971; Gerlach *et al.*, 1974).

4.7. Metabolism of Glucocorticoids in the Brain

Glucocorticoid metabolism by neural tissue has largely been studied *in vitro*. Rat, mouse, dog, and baboon (but not guinea pig) brain tissue has been shown to convert cortisol to cortisone (Eik-Nes and Brizee, 1965; Peterson *et al.*, 1965; Sholiton *et al.*, 1965; Grosser, 1966; Grosser and Bliss, 1966; Grosser and Axelrod, 1968). The enzyme responsible, 11β-hydroxysteroid dehydrogenase (E.C. 1.1.1.146), can also oxidize corticosterone to 11-dehydroxycorticosterone and 11-hydroxyandrostenedione to adrenosterone, although these substrates are converted at a slower rate. The reactions are reversible, NADP catalyzing the oxidation reaction and NADPH catalyzing the reduction (Grosser and Bliss, 1966). In the rat, the rate of conversion of corticosterone to its 11β-reduced metabolite was found to be 10 times greater in the cerebellum and cerebral cortex than in the hypothalamus (Grosser and Bliss, 1966). In the mouse, the rate was 5 times higher in a glial tumor than in normal cerebral cortex (Grosser, 1966). The latter finding raises the interesting possibility that glial cells might participate in the inactivation of steroid hormones as they appear to do in the inactivation of certain neurotransmitters (Beart *et al.*, 1974; Schrier and Thompson, 1974).

Brain tissue from neonatal rats or baboons is also able to form acetylated metabolites of corticosterone, 11-dehydrocorticosterone, cortisol, and cortisone (Grosser and Axelrod, 1967, 1968; Purdy and Axelrod, 1968; Purdy *et al.*, 1968). The enzyme responsible, corticosteroid-21-*O*-acetyltransferase (E.C. 2.3.1.27), is located in the supernatant fraction and uses acetyl CoA as the acetate donor. Although the transferase reaction is essentially irreversible, the acetate groups can be removed by cholinesterase, the latter reaction being blocked by physostigmine. A decrease in the activity of corticosteroid-21-*O*-acetyltransferase with age was found in both the rat and baboon.

The biochemical and physiological importance of these reactions *in vivo* still must be evaluated. Brain perfusion offers one approach to the study of hormone metabolism *in vivo* (Axelrod, 1971). In a preliminary study using a perfusion technique, Axelrod (1971) demonstrated the activity of the 11β-hydroxysteroid dehydrogenase *in vivo*.

4.8. Measurements of Endogenous Glucocorticoids in the Nervous System

Endogenous glucocorticoids have been measured in neural tissue from a number of species. Cortisone and cortisol have been identified in human cerebrospinal fluid, and the latter hormone has been found in human postmortem tissue from the peripheral and central nervous system (Baron and Abelson, 1954; Touchstone *et al.*, 1963, 1966). Henkin *et al.* (1968)

found approximately equal concentrations of corticosterone and cortisol (30 μg/100 g) in the cat brain. The concentrations of the steroids were about 30 times higher in brain than in serum. Much lower levels of corticosterone have been reported for the mouse and rat brain (0.5–2.7 μg/100 g) (Butte *et al.*, 1972). In the latter two species, the concentration of corticosterone was 3–4 times higher in plasma than in brain.

Butte *et al.* (1972) found the endogenous concentrations of corticosterone in the hippocampus, hypothalamus, and brain stem to be about the same. The reason for the discrepancy between these results and those from studies using [^{3}H]corticosterone in adrenalectomized rats can be resolved only by further experimentation. It should be noted, however, that the regional differences in total [^{3}H]corticosterone retained were quite small (McEwen *et al.*, 1968, 1969; Knizley, 1972) and that the large variation found in the measurement of endogenous corticosterone might obscure similar regional differences. The unequal anatomical distribution of bound [^{3}H]corticosterone was much clearer when the nuclear or cytosol fractions were examined, and thus a study of the endogenous level of corticosterone in subcellular fractions from different regions would be useful.

4.9. Correlations Between Corticosterone Binding and Corticosterone Action

The relationship between corticosterone binding and corticosterone action in the brain is not at all obvious at the present time. Based on implantation studies, one might have predicted a concentration of glucocorticoid binding sites in the hypothalamus much as was found for estrogens and androgens. Implants of corticosterone, cortisol, and dexamethasone in the hypothalamus have been shown to inhibit the secretion of ACTH by the pituitary under a number of conditions (for a summary of these studies, see McEwen *et al.*, 1972*b*; Stumpf and Sar, 1973). However, the physiological significance of these implant studies is a matter of some controversy (Kendall, 1971). In addition, corticosterone implants in the hippocampus and amygdala—areas of high corticosterone retention—also affect the pituitary–adrenal axis (Kawakami *et al.*, 1968).

The behavioral effects of corticosterone on extinction of avoidance behavior, suppression of paradoxical sleep, and sensory perception have only recently received much attention and little is known about the areas of the nervous system responsible for these effects (for references, see McEwen, 1973*b*). Thus it is impossible at present to evaluate the possible role of hormone-binding sites in these processes.

Besides implantation, iontophoresis has been used in an attempt to localize glucocorticoid-sensitive cells in the brain. Many cells in the hypothalamus and septum were found to change their firing rate after direct application of dexamethasone phosphate. Cells in the dorsal hippocampus, cortex, and thalamus showed no response (Ruf and Steiner, 1967; Steiner *et al.*, 1969; Steiner, 1971). Since these electrophysiological changes occurred within seconds after administration of dexamethasone, it is quite plausible that they result from an interaction of the steroid with the cell membrane rather than with a cytoplasmic or nuclear binding protein.

Electrophysiological changes have also been detected in neurons in the hypothalamus and limbic systems after systemic administration of glucocorticoids. One result which is particularly intriguing in terms of hormone binding was the finding that a long-lasting inhibition of unit activity occurs in the dorsal hippocampus in hypophysectomized animals beginning 10–40 min after an intraperitoneal injection of corticosterone and lasting for 2 h after the injection (Pfaff *et al.*, 1971). However, since the hormone was administered systemically its site of action is unclear.

From this brief summary, it can be seen that in the development of our knowledge of the effects of corticosterone in the brain a rather complete description of the binding of the hormone has preceded similarly extensive studies on its sites of action. One might hope that in this instance—perhaps more so than in the case of estradiol and testosterone—the biochemical and histochemical data on hormone localization will serve a predictive function to stimulate future behavioral and neuroendocrine work.

5. PROGESTINS

5.1. Regional Differences in the Retention of Progesterone

Progesterone enters the brain rapidly after a peripheral injection, reaching its maximum concentration within 3 min (Laumas and Farooq, 1966; Raisinghani *et al.*, 1968). One hour after administration of labeled progesterone to ovariectomized rats, the highest concentration of radioactivity in the brain was found in the midbrain and in the pontine reticular formation (Whalen and Luttge, 1971*a,b*). The hypothalamus contained less radioactivity per milligram wet weight than these caudal structures, but more than the cerebral cortex (Seiki *et al.*, 1968, 1969; Seiki and Hattori, 1971; Whalen and Luttge, 1971*a,b*). The midbrain also showed high retention of progesterone and its metabolites in ovariectomized guinea pigs, hamsters, and mice (Wade and Feder, 1972*a,b*; Wade *et al.*, 1973; Luttge *et al.*, 1973).

The retention of progesterone differed in the guinea pig and in the rat in three aspects. First, after an injection of labeled progesterone 60–70% of the radioactivity was unmetabolized [^{3}H]progesterone in the guinea pig, while in the rat only 20–30% remained as progesterone (Wade and Feder, 1972*a*; Wade *et al.*, 1973). Second, the guinea pig retained progesterone longer than the rat (Wade *et al.*, 1973). Finally, the guinea pig had a higher concentration of [^{3}H]progesterone in the brain than in the plasma, while the rat did not (Wade and Feder, 1972*a*; Wade *et al.*, 1973).

5.2. Progesterone Metabolism *in Vivo* and *in Vitro*

Following *in vivo* administration of progesterone, 3α-hydroxy-5α-pregnan-20-one has been identified in the rat brain and a metabolite with the chromatographic mobility of pregnanedione (5α-pregnane-3,20-dione) has been found in the guinea pig (Raisinghani *et al.*, 1968; Wade and Feder, 1972*a*). Both metabolites can be formed by rat brain tissue *in vitro* (Karavolas and Herf, 1971; Rommerts and van der Molen, 1971; Snipes and Shore, 1972; Cheng and Karavolas, 1973; Denef *et al.*, 1973). Pregnanedione is the main metabolite found after incubation of medial basal hypothalamus with progesterone, while 3α-hydroxy-5α-pregnane-20-one is more prevalent after incubation of uterine tissue (Karavolas and Herf, 1971; Armstrong and King, 1971).

The percentage of progesterone converted to pregnanedione varied in different brain areas—midbrain tegmentum (12%), hypothalamus (6%), and cerebral cortex (2%) (Snipes and Shore, 1972). Pretreatment with estradiol increased the rate of progesterone metabolism in the uterus of prepubertal rats but had no effect in the brain (Armstrong and King, 1971; Snipes and Shore, 1972; Massa *et al.*, 1972; Cheng and Karavolas, 1973; Iramain and Strott, 1973). Changes in progesterone metabolism have been found in the hypothalamus during the estrus cycle, with pregnanedione formation being higher during diestrus 2 and estrus than during diestrus 1 or proestrus (Cheng and Karavolas, 1973).

The 5α-steroid reductase in the brain responsible for the conversion of progesterone to pregnanedione is probably identical to the enzyme which converts testosterone to dihydrotestosterone. The two enzymatic activities have a similar regional and subcellular distribution, and progesterone interferes with the conversion of testosterone to dihydrotestosterone *in vitro*, probably by competitive inhibition (Rommerts and van der Molen, 1971; Snipes and Shore, 1972; Denef *et al.*, 1973). In the prostrate, where the specificity of the 5α-steroid reductase has been studied in detail, the results also suggest the existence of a single enzyme which can metabolize testosterone, progesterone, and a number of other steroids (Frederiksen and Wilson, 1971). Nonetheless, this question must be examined in each tissue studied since the liver has been shown to contain a variety of 5α-steroid reductases with different specificities (McGuire and Tompkins, 1960).

5.3. Saturability of Progesterone Retention

Although regional differences in the retention of progesterone have been found, there is little biochemical evidence for the existence of saturable binding sites for this hormone. Adrenalectomy in previously ovariectomized rats increased the retention of [^{3}H]progesterone and its metabolites in all brain regions studied, raising the possibility that adrenal progestins were competing for binding sites with exogenously administered hormone (Whalen and Luttge, 1971*a,b*). However, adrenalectomy also raised the plasma concentration of radioactivity, leaving the tissue/plasma ratio essentially unchanged (Whalen and Luttge, 1971*a,b*). In the mouse, adrenalectomy had no effect on progesterone retention (Luttge *et al.*, 1973).

Pretreatment with unlabeled progesterone (1 mg) did not alter the retention of [^{3}H]progesterone in the guinea pig brain (Wade and Feder, 1972*a*). In contrast, [^{3}H]progesterone retention by the uterus was significantly reduced by such treatment (Falk and Bardin, 1970; Wade and Feder, 1972*a*). *In vitro* incubation of different rat brain regions with [^{3}H]progesterone produced similar differences in the retention of radioactivity as seen *in vivo* (Whalen and Luttge, 1971*b*; Luttge and Wallis, 1973). Attempts to saturate the progesterone uptake with a large (10,000 times) excess of unlabeled hormone produced only a small (4%) decrement in the retention of radioactivity in the midbrain.

In an effort to understand the mechanism for the uneven distribution of progesterone in the brain, Wade and Feder (1972*b*) studied the retention of three other steroids: 20α-hydroxy-4-pregnan-3-one, corticosterone, and estradiol. Corticosterone and estradiol were studied under conditions in which their specific binding sites would be saturated ([^{3}H]corticosterone was injected into nonadrenalectomized animals and [^{3}H]estradiol into animals pretreated with a large dose of unlabeled estradiol). Under these conditions, all three steroids had the same regional distribution as progesterone (i.e., midbrain > hypothalamus > cortex). The extent of retention of the compounds in all brain areas was inversely related to their polarity (i.e., progesterone > 20α-hydroxy-4-pregnan-3-one > estradiol > corticosterone).

These results suggest that the high midbrain concentration of progesterone may not be due to the presence of specific binding sites but rather to the more general ability of this brain region to retain nonpolar steroids.

5.4. Subcellular and Cellular Localization of Progesterone

Attempts to demonstrate specific progesterone binding on the subcellular level using biochemical techniques have also proved unsuccessful thus far. No binding of [^{3}H]progesterone was found in cytosol fractions from bovine median eminence or guinea pig hypothalamus (Kahwanago *et al.*,

1970; Alger *et al.*, 1974). While Karavolas and Herf (1971) found that over 90% of the [^{3}H]progesterone retained by the hypothalamus *in vitro* was in a crude nuclear pellet, similar results were found in two control samples—cerebral cortex and boiled hypothalamus.

In contrast to these negative results using biochemical approaches, Sar and Stumpf (1973*d*) have described labeled cells in the medial basal hypothalamus of estrogen-primed guinea pigs after an injection of [^{3}H]progesterone. Labeled cells were found in the periventricular and suprachiasmatic nuclei of the preoptic area and in the arcuate nucleus (particularly its caudal part). A few labeled cells were found in the ventromedial and ventral premammillary nuclei. Labeled cells were absent from the medial preoptic nucleus and the lateral part of the ventromedial nucleus, two areas which contained labeled cells after an injection of [^{3}H]estradiol and [^{3}H]testosterone.

Silver grains were concentrated over the nuclei of labeled cells, although grains were also found over the cytoplasm and extracellular space. Pretreatment with progesterone (500 μg) but not cortisol (1 mg) greatly inhibited the nuclear concentration of radioactivity. When unprimed guinea pigs instead of estrogen-primed animals were studied, only weak cellular labeling was found.

Compared with previous studies on the distribution of labeled cells after injection of [^{3}H]estradiol or [^{3}H]testosterone, fewer cells were labeled after [^{3}H]progesterone and a smaller percentage of the grains were concentrated over cell nuclei (Stumpf, 1970*a*; Sar and Stumpf, 1973*a,d*). It should also be noted that a shorter time interval between injection and sacrifice (15 min) and a higher dose of steroid (1 mg/100 g) were used in the progesterone study than in these earlier studies. The small number of labeled cells may explain why Wade and Feder (1972*a*) did not find saturable progesterone binding in the whole hypothalamus.

5.5. Role of Progesterone in Female Mating Behavior

Although estrogen injections stimulate lordosis behavior in ovariectomized rats and guinea pigs, levels of behavior comparable to those seen in natural heat seem to require both an estrogen and a progestin (Dempsey *et al.*, 1936; Boling and Blandau, 1939; Beach, 1942*b*). The standard procedure for testing female sexual behavior in the rat is to inject ovariectomized animals with estradiol at 0 h and with progesterone at 24 or 48 h and then to test their response to a sexually active male approximately 4 h later. The procedure roughly mimics the sequence of events in the normal estrus cycle, during which the plasma concentration of estradiol reaches its maximum value on the morning of proestrus followed by a peak in plasma progesterone and later by the onset of behavioral receptivity (Feder *et al.*, 1969;

Schwartz, 1969; Uchida *et al.*, 1969*a*; Brown-Grant, 1971) (Fig. 10). The involvement of progesterone in the onset of behavioral receptivity is further supported by the finding that ovariectomy on the morning of proestrus, after the peak in plasma estradiol but before the peak in plasma progesterone, significantly reduces the frequency of lordosis seen that evening (Powers, 1970). When ovariectomy was delayed until the afternoon of proestrus, after the peak in plasma progesterone, the animals behaved normally (Powers, 1970).

Under certain conditions, progesterone can inhibit mating behavior. Thus a single injection of progesterone in an estrogen-primed guinea pig or rat can have a biphasic effect, producing first a period of receptivity and later a refractory period (Zucker, 1966*b*, 1968; Zucker and Goy, 1967; Nadler, 1970). Also, injections of progesterone during the normal cycle of the rat can advance or delay the onset of receptivity depending on the time of injection (Zucker, 1967*a*). Analogous effects of progesterone have been found on the timing of ovulation (Everett, 1961).

5.6. Anatomical and Chemical Specificity of Progesterone Action in the Brain

In perhaps the earliest demonstration that hormones can act in the brain to influence an animal's behavior, Kent and Liberman (1949) showed that progesterone injected into the lateral ventricle facilitated mating behavior in the estrogen-primed female hamster. This effect could be produced by a dose of progesterone which was too low to be effective if injected peripherally. More recently, crystalline progesterone has been implanted in various parts of the brain in an attempt to delineate its site(s) of action. Ross *et al.* (1971) found that unilateral implants in the mesencephalic reticular formation facilitated lordosis in the rat while implants in the preoptic area and medial basal hypothalamus were ineffective. On the other hand, Powers (1972), using biltateral implants, found effective sites in the ventromedial and arcuate nuclei but not in the mesencephalon. However, these two studies are not directly comparable due to differences in the procedures used and in the exanct placement of the implants.

Progesterone can also act in the hypothalamus to regulate the synthesis or secretion of gonadotropin releasing factors. Progesterone pellets placed in the arcuate nucleus–median eminence region blocked ovulation, while similar pellets of cholesterol had no effect (Smith *et al.*, 1969; Labhsetwar and Bainbridge, 1971). Implants both in this region and in the preoptic area are effective in lengthening the estrus cycle and in inducing pseudopregnancy (Pasteels and Ectors, 1971). The preoptic area is also sensitive to progesterone in the hamster (Reuter and Lisk, 1973). The site of action of the stimulatory effects of progesterone on ovulation is unknown (Davidson, 1969).

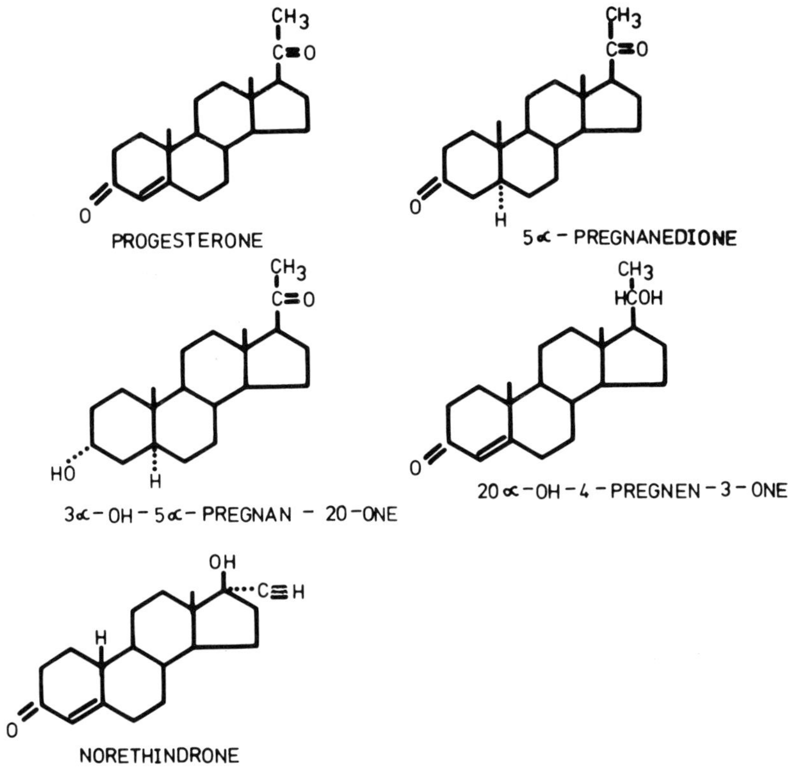

FIG. 23. Chemical structures of progesterone, three metabolites of progesterone (5α-pregnanedione, 3α-hydroxy-5α-pregnan-20-one, and 20α-hydroxypregn-4-en-3-one) and the synthetic progestin norethindrone.

Considerable information is available on the relative ability of different naturally occurring and synthetic steroids to facilitate lordosis in the estrogen-primed rat or guinea pig. 20α-Hydroxy-pregn-4-en-3-one has received particular attention since it is present in plasma at levels comparable to those of progesterone and since there is a peak in the ovarian secretory rate of both hormones prior to the period of behavioral estrus (Uchida *et al.*, 1969*a*) (Fig. 23). In a number of studies, this 20α-hydroxysteroid was found to be either completely ineffective or only weakly effective in stimulating lordosis behavior in the rat (Langford and Hilliard, 1967; Zucker, 1967*b*; Meyerson, 1972; Whalen and Gorzalka, 1972), although it was somewhat more potent in the guinea pig (Zucker and Goy, 1967). The two metabolites of progesterone which have been found in the brain, pregnanedione and 3α-hydroxy-5α-pregnan-20-one, facilitate lordosis behavior to some extent but are weaker than progesterone (Meyerson, 1972; Wade and Feder, 1972*c*; Whalen and Gorzalka, 1972). 17α-Hydroxy-4-pregnan-3-one, a metabolite of progesterone found in plasma, is weakly, if at all, effective (Byrnes and Shipley, 1955; Zucker, 1967*b*; Meyerson, 1972; Wade and Feder, 1972*c*). Of all the other naturally occurring steroids which have been tested, only desoxycorticosterone acetate had any appreciable activity (Kincl, 1964). Thus these results suggest that progesterone itself rather than a metabolite is active in facilitating female reproductive behavior. It is possible, on the other hand, that progesterone metabolites are important in other aspects of the hormone's action in the nervous system (Hilliard *et al.*, 1967).

Of the synthetic compounds tested for their ability to facilitate lordosis behavior, 19-norprogesterone and various 4,9-dihalo derivatives (e.g., 4,9α-dichloro-11β-hydroxyprogesterone) were considerably more potent than progesterone (Kincl, 1964). Medroxyprogesterone (6α-methyl-17α-hydroxyprogesterone) and isopregnenone (6-dehydroretroprogesterone) were about equipotent with progesterone (Meyerson, 1967, 1972). Compounds such as these might be useful in studying the biochemical and electrophysiological effects of progesterone both because of their potency and because of the possibility of dissociating different aspects of progesterone function using different steroids. In this regard, Meyerson (1967) showed that the anesthetic properties of various steroids were not correlated with their ability to facilitate reproductive behavior. For instance, isopregnenone, which facilitates lordosis behavior, does not induce anesthesia (Meyerson, 1967).

Uchida *et al.* (1969*b*, 1970) compared the ability of several progestins to advance the time of ovarian progesterone secretion when injected during the morning of proestrus. Progesterone itself was the most potent compound, while norethindrone (Fig. 23), medroxyprogesterone acetate, and desoxycorticosterone also had a significant effect. 20α-Hydroxypregn-4-en-3-one, medroxyprogesterone, and corticosterone were inactive, as were estradiol and testosterone.

6. CONCLUSION

The binding and metabolism in the central nervous system of estrogens, androgens, glucocorticoids, and progestins have been reviewed. An attempt has been made to relate these findings to what is known of the behavioral and endocrinological effects of the hormones. Each of the four groups of hormones differs in the anatomical distribution and chemical specificity of its binding macromolecules. Obviously the main question is whether or not these "binding macromolecules" are actual "receptors" mediating the hormones' actions in the central nervous system. A firm answer to this question must await a future edition of this handbook.

ACKNOWLEDGMENTS

I should like to thank Pamela Haynes and Chris Rayner for help in preparing this chapter and Bruce McEwen for reading the section on glucocorticoids.

7. REFERENCES

ALGER, M., BAULIEU, E.-E., and MILGRAM, E., 1974, An investigation of progesterone receptors in guinea-pig vagina, uterine cervix, mammary glands, pituitary and hypothalamus, *Endocrinology* **94:**161–167.

ALVAREZ, E., and RAMIREZ, V., 1970, Distribution curves of ^{3}H-testosterone and ^{3}H-estradiol in neonatal female rats, *Neuroendocrinology* **6:**349–360.

ANDERSON, C. H., and GREENWALD, G. S., 1969, Autoradiographic analysis of estradiol uptake in the brain and pituitary of the female rat, *Endocrinology* **85:**1160–1165.

ANDERSON, J. N., PECK, E. J., JR., and CLARK, J. H., 1973, Nuclear receptor complex: Accumulation, retention, and localization in the hypothalamus and pituitary, *Endocrinology* **93:**711–717.

ANDERSON, K. M., and LIAO, S., 1968, Selective retention of dihydrotestosterone by prostatic nuclei, *Nature* **219:**277–279.

APPELGREN, L.-E., 1970, Chromatographic studies and scintillation counting of selected tissues of mice injected with labelled testosterone, *Biol. Reprod.* **3:**128–133.

APPLETON, T. C., 1964, Autoradiography of soluble labelled compounds, *J. Roy. Micros. Soc.* **83:**277–281.

ARAI, Y., and GORSKI, R. A., 1968, Effects of anti-estrogen on steroid induced sexual receptivity in ovariectomized rats, *Physiol. Behav.* **3:**351–353.

ARMSTRONG, D. T., and KING, E. R., 1971, Uterine progesterone metabolism and progestational response: Effects of estrogens and prolactin, *Endocrinology* **89:**191–197.

ATTRAMADAL, A., 1964, Distribution and site of action of oestradiol in the brain and pituitary gland of rat following intramuscular administration, in: *Proceedings of the Second International Congress of Endocrinology*, pp. 612–616, Excerpta Medica International Congress Series No. 83, Amsterdam.

AXELROD, L. R., 1971, The metabolism of corticosteroids by incubated and perfused brain tissues, in: *Influence of Hormones on the Nervous System: Proceedings of the International Society of Psychopharmacology, Brooklyn 1970*, pp. 74–84, Karger, Basel.

BAINBRIDGE, J. G., and LABHSETWAR, A. P., 1971, The role of oestrogens in spontaneous ovulation: Location of site of action of positive feedback of oestrogen by intracranial implantation of the anti-oestrogen, I.C.I. 46474, *J. Endocrinol.* **50:**321–327.

BALL, J., 1940, The effect of testosterone on the sex behaviour of female rats, *J. comp. Psychol.* **29:**151–165.

BARNEA, A., WEINSTEIN, A., and LINDNER, H. R., 1972, Uptake of androgens by the brain of the neonatal female rat, *Brain Res.* **46:**391–402.

BARON, D. N., and ABELSON, D., 1954, Cortisone and hydrocortisone in cerebrospinal fluid, *Nature* **173:**174.

BARRACLOUGH, C. A., and HALLER, E. W., 1970, Positive and negative feedback effects of estrogen on pituitary LH synthesis and release in normal and androgen sterilized female rats, *Endrocinology* **86:**542–551.

BAULIEU, E. E., LASNITZKI, I., and ROBEL, P., 1968, Metabolism of testosterone and action of metabolites on prostate glands grown in organ culture, *Nature* **219:**1155–1156.

BEACH, F. A., 1942*a*, Male and female mating behaviour in prepuberally castrated female rats treated with androgen, *Endocrinology* **31:**673–678.

BEACH, F. A., 1942*b*, Importance of progesterone to induction of sexual receptivity in spayed female rats, *Proc. Soc. Exp. Biol. Med.* **51:**369–371.

BEACH, F. A., 1948, *Hormones and Behaviour: A Survey of Interrelationships Between Endocrine Secretions and Patterns of Overt Response*, Hoeber, New York.

BEACH, F. A., and WESTBROOK, W. H., 1968*a*, Morphological and behavioural effects of an "antiandrogen" in male rats, *J. Endocrinol.* **42:**379–382.

BEACH, F. A., and WESTBROOK, W. H., 1968*b*, Dissociation of androgenic effects on sexual morphology and behaviour in male rats, *Endocrinology* **83:**395–398.

BEART, P. M., KELLY, J. S., and SCHON, F., 1974, γ-Aminobutyric acid in the rat peripheral nervous system, pineal and posterior pituitary, *Biochem. Soc. Trans.* **2:**266–268.

BEYER, C., and KOMISARUK, B., 1971, Effects of diverse androgens on estrous behaviour, lordosis reflex and genital tract morphology in the rat, *Horm. Behav.* **2:**217–225.

BEYER, C., and VIDAL, N., 1971, Inhibitory action of Mer-25 on androgen-induced oestrus behaviour in the ovariectomized rabbit. *J. Endocrinol.* **51:**401–402.

BEYER, C., MCDONALD, P., and VIDAL, N., 1970*a*, Failure of 5α-dihydrotestosterone to elicit estrous behaviour in the ovariectomized rabbit, *Endocrinology* **86:**939–941.

BEYER, C., VIDAL, N., and MAJARES, A., 1970*b*, Probable role of aromatization in the induction of estrous behaviour by androgens in the ovariectomized rabbit, *Endocrinology* **87:**1386–1389.

BEYER, C., MORALI, G., and CRUZ, M. L., 1971*a*, Effect of 5α-dihydrotestosterone on gonadotrophin secretion and estrous behaviour in the female Wistar rat, *Endocrinology* **89:**1158–1161.

BEYER, C., MORALI, G., and VORGAS, R., 1971*b*, Effects of diverse estrogens on estrous behaviour and genital tract development in ovariectomized rats, *Horm. Behav.* **2:**273–277.

BEYER, C., JAFFE, R. B., and GAY, V. L., 1972, Testosterone metabolism in target tissues: Effects of testosterone and dihydrotestosterone injection and hypothalamic implantation on serum LH in ovariectomized rats, *Endocrinology* **91:**1372–1375.

BILLARD, R., and MCDONALD, P. G., 1973, Inhibition of ovulation in the rat by intrahypothalamic implants of an antioestrogen, *J. Endocrinol.* **56:**585–590.

BOLING, J. L., and BLANDAU, R. J., 1939, The estrogen–progesterone induction of mating responses in the spayed female rat, *Endocrinology* **25:**359–364.

BLOCH, G. J., and DAVIDSON, J. M., 1967, Antiandrogen implanted in brain stimulates male reproductive system, *Science* **155:**593–595.

BLOCH, G. J., and DAVIDSON, J. M., 1971, Behavioural and somatic responses to the antiandrogen cyproterone, *Horm. Behav.* **2:**11–25.

BOGDANOVE, E. M., 1963, Direct gonad–pituitary feedback: An analysis of effects of intracranial estrogenic depots on gonadotrophin secretion, *Endocrinology* **73:**696–712.

BOTTOMS, G. D., SMITH, R. D., and BURGEN, R. O., 1969, Distribution of radioactivity in different tissues of pigs after ^{3}H-hydrocortisone injection, *Proc. Soc. Exp. Biol. Med.* **132:**1133–1136.

BROWN-GRANT, K., 1971, The role of steroid hormones in the control of gonadotrophin secretion in adult female mammals, in: *Steroid Hormones and Brain Function* (C. H. Sawyer and R. A. Gorski, eds.), pp. 269–284, University of California Press, Los Angeles.

BROWN-GRANT, K., 1974, Failure of ovulation after the administration of steroid hormones to female rats during the neonatal period, *J. Endocrinol.*, in press.

BROWN-GRANT, K., MUNK, A., NAFTOLIN, F., and SHERWOOD, M. R., 1971, The effects of the administration of testosterone propionate alone or with phenobarbitone and of testosterone metabolites to neonatal female rats, *Horm. Behav.* **2:**173–182.

BRUCHOVSKY, N., and WILSON, J. D., 1968, The conversion of testosterone to 5α-androstan-17β-ol-3-one by rat prostate *in vivo* and *in vitro*, *J. Biol. Chem.* **243:**2012–2021.

BUSH, I. E., 1953, Species differences in adrenocortical secretion, *J. Endocrinol.* **9:**95–100.

BUTTE, J. C., KAKIHANA, R., and NOBLE, E. P., 1972, Rat and mouse brain corticosterone, *Endocrinology* **90:**1091–1100.

BYRNES, W. W., and SHIPLEY, E. G., 1955, Guinea pig copulatory reflex in response to adrenal steroids and similar compounds, *Endocrinology* **57:**5–9.

CALLANTINE, M. R., 1967, Non-steroid estrogen antagonists, *Clin. Obstet. Gynecol.* **10:**74–87.

CALLANTINE, M. R., HUMPHREY, R. R., LEE, S. L., WINDSOR, B. L., SCHOTTIN, N. H., and O'BRIEN, O. P., 1966, Action of an estrogen antagonist on reproductive mechanism in the rat, *Endocrinology* **79:**153–167.

CALLANTINE, M. R., CLEMENS, L. E., and SHIH, Y., 1968, Displacement of 17β-estradiol from uterine receptor sites by an estrogen antagonist, *Proc. Soc. Exp. Biol. Med.* **128:**382–386.

CHADER, G. J., 1973, Some factors affecting the uptake, binding and retention of ^{3}H-cortisol by the chick embryo retina as related to enzyme induction, *J. Neurochem.* **21:**1525–1532.

CHADER, G. J., and VILLEE, C. A., 1970, Uptake of oestradiol by the rabbit hypothalamus: Specificity of binding by nuclei *in vitro*, *Biochem. J.* **118:**93–97.

CHADER, G. J., and VILLEE, C. A., 1971, Estrogen receptors in the hypothalamus, in: *Influence of Hormones on the Nervous System: Proceedings of the International Society of Psychoneuroendocrinology, Brooklyn, 1970* (D. H. Ford, ed.), pp. 17–24, Karger, Basel.

CHAMBERS, W. F., and HOWE, G., 1968, A study of estrogen-sensitive hypothalamic centers using a technique for rapid application and removal of estradiol, *Proc. Soc. Exp. Biol. Med.* **128:**292–294.

CHENG, Y., and KARAVOLAS, H. J., 1973, Conversion of progesterone to 5α-pregnane-3,20-dione and 3α-hydroxy-5α-pregnane-20-one by rat medial basal hypothalami and the effects of estradiol and stage of estrous cycle on conversion, *Endocrinology* **93:**1157–1162.

CHYTIL, F., and TOFT, D., 1972, Corticoid binding component in rat brain, *J. Neurochem.* **19:**2877–2880.

CLARK, J. H., CAMPBELL, P. S., and PECK, E. J., 1972, Receptor estrogen complex in the nuclear fraction of the pituitary and hypothalamus of male and female immature rats, *Neuroendocrinology* **77:**218–228.

DAVIDSON, J. M., 1966, Activiation of the male rat's sexual behaviour by intracerebral implantation of androgen, *Endocrinology* **79:**783–794.

DAVIDSON, J. M., 1969, Feedback control of gonadotrophin secretion, in: *Frontiers in Neuroendocrinology* (W. F. Ganong and L. Martini, eds.), pp. 343–388, Oxford University Press, New York.

DAVIDSON, J. M., and BLOCH, G. J., 1969, Neuroendocrine aspects of male reproduction, *Biol. of Reprod.* **1:**67–92 (Suppl. 1).

DE KLOET, E. R., WALLACH, G., and MCEWEN, B. S., 1974, Differences in glucocorticosteroid binding to macromolecules in rat brain regions and pituitary, Fifty-sixth Meeting of the Endocrine Society, p. A-203 (abst.).

DEMPSEY, E. W., HERZ, R., and YOUNG, W. C., 1936, The experimental induction of oestrus (sexual receptivity) in the normal and ovariectomized guinea-pig, *Am. J. Physiol.* **116:**201–209.

DENEF, C., MAGNUS, C., and MCEWEN, B. S., 1973, Sex differences and hormonal control of testosterone metabolism in rat pituitary and brain, *J. Endocrinol.* **59:**605–621.

DIAMOND, H., and DALE, E., 1967, Distribution of radiolabelled steroid after administration to the neonatal rat, *Anat. Rec.* **157:**234 (abst.).

DORFMAN, R. I., and SHIPLEY, R. A., 1956, *Androgens, Biochemistry, Physiology, and Clinical Significance*, Wiley, New York.

DUNCAN, G. W., LYSTER, S. C., CLARK, J. J., and LEDNICER, D., 1963, Antifertility activities of two diphenyl-dihydronaphthalene derivatives, *Proc. Soc. Exp. Biol. Med.* **112:**439–442.

EDWARDS, D. A., and THOMPSON, M. L., 1970, Neonatal androgenization and estrogenization and the hormonal induction of sexual receptivity in rats, *Physiol. Behav.* **5:**1115–1119.

EIK-NES, K. B., and BRIZEE, K. R., 1965, Concentration of tritium in brain tissue of dogs given (1,2-^{3}H) cortisol intravenously, *Biochim. Biophys. Acta* **97:**320–333.

EISENFELD, A. J., 1967, Computer analysis of the distribution of [^{3}H] estradiol, *Biochim. Biophys. Acta* **136:**498–507.
EISENFELD, A. J., 1969, Hypothalamic estradiol binding macromolecules, *Nature* **224:**1202–1203.
EISENFELD, A. J., 1970, ^{3}H-estradiol: *In vivo* binding to macromolecules from the rat hypothalamus, anterior pituitary and uterus, *Endocrinology* **86:**1313–1318.
EISENFELD, A. J., 1972, Interaction of estrogens, progestational agents and androgens with brain and pituitary and their role in the control of ovulation, in: *Perspectives in Neuropharmacology* (S. H. Snyder, ed.), pp. 113–142, Oxford University Press, Oxford.
EISENFELD, A. J., and AXELROD, J., 1965, Selectivity of estrogen distribution in tissues, *J. Pharmacol. Exp. Ther.* **150:**469–475.
EISENFELD, A. J., and AXELROD, J., 1966, Effect of steroid hormones, ovariectomy, estrogen pretreatment, sex and immaturity on the distribution of ^{3}H-estradiol, *Endocrinology* **79:**38–42.
EISENFELD, A. J., and AXELROD, J., 1967, Evidence for estradiol binding in the hypothalamus—The effects of drugs, *Biochem. Pharmacol.* **16:**1781–1785.
ENGLAND, J. M., ROGERS, A. W., and MILLER, R. G., 1973, The identification of labelled structures on autoradiographs, *Nature* **242:**612–613.
EVERETT, J. W., 1961, The mammalian female reproductive cycle and its controlling mechanisms, in: *Sex and Internal Secretions*, Vol. 1, 3rd ed. (W. C. Young, ed.), pp. 497–555, Williams and Wilkins, Baltimore.
FALK, R. J., and BARDIN, C. W., 1970, Uptake of tritiated progesterone by the uterus of the ovariectomized guinea-pig, *Endocrinology* **86:**1059–1063.
FEDER, H. H., 1971, The comparative actions of testosterone propionate and 5α-androstan-17β-ol-3-one propionate on the reproductive behaviour, physiology and morphology of male rats, *J. Endocrinol.* **51:**241–252.
FEDER, H. H., BROWN-GRANT, K., CORKER, C. S., and EXLEY, D., 1969, Systemic plasma progesterone levels during the pro-oestrus critical period in rats, *J. Endocrinol.* **43:**XXIX (abst.).
FEDER, H. H., NAFTOLIN, F., and RYAN, K. J., 1974, Male and female sexual responses in male rats given estradiol benzoate and 5α-androstan-17β-ol-3-one propionate, *Endocrinology* **94:**136–141.
FERIN, M., TEMPONE, A., ZIMMERING, P. E., and VANDE WIELE, R. L., 1969, Effect of antibodies to 17β-estradiol and progesterone on the estrous cycle of the rat, *Endocrinology* **85:**1070–1078.
FLERKO, B., and MESS, B., 1968, Reduced oestradiol-binding of androgen-sterilized rats, *Acta Biol. Acad. Sci. Hung.* **33:**111–113.
FLERKO, B., MESS, B., and ILLEI-DONHOFFER, A., 1969, On the mechanism of androgen sterilization, *Neuroendocrinology* **4:**164–169.
FLERKO, B., ILLEI-DONHOFFER, A., and MESS, B., 1971, Oestradiol-binding capacity in neural and non-neural target tissues of neonatally androgenized female rats, *Acta Biol. Acad. Sci. Hung.* **22:**125–130.
FLORES, F., NAFTOLIN, F., RYAN, K. J., and WHITE, R. J., 1973, Estrogen formation by the isolated perfused monkey brain, *Science* **180:**1074–1075.
FONTANA, J. A., WALKER, M. D., CASPER, A. G. T., MERET, S., and HENKIN, R. I., 1970, Sequential subcellular localization of cortisol in cat brain, *Endocrinology* **86:**1469–1471.
FREDERIKSEN, D. W., and WILSON, J. D., 1971, Partial characterization of the nuclear reduced nicotinamide adenine dinucleotide phosphate: Δ^4-3-Ketosteroid 5α-oxidoreductase of rat prostate, *J. Biol. Chem.* **246:**2584–2593.
GERLACH, J. L., and MCEWEN, B. S., 1972, Rat brain binds adrenal steroid hormone: Radioautography of hippocampus with corticosterone, *Science* **175:**1133–1136.
GERLACH, J. L., MCEWEN, B. S., PFAFF, D. W., FERIN, M., CARMEL, P. W., 1974, Rhesus monkey brain binds radioactivity from ^{3}H-estradiol and ^{3}H-corticosterone, demonstrated by nuclear isolation and radioautography, Fifty-sixth Meeting of the Endocrine Society, p. A-240 (abst.).

GERALL, A. A., and KENNEY, A. MCM., 1970, Neonatally androgenized females' responsiveness to estrogen and progesterone, *Endocrinology* **87:**560–566.

GLASCOCK, R. F., and MICHAEL, R. P., 1962, Localization of oestrogen in a neurological system in the brain of the female cat, *J. Physiol.* **163:**38P–39P.

GOGAN, F., 1968, Sensibilité hypothalamique à la testosterone chez le Canard, *Gen. Comp. Endocrinol.* **11:**316–327.

GORDON, A. S., ZANJANI, E. D., LEVERE, R. D., and KAPPAS, A., 1970, Stimulation of mammalian erythropoiesis by 5β-H steroid metabolites, *Proc. Natl. Acad. Sci.* **65:**919–924.

GORSKI, R. A., 1963, Modification of ovulatory mechanism by postnatal administration of estrogen to the rat, *Am. J. Physiol.* **205:**842–844.

GREEN, J. D., CLEMENTE, C. D., and DE GROOT, J., 1957, Rhinencephalic lesions and behavior in cats: An analysis of the Kluver-Bucy syndrome with particular reference to normal and abnormal sexual behaviour. *J. Comp. Neurol.* **108:**505–536.

GREEN, R., LUTTGE, W. G., and WHALEN, R. E., 1969, Uptake and retention of tritiated estradiol in brain and peripheral tissues of male, female and androgenized female rats, *Endocrinology* **85:**373–378.

GREEN, R., LUTTGE, W. G., and WHALEN, R. E., 1970, Induction of receptivity in ovariectomized rats by a single intravenous injection of estradiol-17β, *Physiol. Behav.* **5:**137–141.

GROSSER, B. I., 1966, 11β-Hydroxy steroid metabolism by mouse brain and glioma 261, *J. Neurochem.* **13:**475–478.

GROSSER, B. I., and AXELROD, L. R., 1967, Acetylation of cortisol by neonatal rat brain *in vitro*, *Steroids* **9:**229–234.

GROSSER, B. I., and AXELROD, L. R., 1968, Conversion of cortisol to cortisol acetate, cortisone acetate, and cortisone by the developing primate brain, *Steroids* **11:**827–836.

GROSSER, B. I., and BLISS, E. L., 1966, Metabolism of 11-hydroxysteroids by cerebral tissues *in vitro*, *Steroids* **8:**915–928.

GROSSER, B. I., STEVENS, W., BRUENGER, F. W., and REED, D. J., 1971, Corticosterone binding in rat brain cytosol, *J. Neurochem.* **18:**1725–1732.

GROSSER, B. I., STEVENS, W., and REED, D. J., 1973, Properties of corticosterone binding macromolecules from rat brain cytosol, *Brain Res.* **57:**387–395.

GUAL, C., MORATO, T., HAYANO, M., GUT, M., and DORFMAN, R. I., 1962, Biosynthesis of estrogens, *Endocrinology* **71:**920–925.

HAMILTON, T. H., 1968, Control by estrogen of genetic transcription and translation, *Science* **161:**649–660.

HARPER, M. J. K., and WALPOLE, A. L., 1967, A new derivative of triphenylethylene: Effect on implantation and mode of action in rats, *J. Reprod. Fertil.* **13:**101–119.

HARRIS, G. W., and MICHAEL, R. P., 1964, The activation of sexual behaviour by hypothalamic implants of oestrogen, *J. Physiol.* **171:**275–301.

HARRIS, G. W., MICHAEL, R. P., and SCOTT, P. P., 1958, Neurological site of action of stilboestrol in eliciting sexual behaviour, in: *Ciba Foundation Symposium on the Neurological Basis of Behaviour* (G. E. W. Wolstenholme and C. M. O'Connor, eds.), pp. 236–251, Churchill, London.

HART, B. L., 1967, Testosterone regulation of sexual reflexes in spinal male rats, *Science* **155:**1283–1284.

HART, B. L., 1968, Alteration of quantitative aspects of sexual reflexes in spinal male dogs by testosterone, *J. Comp. Physiol. Psychol.* **66:**726–730.

HART, B. L., 1969, Gonadal hormones and sexual reflexes in the female rat, *Horm. Behav.* **1:**65–71.

HART, B. L., 1970, Mating behaviour in the female dog and the effects of estrogen on sexual reflexes, *Horm. Behav.* **1:**93–104.

HART, B. L., and HAUGEN, C. M., 1968, Activation of sexual reflexes in male rats by spinal implantation of testosterone, *Physiol. Behav.* **3:**735–738.

HEFFNER, L. J., and VAN TIENHOVEN, A., 1973, Effects of progesterone on uptake and retention of ^{3}H-testosterone in the neonatal female rat, *Neuroendocrinology* **12:**129–141.

HENKIN, R. A., CASPER, A., BROWN, R., HORLAN, A., and BARTER, F., 1968, Presence of corticosterone and cortisol in the central and peripheral nervous system of the cat, *Endocrinology* **82:**1058–1061.

HILLIARD, J., PENARD, R., and SAWYER, C. H., 1967, A functional role for 20α-hydroxypregn-4-en-3-one in the rabbit, *Endocrinology* **80:**901–909.

HOLTKAMP, D. E., GRESLIN, J. G., ROOT, C. A., and LERNER, L. J., 1960, Gonadotrophin inhibiting and anti-fecundity effects of chloramiphene, *Proc. Soc. Exp. Biol. Med.* **105:**197–201.

HUTCHISON, J. B., 1970, Influence of gonadal hormones on the hypothalamic integration of courtship behaviour in the Barbary dove, *J. Reprod. Fertil. Suppl.* **11:**15–41.

HUTCHISON, J. B., 1975, Hypothalamic mechanisms of sexual behaviour, with special reference to birds, in: *Advances in the Study of Behaviour*, Vol. 6 (J. S. Rosenblatt, R. A. Hinde, E. Shaw, and C. Beer, eds), Academic Press, New York, in press.

IRAMAIN, C. A., and STROTT, C. A., 1973, Uptake and regional distribution of progesterone in the female guinea pig brain and adenohypophysis: A comparison with known target (uterus) and non-target (muscle) tissues, *Fifty-fifth Meeting of the Endocrine Society*, p. A117 (abst.).

JAFFE, R. B., 1969, Testosterone metabolism in target tissues: Hypothalamic and pituitary tissues of the adult rat and human fetus and the immature rat epiphysis, *Steroids* **14:**483–498.

JENSEN, E. V., 1966, Mechanism of estrogen action in relation to carcinogenesis, *Canad. Cancer Conf.* **6:**143–165.

JENSEN, E. V., and DE SOMBRE, E. R., 1973, Estrogen–receptor interaction, *Science* **182:**126–134.

JENSEN, E. V., and JACOBSON, H. I., 1962, Basic guides to the mechanism of estrogen action, *Rec. Prog. Horm. Res.* **18:**387–408.

JOHNSTON, P., and DAVIDSON, J. M., 1972, Intracerebral androgens and sexual behaviour in the male rat, *Horm. Behav.* **3:**345–357.

JOUAN, P., SAMPEREZ, S., THIEULANT, M. L., and MERCIER, L., 1971, Étude du recepteur cytoplasmique de la [1,2-^{3}H]testosterone dans l'hypophyse anterieure et l'hypothalamus du rat, *J. Steroid Biochem.* **2:**223–236.

JUNG, I., and BAULIEU, E. E., 1972, Testosterone cytosol "receptor" in the rat levator ani muscle, *Nature New Biol.* **237:**24–26.

KAHWANAGO, I., HEINRICHS, W. L., and HERRMANN, W. L., 1969, Isolation of oestradiol receptors from bovine hypothalamus and anterior pituitary gland, *Nature* **223:**313–314.

KAHWANAGO, I., HEINRICHS, W. L., and HERRMANN, W. L., 1970, Oestradiol "receptors" in the hypothalamus and anterior pituitary gland: Inhibition of estradiol binding by SH group blocking agents and clomiphene citrate, *Endocrinology* **86:**1319–1326.

KARAVOLAS, H. J., and HERF, S. H., 1971, Conversion of progesterone by rat medial basal hypothalamic tissue to 5α-pregnane-3,20-dione, *Endocrinology* **89:**940–942.

KATO, J., 1970, *In vitro* uptake of tritiated oestradiol by the rat anterior hypothalamus during the oestrous cycle, *Acta Endocrinol. (Copenhagen).* **63:**577–584.

KATO, J., and VILLEE, C. A., 1967*a*, Preferential uptake of estradiol by the hypothalamus of the rat, *Endocrinology* **80:**567–575.

KATO, J., and VILLEE, C. A., 1967*b*, Factors affecting the uptake of estradiol-6,7-^{3}H by the hypophysis and hypothalamus, *Endocrinology* **80:**1133–1138.

KATO, J., KOBAYASHI, T., and VILLEE, C. A., 1968, Effect of clomiphene on the uptake of estradiol by the anterior hypothalamus and hypophysis, *Endocrinology* **82:**1049–1052.

Kato, J., Inaba, M., and Kobayashi, T., 1969, Variable uptake of tritiated oestradiol by the anterior hypothalamus of postpubertal female rats, *Acta Endocrinol. (Copenhagen).* **61:**585–591.

Kato, J., Sugimara, N., and Kobayashi, T., 1971*a*, Changing patterns of the uptake of estradiol by the anterior hypothalamus, the median eminence and the hypophysis in the developing female rat, in: *Hormones in Development* (M. Hamburgh and E. J. W. Barrington, eds.), pp. 689–703, Appleton-Century-Crofts, New York.

Kato, J., Atsumi, Y., and Inaba, M., 1971*b*, Development of oestrogen receptor in rat hypothalamus, *J. Biochem.* **70:**1051–1053.

Kawakami, M., Seto, K., and Yoshida, K., 1968, Influence of corticosterone implantation in limbic structures upon biosynthesis of adrenocortical steroid, *Neuroendocrinology* **3:**349–354.

Keefer, D. A., Stumpf, W. E., and Sar, M., 1973, Estrogen-topographical localization of estrogen-concentrating cells in the rat spinal chord following ^{3}H-estradiol administration, *Proc. Soc. Exp. Biol. Med.* **143:**414–417.

Kendall, J. W., 1971, Feedback control of adrenocorticotrophic hormone secretion, in: *Frontiers in Neuroendocrinology* (L. Martini and W. F. Ganong, eds.), pp. 177–207, Oxford University Press, New York.

Kent, G. C., and Liberman, M. J., 1949, Induction of psychic estrus in the hamster with progesterone administered via the lateral brain ventricle, *Endocrinology* **45:**29–32.

Kincl, F. A., 1964, Copulatory reflex response to steroids, in: *Methods in Hormone Research,* Vol. 3 (R. I. Dorfman, ed.), pp. 477–484, Academic Press, New York.

Kincl, F., 1970, Neonatal sterilization of rodents with steroid hormones. I. The uptake of radioactivity from injected estradiol or testosterone propionate in various organs of 5-day old male and female rats, *Endocrinol. Exp.* **4:**139–141.

Knizley, H., 1972, The hippocampus and septal area as primary target sites for corticosterone, *J. Neurochem.* **19:**2737–2745.

Komisaruk, B. R., and Beyer, C., 1972, Differential antagonism, by Mer-25 of behavioral and morphological effects of estradiol benzoate in rats, *Horm. Behav.* **3:**63–70.

Kulin, H. E., and Reiter, E. O., 1972, Ontogeny of the *in vitro* uptake of tritiated estradiol by the hypothalamus of the female rat, *Endocrinology* **90:**1371–1374.

Labhsetwar, A. P., 1970*a*, The role of oestrogens in spontaneous ovulation: Evidence for positive oestrogen feedback in the 4-day oestrous cycle, *J. Endocrinol.* **47:**481–493.

Labhsetwar, A. P., 1970*b*, The role of oestrogen in spontaneous ovulation as revealed by the use of oestrogen-antagonist, I.C.I. 46,474, *Nature* **225:**80–81.

Labhsetwar, A. P., 1970*c*, Role of oestrogens in ovulation: A study using the oestrogen-antagonist, I.C.I. 46,474, *Endocrinology* **87:**542–551.

Labhsetwar, A. P., and Bainbridge, J. G., 1971, Inhibition of ovulation by intracranial implantation of progesterone in the 4-day cyclic rat, *J. Reprod. Fertil.* **27:**445–449.

Langford, J., and Hilliard, J., 1967, Effect of 20α-hydroxypregn-4-en-3-one on mating behavior in spayed female rats, *Endocrinology* **80:**381–383.

Laumas, K. R., and Farooq, A., 1966, The uptake *in vivo* of [1,2-^{3}H]progesterone by the brain and genital tract of the rat, *J. Endocrinol.* **36:**95–96.

Lemaire, I., Dupont, A., Bastarache, E., Labrie, F., and Fortier, C., 1974, Some corticosterone-binding characteristics of the dorsal hippocampus and of the adenohypophysis in the rat, *Can. J. Physiol. Pharmacol.* **52:**451–457.

Lerner, L. J., Holthaus, F. J., Jr., and Thomas, C. R., 1958, A non-steroidal estrogen antagonist 1-(*p*-2-diethylaminoethoxyphenyl)-1-phenyl-2-*p*-methoxyphenyl ethanol, *Endocrinology* **63:**295–318.

Levere, R. D., Kappas, A., and Granick, S., 1967, Stimulation of hemoglobin synthesis in chick blastoderms by certain 5β androstane and 5β pregnane steroids, *Proc. Natl. Acad. Sci.* **58:**985–990.

LIAO, S., and FANG, S., 1969, Receptor-proteins for androgens and the mode of action of androgens on gene transcription in ventral prostate, *Vitam. Horm.* **27:**17–90.

LISK, R. D., 1962, Diencephalic placement of estradiol and sexual receptivity in the female rat, *Am. J. Physiol.* **203:**493–496.

LISK, R. D., 1967, Neural localization for androgen activation of copulatory behavior in the male rat, *Endocrinology* **80:**754–761.

LØVTRUP-REIN, H., and MCEWEN, B. S., 1966, Isolation and fractionation of rat brain nuclei, *J. Cell Biol.* **30:**405–415.

LUTTGE, W. G., 1972*a*, The estrous cycle of the rat: Effects on the accumulation of estrogenic metabolites in brain and peripheral tissues, *Brain Res.* **38:**315–325.

LUTTGE, W. G., 1972*b*, Activation and inhibition of isolation induced intermale fighting behavior in castrate male CD-1 mice treated with steroidal hormones, *Horm. Behav.* **3:**71–81.

LUTTGE, W. G., and WALLIS, C. J., 1973, *In vitro* accumulation and saturation of ^{3}H-progestins in selected brain regions and in the adenohypophysis, uterus and pineal of the female rat, *Steroids* **22:**493–502.

LUTTGE, W. G., and WHALEN, R. E., 1970*a*, Regional localization of estrogenic metabolites in the brain of male and female rats, *Steroids* **15:**605–612.

LUTTGE, W. G., and WHALEN, R. E., 1970*b*, Dihydrotestosterone, androstenedione, testosterone: Comparative effectiveness in masculinizing and defeminizing reproductive systems in male and female rats, *Horm. Behav.* **1:**265–281.

LUTTGE, W. G., and WHALEN, R. E., 1972, The accumulation, retention and interaction of oestradiol and oestrone in central neural and peripheral tissues of gonadectomized female rats, *J. Endocrinol.* **52:**379–395.

LUTTGE, W. G., CHRONISTER, R. B., and HALL, N. R., 1973, Accumulation of ^{3}H-progestins in limbic, diencephalic and mesencephalic regions of mouse brain, *Life Sci.* **12:**419–424.

MAINWARING, W. I. P., 1969, A soluble androgen receptor in the cytoplasm of rat prostate, *J. Endocrinol.* **45:**531–541.

MASSA, R., STUPNICKA, E., KNIEWALD, Z., and MARTINI, L., 1972, The transformation of testosterone into dihydrotestosterone by the brain and the anterior pituitary, *J. Steroid Biochem.* **3:**385–399.

MAURER, R., and WOOLEY, D., 1971, Distribution of ^{3}H-estradiol in clomiphene treated and neonatally androgenized rats, *Endocrinology* **88:**1281–1287.

MCDONALD, P. G., 1971, Some biological actions of dihydrotestosterone (DHT), *J. Reprod. Fertil.* **25:**309–310 (abst.).

MCDONALD, P. G., and DOUGHTY, C., 1972*a*, Comparison of the effect of neonatal administration of testosterone and dihydrotestosterone in the female rat, *J. Reprod. Fertil.* **30:**55–62.

MCDONALD, P. G., and DOUGHTY, C., 1972*b*, Inhibition of androgen-sterilization in the female rat by administration of an anti-oestrogen, *J. Endocrinol.* **55:**455–456.

MCDONALD, P. G., VIDAL, N., and BEYER, C., 1970*a*, Sexual behavior in the ovariectomized rabbit after treatment with different amounts of gonadal hormones, *Horm. Behav.* **1:**161–172.

MCDONALD, P., BEYER, C., NEWTON, F., BRIEN, B., BAKER, R., TAN, H. S., SAMPSON, C., KITCHING, P., GREENHILL, R., and PRITCHARD, D., 1970*b*, Failure of 5α-dihydrotestosterone to initiate sexual behavior in the castrated male rat, *Nature* **227:**964–965.

MCEWEN, B. S., 1973*a*, Glucocorticoid binding sites in rat brain: Subcellular and anatomical localizations, *Prog. Brain Res.* **39:**87–96.

MCEWEN, B. S., 1973*b*, Adrenal steroid binding to presumptive receptors in the limbic brain of the rat, *Neuroendocrinologie de l'axe corticotrope (Brain-Adrenal Interactions)*, Les Colloques de l'Institut National de la Sante et de la Recherche Medicale (P. Dell, ed.), pp. 41–62, INSERM, Paris.

McEwen, B. S., and Pfaff, D. W., 1970, Factors influencing sex hormone uptake by rat brain regions. I. Effects of neonatal treatment, hypophysectomy, and competing steroid on estradiol uptake, *Brain Res.* **21:**1–16.

McEwen, B. S., and Pfaff, D. W., 1973, Chemical and physiological approaches to neuroendrocrine mechanisms: Attempts at integration, in: *Frontiers in Neuroendocrinology* (L. Martini and W. F. Ganong, eds.), pp. 267–335, Oxford University Press, New York.

McEwen, B. S., and Plapinger, L., 1970, Association of corticosterone-1,2-^{3}H with macromolecules extracted from brain cell nuclei, *Nature* **226:**263–264.

McEwen, B. S., and Wallach, G., 1973, Corticosterone binding to hippocampus: Nuclear and cytosol binding *in vitro*, *Brain Res.* **57:**373–386.

McEwen, B. S., and Zigmond, R. E., 1972, Isolation of brain cell nuclei, in: *Research Methods in Neurochemistry*, Vol. 1 (N. Marks and R. Rodnight, eds.), pp. 139–161, Plenum Press, New York.

McEwen, B. S., Weiss, J. M., and Schwartz, L. S., 1968, Selective retention of corticosterone by limbic structures in rat brain, *Nature* **220:**911–912.

McEwen, B. S., Weiss, J. M., and Schwartz, L. S., 1969, Uptake of corticosterone by rat brain and its concentration by certain limbic structures, *Brain Res.* **16:**227–241.

McEwen, B. S., Pfaff, D. W., and Zigmond, R. E., 1970*a*, Factors influencing sex hormone uptake by rat brain regions. II. Effects of neonatal treatment and hypophysectomy on testosterone uptake, *Brain Res.* **21:**17–28.

McEwen, B. S., Pfaff, D. W., and Zigmond, R. E., 1970*b*, Factors influencing sex hormone uptake by rat brain regions. III. Effects of competing steroids on testosterone uptake, *Brain Res.* **21:**29–38.

McEwen, B. S., Weiss, J. M., and Schwartz, L. S., 1970*c*, Retention of corticosterone by cell nuclei from brain regions of adrenalectomized rats, *Brain Res.* **17:**471–482.

McEwen, B. S., Zigmond, R. E., Azmitia, E. C., Jr., and Weiss, J. M., 1970*d*, Steroid hormone interaction with specific brain regions, in: *Biochemistry of the Brain and Behavior* (R. E. Bowman and S. P. Data, eds.), pp. 123–167, Plenum Press, New York.

McEwen, B. S., Magnus, C., and Wallach, G., 1971, Biochemical studies of corticosterone binding to cell nuclei and cytoplasmic macromolecules in specific regions of the brain, in: *Steroid Hormones and Brain Function* (C. H. Sawyer and R. A. Gorski, eds.), pp. 247–258, UCLA Forum Med. Sci. No. 15, University of California Press, Los Angeles.

McEwen, B. S., Magnus, C., and Wallach, G., 1972*a*, Soluble corticosterone-binding macromolecules extracted from rat brain, *Endocrinology* **90:**217–226.

McEwen, B. S., Zigmond, R. E., and Gerlach, J. L., 1972*b*, Sites of steroid binding and action in the brain, in: *Structure and Function of the Nervous System*, Vol. 5, (G. H. Bourne, ed.), pp. 205–291, Academic Press, New York.

McEwen, B. S., Wallach, G., and Magnus, C., 1974*a*, Corticosterone binding to hippocampus: Immediate and delayed influence of the absence of adrenal secretion, *Brain Res.* **70:**321–334.

McEwen, B. S., Denef, C. J., Gerlach, J. L., and Plapinger, L., 1974*b*, Chemical studies of the brain as a steroid hormone target tissue, in: *The Neurosciences: Third Study Program* (F. O. Schmitt and F. G. Worden, eds.), pp. 599–620, M.I.T. Press, Cambridge, Mass.

McGuire, J. L., and Lisk, R. D., 1968, Estrogen receptors in the intact rat, *Proc. Natl. Acad. Sci.* **61:**497–503.

McGuire, J. L., and Lisk, R. D., 1969, Localization of estrogen receptors in the rat hypothalamus, *Neuroendocrinology* **4:**289–295.

McGuire, J. S., Jr., and Tompkins, G. H., 1960, The heterogeneity of Δ^4-3-ketosteroid reductases, *J. Biol. Chem.* **235:**1634–1638.

Meyer, C. C., 1973, Testosterone concentration in the male chick brain: An autoradiographic survey, *Science* **180:**1381–1383.

MEYERSON, B. J., 1967, Relationship between the anaesthetic and gestagenic action and estrous behavior-inducing activity of different progestins, *Endocrinology* **81:**369–374.

MEYERSON, B., 1972, Latency between intravenous injection of progestins and the appearance of estrous behavior in estrogen-treated ovariectomized rats, *Horm. Behav.* **3:**1–9.

MEYERSON, B. J., and LINDSTROM, L., 1968, Effects of an oestrogen antagonist ethamoxytripetol (MER-25) on oestrous behavior in rats, *Acta Endocrinol.* **59:**41–48.

MEYERSON, B. J., NORDSTRÖM, E.-B., and AGMO, A., 1971, Sexual behavior and testosterone in the female rat, *Acta. Pharmacol. Toxicol.* **29:**38 (abst.) (Suppl. 4).

MICHAEL, R. P., 1961, An investigation of the sensitivity of circumscribed neurological areas to hormonal stimulation by means of the application of oestrogens directly to the brain of the cat, in: *Regional Neurochemistry* (S. Kety and J. Elkes, eds.), pp. 465–480, Pergamon Press, Oxford.

MICHAEL, R. P., 1962, Estrogen-sensitive neurons and sexual behavior in female cats, *Science* **136:**322–323.

MICHAEL, R. P., 1964, Action of hormones on the cat brain, in: *Brain and Behavior*, Vol. III (R. A. Gorski and R. E. Whalen, eds.), pp. 82–98, University of California Press, Los Angeles.

MICHAEL, R. P., 1965*a*, The selective accumulation of estrogens in the neural and genital tissues of the cat, in: *Hormonal Steroids*, Vol. 2 (L. Martini and A. Pecile, eds.), pp. 469–480, Academic Press, New York.

MICHAEL, R. P., 1965*b*, Oestrogens in the central nervous system, *Brit. Med. Bull.* **21:**87–90.

MICHAEL, R. P., 1966, Action of hormones on the cat brain, in: *Brain and Behavior*, Vol. III: *The Brain and Gonadal Function* (R. A. Gorski and R. E. Whalen, eds.), pp. 82–98, University of California Press, Los Angeles.

MOWLES, T. F., ASHKANAZY, G., MIX, E., and SHEPPARD, M., 1971, Hypothalamic and hypophyseal estradiol binding complexes, *Endocrinology* **89:**484–491.

NADLER, R. D., 1970, A biphasic influence of progesterone on sexual receptivity of spayed female rats, *Physiol. Behav.* **5:**95–97.

NADLER, R. D., 1973, Further evidence on the intra-hypothalamic locus for androgenization of female rats, *Neuroendocrinology* **12:**110–119.

NAFTOLIN, F., RYAN, K. J., and PETRO, Z., 1971*a*, Aromatization of androstenedione by the diencephalon, *J. Clin. Endocrinol.* **33:**368–370.

NAFTOLIN, F., RYAN, K. J., and PETRO, Z., 1971*b*, Aromatization of androstenedione by limbic system tissue from human foetuses, *J. Endocrinol.* **51:**795–796.

NAFTOLIN, F., RYAN, K. J., and PETRO, Z., 1972, Aromitization and androstenedione by the anterior hypothalamus of adult male and female rats, *Endocrinology* **90:**295–298.

NAFTOLIN, F., RYAN, K. J., DAVIS, I. J., PETRO, Z., and KUHN, M., 1974, The formation and metabolism of estrogens in brain tissue, *Advan. Biosci.*, in press.

NEQUIN, L. G., and SCHWARTZ, N. B., 1971, Adrenal participation in the timing of mating and LH release in the cyclic rat, *Endocrinology* **88:**325–331.

NUNEZ, E., ENGELMANN, F., BENASSAYAG, C., and JAYLE, M.-F., 1971, Identification et purification préliminaire de la foeto-protéine liant les oestrogenes dans le serum de rats nouveau-nés, *C. R. acad. Sci. Paris* **273:**831–834.

PALKA, Y. S., and SAWYER, C. H., 1966*a*, The effect of hypothalamic implants of ovarian steriods on oestrous behaviour in rabbits, *J. Physiol.* **185:**251–269.

PALKA, Y. S., and SAWYER, C. H., 1966*b*, Induction of estrous behaviour in rabbits by hypothalamic implants of testosterone, *Am. J. Physiol.* **211:**225–228.

PALKA, Y. S., RAMIREZ, V. D., and SAWYER, C. H., 1966, Distribution and biological effects of tritiated estradiol implanted in the hypothalamus hypophyseal region of female rats, *Endocrinology* **78:**487–499.

PASTEELS, J. L., and ECTORS, F., 1971, Identical localization of oestrogen- and progestogen-sensitive hypothalamic areas, in: *Basic Actions of Sex Steroids on Target Organs* (P. O. Hubinont, F. Leroy, and P. Galand, eds.), pp. 200–207, Karger, Basel.

PENG, M.-T., and PENG, Y.-M., 1973, Changes in the uptake of tritiated estradiol in the hypothalamus and adenohypophysis of old female rats, *Fert. Steril.* **24:**534–539.

PERETZ, E., 1968, Estrogen dose and the duration of the mating in cats, *Physiol. Behav.* **3:**41–43.

PEREZ-PALACIOS, G., CASTANEDA, E., GOMEZ-PEREZ, F., PEREZ, A. E., and GUAL, C., 1970, *In vitro* metabolism of androgens in dog hypothalamus, pituitary and limbic system, *Biol. Reprod.* **3:**205–213.

PETERSON, N. A., and CHAIKOFF, I. L., 1963, Uptake of intravenously-injected [4-^{14}C]cortisol by adult rat brain, *J. Neurochem.* **10:**17–23.

PETERSON, N. A., CHAIKOFF, I. L., and JONES, C., 1965, The *in vitro* conversion of cortisol to cortisone by subcellular brain fractions of young and adult rats, *J. Neurochem.* **12:**273–278.

PETRUSZ, P., and NAGY, E., 1967, On the mechanism of sexual differentiation of the hypothalamus: Decreased hypothalamic oestrogen sensitivity in androgen-sterilized female rats, *Acta Biol. Acad. Sci. Hung.* **18:**21–26.

PFAFF, D. W., 1968, Autoradiographic localization of radioactivity in the rat brain after injection of tritiated sex hormones, *Science* **161:**1355–1356.

PFAFF, D. W., 1970*a*, Nature of sex hormone effects on rat sex behaviour: Specificity of effects of individual patterns of response, *J. Comp. Physiol. Psychol.* **73:**349–358.

PFAFF, D. W., 1970*b*, Synergistic and antagonistic effects of sex hormones on rat sexual behaviour, *Am. Zoologist* **10:** (abst.).

PFAFF, D. W., 1971, Steroid sex hormones in the rat brain: Specificity of uptake and physiological effects, in: *Steroid Hormones and Brain Function* (C. H. Sawyer and R. A. Gorski, eds.), pp. 103–110, University of California Press, Los Angeles.

PFAFF, D. W., and KEINER, M., 1972, Estradiol-concentrating cells in the rat amygdala as part of a limbic hypothalamic hormone-sensitive system, in: *The Neurobiology of the Amygdala* (B. Eleftheriou, ed.), pp. 775–785, Plenum Press, New York.

PFAFF, D. W., and KEINER, M., 1973, Atlas of estradiol concentrating cells in the central nervous system of the female rat, *J. Comp. Neurol.* **151:**121–158.

PFAFF, D. W., and ZIGMOND, R. E., 1971, Neonatal androgen effects on sexual and nonsexual behaviour of adult rats tested under various hormone regimes, *Neuroendocrinology* **7:**129–145.

PFAFF, D. W., SILVA, M. T. A., and WEISS, J. H., 1971, Telemetered recording of hormone effects on hippocampal neurons, *Science* **172:**394–395.

PFAFF, D. W., DIAKOW, C., ZIGMOND, R. E., and KOW, L.-M., 1974, Neural and hormonal determinants of female mating behaviour in rats, in: *The Neurosciences*, Vol. III (F. O. Schmitt and F. G. Worden, eds.), pp. 621–646, M.I.T. Press, Boston.

PHOENIX, C. H., 1973, The role of testosterone in the sexual behaviour of laboratory male rhesus, in: *Symposium of the Fourth International Congress of Primatology*, Vol. 2: *Primate Reproductive Behaviour*, pp. 99–122, Karger, Basel.

PLAPINGER, L., and MCEWEN, B. S., 1973, Ontogeny of estradiol-binding sites in rat brain. I. Appearance of presumptive adult receptors in cytosol and nuclei, *Endocrinology* **93:**1119–1128.

PLAPINGER, L., MCEWEN, B. S., and CLEMENS, L. E., 1973, Ontogeny of estradiol-binding sites in rat brain. II. Characteristics of a neonatal binding macromolecule, *Endocrinology* **93:**1129–1139.

POTASH, L. M., 1970, Neuroanatomical regions relevant to production and analysis of vocalization within the avian, *Torus semicircularis, Experientia* **26:**1104–1105.

POWERS, J. B., 1970, Hormonal control of sexual receptivity during the estrous cycle of the rat, *Physiol. Behav.* **5:**831–835.

POWERS, J. B., 1972, Facilitation of lordosis in ovariectomized rats by intracerebral progesterone implants, *Brain Res.* **48:**311–325.

PRESL, J., RÖHLING, S., HORSKÝ, J., and HERZMANN, J., 1970, Changes in uptake of ^{3}H-estradiol by the female rat brain from birth to maturity, *Endocrinology* **86:**899–902.

PURDY, R. H., and AXELROD, L. R., 1968, Properties of corticosteroid-21-*O*-acetyltransferase from the baboon brain, *Steroids* **11:**851–862.

PURDY, R. H., GROSSER, B. I., and AXELROD, L. R., 1968, The distribution of corticosteroid-21-*O*-acetyltransferase in the baboon brain, *Steroids* **11:**837–850.

RAISINGHANI, K. H., DORFMAN, R. I., FORCHIELLI, L., GYERNEK, L., and GEUTLER, G., 1968, Uptake of intravenously administered progesterone, pregnanedione and pregnanolone by the rat brain, *Acta Endocrinol. (Copenhagen)* **57:**393–404.

RAYNAUD, J.-P., MERCIER-BODARD, C., and BAULIEU, E. E., 1971, Rat estradiol plasma protein, *Steroids* **18:**767–788.

REDDY, V. V. R., NAFTOLIN, F., and RYAN, K. J., 1973, Aromatization in the central nervous system of rabbits: Effects of castration and hormone treatment, *Endocrinology* **92:**589–594.

REDDY, V. V. R., NAFTOLIN, F., and RYAN, K. J., 1974, Conversion of androstenedione to estrone by neural tissues irom fetal and neonatal rats, *Endocrinology* **94:**117–121.

RESKO, J. A., GOY, R. W., and PHOENIX, C. H., 1967, Uptake and distribution of exogenous testosterone-1,2-^{3}H in neural and genital tissues of castrate guinea-pig, *Endocrinology* **80:**490–498.

REUTER, L. A., and LISK, R. D., 1973, Progesterone-sensitive loci for blockade of ovulation in the hamster, *Neuroendocrinology* **12:**17–29.

RHEES, R. W., ABEL, J. H., JR., and HAACK, D. W., 1972, Uptake of tritiated steroids in the brain of the duck (*Anas platyrhynchos*): An autoradiographic study, *Gen. Comp. Endocrinol.* **18:**292–300.

ROBEL, P., CORPÉCHOT, C., and BAULIEU, E. E., 1973, Testosterone and androstanolone in rat plasma and tissues, *FEBS Letters* **33:**218–220.

RODGERS, C. H., 1970, Timing of sexual behaviour in the female rat, *Endocrinology* **86:**1181–1183.

ROGERS, A. W., 1973, *Techniques of Autoradiography*, Elsevier, Amsterdam.

ROMMERTS, F. F. G., and VAN DER MOLEN, H. J., 1971, Occurrence and localization of 5α-steroid reductase, 3α- and 17β-hydroxysteroid dehydrogenases in hypothalamus and other brain tissues of the male rat, *Biochim. Biophys. Acta* **248:**489–502.

ROSS, J., CLAYBAUGH, C., CLEMENS, L. G., and GORSKI, R. A., 1971, Short latency induction of estrous behaviour with intracerebral gonadal hormones in ovariectomized rats, *Endocrinology* **89:**32–38.

ROSS, J. W., SHRYNE, J., GORSKI, R. A., and MARSHALL, J. R., 1973*a*, Effect of clomiphene citrate and its isomers on sexual behaviour in ovariectomized rats, *Endocrinology* **92:**1079–1083.

ROSS, J. W., PAUP, D. C., BRANT-ZAWADZKI, M., MARSHALL, J. R., and GORSKI, R. A., 1973*b*, Effects of *cis* and *trans*-clomiphene in the induction of sexual behaviour, *Endocrinology* **93:**681–685.

ROTH, L. J., and STUMPF, W. E. (eds.), 1969, *Autoradiography of Diffusable Substances*, Academic Press, New York.

ROTSZTEJN, W. H., 1973, Recherches sur le rôle et la régulation des récepteurs à l'oestradiol dans le système nerveux central et l'hypophyse, Thesis, University of Paris.

ROY, S. K., and LAUMAS, K. R., 1969, [1,2-^{3}H]Testosterone: Distribution and uptake in neural and genital tissues of intact male, castrate male and female rats, *Acta Endocrinol. (Copenhagen)* **61:**629–646.

ROY, S., MAHESH, V. B., and GREENBLATT, R. B., 1964, Effects of clomiphene on the physiology of reproduction in the rat. III. Inhibition of uptake of radioactive oestradiol by the uterus and the pituitary gland on immature rat, *Acta Endocrinol. (Copenhagen)* **47:**669–675.

RUF, K., and STEINER, F. A., 1967, Steroid-sensitive single neurons in rat hypothalamus and midbrain: Identification by microelectrophoresis, *Science* **156:**667–669.

RYAN, K. J., 1960, Estrogen formation by the human placenta: Studies on the mechanisms of steroid aromatization by mammalian tissues, *Acta Endocrinol. (Copenhagen)* **35:**697–698 (abst.) (Suppl. 51).

RYAN, K. J., NAFTOLIN, R., REDDY, V., FLORES, F., and PETRO, Z., 1972, Estrogen formation in the brain, *Am. J. Obstet. Gynecol.* **114:**454–460.

SAR, M., and STUMPF, W. E., 1972, Cellular localization of androgen in the brain and pituitary after the injection of tritiated testosterone, *Experientia* **28:**1364–1366.

SAR, M., and STUMPF, W. E., 1973*a*, Autoradiographic localization of radioactivity in the rat brain after the injection of 1,2-^{3}H-testosterone, *Endocrinology* **92:**251–256.

SAR, M., and STUMPF, W. E., 1973*b*, Cellular and subcellular localization of radioactivity in the rat pituitary after injection of 1,2-^{3}H-testosterone using dry autoradiography, *Endocrinology* **92:**631–635.

SAR, M., and STUMPF, W. E., 1973*c*, Effects of progesterone or cyproterone acetate on androgen uptake in the brain, pituitary and peripheral tissue, *Proc. Soc. Exp. Biol. Med.* **144:**26–29.

SAR, M., and STUMPF, W. E., 1973*d*, Neurons of the hypothalamus concentrate [^{3}H]progesterone or its metabolites, *Science* **182:**1266–1268.

SAUCIER, R., BANERJEE, R. C., BRAZEAU, P., and HUSAIN, S. M., 1970, Effects of norethynodrel on the tissue distribution of ^{3}H-estradiol-17β in ovariectomized rats, *Steroids* **16:**463–470.

SAWYER, C. H., 1972, Functions of the amygdala related to the feedback actions of gonadal steroid hormones, in: *The Neurobiology of the Amygdala* (B. E. Eleftheriou, ed.), pp. 745–762, Plenum Press, New York.

SAWYER, C. H., and GORSKI, R. A., eds., *Steroid Hormones and Brain Function*, UCLA Form. Med. Sci., No. 15, University of California Press, Los Angeles.

SAYLER, A., 1970, The effect of anti-androgens on aggressive behaviour in the gerbil, *Physiol. Behav.* **5:**667–671.

SCHRIER, B. K., and THOMPSON, E. J., 1974, On the role of glial cells in the mammalian nervous system: Uptake, excretion, and metabolism of putative neurotransmitters by cultured glial tumor cells, *J. Biol. Chem.* **249:**1769–1780.

SCHWARTZ, N. B., 1969, A model for the regulation of ovulation in the rat, *Rec. Prog. Horm. Res.* **25:**1–43.

SCHWARTZ, N. B., and TALLEY, W. L., 1965, Effect of acute ovariectomy on mating in the cyclic rat, *J. Reprod. Fertil.* **10:**463–466.

SEIKI, M., and HATTORI, R., 1971, A more extensive study of the uptake of labelled progesterone by the hypothalamus and pituitary gland of rats. *J. Endocrinol.* **51:**793–794.

SEIKI, K., HIGASHIDA, M., IMANISHI, Y., MIYAMOTO, M., KITAGAWA, T., and KOTAMI, M., 1968, Radioactivity in the rat hypothalamus and pituitary after the injection of labelled progesterone, *J. Endocrinol.* **41:**109–110.

SEIKI, M., MIYAMOTO, M., YAMASHITA, A., and KOTAMI, M., 1969, Further studies on the uptake of labelled progesterone by the hypothalamus and pituitary of rats, *J. Endocrinol.* **43:**129–130.

SHERATT, M., EXLEY, D., and ROGERS, A. W., 1969, Failure to demonstrate uptake of ^{3}H-testosterone by the hypothalamus of young rats, *Neuroendocrinology* **4:**374–376.

SHERIDAN, P. J., SAR, M., and STUMPF, W. E., 1973, Localization of ^{3}H-estradiol or its metabolites in the CNS of the neonatal female rat, *Fifty-fifth Meeting of the Endocrine Society*, p. A67 (abst.).

SHERINS, R. J., and LORIAUX, D. L., 1973, Studies on the role of sex steroids in the feedback control of FSH concentrations in men, *J. Clin. Endocrinol. Metab.* **36:**886–893.

SHIRLEY, B., WOLINSKY, J., and SCHWARTZ, N. B., 1968, Effects of a single injection of an estrogen antagonist on the estrous cycle of the rat, *Endocrinology* **82:**959–968.

SHOLITON, L. J., and WERK, E. E., 1969, The less-polar metabolites produced by incubation of testosterone 4-^{14}C with rat and bovine brain, *Acta Endocrinol. (Copenhagen)* **61:**641–648.

SHOLITON, L. J., WERK, E. E., and MACGEE, J., 1965, Metabolism of cortisol-4-C^{14} and cortisone-4-C^{14} by rat brain homogenates, *Metabolism* **14:**1122–1127.

SHOLITON, L. J., HALL, I. L., and WERK, E. E., 1970, The iso-polar metabolites produced by incubation of [4-^{14}C]testosterone with rat and bovine brain, *Acta Endocrinol. (Copenhagen)* **63:**512–518.

SHOLITON, L. J., JONES, C. E., and WERK, E. E., 1972, The uptake and metabolism of (1,2-^{3}H)-testosterone by the brain of functionally hepatectomized and totally eviscerated male rats, *Steroids* **20:**399–415.

SMITH, E. R., and DAVIDSON, J. M., 1967, Testicular maintenance and its inhibition in pituitary transplanted rats, *Endocrinology* **80:**725–734.

SMITH, E. R., WEICK, R. F., and DAVIDSON, J. M., 1969, Influence of intracerebral progesterone on the reproductive system of female rats, *Endocrinology* **85:**1129–1136.

SNIPES, C. A., and SHORE, L. S., 1972, Metabolites of progesterone *in vitro* by neural and uterine tissues, *Fed. Proc.* **31:**236 (abst.).

STEGGLES, A. W., and KING, R. J. B., 1970, The use of protamine to study [6,7-^{3}H]oestradiol-17β binding in rat uterus, *Biochem. J.* **118:**695–701.

STEINER, F. A., 1971, Local effects of adrenal steroids on cerebral neurons, in: *Steroid Hormones and Brain Function* (C. H. Sawyer and R. A. Gorski, eds.), pp. 43–47, University of California Press, Berkeley.

STEINER, F. A., RUF, K., and AKERT, F., 1969, Steroid-sensitive neurones in rat brain: Anatomical localization and responses to neurohumours and ACTH, *Brain Res.* **12:**74–85.

STERN, J. M., 1972, Androgen accumulation in hypothalamus and anterior pituitary of male ring doves; influence of steroid hormones, *Gen. Comp. Endocrinol.* **18:**439–449.

STERN, J. M., and EISENFELD, A., 1969, Androgen accumulation as binding to macromolecules in seminal vesicles: Inhibition by cyproterone, *Science* **166:**233–235.

STERN, J. M., and EISENFELD, A., 1971, Distribution and metabolism of ^{3}H-testosterone in castrated male rats; effects of cyproterone, progesterone and unlabelled testosterone, *Endocrinology* **88:**1117–1125.

STETSON, M. H., 1972, Feedback regulation of testicular function in Japanese quail: Testosterone implants in the hypothalamus and adenohypophysis, *Gen. Comp. Endocrinol.* **19:**37–47.

STEVENS, W., GROSSER, B. I., and REED, D. J., 1971, Corticosterone-binding molecules in rat brain cytosols: Regional distribution, *Brain Res.* **35:**602–607.

STEVENS, W., REED, D. J., ERICKSON, S., and GROSSER, B. I., 1973, The binding of corticosterone to brain proteins: Diurnal variation, *Endocrinology* **93:**1152–1156.

STUMPF, W. E., 1968*a*, Estradiol concentrating neurons: Topography in the hypothalamus by dry-mount autoradiography, *Science* **162:**1001–1003.

STUMPF, W. E., 1968*b*, Cellular and subcellular ^{3}H-estradiol localization in the pituitary by autoradiographs, *Z. Zellforsch.* **92:**23–33.

STUMPF, W. E., 1970*a*, Estrogen-neurons and estrogen-neuron systems in the periventricular brain, *Am. J. Anat.* **129:**207–218.

STUMPF, W. E., 1970*b*, Localization of hormones by autoradiography and other histochemical techniques: A critical review, *J. Histochem. Cytochem.* **18:**21–29.

STUMPF, W. E., 1971, Hypophysiotropic neurons in the periventricular brain: Topography of estradiol concentrating neurons, in: *Steroid Hormones and Brain Function* (C. H. Sawyer and R. A. Gorski, eds.), pp. 215–223, University of California Press, Los Angeles.

STUMPF, W. E., 1972, Estrogen, androgen and glucocorticoid concentrating neurons in the amygdala, studied by dry autoradiography, in: *The Neurobiology of the Amygdala* (B. E. Eleftheriou, ed.), pp. 763–774, Plenum Press, New York.

STUMPF, W. E., and ROTH, L. J., 1965, Thin sections cut at temperatures of −70° to −90 °C, *Nature* **205:**712–713.

STUMPF, W. E., and ROTH, L. J., 1966, High resolution autoradiography with dry-mounted freeze-dried frozen sections, *J. Histochem. Cytochem.* **14:**274–287.

STUMPF, W. E., and ROTH, L. J., 1967, Freeze-drying of small tissue samples and thin frozen sections below −60°C: A simple method of cryosorption pumping, *J. Histochem. Cytochem.* **15:**243–251.

STUMPF, W. E., and SAR, M., 1973, Hormonal inputs to releasing factor cells, feedback sites, in: *Drug Effects on Neuroendocrine Regulation* Vol. 39 of *Progress in Brain Research*, pp. 53–70, Elsevier, Amsterdam.

SULMAN, F. G., 1958, The mechanism of the push and pull principle. I. Pharmacological effect of oestrogenic hormone on the cells of the pituitary anterior lobe, *Arch. Int. Pharmacodyn.* **115:**354–359.

SWANECK, G. E., HIGHLAND, E., and EDELMAN, I. S., 1969, Stereospecific nuclear and cytosol aldosterone-binding proteins of various tissues, *Nephron* **6:**297–316.

THIESSEN, D. D., YAHR, P. I., and OWEN, K., 1973, Regulatory mechanisms of territorial marking in the Mongolian gerbil, *J. Comp. Physiol. Psychol.* **82:**382–393.

THOMAS, P. J., 1968, Cortisol acetyltransferase from baboon brain, *Biochem. J.* **109:**695–696.

TOUCHSTONE, J. C., GRIFFIN, J. E., and KASPAROW, M., 1963, Cortisol from human nerve, *Science* **141:**1275–1276.

TOUCHSTONE, J. C., KASPAROW, M., HUGHES, M. A., and HAROWITZ, M. R., 1966, Corticosteroids in human brain, *Steroids* **7:**205–211.

TUOHIMAA, P., 1971, The radioautoragraphic localization of exogenous tritiated dihydrotestosterone, testosterone, and oestradiol in the target organs of female and male rats, in: *Basic Actions of Sex Steroids on Target Organs* (P. O. Hubinot, F. Leroy, and P. Galand, eds.), pp. 208–214, Karger, Basel.

TUOHIMAA, P., and JOHANSSON, R., 1971, Decreased oestradiol binding in the uterus and anterior hypothalamus of androgenized female rats, *Endocrinology* **88:**1159–1164.

TUOHIMAA, P., and NIEMI, M., 1972*a*, Uptake of sex steroids by the hypothalamus and anterior pituitary of pre- and neonatal rats, *Acta Endocrinol. (Copenhagen)* **71:**37–44.

TUOHIMAA, P., and NIEMI, M., 1972*b*, *In vitro* uptake of tritiated sex steroids by the hypothalamus of adult rats treated neonatally with an anti-androgen (cyproterone), *Acta Endocrinol. (Copenhagen)* **71:**45–54.

UCHIDA, K., KADOWAKI, M., and MIYAKE, T., 1969*a*, Ovarian secretion of progesterone and 20α-hydroxypregn-4-en-3-one during rat estrous cycle in chronological relation to pituitary release of luteinizing hormone, *Endocrinol. Jap.* **16:**227–237.

UCHIDA, K., KADOWAKI, M., and MIYAKE, T., 1969*b*, Effect of exogenous progesterone on the preovulatory progesterone secretion in the rat, *Endocrinol. Jap.* **16:**485–491.

UCHIDA, K., KADOWAKI, M., and MIYAKE, T., 1970, Further studies on the effect of exogenous progesterone and related compounds on the preovulatory progesterone secretion in the rat, *Endocrinol. Jap.* **17:**99–106.

VON BERSWORDT-WALLRABE, R., and NEUMANN, F., 1967, Influence of a testosterone antagonist (cyproterone) on pituitary and serum FSH-content in juvenile male rats, *Neuroendocrinology* **2:**107–112.

VERTES, M., and KING, R. J. B., 1971, The mechanism of oestradiol binding in rat hypothalamus: Effect of androgenization, *J. Endocrinol.* **51:**271–282.

VERTES, M., BARNES, A., LINDNER, H. R., and KING, R. J. B., 1973, Studies on androgen and estrogen uptake by rat hypothalamus, in: *Receptors for Reproductive Hormones*, Vol. 36 st. *Advances in Experimental Medicine and Biology* (B. W. O'Malley and A. R. Means, eds.), pp. 137–173, Plenum Press, New York.

WADE, G. N., and FEDER, H. H., 1972*a*, [1,2-^{3}H]Progesterone uptake by guinea-pig brain and uterus: Differential localization, time-course of uptake and metabolism and effects of age, sex, estrogen-priming and competing steroids, *Brain Res.* **45:**525–543.

WADE, G. N., and FEDER, H. H., 1972*b*, Uptake of [1,2-^{3}H]20α-hydroxypregn-4-en-3-one, [1,2-^{3}H]corticosterone, and [6,7-^{3}H]estradiol-17β by guinea pig brain and uterus: Comparison with uptake of [1,2-^{3}H]progesterone, *Brain Res.* **45:**545–554.

WADE, G. N., and FEDER, H. H., 1972*c*, Effects of several pregnane and pregnene steroids on estrous behaviour in ovariectomized estrogen-primed guinea pigs, *Physiol. Behav.* **9:**773–775.

WADE, G. N., HARDING, C. F., and FEDER, H. H., 1973, Neural uptake of [1,2-^{3}H]progesterone in ovariectomized rats, guinea pigs and hamsters: Correlation with species differences in behavioural responsiveness, *Brain Res.* **61:**357–367.

WAREMBOURG, M., 1970*a*, Fixation de l'oestradiol ^{3}H dans le telencephale et le diencephale chez la souris femelle, *C. R. Soc. Biol.* **164:**126–129.

WAREMBOURG, M., 1970*b*, Fixation de l'oestradiol ^{3}H au niveau des noyaux amygdaliens, septaux et du système hypothalamo-hypophysaire chez la souris femelle, *C. R. Acad. Sci. Paris* **270:**152–154.

WAREMBOURG, M., 1971, Étude historadioautographique des rétroactions hormonales gonado-hypothalamiques, *Lille Med.* **16:**507–514.

WAREMBOURG, M., 1973, Études radioautographique des retroactions centrales des corticosteroides ^{3}H chez le rat et le cobaye, *Neuroendocrinologie de l'Axe Corticotrope (Brain-Adrenal Interactions)* Les Colloques de l'Institut National de la Sante et de la Recherche Medicale (P. Dell, ed.), pp. 79–94, INSERM, Paris.

WEISZ, J., and PHILPOTT, J., 1971, Uptake and metabolism of testosterone by the brain of the newborn rat, in: *Influence of Hormones on the Nervous System: Proceedings of the International Society of Psychoneuroendocrinology, Brooklyn 1970,* pp. 282–295, Karger, Basel.

WHALEN, R. E., and EDWARDS, D. A., 1969, Effects of the anti-androgen cyproterone acetate on mating behaviour and seminal vesicle tissue in male rats, *Endocrinology* **84:**155–156.

WHALEN, R. E., and GORZALKA, B. B., 1972, The effects of progesterone and its metabolites on the induction of sexual receptivity in rats, *Horm. Behav.* **3:**221–226.

WHALEN, R. E., and GORZALKA, B. B., 1973, Effects of an estrogen antagonist on behaviour and on estrogen retention in neural and peripheral target tissues, *Physiol. Behav.* **10:**35–40.

WHALEN, R. E., and HARDY, D. F., 1970, Induction of receptivity in female rats and cats with estrogen and testosterone, *Physiol. Behav.* **5:**529–533.

WHALEN, R. E., and LUTTGE, W. G., 1971*a*, Differential localization of progesterone uptake in brain: Role of sex, estrogen pretreatment and adrenalectomy, *Brain Res.* **33:**147–155.

WHALEN, R. E., and LUTTGE, W. G., 1971*b*, Role of the adrenal in the preferential accumulation of progestin by mesencephalic structures, *Steroids* **18:**141–146.

WHALEN, R. E., and LUTTGE, W. G., 1971*c*, Testosterone, androstenedione, and dihydrotestosterone: Effects on mating behaviour of male rats, *Horm. Behav.* **2:**117–125.

WHALEN, R. E., and REZEK, D. L., 1972, Localization of androgenic metabolites in the brain of rats administered testosterone or dihydrotestosterone, *Steroids* **20:**717–725.

WHALEN, R. E., LUTTGE, W. G., and GREEN, R., 1969, Effects of the anti-androgen cyproterone acetate on the uptake of 1,2-^{3}H testosterone in neural and peripheral tissues of the castrate male rat, *Endocrinology* **84:**217–222.

WHALEN, R. E., LUTTGE, W. G., and GORZALKA, B. B., 1971, Neonatal androgenization and the development of estrogen responsivity in male and female rats, *Horm. Behav.* **2:**83–90.

WHALEN, R. E., BATTIE, C., and LUTTGE, W. G., 1972, Anti-estrogen inhibition of androgen induced sexual receptivity in rats, *Behav. Biol.* **7:**311–320.

WHITSETT, J. H., BRONSON, F. H., PETERS, P. J., and HAMILTON, T. H., 1972, Neonatal organization of aggression in mice: Correlation of critical period with uptake of hormone, *Horm. Behav.* **3:**11–21.

WILSON, F. E., 1970, The tubero-infundibular neuron region of the hypothalamus: A focus of testosterone sensitivity in male tree sparrows (*Spizella arborea*), in: *Aspects of Neuroendocrinology* (W. Bargmann and B. Scharrer, eds.), pp. 274–286, Springer-Verlag, Heidelberg.

WILSON, J. D., and GLOYNA, R. E., 1970, The intranuclear metabolism of testosterone in the accessory organs of reproduction, *Rec. Prog. Horm. Res.* **26:**309–330.

WILSON, J. D., BRUCHOVSKY, N., and CHATFIELD, J. N., 1969, Intranuclear localization of testosterone-1,2-^{3}H in rat prostate, in: *Progress in Endocrinology: Proceedings of the Third International Congress of Endocrinology, Mexico 1968,* pp. 17–23, Excerpta Medica Foundation, Amsterdam.

WOOLEY, D. E., HOLINKA, C. F., and TIMIRAS, D. E., 1969, Changes in ^{3}H-estradiol distribution with development in the rat, *Endocrinology* **84:**157–161.

WYSS, K. H., KARSZNIA, K., HEINRICHS, W. L., and HERRMANN, W. L., 1968, Inhibition of uterine receptor binding of estradiol by antiestrogens (clomiphene and CL-868), *J. Clin. Endocrinol.* **28:**1824–1828.

ZIGMOND, R. E., 1971, Anatomical and chemical specificity of gonadal hormone retention in the rat brain, Thesis, Rockefeller University, New York.

ZIGMOND, R. E., and MACKAY, A. V. P., 1974, Dissociation of stimulatory and synthetic phases in the induction of tyrosine hydroxylase, *Nature* **247:**112–113.

ZIGMOND, R. E., and MCEWEN, B. S., 1970, Selective retention of estradiol by brain cell nuclei in specific regions of the ovariectomized rat, *J. Neurochem.* **17**:889–899.

ZIGMOND, R. E., STERN, J. M., and MCEWEN, B. S., 1972*a*, Retention of radioactivity by brain cell nuclei in the ring dove after injection of ^{3}H-testosterone, *Gen. Comp. Endocrinol.* **18**:450–453.

ZIGMOND, R. E., NOTTEBOHM, F., and PFAFF, D. W., 1972*b*, Distribution of androgen-concentrating cells in the brain of the chaffinch, in: *Proceedings of the Fourth International Congress of Endocrinology, Washington 1972*, Excerpta Medica Foundation, Amsterdam (abst.).

ZIGMOND, R. E., NOTTEBOHM, F., and PFAFF, D. W., 1973, Androgen-concentrating cells in the midbrain of a songbird, *Science* **179**:1005–1007.

ZIGMOND, R. E., MACKAY, A. V. P., and IVERSEN, L. L., 1974, Minimum duration of trans-synaptic stimulation required for the induction of tyrosine hydroxylase by reserpine in the rat superior cervical ganglion, *J. Neurochem.* **23**:355–358.

ZUCKER, I., 1966*a*, Effects of an antiandrogen on the mating behaviour of male guinea pigs and rats, *J. Endocrinol.* **35**:209–210.

ZUCKER, I., 1966*b*, Facilitatory and inhibitory effects of progesterone on sexual responses of spayed guinea pigs, *J. Comp. Physiol. Psychol.* **62**:376–381.

ZUCKER, I., 1967*a*, Progesterone in the experimental control of the behavioural sex cycle in the female rat, *J. Endocrinol.* **38**:269–277.

ZUCKER, I., 1967*b*, Actions of progesterone in the control of sexual receptivity of the spayed female rat, *J. Comp. Physiol. Psychol.* **63**:313–316.

ZUCKER, I., 1968, Biphasic effects of progesterone on sexual receptivity in the female guinea pig, *J. Comp. Physiol. Psychol.* **65**:472–478.

ZUCKER, I., and GOY, R. W., 1967, Sexual receptivity in the guinea pig: Inhibitory and facilitatory actions of progesterone and related compounds, *J. Comp. Physiol. Psychol.* **64**:378–383.

6

OPIATE RECEPTOR MECHANISMS

Solomon H. Snyder, Gavril W. Pasternak, and Candace B. Pert

1. INTRODUCTION

Research directed at identifying mechanisms whereby drugs exert their therapeutic actions is inherently difficult. It is easy for pharmacologists to describe many "effects" of drugs on physiological and biochemical processes. Uncertainties crop up when one endeavors to conclude that a particular effect represents the mechanism of action of the drug. Opiates, like most other drugs, produce myriad effects on biological organisms, on energy metabolism, protein synthesis, nucleic acid disposition, neuronal firing patterns, and neurotransmitter disposition. Some of these effects are clearly irrelevant pharmacologically, because they are elicited by drugs that have no opiate-like pharmacological actions. However, even for effects which correlate with the relative pharmacological potency of various opiates, one cannot readily ascertain whether the effects are primary or are simply secondary consequences of some other, more fundamental drug action.

If pharmacological actions of opiates are consequent to a selective interaction of these drugs with discrete receptor sites and if it were

---

Solomon H. Snyder, Gavril W. Pasternak, and Candace B. Pert • Departments of Pharmacology and Experimental Therapeutics and Psychiatry and Behavioral Sciences. The Johns Hopkins University School of Medicine, Baltimore, Maryland. Work supported by USPHS Drug Abuse Research Center Grant DA-00266, Scottish Rite and Medical Life Insurance fellowships to C. B. P. and G. W. P., respectively, and NIMH RSDA Award MH 33128 to S. H. S.

possible to label biochemically these receptor sites, one might readily answer major questions about opiate actions. For instance, much is known about the roles of various brain areas in mediating pain. A selective localization of opiate receptors to particular "pain centers" in the brain might explain how the drugs elicit analgesia. Much research has focused on interactions of opiates and biogenic amine neurotransmitters. If the opiate receptor were selectively localized to neurons using a particular neurotransmitter, one could conclude that such neurons represented the initial critical site of opiate action. Most tantalizing is the possibility that understanding of opiate receptor mechanisms might elucidate the nature of tolerance to and physical dependence on opiates.

An abundance of pharmacological data suggests that opiates do act on discrete receptors. There are striking commonalities in the chemical structures of most opiates (Fig. 1 and Table 1). Although some opiates such as meperidine and methadone at first glance seem to lack the basic morphine-like formula, molecular models indicate that they readily assume a conformation mimicking the basic elements of the morphine structure. These are (1) a quaternary carbon atom, (2) an aromatic nucleus linked to this carbon, (3) a tertiary amino group two saturated carbon atoms away from the quaternary carbon atom, and (4) a phenolic hydroxyl group *meta* to the quaternary carbon, if the tertiary nitrogen is part of a fused piperidine ring.

Besides similar chemical structures, the marked stereospecificity of opiate actions strongly favors highly selective stereospecific receptor sites. For most opiates, the (−)-isomer contains essentially all pharmacological

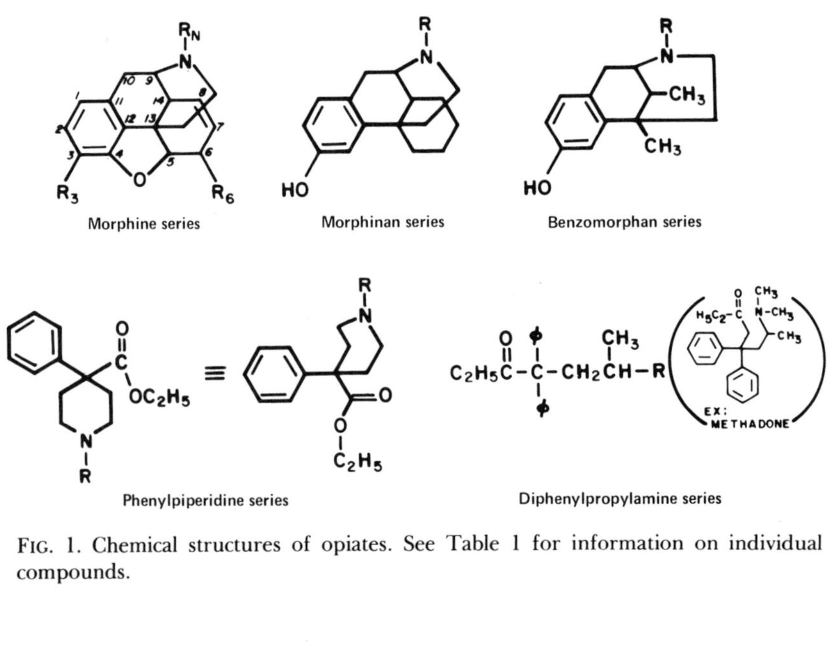

FIG. 1. Chemical structures of opiates. See Table 1 for information on individual compounds.

TABLE 1

Chemical Structures of Opiates (see Fig. 1)

Name	R_3	R_6	R_N	C_{14}	C_7–C_8 bond	Other
Morphine series						
Morphine	$-OH$	$-OH$	$-CH_3$	$-H$	Double	—
Heroin	$-OCOCH_3$	$-OCOCH_3$	$-CH_3$	$-H$	Double	—
Codeine	$-OCH_3$	$-OH$	$-CH_3$	$-H$	Double	—
Normorphine	$-OH$	$-OH$	$-H$	$-H$	Double	—
Nalorphine	$-OH$	$-OH$	$-CH_2CH{=}CH_2$	$-H$	Double	—
Dihydromorphine	$-OH$	$-OH$	$-CH_3$	$-H$	Single	—
Thebaine	$-OCH_3$	$-OCH_3$	$-CH_3$	—	Single	Double bonds at C_8–C_{14} and C_6–C_7
Hydromorphone	$-OH$	$=O$	$-CH_3$	$-H$	Single	—
Metopon	$-OH$	$=O$	$-CH_3$	$-H$	Single	$-CH_3$ at C_5
Oxymorphone	$-OH$	$=O$	$-CH_3$	$-OH$	Single	—
Oxycodone	$-OCH_3$	$=O$	$-CH_3$	$-OH$	Single	—
Naloxone	$-OH$	$=O$	$-CH_2CH{=}CH_2$	$-OH$	Single	—
Naltrexone	$-OH$	$=O$	$-CH_2-CH\begin{smallmatrix}CH_2\\ \vert\\ CH_2\end{smallmatrix}$	$-OH$	Single	—
Etorphine	$-OH$	$-OCH_3$	$-CH_3$	—	Single	Add $C_{14}-CH{=}CH-C_6$ bridge; add $-\overset{OH}{\underset{CH_3}{C}}C_3H_7$ at C_7
Diprenorphine	$-OH$	$-OCH_3$	$-CH_2-CH\begin{smallmatrix}CH_2\\ \vert\\ CH_2\end{smallmatrix}$	—	Single	Add $C_{14}-CH{=}CH-C_6$ bridge; add $-\overset{OH}{C}(CH_3)_2$ at C_7

TABLE 1—*contd.*

Name	R
Morphinan series	
Levorphanol	$-CH_3$
Levallorphan	$-CH_2CH{=}CH_2$
Cyclorphan	$-CH_2-CH\begin{smallmatrix}CH_2\\ \vert \\ CH_2\end{smallmatrix}$
	R
Benzomorphan series	
Metazocine	$-CH_3$
Phenazocine	$-CH_2CH_2$-phenyl
Pentazocine	$-CH_2CH{=}C(CH_3)_2$
Cyclazocine	$-CH_2CH\begin{smallmatrix}CH_2\\ \vert \\ CH_2\end{smallmatrix}$
	R
Phenylpiperidine series	
Meperidine	$-CH_3$
Anileridine	$-CH_2CH_2$-phenyl-*p*-NH_2
Piminodine	$-CH_2CH_2CH_2NH$-phenyl
Phenoperidine	$-CH_2CH_2CHOH$-phenyl
α-Prodine	$-CH_3$
	Replace $-OCOC_2H_5$ with $-COOC_2H_5$

	R
Diphenylpropylamine series	
Methadone	$-N(CH_3)_2$
Phenadoxone	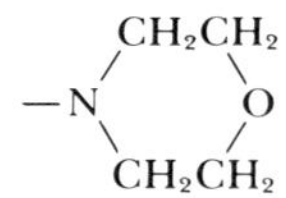
Dipipanone	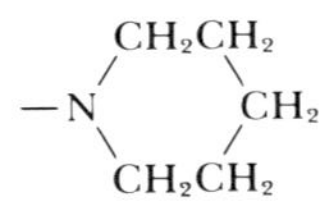

activity of the drug, the (+)-form being virtually inactive. The cross-tolerance among all opiates examined also argues for specific receptors.

2. BIOCHEMICAL IDENTIFICATION OF OPIATE–RECEPTOR BINDING

Most attempts to identify opiate–receptor binding have made use of the stereospecific character of opiate actions. Opiate–receptor binding is suggested by the extent to which the (−)-isomer exhibits greater binding than the (+)-isomer. Several studies of the accumulation by the brain of radioactive opiates administered either *in vivo* or *in vitro* failed to discriminate between (+)- and (−)-isomers or opiates of different pharmacological potencies and presumably did not represent selective accumulation by opiate receptor sites (Ingoglia and Dole, 1970; Berkowitz and Way, 1971; Hug and Oka, 1971; Navon and Lajtha, 1970; Seeman *et al.*, 1972; Clouet and Williams, 1973). Goldstein *et al.* (1971) examined the binding of radioactive levorphanol to mouse brain homogenates and determined the extent to which nonradioactive levorphanol or its (+)-isomer, dextrorphan, prevented levorphanol binding. Only 2% of levorphanol binding was displaced to a greater extent by levorphanol than by dextrorphan. Presumably because stereospecific binding was so limited, displacement by a variety

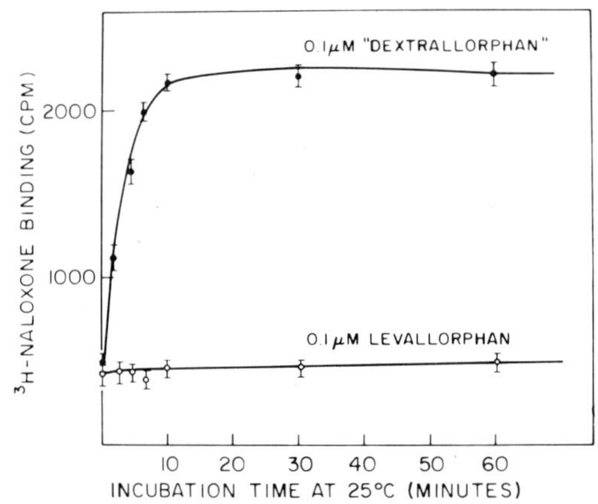

FIG. 2. Time course of [^{3}H]naloxone binding. Standard rat brain homogenate was incubated from 0 to 60 min in the presence of [^{3}H]naloxone (1.5 nM) and either (−)-3-hydroxy-*N*-allylmorphinan (levallorphan) or (+)-3-hydroxy-*N*-allylmorphinan (dextrallorphan) at a concentration of 0.1 μM.

TABLE 2

Glass Fiber Filter Binding of [^{3}H]Naloxone[a]

	[^{3}H]Naloxone bound (counts/min)			
	No drug	Levorphanol	Dextrorphan	Stereo-specific
"Solubilized receptor"	815 ± 40	680 ± 15	862 ± 23	178 ± 27
"Solubilized receptor" from trypsinized tissue	834 ± 24	603 ± 32	893 ± 53	293 ± 62
Buffer only	1101 ± 51	597 ± 12	872 ± 30	293 ± 32

[a] Rat brains were homogenized in 10 vol 0.32 M sucrose and the supernatant from a 1000 *g* 10-min centrifugation was divided into equal portions. One was treated with trypsin (1 mg/ml) at 25 °C for 20 min (when the treated homogenate was tested there was no stereospecific particulate binding remaining). The treated and control tissue homogenates were then centrifuged at 49,000 *g* for 20 min and the pellets were extracted with deoxycholate (1%), centrifuged at 100,000 *g* for 2 h, and extensively dialyzed. The precipitates which formed following the dialyses were then tested for stereospecific [^{3}H]naloxone binding in a typical assay (Pasternak and Snyder, 1974) with either levorphanol or dextrorphan present at 0.1 μM and filtered over Whatman glass fiber filters (B). The values reported are the means ± SE of triplicate samples.

of opiates was not examined to establish whether the stereospecific binding was pharmacologically relevant. Such experiments are crucial because stereospecific binding might involve some tissue component which is unrelated to the pharmacological opiate receptor but which exhibits sufficient conformational symmetry so as to bind levorphanol in a stereospecific fashion.

Using [^{3}H]naloxone of high specific activity (6 Ci/mmol), we identified stereospecific opiate–receptor binding (Pert and Snyder, 1973*a,b*), findings confirmed by others (Terenius, 1973, 1974; Simon *et al.*, 1973; Wong and Horng, 1973; Hitzemann and Loh, 1973; Klee and Streaty, 1974). The majority of [^{3}H]naloxone binding by brain homogenates could be displaced by levorphanol but not by dextrorphan so that the ratio of "experimental" to "blank" values was about 2.5 : 1 (Fig. 2). More recently, using [^{3}H]opiates of greater specific activity, we found 90% of the binding to be stereospecific.

However, stereospecific binding, while necessary, is not a sufficient criterion for the opiate receptor. This became fairly evident to us in the course of the experiments in which we felt we had "solubilized" the opiate receptor. Membrane fractions from the brain had been treated with detergents to solubilize the receptor. After the detergent had been dialyzed away, the reprecipitated "soluble" fraction was incubated with radioactive opiates in the presence of nonradioactive levorphanol or dextrorphan, and the mixture filtered rapidly on glass filters. Definite stereospecific binding was obtained. But when we repeated the same experiment omitting brain tissue, we also obtained stereospecific binding. Clearly the filters themselves were capable of binding opiates in a stereospecific fashion (Table 2). Stereospecific opiate binding occurs with some filters but not with others.

If glass filters can bind opiates stereospecifically, might not certain macromolecular brain constituents also exhibit stereospecific opiate binding, which, like the glass filters, is not related to the pharmacological actions of opiates? Lowney *et al.* (1974) described the solubilization and purification of a lipid-rich brain substance that binds levorphanol stereospecifically and saturably. Loh *et al.* (1974) showed that this binding could be accounted for by cerebrosides, which may or may not be related to the opiate receptor.

One must be cautious about equating tissue binding with receptor function even if the binding examined is saturable at low concentrations. Hollenberg and Cuatrecasas (personal communication) observed that insulin binding to glass saturates at extremely low concentrations, similar to the affinity of the true insulin receptor for insulin.

To ensure that stereospecific [^{3}H]naloxone binding to brain homogenates represents true opiate–receptor binding, we evaluated a wide range of drugs (Table 3). The pharmacological potencies of a variety of opiates and opiate antagonists are related proportionally to their ability to compete with [^{3}H]naloxone for binding to the opiate receptor. Etorphine, one of the most potent known analgesics, has 20 times the affinity of morphine, with an ED_{50} value of about 0.3 nM. Etonitazene, an opiate whose potency *in vivo* is similar to that of etorphine, is almost as potent as etorphine in displacing [^{3}H]-naloxone binding. Levorphanol has 4000 times the affinity of dextrorphan,

TABLE 3

Relative Potencies of Drugs in Reducing Stereospecific [^{3}H]Naloxone Binding to Rat Brain Homogenate[a]

Drug	ED_{50} (nM)	No effect at 0.1 mM
(−)-Etorphine	0.3	Phenobarbital
(−)-Etonitazene	0.5	Norepinephrine
Levallorphan	1	Atropine
Levorphanol	2	Pilocarpine
(−)-Nalorphine	3	Arecholine
(−)-Morphine	7	Colchicine
(−)-Cyclazocine	10	γ-Aminobutyric acid
(−)-Naloxone	10	Bicuculline
(−)-Hydromorphine	20	Serotonin
(−)-Methadone	30	Carbamylcholine
(±)-Pentazocine	50	Neostigmine
(+)-Methadone	300	Hemicholinium
Meperidine	1,000	Histamine
(±)-Propoxyphene	1,000	Glycine
(+)-3-Hydroxy-*N*-allylmorphinan	7,000	Glutamic acid
Dextrorphan	8,000	Δ^9-Tetrahydrocannabinol
(−)-Codeine	20,000	Acetylsalicylic acid
(−)-Oxycodone	30,000	Caffeine

[a]From Pert and Snyder (1973*b*).

its analgesically inactive enantiomer. Similarly, levallorphan, the opiate antagonist derived from levorphanol, is 7000 times more potent than its (+)-enantiomer. (−)-Methadone, the more analgesically active form of methadone, is only about 10 times as potent as (+)-methadone, perhaps because it has greater conformational mobility than levorphanol. Codeine, which is analgesically about one-fifth as potent as morphine, displays less than 1/3000 the receptor affinity of morphine. This apparent lack of correlation between affinity for opiate receptor binding sites and pharmacological activity does not represent a true discrepancy. Instead, it is consistent with pharmacological studies which indicate that codeine has no analgesic activity itself, but acts only after *O*-demethylation by liver microsomal enzymes to morphine (Way and Alder, 1962). Thus while codeine is an effective analgesic when administered parenterally, it is inactive when injected directly into the brain. Propoxyphene, a weak analgesic, has only 1/200 the affinity of morphine for receptor sites.

Since these opiates differ in their accessibility to the brain and their metabolic rate, we sought a series of opiate homologues which presumably enter the brain to a similar extent. The ketobemidones all have the same basic structure, differing only in the *N* substituent, yet have markedly discrepant analgesic potencies (Table 4). The pharmacological potency of these drugs correlates very closely with affinity for the opiate receptor.

Despite the impressive correlation between pharmacological potency and affinity for [^{3}H]naloxone binding sites, one could argue that if these sites were to interact with a large number of other drugs they might not be truly

TABLE 4

Ketobemidones: Correlations of Analgesic Potency and Opiate Receptor Affinity

Compound	Analgesic potency ED_{50} mg/kg	ED_{50} (nM) no sodium
Norketobemidone	Not tested	7–8
Ketobemidone	0.8	7–10
Ethyl-	23.0	400
Propyl-	5.7	200
Butyl-	1.7	50
Pentyl-	0.3	8
Hexyl-	3.0	20
Heptyl	3.7	20
Octyl	15–20	200
Nonyl-	15–20	700
Decyl-	Inactive	500

From Wilson *et al.* (1975).

TABLE 5

Drugs Ineffective in Altering [³H]Dihydromorphine Binding[a]

Acetyl-β-methylcholine	Doxepin	Phenelzine
Acetylsalicylic aid	Ecolid	Neostigmine
γ-Aminobutyric acid	Ephedrine	Nialamide
Arecoline	Epinephrine	Nicotine
Atropine	Ethosoximide	Nortriptyline
Bicuculline	Fenfluramine	Octopamine
Bretylium	Glutamic acid	Ornithine
Brocresine	Glycine	Orphenadrine
Bromodiphenhydramine	Hemicholinium-3	Pargyline
3α-(5*H*-Dibenzo[*a, d*]-cyclohepten-*S*-yl)	Histamine	Peganone
Oxytropane	Hydroxyamphetamine	Promethazine
Bulbocapnine	Hydroxychloroquine	Phenobarbital
Butylcholine	Hydroxyzine	Phenylpropanolamine
Caffeine	Hyoscine	Pilocarpine
Carbamylcholine	Imipramine	Serotonin
Carbinoxamine	Iprindole	Taurine
Chlordiazepoxide	Isoproteronol	Tetrabenazine
Chlorpheniramine	Leucine	Δ^9-Tetrahydrocannabinol
Cobefrin	Mecamylamine	β-(2-Thienyl)isopropylamine
Colchicine	Methergine	Threonine
Cycramine	Methdilazine	Tranylcypromine
Decamethonium	3-Methoxytyramine	Trifluoperazine
Desipramine	3-Methoxy-4-hydroxy-mandelic acid	Triprolidine
Diethylpropion	α-Methyldopa	Tryptamine
Dopamine	Pentylenetetrazole	Tryptophan
		3-Iodo-L-tyrosine
		Urecholine
		Valine

[a] Drugs at a final concentration of 3×10^{-5} M were preincubated with rat brain homogenate in the standard binding assay using [³H]dihydromorphine (1 nM) as previously described (Pert and Snyder, 1973*b*). None of the listed compounds produces significant inhibition of stereospecific [³H]dihydromorphine binding at 3×10^{-5} M.

specific "opiate receptors." To examine this possibility, we examined a large number of nonopiates. All displayed negligible affinity for naloxone binding sites (Table 5).

3. LOCALIZATION OF THE OPIATE RECEPTOR TO SYNAPTIC MEMBRANES

To ascertain what types of tissue might contain opiate receptors, we evaluated a range of organs (Table 6). Receptor binding appears largely restricted to tissues that contain a significant innervation and is absent from

TABLE 6

Tissue Distribution of Stereospecific [^{3}H]Naloxone Binding[a]

Source	Weight of tissue (g)	Stereospecific binding (counts/min)
Rat brain	0.016	623
Guinea pig kidney	0.168	1400
Rat kidney	0.165	N.D.
Guinea pig heart	0.143	N.D.
Rat liver	0.060	N.D.
Guinea pig liver	0.140	N.D.
Guinea pig small intestine:		
Myenteric plexus and longitudinal muscle	0.070	706
Longitudinal muscle only	0.070	N.D.
Rat intestine:		
Myenteric plexus and longitudinal muscle	0.060	N.D.
Human erythrocytes	0.110	N.D.
Baker's yeast	0.040	N.D.

[a][^{3}H]Naloxone (8 nM) binding was assessed by the standard binding assay or centrifugation. N.D., Not detectable. The lower limit of reliable detection is about 50 counts/min. In part from Pert and Snyder (1973*a*).

tissues such as red blood cells, yeast, and liver, which are largely nonnervous. The guinea pig ileum responds pharmacologically to opiates in a fashion which correlates closely with the relative analgesic activities of these drugs (Paton, 1957; Kosterlitz *et al.*, 1973). Guinea pig ileum displays substantial amounts of opiate–receptor binding, as does the brain. Removal of the myenteric plexus of nerves from the intestine abolishes receptor binding despite the fact that the nervous plexus by weight is only a miniscule fraction of total tissue mass. Thus in the guinea pig ileum the opiate receptor is restricted to nervous tissue. The rat intestine, which does not respond pharmacologically to opiates (H. Kosterlitz, personal communication), also has no detectable opiate–receptor binding. Binding is abundant in guinea pig kidney but not in rat kidney.

Within the brain, an important question relates to the subcellular localization of the opiate receptor. Many theories postulate that opiates act at synapses in the brain. Techniques are currently available which enable one to isolate in fairly pure fashion synaptosomes, or pinched-off nerve endings. The synaptosomes can be hypotonically lysed and the mixture further fractionated to produce preparations of synaptic vesicles, synaptic membranes, mitochondria, and other membranes. When brains of rats are subjected to such fractionation procedures (Pert *et al.*, 1974*a*), opiate–receptor binding is highly localized to the synaptosome fraction purified from the crude mitochondrial pellet of rat brain homogenates (Table 7). When the crude mitochondrial pellet is subjected to hypotonic lysis and the mixture centrifuged on a sucrose grandient, the majority of

TABLE 7

Subcellular Localization of the Opiate Receptor: Subfractions of Unlysed P_2 and P_1[a]

	[^{3}H]Dihydromorphine specifically bound (fmol/mg protein)	Activity (% of total) Opiate receptor
Whole homogenate	20.6	
P_1 (1000 *g*, 10 min)	6.9	31
P_2 (17,500 *g*, 20 min)	29.6	52
S_2	11.8	17
Subfractionation of P_2 (0.32 M)	2	0
A (0.32–0.8 M), myelin, etc.	19.7	11
B (0.8–1.2 M), synaptosomes	45.1	67
C (1.2 M), mitochondria	25.8	22
Subfractionation of P_1		
A (0.32–1.5 M)	6.8	95
B (1.8 M), nuclear pellet	3.9	5

[a] Stereospecific [^{3}H]dihydromorphine binding to various subfractions of rat brain homogenate was determined after differential centrifugation on a discontinuous sucrose gradient. About 1.5 mg of protein was incubated in triplicate with 1 nM [^{3}H]dihydromorphine for 30 min at 25 °C in the presence of dextrorphan or levorphanol (100 nM). Values are the means of three experiments which varied less than 15%. Mean recovery of the total activity of the whole homogenate was 104%, while 94% of the total activity of P_2 could be recovered in fractions A, B, and C. In some experiments, when stereospecific [^{3}H]naloxone (1.5 nM) was assessed in parallel almost identical distribution of enrichment and activity among fractions as with [^{3}H]dihydromorphine was found. Adapted from Pert *et al.* (1974*a*).

opiate–receptor binding is recovered in fractions enriched in synaptic membranes (Table 8). Virtually no opiate–receptor binding is detected in the synaptic vesicle fraction and very little appears in the fraction containing intact mitochondria. Localization of opiate–receptor binding to synaptic membranes does not establish whether the membranes involved are presynaptic or postsynaptic. However, it does suggest that opiates exert their primary pharmacological effects by altering synaptic function.

4. REGIONAL DISTRIBUTION OF OPIATE–RECEPTOR BINDING

Mechanisms mediating pain involve diverse brain areas. Rapidly conducting somatosensory projection pathways involved in fine sensory discrimination with the brain are localized, in part, in the medial lemniscus in the midbrain, in the ventrobasal complex of the thalamus, and in the parietal region of the

TABLE 8

Subcellular Localization of the Opiate Receptor: Subfractionation of Lysed P_2[a]

	[³H]Dihydromorphine specifically bound (fmol/mg protein)	Activity (% of total)		
		Opiate receptor	MAO	K
Whole homogenate	23.9			
P_1	7.2	15	26	4
S_2	6.3	18	8	76
Lysed P_2, 10,000 *g* supernatant fluid	25.7	32	11	17
Lysed P_2, 10,000 *g* pellet	26.6	35	55	3
Subfractionation of lysed P_2, 10,000 *g* supernatant fluid				
Lysate (0), no organized structures	<2	0	11	73
D (0–0.4 M), synaptic vesicles	2.6	10	13	19
E (0.4–0.6 M), microsomes, etc.	25.2	6	10	4
F (0.6–0.8 M), synaptosome ghosts, membrane fragments	87.3	32	25	2
G (0.8–1.0 M), same as F	96.1	36	27	1
H (1.0–1.2 M), damaged synaptosomes	50.8	21	3	0
I (1.2 M), small mitochondria, shrunken synaptosomes	21.0	4	11	0

[a] Stereospecific [^{3}H]dihydromorphine binding to various subfractions of rat brain homogenate was determined after lysis and differential centrifugation of the crude synaptosomal–mitochondrial pellet (P_2) on a discontinuous sucrose gradient. Values are the means of three experiments which varied less than 15%. Mean recovery of the total activity of the homogenate was 87%. When stereospecific [^{3}H]naloxone (1.5 nM) was assessed in parallel, almost identical distribution of enrichment and activity among fractions as with [^{3}H]dihydromorphine was found. Recovery of lysed P_2 activity was 96%. Adapted from Pert *et al.* (1974*a*).

cerebral cortex. The more slowly conducting somato-sensory projection pathways are somewhat more diffusely localized throughout the brain and include the periaqueductal gray of the midbrain, the intralaminar and medial nuclei of the thalamus, hence the more medial portions of the thalamus, and the frontal portion of the cerebral cortex. The system also possesses intimate connections with all regions of the limbic system such as the olfactory areas of the brain, the amygdala, and the septum. These more slowly conducting pathways are thought to be more intimately involved in pain perception itself than the rapid pathways. Certainly, knowing which parts of the brain are richest in opiate–receptor binding might help to elucidate the effect of opiates on pain. To clarify some of the questions, we examined opiate–receptor binding in numerous regions of monkey and human brain (Kuhar *et al.*, 1973*a*) (Table 9).

Opiate–receptor binding varies dramatically throughout the monkey brain. The amygdala contains the greatest amount of binding, with the

TABLE 9

Opiate–Receptor Binding in Regions of Monkey Brain[a]

Region	Stereospecific dihydromorphine binding (fmol/mg protein)		Region	Stereospecific dihydromorphine binding (fmol/mg protein)	
Cerebral hemispheres			Hypothalamus		
Frontal pole	11.9 ± 1.4	(4)	Medial hypothalamus	24.2 ± 3.2	(4)
Superior temporal gyrus	10.8 ± 2.5	(3)	Anterior hypothalamus	24.3 ± 3.7	(3)
Middle temporal gyrus	7.1	(1)	Posterior hypothalamus	24.7 ± 1.4	(3)
Inferior temporal gyrus	6.0	(1)	Hypothalamus	32.2	(1)
Precentral gyrus	3.4	(2)	Mammillary bodies	5.0	(1)
Postcentral gyrus	2.8	(2)			
Occipital pole	2.3 ± 0.5	(4)			
White matter areas			Thalamus		
Corpus callosum	< 2	(2)	Medial thalamus	24.6 ± 1.6	(3)
Corona radiata	≤ 2	(2)	Lateral thalamus	7.8	(2)
Anterior commissure	5.4	(2)			
Fornix	< 2	(2)	Extrapyramidal areas		
Optic chiasm	< 2	(2)	Caudate nucleus (head)	19.4 ± 2.3	(4)
			Caudate nucleus (body)	9.0 ± 1.2	(3)
Limbic cortex			Caudate nucleus (tail)	8.9 ± 3.0	(3)
Anterior amygdala	65.1 ± 21	(4)	Putamen	11.7 ± 1.9	(6)
Posterior amygdala	34.1 ± 4.2	(4)	Globus pallidus	7.7	(2)
Hippocampus	12.5 ± 2.2	(4)	Internal capsule	5.4	(2)

Midbrain			Cerebellum–lower brain stem—*cont.*		
Superior colliculi	10.6 ± 2.0	(3)	Dentate nucleus	1.9	(2)
Inferior colliculi	6.7 ± 0.7	(3)	Floor of fourth ventricle	6.3 ± 1.3	(3)
Interpeduncular nucleus area	13.7 ± 1.5	(4)	Pyramidal tract	3.0	(2)
Raphe area	8.2	(2)	Lower medulla	5.8	(2)
Periaqueductal gray	31.1 ± 4.6	(4)			
			Spinal cord (thoracic)		
Cerebellum–lower brain stem			Dorsal column (white)	3.1	(2)
Pons (ventral)	1.4	(2)	Lateral cord (white)	3.3	(1)
Cerebellar cortex	< 2	(2)	Gray matter	8.8	(2)

[a] Values represent means ± SEM followed in parentheses by the number of determinations. Each determination was calculated from triplicate incubations with 1 nM [^{3}H]dihydromorphine in the presence of 100 nM levorphanol or dextrorphan. Five rhesus monkeys (*Macaca mulatta*) were decapitated 2 h after anesthesia with 30–45 mg/kg i.p. of sodium pentobarbital, The brain was removed within 5 min and dissected rapidly on ice. Adapted from Kuhar *et al.* (1973*a*).

anterior portion displaying almost twice as much binding as the posterior amygdala. Binding in the periaqueductal area of the midbrain is about the same as that in the posterior amygdala. The hypothalamus and the medial thalamus, the next highest areas, display only about 40% of the binding of the anterior amygdala. No regional variations are detected within the hypothalamus, while the medial thalamus possesses about 3 times as much binding as the lateral thalamus. In the head of the caudate, receptor binding is about 80% of that in hypothalamus and medial thalamus, double that of the body and tail of the caudate, and 1.7 times binding in the putamen. Levels of binding in the putamen are similar to those of the hippocampus, the superior colliculi, the interpeduncular nucleus area and the frontal pole and superior temporal gyrus of the cerebral cortex.

Within the cerebral cortex, there are marked regional variations. Thus binding in the precentral gyrus, postcentral gyrus, and occipital pole is less than a quarter of that in the frontal cortex. Receptor binding is very low or not detectable in white matter areas such as the corpus callosum, corona radiata, fornix, and optic chiasm.

As observed before in the rat brain (Pert and Snyder, 1973*a*), opiate–receptor binding in monkey is quite low in the cortex and dentate nucleus of the cerebellum and in the lower brain stem and spinal cord. Within the spinal cord, binding is greater in gray than in white matter.

Kinetic analysis of receptor binding indicates that regional differences in stereospecific binding reflect variations in the total number of receptor sites rather than in their affinity.

Regional differences in opiate–receptor binding in the human brain grossly resemble those in the monkey (Kuhar *et al.*, 1973*a*; Hiller *et al.*, 1973). The greatest amount of binding occurs in the amygdala and the thalamus. The thalamic sample analyzed predominantly represents medial portions of this brain area. The concentration of opiate receptors is next highest in the human in the head of the caudate and the hypothalamus. In the human as in the monkey, the periaqueductal area of the midbrain and the putamen display high levels of binding while negligible binding is detected in the cerebellar cortex. Also, as in the monkey, binding varies within the human cerebral hemisphere, with 5 times as much binding in the frontal pole as in the occipital pole and negligible binding in the corona radiata. Hiller *et al.* (1973) also report high levels of binding in the human olfactory trigone and the septum.

How does this distribution compare with the relative roles of various brain areas in mediating opiate-induced analgesia? In experiments in which morphine was injected stereotaxically into numerous sites of rhesus monkey brain, analgesic responses were found to be limited to the mesencephalic and ventral diencephalic areas surrounding the third and fourth ventricles (Pert and Yaksh, 1974). Similar experiments with rats and mice also suggest that these areas are critical for eliciting analgesia (Tsou and Jang, 1964; Herz and Teschemacher, 1971). Following the application of naloxone crystals in the rat brain, abstinence signs in opiate-addicted animals are most frequently elicited in the medial thalamus and in medial areas of the diencephalic–mesencephalic junctures (Wei *et al.*, 1973), which are among the richest in opiate–receptor binding. The periaqueductal gray, second highest in opiate–receptor binding, appears to be critical in pain relief since lesions in it elicit analgesia.

One feature common to areas rich in opiate–receptor binding is that all are portions of the limbic system (Nauta, 1957). In our dissection, the head of the caudate, with more than twice the receptor binding of other parts of the corpus striatum, contains the nucleus accumbens, a component of the limbic system. The frontal and superior temporal cerebral cortices, more closely associated with the limbic system than other areas of the cerebral cortex, contain 4–5 times more receptor binding than other parts of the cerebral cortex. Opiate–receptor binding is, however, not uniformly high throughout the limbic system, since the mammillary bodies and hippocampus, respectively, possess low and moderate binding activity. Opiate–receptor distribution corresponds well with the medially located paleospinothalamic and spinoreticulodiencephalic pain-conducting pathways. These pathways regulate the motivational–affective features of pain responses. Interestingly, morphine affects emotional aspects of pain more than pain sensation (Beecher, 1957).

5. EFFECT OF DESTRUCTION OF NOREPINEPHRINE, SEROTONIN, ACETYLCHOLINE, AND DOPAMINE TRACTS ON OPIATE–RECEPTOR BINDING

Most brain biochemicals are distributed fairly uniformly throughout the brain. The striking heterogeneity of opiate–receptor distribution reminds one of the large regional differences found for concentrations of neurotransmitters.

Because initial regional studies in the rat brain suggested an association with cholinergic neuronal systems, samples from monkey brain regions were also assayed for choline acetyltransferase (Kuhar *et al.*, 1973*a*). Both similarities and differences exist in the regional distributions of choline acetyltransferase and the opiate receptor (Table 9). Thus while both choline acetyltransferase and opiate–receptor binding in the monkey are high in the caudate, the putamen contains the highest choline acetyltransferase values but only moderate opiate–receptor binding. The periaqueductal area of the midbrain, the second highest in opiate–receptor values, possesses only moderate choline acetyltransferase activity.

Regional variations in γ-aminobutyric acid (GABA) content in rhesus monkey brain (Fahn and Côté, 1968) also display both similarities to and differences from that of the opiate-receptor. Thus, while the hypothalamus is rich in GABA and opiate-receptor binding, the globus pallidus, which contains one of the highest GABA concentrations in the brain, is relatively low in opiate-receptor binding. The occipital cortex contains more GABA than the frontal cortex, while their relationship is reversed for opiate-receptor binding.

Regional differences in tyrosine hydroxylase activity (Côté and Fahn, 1967) should provide some index of the relative density of dopamine and norepinephrine neurons. Like the opiate-receptor, high tyrosine hydroxylase activity occurs in the caudate. Although the putamen is as active in tyrosine hydroxylase as is the caudate, it contains only half the opiate-receptor binding of the caudate. The hypothalamus and periaqueductal gray are relatively rich in tyrosine hydroxylase and also contain high levels of opiate-receptor binding. While the medial thalamus contains much more opiate-receptor binding than the lateral thalamus, the reverse situation occurs for tyrosine hydroxylase activity. Within the corpus striatum, the relative amounts of tyrosine hydroxylase in caudate nucleus and globus pallidus are similar to the relative proportions of opiate-receptor binding.

To determine more directly whether the opiate receptor might be localized on or within neurons utilizing particular transmitters, we made lesions to destroy specific cholinergic, noradrenergic, dopaminergic, and serotoninergic tracts. Lesions of the septal area of the rat brain destroy cholinergic projections to the hippocampus, as indicated by a profound reduction in hippocampal acetylcholine, choline acetyltransferase, and high-affinity choline uptake (Table 10). At various intervals between 4 and 49 days after such lesions, there is no alteration in opiate-receptor binding in the hippocampus. Electrolytic lesions of the locus coeruleus destroy ascending noradrenergic projections, causing a 70% decrease in endogenous norepinephrine in the ipsilateral cerebral cortex.

[^{3}H]Norepinephrine uptake is reduced in brain regions where norepinephrine neurons are destroyed, but there is no associated change in opiate-receptor binding 21 days after placement of the lesion. Electrolytic destruction of the midbrain raphe nuclei produces a 70–80% decrease in high-affinity serotonin uptake and endogenous serotonin and tryptophan hydroxylase activity in the forebrain, but no change in opiate-receptor binding is apparent in the forebrain 15 days after the lesion. Lesions of the nigrostriatal dopamine pathway with 6-hydroxydopamine do not alter striatal opiate-receptor binding (Creese and Snyder, in preparation).

The lesioning experiments indicate that the opiate receptor is not a unique component of axons or nerve endings of any one of these tracts. Because considerable amounts of opiate-receptor binding are detected in

TABLE 10

Effect of Destruction of Noradrenergic, Serotoninergic, and Cholinergic Tracts on Opiate–Receptor Binding[a]

Neurotransmitter	Lesion area	Assay area	Assay (control/lesion): Days after lesion	Uptake	Opiate receptor (fmol/mg protein)
Norepinephrine (NE)	Locus coeruleus	Ipsilateral cerebral cortex	21	0.88/0.37	4.0 ± 0.2/4.1 ± 0.2
Serotonin (5-HT)	Midbrain raphe nuclei	Forebrain	15	3.4/1.0	1.9 ± 0.3/2.2 ± 0.3
				Choline acetyltransferase	
Acetylcholine	Medial septum	Hippocampus	4	3.4/0.68	16.5 ± 2.0/17.4 ± 2.2
			7	—	21.3 ± 2.1/22.2 ± 1.9
			15	3.9/0.65	17.8 ± 2.8/19.0 ± 1.9
			49	—	18.6 ± 0.9/17.0 ± 1.2

[a] Lesioned animals were prepared as described in the text. Synaptosomal uptake and choline acetyltransferase assays were performed as previously described (Kuhar *et al.*, 1973*a,b*; Uretsky and Iversen, 1970). Placement of lesions was verified by histological examination in all cases, and uptake and enzyme assays were used with some animals from each group to further verify tract degeneration. Incubation media concentrations of NE and 5-HT were 0.1 μM and 10 nM, respectively. Uptake results are mean values from three animals and are expressed as pmol/4 min/1.8 mg protein. Choline acetyltransferase activity is expressed as μ mol/h/g. Values represent the means ± SEM of five experimental determinations and their five controls. Each determination was calculated from triplicate incubations with 1 nM [^{3}H]dihydromorphine in the presence of 100 nM levorphanol or dextrophan.

forebrain areas lacking serotonin or norepinephrine cell bodies, it is unlikely that the opiate receptor is associated exclusively with cell bodies of these neuronal systems. We cannot exclude the possibility that opiate receptor sites are associated with postsynaptic elements of these tracts or with more than one neurotransmitter system.

6. PHYLOGENETIC DISTRIBUTION OF THE OPIATE RECEPTOR

Although in animals the "function" of the opiate receptor is to mediate pharmacological responses to opiates, presumably these highly specific receptors play some role in normal brain function. Their strict structural requirements suggest that opiate receptors normally interact with some naturally occurring "endogenous ligand" for which morphine and its congeners provide structural analogues. Examining the phylogenetic distribution of opiate–receptor binding might provide insight into the relative importance of the normal neurobiological functions of opiate receptors throughout the animal kingdom.

While pharmacological actions of opiates have been studied in mammals (Martin, 1963) and birds (McMillan *et al.*, 1970), we are unaware of studies describing specific opiate effects in other vertebrates and invertebrates. We measured opiate–receptor binding in several vertebrate and invertebrate species (Pert *et al.*, 1974*b*) (Table 11). Substantial amounts of stereospecific opiate–receptor binding are present in brains of all vertebrates examined. There does not appear to be any evolutionary trend in the total amount of stereospecific binding. Thus slime hags, the most primitive extant vertebrates, display more binding than the four mammals examined, including mice, rats, monkeys, and humans. While the spiny dogfish contains less than half the receptor binding of goldfish and slime hags, its close relative the smooth dogfish contains more than twice as much receptor binding as the spiny dogfish. Strikingly, no opiate–receptor binding can be detected in any of the invertebrates examined. In mosquitoes, cockroaches, and schistosomes, the entire head region was examined so that it is conceivable that nonneuronal tissue might interfere with receptor binding of the brain. However, for all other invertebrates studied the head ganglion was dissected free of surrounding tissue and assayed for opiate–receptor binding.

Conceivably receptor binding measured at a single concentration of an opiate may not reflect the relative total number of receptor sites if different species have markedly varying affinities. Accordingly, we measured specific [^{3}H]dihydromorphine binding over a wide range of concentrations in four different vertebrate species in order to estimate affinity constants. The

TABLE 11

Phylogenetic Distribution of Stereospecific [^3H]Dihydromorphine Binding[a]

	Stereospecific binding (fmol/mg tissue)
Invertebrate	
Platyhelminths	
Schistosoma mansoni	<0.2
Schistosoma japonicum	<0.2
Mollusca	
Gastropoda (snail)	<0.2
Cephalopoda (squid)	<0.2
Arthropoda	
Crustacea	
(crayfish)	<0.2
(crab)	<0.2
Insecta	
(mosquito)	<0.2
(cockroach)	<0.2
Arachnida	
(tarantula)	<0.2
Vertebrate	
Pisces	
Agnatha (*Bdellostema*, slime hags)	3.9
Chondrichthyes	
(spiny dogfish)	0.8
(smooth dogfish, forebrain)	1.8
Osteichthyes (goldfish)	2.0
Tetrapoda	
Amphibia (toad)	1.3
Reptilia (turtle)	2.9
Aves (chick)	0.8
Mammalia	
(rat)	2.5
(mouse)	1.6
(monkey, frontal pole)	1.2
(human, frontal pole)	1.5

[a] Nervous tissue was dissected free from surrounding tissue and homogenized immediately in 100 vol (w/v) of 0.05 M tris buffer, pH 7.4, at 37 °C. In schistosomes, cockroaches, and mosquitoes, the entire head region was removed and homogenized. Homogenates were assayed in quadruplicate in the presence of levorphanol and dextrorphan (0.1 μM) with [^{3}H]dihydromorphine (1 nM final concentration). Values are the means of quadruplicate determinations which varied less than 10%. Adapted from Pert *et al.* (1974*b*).

calculated K_D values for stereospecific [^{3}H]dihydromorphine binding in the spiny dogfish, turtle, 2-day-old chick, and adult mouse are all between 2 and 3 nM. Thus the affinity of the opiate receptor for dihydromorphine is similar in four species which range from very primitive to very advanced vertebrate development.

To determine if stereospecific [^{3}H]dihydromorphine binding in various vertebrates involves a receptor with the same characteristics as the mammalian opiate receptor, we compared the ability of nine opiates and their antagonists to inhibit binding in brain homogenates of mice, fish, and turtles (Table 12). The relative potency of various drugs in inhibiting [^{3}H]dihydromorphine binding is essentially the same in these three widely divergent species.

Since various brain areas assume different functions as species evolve, we wondered whether regional variations in receptor binding described in monkeys and humans might also occur in more primitive species (Table 13). Marked regional variations in opiate–receptor binding do occur in the chick, goldfish, and smooth dogfish. As is the case in monkey, human, and rat, there is little or no stereospecific binding in the cerebellum. The olfactory bulbs of goldfish and chick are highly enriched in opiate receptor sites, as is the olfactory trigone in humans. The archistriatum of chick brain, which is the analogous precursor to the mammalian amygdala (Papez, 1967), is highly enriched in opiate–receptor binding, while the remainder of chick striatum is relatively poor in binding. In the goldfish, the ventral midbrain (tegmentum) is also enriched in opiate–receptor binding. In the dogfish, however, most of the brain's opiate receptor content is localized in the

TABLE 12

Inhibition of Stereospecific [^{3}H]Dihydromorphine Binding by Opiates in Mouse, Turtle, and Fish Brain Homogenates[a]

	ED_{50} concentration (nM)		
	Mouse	Fish	Turtle
Etonitazene	0.7–0.9	0.7–1.0	0.9–1.5
Naloxone	0.3–0.6	0.7–1.0	0.5–0.8
(−)-3-Hydroxy-*N*-allylmorphinan (levallorphan)	1.5–3.0	2–3	0.7–1.0
(+)-3-Hydroxy-*N*-allylmorphinan (dextrallorphan)	6000–9000	1500–2500	2500–3000
Levorphanol	1–2	3–6	1.8–2.3
Dextrorphan	6000–9000	3000–5000	2500–5000
(−)-Methadone	20–30	20–30	7–10
(+)-Methadone	200–300	400–500	100–110
Meperidine	1000–3750	900–1300	1100–1300

[a] Homogenates of mouse, fish, or turtle brain (100 vol, w/v) were included with 1 nM[^{3}H]dihydromorphine and 3–6 concentrations of nonradioactive opiates. The concentration of each nonradioactive opiate required to inhibit 50% of the stereospecific [^{3}H]dihydromorphine binding (ED_{50}) was determined by log-probit analysis. Values represent the range obtained in two or three separate experiments. Adapted from Pert *et al.* (1974*b*).

TABLE 13

Regional Distribution of Opiate–Receptor Binding in Dogfish, Goldfish, and Chick[a]

	Opiate receptor binding		
	Smooth dogfish	Goldfish	Chick
Spinal cord	*b*		
Hindbrain (medulla)	*b*	1	1
Cerebellum	1	*b*	*b*
Tectum (optic lobes)	1	1	4
Ventral midbrain		3	
Olfactory bulbs			5
Archistriatum			7
Forebrain	4	1	1
Cortex			1
Striatum			1
Brainstem anterior to infundibulum			1
Brainstem posterior to infundibulum			1

[a] Brains were dissected and each region was homogenized in 100–200 vol (w/v) 0.05 M tris-HCl buffer. Regions were assayed in triplicate with [^{3}H]naloxone (1 nM) in the presence of levallorphan or dextrallorphan [(+)-3-hydroxy-*N*-allylmorphinan]. Values are expressed as the ratio of stereospecific binding per milligram of tissue in a given region to that of the brain region of poorest receptor enrichment (arbitrary value of 1), whose binding was 0.24, 0.28, and 0.42 fmol stereospecific [^{3}H]naloxone binding per milligram of tissue in the dogfish, goldfish, and chick, respectively. Data are the mean of three or four determinations which varied less than 20%.

[b] No significant stereospecific binding detected. Adapted from Pert *et al.* (1974*b*).

forebrain, which is almost wholly an olfactory organ. The limbic system of mammals is believed to have evolved from brain areas concerned with olfaction in more primitive vertebrates (MacLean, 1949). It is therefore quite striking that enrichment of opiate–receptor binding sites is associated with olfactory regions of shark, fish, and chick brains just as the limbic system of monkeys and humans contains the highest receptor binding.

What might be the function of opiate receptors in various brain regions of primitive vertebrates? Perhaps in primitive vertebrates the opiate receptor "marks" brain regions which integrate painful stimuli. Alternatively, perhaps in primitive vertebrates opiates produce pharmacological actions other than analgesia that depend on which brain areas contain the highest density of receptors.

The apparent absence of opiate receptors in brains of invertebrates suggests that these drugs do not elicit specific pharmacological responses in invertebrates. Thus investigators should be cautious about using invertebrates in studies of opiate actions.

7. EFFECT OF SODIUM ON OPIATE–RECEPTOR BINDING

One of the most perplexing features of our initial opiate receptor studies was the fact that opiates and their corresponding antagonists had essentially the same affinity for the receptor, whereas pharmacologically antagonists are much more potent than agonists. Initial receptor studies had been performed with buffers containing no sodium. With physiological concentrations of sodium, binding of the opiate antagonist [^{3}H]naloxone is increased while binding of the agonist [^{3}H]dihydromorphine is markedly depressed (Fig. 3). The binding of other ^{3}H-labeled agonists such as oxymorphone and levorphanol is also reduced by sodium, while the binding of other ^{3}H-labeled antagonists such as nalorphine and levallorphan is enhanced by sodium (Pert *et al.*, 1973; Pert and Snyder, 1974). As little as 0.5 mM sodium chloride markedly enhances [^{3}H]naloxone binding, and maximal increase occurs at

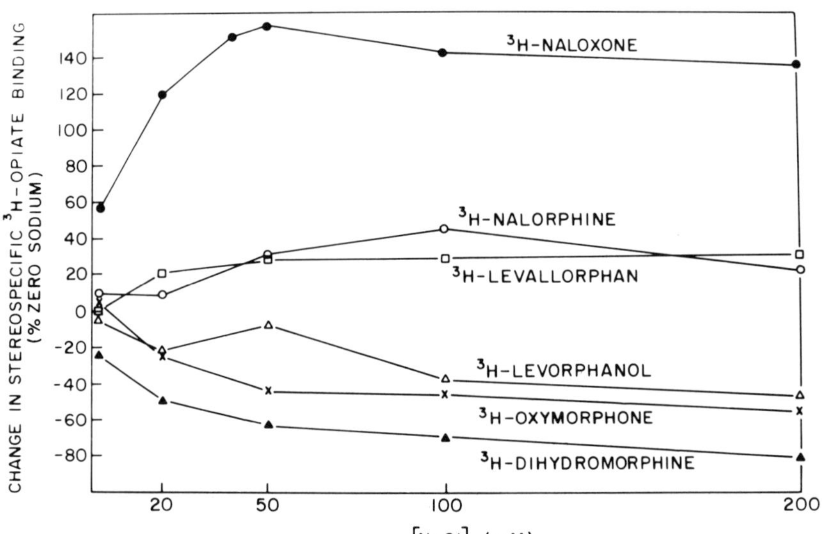

FIG. 3. Effect of five monovalent cations on stereospecific [^{3}H]naloxone and [^{3}H]dihydromorphine binding. [^{3}H]Naloxone (1.5 nM) and [^{3}H]dihydromorphine (1 nM) were incubated with 100 nM levorphanol, levallorphan, dextrorphan, or dextrallorphan in the standard binding assay with rat brain homogenate which had been "washed" once. Seven concentrations (1–150 mM) of each monovalent cation were incubated in triplicate with [^{3}H]naloxone and [^{3}H]dihydromorphine. Control stereospecific binding values were 1096 ± 102 counts/min for [^{3}H]naloxone and 2120 ± 201 counts/min for [^{3}H]dihydromorphine. Nonspecific binding values, whether determined in the presence of levorphanol or levallorphan, were the same and were unaffected by the cations. Binding values in the presence of dextrallorphan, dextrorphan, or no nonradioactive opiate were not significantly different. Bars denote SEM. * $p < 0.005$. From Pert and Snyder (1974).

concentrations of around 100 mM. Double-reciprocal analysis indicates that sodium increases the number of binding sites with no change in affinity for naloxone. The decrease of [^{3}H]dihydromorphine binding is significant in 5 mM sodium, with the greatest decrease at 150 mM.

The influence of sodium on opiate–receptor binding appears to be highly specific. Lithium, whose atomic radius and biological activity are similar to those of sodium, is the only other ion which can mimic the actions of sodium. It increases naloxone binding somewhat less than does sodium but is similarly effective in reducing dihydromorphine binding. By contrast, potassium, rubidium, and cesium, which have different atomic radii and biological properties, do not discriminate between agonists and antagonists. These other ions decrease the binding of both naloxone and dihydromorphine.

To evaluate the influence of sodium on receptor interactions of numerous opiates, it would be desirable to perform studies with nonradioactive drugs. This can be accomplished by measuring the ability of drugs to inhibit stereospecific [^{3}H]naloxone binding in the presence or absence of sodium (Fig. 4). The ability of nonradioactive naloxone to inhibit [^{3}H]naloxone binding is not affected by sodium, because this experiment simply involves isotope dilution. The influence of sodium of the ability of drugs to inhibit [^{3}H]naloxone binding seems to differentiate antagonists in terms of their relative "purity." Pure antagonists are those like naloxone which do not display any agonist activity such as analgesia or euphoria. The ability of relatively pure antagonists such as naloxone, naltrexone, and diprenorphrine to inhibit naloxone binding is unaffected by sodium. By contrast, antagonists which are "contaminated" with some agonist activity (cyclazocine, levallorphan, and nalorphine) become less potent in the

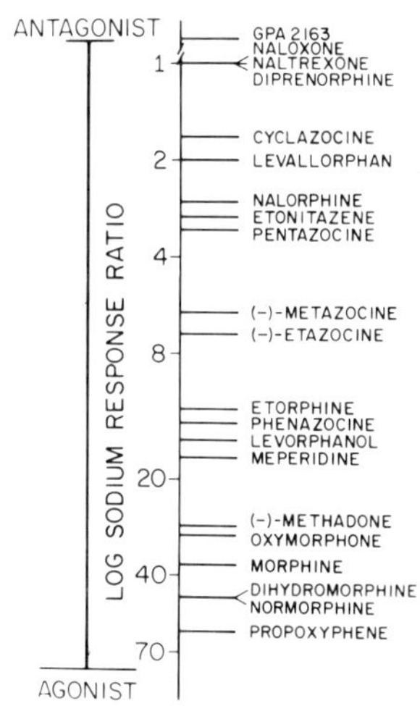

FIG. 4. Differential influence of sodium on inhibition of [^{3}H]naloxone binding by opiate agonists, antagonists, and mixed agonist–antagonists. The sodium response ratio is the ratio of the ED_{50} (concentration of drug to inhibit [^{3}H]naloxone binding 50%) of a drug in the presence of sodium to its ED_{50} in the absence of sodium. From Pert (1974).

presence of sodium. GPA-2163, the propargyl derivative of benzazocine, a reportedly "pure" antagonist, actually becomes 5 times as potent in inhibiting [^{3}H]naloxone binding in the presence of sodium. Thus GPA-2163 behaves like a "superantagonist," 5 times as "pure" an antagonist as naloxone. It is unclear just what pharmacological properties might be anticipated of an opiate antagonist which is "purer" than naloxone.

Opiate agonists are also affected differentially by sodium. The decreased binding of opiate agonists in the presence of sodium is profound. The ability of agonists to inhibit naloxone binding is decreased between twelve-fold and sixty-fold. We do not know what accounts for this five-fold variation in the ability of sodium to depress the binding of opiate agonists to the receptor. The extremely potent opiate etorphine is least sensitive to sodium, while morphine and propoxyphene are most affected. One might speculate that just as resistance to sodium is correlated with the "purity" of antagonists, perhaps the drugs whose receptor binding is reduced most by sodium are "purer" agonists. In the guinea pig ileum, Kosterlitz *et al.* (1973) found antagonist properties for all opiates including morphine. Those which we would label as "pure" agonists, on the basis of their response to sodium, have the least antagonist properties. Conceivably "pure" agonists may be drugs with the greatest fundamental addictive potential.

Mixed agonist–antagonist drugs are affected by sodium in an intermediate fashion. Pentazocine, a mixed agonist–antagonist benzomorphan employed clinically as a relatively nonaddicting analgesic, displays a reduction of about 3.3-fold in its ability to inhibit naloxone binding in the presence of sodium. Other benzomorphan mixed agonist–antagonist drugs become between 4 and 7 times less potent in the presence of sodium (Pert *et al.*, 1974*c*). Since combination opiate agonist–antagonists offer great therapeutic potential as relatively nonaddicting analgesics, the opiate receptor's sodium sensitivity can predict new, potentially less abusable analgesics.

What may account for the ability of sodium to discriminate agonists and antagonists? Conceivably, the opiate receptor can assume different conformations: one in the presence of sodium which binds antagonists more efficiently and another in the absence of sodium which binds agonists more efficiently. Presumably sodium allosterically transforms the receptor between the two conformations (Pert and Snyder, 1975).

We obtained direct evidence that there exist two forms of the opiate receptor. The protein-modifying reagent iodoacetamide markedly reduces receptor binding of the agonist [^{3}H]dihydromorphine in low concentrations, but does not affect binding of the antagonist naloxone (Table 14). This effect is not restricted to dihydromorphine and naloxone. The same results are observed with a series of ^{3}H-labeled agonists and ^{3}H-labeled antagonists. A large number of opiate agonists and antagonists can be evaluated in a nonradioactive form by assessing their ability to inhibit [^{3}H]naloxone binding by membranes with or without iodoacetamide treatment.

TABLE 14

Effect of Iodoacetamide on [^{3}H]Opiate Binding

Opiate	Stereospecific opiate binding (counts/min)		Percent change
	Control	Iodoacetamide	
Antagonists			
[^{3}H]Naloxone	1040	1092	+5
[^{3}H]Levallorphan	1551	1672	+8
Agonists			
[^{3}H]Oxymorphone	719	401	−44
[^{3}H]Levorphanol	1228	827	−36
[^{3}H]Dihydromorphine	1871	878	−53

[a] A rat brain was homogenized in 30 ml standard tris buffer (50 mM, pH 7.7, at 25 °C) and centrifuged at 50,000 *g* for 15 min. The pellet was resuspended in 150 ml of standard tris buffer and equal volumes were incubated in the presence and absence of 20 mM iodoacetamide for 20 min at 25 °C. The homogenates were then spun down as before, resuspended in their original volumes, and assayed with either (+)-levallorphan or (−)-levallorphan at 200 nM and the appropriate [^{3}H]opiate as previously described (Pasternak *et al.*, in preparation). The following concentrations of [^{3}H]opiates were used: [^{3}H]naloxone 1.7 nM, [^{3}H]levallorphan 2.8 nM, [^{3}H]oxymorphone 37.0 nM, [^{3}H]levorphanol 4 nM, and [^{3}H]dihydromorphine 0.7 nM.

Iodoacetamide reduces the ability of opiate agonists to inhibit naloxone binding without affecting the inhibitory potency of antagonists (Pasternak *et al.*, 1975*a*; Wilson *et al.*, 1975).

Thus the opiate receptor can assume two conformations, one favoring antagonists and one favoring agonists. The agonist conformation appears to be more labile. Proteolytic enzymes inhibit agonist binding more than antagonist binding (Pasternak and Snyder, 1975*b*), while divalent cations have opposite effects (Pasternak *et al.*, 1975*a*).

8. TOWARD A THEORY OF ADDICTION

Scientifically and practically, the most tantalizing question in the field of opiate research is "What is the nature of addiction?" In animals, the two major components of the addictive process are tolerance, whereby progressively larger doses of opiates are required to elicit analgesia, and physical dependence, in which addicted animals undergo abstinence symptoms when opiates are withdrawn or when antagonists are administered. Since tolerance and physical dependence are intimately related (Way *et al.*, 1969), numerous theories have been offered to explain addiction in terms of these two components (Goldstein and Goldstein, 1968; Maynert and Kingman, 1962; Gunne, 1963; Cochin and Kornetsky, 1964; Way *et al.*, 1968, 1969;

Collier, 1966; Jaffe and Sharpless, 1968; Martin, 1968; Seevers and Deneau, 1963). Some of these theories involve alterations in the number of opiate receptors. When we measure opiate–receptor binding in animals treated chronically with morphine, we detect increases of 50–100% (Pert *et al.*, 1973). However, these increases occur as soon as 5 min after injection of an opiate, while tolerance and physical dependence are not demonstrable for at least 12–24 h. Moreover, opiate antagonists are much more potent than agonists in eliciting this increase, whereas tolerance and physical dependence do not develop to pure antagonists. Hence this increased receptor binding is not causally related to addiction.

However, it is possible to conceptualize alterations in the opiate receptor which could account for tolerance and physical dependence. As animals or humans become progressively more dependent on opiates, the dose of an antagonist required to precipitate abstinence symptoms becomes progressively lower by up to 2 orders of magnitude. This is especially remarkable since one would expect that a larger dose of an antagonist would be required to compete with the larger amount of opiate present in the body of an addicted organism.

Thus the addicted state is associated with increased sensitivity to antagonists. Similarly, tolerance can be described simply as decreased sensitivity to opiate agonists. These two phenomena, increased sensitivity to antagonists and decreased sensitivity to agonists, are strikingly reminiscent of the influence of sodium on the opiate receptor. Sodium transforms the receptor into a state in which it is more sensitive to antagonists and less sensitive to agonists. Antagonists themselves transform the receptor into the "antagonist" conformation, while agonists "push" it into the "agonist" conformation.

We speculate that tolerance and physical dependence are caused by a progressive alteration of the opiate receptor's conformation so that it assumes the "antagonist" conformation to a greater extent than in nonaddicted organisms. In the new conformation it will require higher concentrations of agonists to produce effects elicited by smaller amounts of agonists in nonaddicted organisms.

Changes in the conformation of the opiate receptor posited by this theory may not be detected readily experimentally. Alterations in receptor conformation which occur when an animal is killed and its brain homogenized and incubated with drugs in varying ionic media may very well "wash out" altered receptor conformations.

Whether or not this particular theory is valid, it provides specific predictions which can be tested experimentally. Besides offering an approach to studies of addiction mechanisms, biochemical identification of the opiate receptor may furnish a means to explore other important aspects of opiate action. What is the endogenous ligand for the opiate receptor? The fact that the stringent structural specifications of the opiate receptor have remained the same throughout vertebrate evolution argues for the presence of an endogenous ligand; if the opiate receptor were only some structural curiosity of central nervous membranes which fortuitously interacts with opiates, one would have anticipated it to undergo changes in its structure during the course of evolution. Examination of brain extracts for an endogenous substance which might interact with the opiate receptor should provide a means of identifying such an endogenous ligand, and this has been recently accomplished (Hughes, 1975; Pasternak *et al.*, 1975*a*). Autoradiographic visualization of the detailed distribution of opiate receptor sites in rat brain (Pert *et al.*, 1975) may elucidate the natural function of the opiate receptor and its ligand.

9. REFERENCES

BEECHER, H. K., 1957, The measurement of pain, *Pharmacol. Rev.* **9:**59–209.

BERKOWITZ, B. A., and WAY, E. L., 1971, Analgesic activity and central nervous system distribution of the optical isomers of pentazocine in the rat, *J. Pharmacol. Exp. Ther.* **177:**500–508.

CLOUET, D. H., and WILLIAMS, N., 1973, Localization in brain particulate fractions of narcotic analgesic drugs administered intracisternally to rats, *Biochem. Pharmacol.* **22:**1283–1293.

COCHIN, J., and KORNETSKY, C., 1964, Development and loss of tolerance to morphine in the rat after single and multiple injections, *J. Pharmacol. Exp. Ther.* **145:**1–10.

COLLIER, H. O. J., 1966, Tolerance, physical dependence and receptors: A theory of the genesis of tolerance and physical dependence through drug-induced changes in the number of receptors, *Advan. Drug Res.* **3:**171–188.

CÔTÉ, L., and FAHN, S., 1967, Some aspects of the biochemistry of the substantia nigra of the rhesus monkey, in: *Progress in Neurogenetics*, Vol. 1, pp. 311–317, Excerpta Medica International Congress Series, Amsterdam.

FAHN, S., and CÔTÉ, L. J., 1968, Regional distribution of gamma-aminobutyric acid (GABA) in brain of the rhesus monkey, *J. Neurochem.* **15:**209–213.

GOLDSTEIN, A., and GOLDSTEIN, D. B., 1968, Enzyme expansion theory of drug tolerance and physical dependence, *Proc. Assoc. Res. Nerv. Ment. Dis.* **46:**265–267.

GOLDSTEIN, A., LOWNEY, L. I., and PAL, B. K., 1971, Stereospecific and nonspecific interactions of the morphine congener levorphanol in subcellular fractions of the mouse brain, *Proc. Natl. Acad. Sci.* **68:**1742–1747.

GUNNE, L. M., 1963, Catecholamines and 5-hydroxytryptamine in morphine tolerance and withdrawal, *Acta Physiol. Scand.* **58:**85–91 (Suppl. 204).

HERZ, A., and TESCHEMACHER, H.-J., 1971, Activities and sites of antinociceptive action of morphine-like analgesics, *Advan. Drug Res.* **6:**29–119.

HILLMAN, J. M., PEARSON, J., and SIMON, E. J., 1973, Distribution of stereospecific binding of the potent narcotic analgesic etorphine in the human brain: Predominance in the limbic system, *Res. Commun. Chem. Pathol. Pharmacol.* **6:**1052–1061.

HITZEMANN, R. J., and LOH, H. H., 1973, Characteristics of the binding of ^{3}H-naloxone in the mouse brain, *Proc. Soc. Neurosci.* **3:**350.

HUG, C. C., JR., and OKA, T., 1971, Uptake of dihydromorphine-^{3}H by synaptosomes, *Life Sci.* **10:**201–213.

HUGHES, J., 1975, Isolation of an endogenous compound from the brain with pharmacological properties similar to morphine, *Brain Res.* **88:**295–308.

INGOGLIA, N. A., and DOLE, V. P., 1970, Localization of *d*- and *l*-methadone after ventricular injection into rat brains, *J. Pharmacol. Exp. Ther.* **175:**84–87.

JAFFE, J. H., and SHARPLESS, S. K., 1968, Pharmacological denervation supersensitivity in the central nervous system: A theory of physical dependence, *Proc. Assoc. Res. Nerv. Ment. Dis.* **46:**226–246.

KLEE, W. A., and STREATY, R. A., 1974, Narcotic receptor sites in morphine-dependent rats, *Nature* **248:**61–63.

KOSTERLITZ, H. W., LORD, J. A. H., and WATT, A. J., 1973, Morphine receptor in the myenteric plexus of the guinea-pig ileum, in: *Agonist and Antagonist Actions of Narcotic Analgesic Drudgs* (H. W. Kosterlitz, H. O. J. Collier, and J. E. Villarreal, eds.), pp. 45–61, University Park Press, University Park, Pa.

KUHAR, M. J., PERT, C. B., and SNYDER, S. H., 1973*a*, Regional distribution of opiate receptor binding in monkey and human brain, *Nature* **245:**447–451.

KUHAR, M. J., SETHY, V. H., ROTH, R. H., and AGHAJANIAN, G. K., 1973*b*, Choline: Selective accumulation by central cholinergic neurons, *J. Neurochem.* **20:**581–593.

LOH, H. H., CHO, T. M., WU, Y.-C., and WAY, E. L., 1974, Stereospecific binding of narcotics to brain cerebrosides. *Life Sci.*, in press.

LOWNEY, L. I., SCHULZ, K., LOWERY, P. J., and GOLDSTEIN, A., 1974, Partial purification of an opiate receptor from mouse brain, *Science* **183:**749–753.

MACLEAN, P. D., 1949, Psychosomatic disease and the "visceral brain," *Psychosom. Med.* **11:**338–353.

MARTIN, W. R., 1963, Analgesic and antipyretic drugs—Strong analgesics, in: *Physiological Pharmacology*, Vol. 1: *The Nervous System*, Part A: Central Nervous System Drugs (W. S. Root and F. G. Hoffman, eds.), pp. 275–312, Academic Press, New York.

MARTIN, W. R., 1968, A homeostatic and redundancy theory of tolerance to and dependence on narcotic analgesics, *Proc. Assoc. Res. Nerv. Ment. Dis.* **46:**206–225.

MAYNERT, E. W., and KINGMAN, G. I., 1962, Tolerance to morphine. I. Effects of catecholamines in the brain and adrenal glands, *J. Pharmacol. Exp. Ther.* **135:**285–295.

MCMILLAN, D. E., WOLF, P. S., and CARCHMAN, R. A., 1970, Antagonism of the behavioural effects of morphine and methadone by narcotic antagonists in the pigeon, *J. Pharmacol. Exp. Ther.* **175:**443–458.

NAUTA, W. J. H., 1957, Some neural pathways related to the limbic system, in: *Electrical Studies on the Unanaesthetized Brain* (E. k. Ramey and D. S. O'Doherty, eds.), pp. 1–16, Hoeber, New York.

NAVON, S., and LAJTHA, A., 1970, Uptake of morphine in particulate fractions from rat brain, *Brain Res.* **24:**534–536.

PAPEZ, J. W., 1967, *Comparative Neurology*, pp. 429–474, Hafner, New York.

PASTERNAK, G. W., and SNYDER, S. H., 1974, Opiate receptor binding: Effects of enzymatic treatments, *Mol. Pharmacol.* **10:**183–193.

PASTERNAK, G. W., and SNYDER, S. H., 1975*a*, Identification of novel high affinity opiate receptor binding in rat brain, *Nature* **253:**563–565.

PASTERNAK, G. W., and SNYDER, S. H., 1975*b*, Opiate receptor binding: Enzymatic treatments discriminate between agonist and antagonist interactions, *Mol. Pharmacol.*, in press.

PASTERNAK, G. W., GOODMAN, R., and SNYDER, S. H., 1975*a*, An endogenous morphine-like factor in mammalian brain, *Life Sciences*, in press.

PASTERNAK, G. W., SNOWMAN, A., and SNYDER, S. H., 1975*b*, Selective enhancement of [^{3}H]opiate agonist binding by divalent cations, *Mol. Pharmacol.*, in press.

PASTERNAK, G. W., WILSON, H. A., and SNYDER, S. H., 1975*c*, Differential effects of protein modifying reagents on receptor binding of opiate agonists and antagonists, *Mol. Pharmacol.*, in press.

PATON, W. D. M., 1957, The action of morphine and related substances on contraction and on acetylcholine output of coaxially-stimulated guinea-pig ileum, *Brit. J. Pharmacol. Chemother.* **12:**119–127.

PERT, C. B., 1974, The opiate receptor: Its demonstration, properties and distribution. Doctoral Dissertation, The Johns Hopkins University, Baltimore, Maryland.

PERT, C. B., and YAKSH, T. L., 1974, Sites of morphine induced analgesia in the primate brain: Relation to pain pathways, *Brain Res.* **80:**125–140.

PERT, C. B., and SNYDER, S. H., 1973*a*, Opiate receptor: Demonstration in nervous tissue, *Science* **179:**1011–1014.

PERT, C. B., and SNYDER, S. H., 1973*b*, Properties of opiate-receptor binding in rat brain, *Proc. Natl. Acad. Sci.* **70:**2243–2247.

PERT, C. B., and SNYDER, S. H., 1974, Opiate-receptor binding of agonists and antagonists affected differentially by sodium, *Mol. Pharmacol.*, **10:**868–879.

PERT, C. B., and SNYDER, S. H., 1975, Differential interactions of agonists and antagonists with the opiate receptor, in: *Opiate Receptor Mechanisms* (S. H. Snyder and S. Matthysse, eds.), *Neurosci. Res. Prog. Bull.*, pp. 73–79.

PERT, C. B., and SNYDER, S. H., 1975, Identification of opiate receptor binding in intact animals, *Life Sciences*, in press.

PERT, C. B., PASTERNAK, G., and SNYDER, S. H., 1973, Opiate agonists and antagonists discriminated by receptor binding in brain, *Science* **182:**1359–1361.

PERT, C. B., SNOWMAN, A. M., and SNYDER, S. H., 1974*a*, Localization of opiate receptor binding in synaptic membranes of rat brain, *Brain Res.* **70:**184–188.

PERT, C. B., APOSHIAN, D., and SNYDER, S. H., 1974*b*, Phylogenetic distribution of opiate receptor binding, *Brain Res.*, **75:**356–361.

PERT, C. B., SNYDER, S. H., and MAY, E. L., 1974*c*, Opiate receptor interactions of benzomorphans in rat brain homogenates, *J. Pharmacol. Exp. Ther.*, in press.

PERT, C. B., KUHAR, M. J., and SNYDER, S. H., 1975, Autoradiographic localization of the opiate receptor in rat brain, *Life Sciences*, in press.

SEEMAN, P., CHAN-WONG, M., and MOYYEN, S., 1972, The membrane binding of morphine, diphenylhydantoin, and tetrahydrocannabinol, *Canad. J. Physiol. Pharmacol.* **5:**1181–1192.

SEEVERS, M. H., and DENEAU, G. A., 1963, Physiological aspects of tolerance and physical dependence, in: *Physiological Pharmacology*, Vol. 1 (W. S. Root and F. G. Hoffman, eds.), pp. 565–640, Academic Press, New York.

SIMON, E. J., HILLER, J. M., and EDELMAN, I., 1973, Stereospecific binding of the patent narcotic analgesic [^{3}H]etorphine to rat brain homogenate, *Proc. Natl. Acad. Sci.* **70:**1947–1949.

TERENIUS, L., 1973, Characteristics of the "receptor" for narcotic analgesics in synaptic plasma membrane fraction from rat brain, *Acta Pharmacol. Toxicol.* **33:**377–384.

TERENIUS, L., 1974, A rapid assay for the narcotic receptor in rat brain: Application to methadone analogues, *Acta Pharmacol. Toxicol.* **34:**88–91.

TSOU, K., and JANG, C. S., 1964, Studies on the site of analgesic action of morphine by intracerebral micro-injection, *Sci. Sinica* **7:**1099–1109.

URETSKY, N. J., and IVERSEN, L. L., 1970, Effects of 6-hydroxydopamine on catecholamine containing neurones in the rat brain, *J. Neurochem.* **17:**269–278.

WAY, E. L., and ADLER, T. K., 1962, The biological disposition of morphine and its surrogates, *Bull. WHO* **27:**359–394.

WAY, E. L., LOH, H. H., and SHEN, F., 1968, Morphine tolerance, physical dependence and synthesis of brain 5-hydroxy tryptamine, *Science* **162:**1290–1292.

WAY, E. L., LOH, H. H., and SHEN, F.-H., 1969, Simultaneous quantitative assessment of morphine tolerance and physical dependence, *J. Pharmacol. Exp. Ther.* **167:**1–7.

WEI, E., LOH, H. H., and WAY, E. L., 1973, Brain sites of precipitated abstinence in morphine-dependent rats, *Pharmacol. Exp. Ther.* **185:**108–115.

WILSON, H. A., PASTERNAK, G. W., and SNYDER, S. H., 1975, Differentiation of opiate agonist and antagonist binding by protein reagents, *Nature* **253:**448–450.

WILSON, R. S., ROGERS, M. E., PERT, C. B., and SNYDER, S. H., 1975, Homologous *N*-alkylnor ketobeminidones. Correlation of receptor binding with analgesic potency, *J. Med. Chem.* **18:**240–242.

WONG, D. T., and HORNG, J. S., 1973, Stereospecific interaction of opiate narcotics in binding of ^{3}H-dihydromorphine to membranes of rat brain, *Life Sci.* **13:**1543–1556.

ADDENDUM

TO ROLE OF CYCLIC NUCLEOTIDES IN THE NERVOUS SYSTEM

John Daly

1. Reviews

BURKARD, W. P., 1975, Adenylate cyclase in the central nervous system, in *Progress in Neurobiology*, Vol. 4 (G. A. Kerkut, and J. W. Phillis, eds.), pp. 241–267, Pergamon Press, New York.

DALY, J. W., 1975, Cyclic adenosine 3′,5′-monophosphate role in the physiology and pharmacology of the central nervous system, *Biochem. Pharmacol.* **24:**159–164.

DRUMMOND, G. I., and MA, Y., 1973, Metabolism and functions of cyclic AMP in nerve, in *Progress in Neurobiology* (G. W. Kerkut, and J. W. Phillis, ed.), pp. 119–176, Pergamon Press, Oxford and New York.

SCHORDERET, M., 1974, AMP cyclique et système nerveux, *J. Physiol.* (Paris) **68:**471–505.

VON HUNGEN, K. and ROBERTS, S., 1974, Neurotransmitter-sensitive adenylate cyclase systems in the brain, in *Reviews of Neuroscience*, Vol. 1 (S. Ehrenpreis, and I. J. Kopin, eds.), pp. 231–281, Raven Press, New York.

2.1. Adenylate Cyclases

BROSTROM, C. O., HUANG, Y-C., BRECKENRIDGE, B. MCL., and WOLFF, D. J., 1975, Identification of a calcium-binding protein as a calcium-dependent regulator of brain adenylate cyclase, *Proc. Nat. Acad. Sci.* **72:**64–68.

CLEMENT-CORMIER, Y. C., KEBABIAN, J. W., PETZOLD, G. L., and GREENGARD, P., 1974, Dopamine-sensitive adenylate cyclase in mammalian brain: A possible site of action of antipsychotic drugs, *Proc. Nat. Acad. Sci.* **17:**1113–1117.

COLLIER, J. O. J., and ROY, A. C., Hypothesis inhibition of E-prostaglandin-sensitive adenyl cyclase as the mechanism of morphine analgesia, *Prostaglandins* **7:**361–376.

DRUMMOND, G. I., SEVERSON, D. L., and DUNCAN, L., 1971, Adenyl cyclase: Kinetic properties and fluoride and hormone stimulation, *J. Biol. Chem.* **246:**4166–4173.

DUFFY, M. J., and POWELL, D., 1975, Stimulation of brain adenylate cyclase activity by the undecapeptide substance P and its modulation by the calcium ion, *Biochim. Biophys. Acta* **385:**275–280.

FRANKS, D. J., PERRIN, L. S., and MALAMUD, D., 1974, Calcium ion: A modulator of parotid adenylate cyclase activity, *FEBS Letters* **42:**267–270.

HORN, A. S., CUELLO, A. C., and MILLER, R. J., 1974, Dopamine in the mesolimbic system of the rat brain: Endogenous levels and the effects of drugs on the uptake mechanism and stimulation of adenylate cyclase activity, *J. Neurochem.* **22:**265–270.

KAROBATH, M. E., 1975, Tricyclic antidepressive drugs and dopamine-sensitive adenylate cyclase from rat brain striatum, *Europ. J. Pharmacol.* **30:**159–163.

KAROBATH, M., and LEITICH, H., 1974, Antipsychotic drugs and dopamine-stimulated adenylate cyclase prepared from corpus striatum of rat brain, *Proc. Nat. Acad. Sci.* **71:**2915–2918.

LIPPMANN, W., PUGSLEY, T., and MERKER, J., 1975, Effect of butaclamol and its enantiomers upon striatal homovanillic acid and adenyl cyclase of olfactory tubercle in rats, *Life Sci.* **16:**213–224.

MACDONALD, I. A., 1974, A convenient colorimetric method for routine assay of brain adenylate cyclase, *Experientia* **30:**1485–1486.

MENON, K. M. J., GIESE, S., and JAFFE, R. B., 1973, Hormone- and fluoride-sensitive adenylate cyclases in human fetal tissues, *Biochim. Biophys. Acta* **304:**203–209.

MILLER, R. J., and IVERSEN, L. L., 1974, Stimulation of a dopamine-sensitive adenylate cyclase in homogenates of rat striatum by a metabolite of piribedil (ET 495), *Naunyn-Schmiedeberg's Arch. Pharmacol.* **282:**213–216.

MILLER, R. J., HORN, A. S., and IVERSEN, L. L., 1975, Effect of butaclamol on dopamine-sensitive adenylate cyclase in the rat striatum, *J. Pharm. Pharmacol.* **27:**212–213.

MILLER, R. J., HORN, A. S., and IVERSEN, L. L., 1974, The action of neuroleptic drugs on dopamine-stimulated adenosine cyclic 3′,5′-monophosphate production in rat neostriatum and limbic forebrain, *Mol. Pharmacol.* **10:**759–766.

PALMER, G. C., and MANIAN, A. A., 1973, Inhibition of the catalytic site of adenylate cyclase in the central nervous system by phenothiazine derivatives, *Neuropharmacology* **13:**651–664.

PIERI, L., PIERI, M., and HAEFELY, W., 1974, LSD as an agonist of dopamine receptors in the striatum, *Nature* **252:**586–688.

PINDER, R., 1974, Effects of dopamine-like drugs on rat striatal adenyl cyclase have implications for CNS dopamine receptor topography, *Nature* **250:**238–241.

PRASAD, K. N., 1974, Manganese inhibits adenylate cyclase activity and stimulates phosphodiesterase activity in neuroblastoma cells: Its possible implication in manganese-poisoning, *Exp. Neurol.* **3:**554–557.

SHEPPARD, H., and BURGHARDT, C. R., 1974, Effects of tetrahydroisoquinoline derivatives on the adenylate cyclases of the caudate nucleus (dopamine-type) and erythrocyte (β-type) of the rat, *Res. Comm. Chem. Path. Pharmacol.* **3:**527–534.

SHEPPARD, H., and BURGHARDT, C. R., 1974, The dopamine-sensitive adenylate cyclase of rat caudate nucleus. I. Comparison with the isoproterenol-sensitive adenylate cyclase (beta receptor system) of rat erythrocytes in response of dopamine derivatives, *Mol. Pharmacol.* **10:**721–726.

SHIMIZU, H., ICHISHITA, H., and MIAOKAMI, Y., 1975, Stimulation of the cell-free adenylate cyclase from guinea pig cerebral cortex by acidic amino acids and veratridine, *J. Cyclic Nucleotide Research* **1:**61–67.

SUTHERLAND, E. W., RALL, T. W., and MENON, T., 1962, Adenyl cyclase. I. Distribution preparation and properties, *J. Biol. Chem.* **237:**1220–1227.

VON HUNGEN, K., ROBERTS, S., and HILL, D. F., 1973, Developmental and regional variations in neurotransmitter-sensitive adenylate cyclase systems in cell-free preparations from rat brain, *J. Neurochem.* **22:**811–819.

VON HUNGEN, K., ROBERTS, S., and HILL, D. F., 1975, Serotonin-sensitive adenylate cyclase activity in immature rat brain, *Brain Res.* **84:**257–268.

ZIMMERMAN, I., and BERG, A., 1973, Levels of adenosine 3′,5′ cyclic monophosphate in the cerebral cortex of aging rats, *Mech. Ageing and Devel.* **3:**33–36.

2.2. Guanylate Cyclases

GORIDIS, C., MASSARELLI, R., SENSENBRENNER, M., and MANDEL, P., 1974, Guanyl cyclase in chick embryo brain cell cultures: Evidence of neuronal localization, *J. Neurochem.* **23:**135–138.

NAKAZAWA, K., and SANO, M., 1974, A new assay method for guanylate cyclase and properties of the cyclase from rat brain, *J. Biol. Chem.* **249:**4207–4211.

2.3. Phosphodiesterases

ADINOLFI, A. M., and SCHMIDT, S. Y., 1974, Cytochemical localization of cyclic nucleotide phosphodiesterase activity of developing synapses, *Brain Res.* **76:**21–31.

AMER, M. S., and KREIGHBAUM, W. E., 1975, Cyclic nucleotide phosphodiesterases: Properties, activators, inhibitors, structure-activity relationships, and possible role in drug development, *J. Pharmaceut. Sciences* **64:**1–37.

BROSTROM, C. O., and WOLFF, D. J., 1974, Calcium-dependent cyclic nucleotide phosphodiesterase from glial tumor cells, *Arch. Biochem. Biophys.* **165:**715–727.

BUBLITZ, C., 1973, Effects of lipids on cyclic-nucleotide phosphodiesterases, *Biochem. Biophys. Res. Commun.* **52:**173–180.

BUTCHER, R. W., and SUTHERLAND, E. W., 1962, Adenosine 3′,5′-phosphate in biological materials. I. Purification and properties of cyclic 3′,5′-nucleotide phosphodiesterase and use of this enzyme to characterize adenosine 3′,5′-phosphate in human urine, *J. Biol. Chem.* **237:**1244–1250.

DRUMMOND, G. I., GILGAN, M. W., REINER, E. J., and SMITH, M., 1964, Deoxyribonucleoside-3′,5′-cyclic phosphates. Synthesis and acid catalyzed and enzymic hydrolysis, *J. Am. Chem. Soc.* **86:**1626–1630.

GADD, R. E. A., CLAYMAN, S., and HEBERT, D., 1973, Inhibition of cyclic 3′,5′-nucleotide phosphodiesterase activity by diuretics and other agents, *Experientia* **29:**1217–1219.

HO, R. J., RUSSELL, T. R., ASAKAWA, T., and HUCKS, M. W., 1975, Inhibition of cyclic nucleotide phosphodiesterase activity by an endogenous factor, *J. Cyclic Nucleotide Res.* **1:**81–88.

KAKIUCHI, S., YAMAZAKI, R., TESHIMA, Y., UENISHI, K., and MIYAMOTO, E., 1975, Multiple cyclic nucleotide phosphodiesterase activities from rat tissues and occurrence of calcium plus-magnesium-ion-dependent phosphodiesterase and its protein activator, *Biochem. J.* **146:**109–120.

LIN, Y. M., LIU, Y. P., and CHEUNG, W. Y., 1975, Cyclic 3′,5′-nucleotide phosphodiesterase Ca^{++}-dependent formation of bovine brain enzyme-activator complex, *FEBS Letters* **49:**356–360.

PLEDGER, W. J., STANCEL, G. M., THOMPSON, W. J., and STRADA, S. J., 1974, Separation of multiple forms of cyclic nucleotide phosphodiesterases from rat brain by isoelectrofocusing, *Biochim. Biophys. Acta* **37:**242–248.

SMOAKE, J. A., SONG, S.-Y., and CHEUNG, W. Y., 1974, Cyclic 3′,5′-nucleotide phosphodiesterase. Distribution and developmental changes of the enzyme and its protein activator in mammalian tissues and cells, *Biochim. Biophys. Acta* **341:**402–411.

STEFANOVICH, V., 1974, Concerniñg specificity of the influence of pentoxifylline on various cyclic AMP phosphodiesterases, *Res. Comm. Chem. Path. Pharmacol.* **8:**673–680.

STRADA, S. J., UZUNOV, P., and WEISS, B., 1974, Ontogenetic development of a phosphodiesterase activator and the multiple forms of cyclic AMP phosphodiesterase of rat brain, *J. Neurochem.* **23:**1097–1104.

TESHIMA, Y., YAMAZAKI, R., and KAKIUCHI, S., 1974, Effects of ATP on the activity of nucleoside 3′,5′-cyclic monophosphate phosphodiesterase from brain, *J. Neurochem.* **22:**789–791.

WEISS, B., FERTEL, R., FIGLIN, R., and UZUNOV, P., 1974, Selective alteration of the activity of the multiple forms of adenosine 3′,5′-monophosphate phosphodiesterase of rat cerebrum, *Mol. Pharmacol.* **19:**615–625.

UZUNOV, P., SHEIN, H. M., and WEISS, B., 1974, Multiple forms of cyclic 3′,5′-AMP phosphodiesterase of rat cerebrum and cloned astrocytoma and neuroblastoma cells, *Neuropharmacology* **13:**377–392.

WOLFF, D. J., and BROSTROM, C. O., 1974, Calcium-binding phosphoprotein from pig brain: Identification as a calcium-dependent regulator of brain cyclic nucleotide phosphodiesterase, *Arch. Biochem. Biophys.* **163:**349–358.

2.4. Protein Kinases

AGREN, G., and RONQUIST, G., 1974, (^{32}P)Phosphoryl transfer by endogenous protein kinase at the glia and glioma cell membranes, *Acta Physiol. Scand.* **92:**430–432.

ALBIN, E. E., and NEWBURGH, R. W., 1975, Cyclic nucleotide-stimulable protein kinases in the central nervous system of *Manduca sexta, Biochim. Biophys. Acta* **377:**389–401.

CASNELLIE, J. E., and GREENGARD, P., 1974, Guanosine 3′,5′-cyclic monophosphatedependent phosphorylation of endogeneous substrate proteins in membranes of mammalian smooth muscle, *Proc. Nat. Acad. Sci.* **71:**1891–1895.

CASOLA, L., MATTEO, G., and AUGUSTI-TOCCO, G., 1974, Neuroblastoma cells in culture: ^{32}P-phosphoprotein labeling and protein kinase activity, *Exp. Neurol.* **44:**417–423.

EHRLICH, Y. H., and ROUTTENBERG, A., 1974, Cyclic AMP regulates phosphorylation of three protein components of rat cerebral cortex membranes for thirty minutes, *FEBS Letters* **45:**237–243.

KUO, J. F., 1974, Guanosine 3′,5′-monophosphate-dependent protein kinases in mammalian tissue, *Proc. Nat. Acad. Sci.* **71:**4037–4041.

KUO, J. F., MIYAMOTO, E., and REYES, P. L., 1974, Activation and dissociation of adenosine 3′,5′-monophosphate-dependent and guanosine 3′,5′-monophosphate-dependent protein kinases by various cyclic nucleotide analogs, *Biochem. Pharmacol.* **23:**2011–2021.

LETERRIER, J. F., RAPPAPORT, L., and NUNEZ, J., 1974, Neurotubulin polymerization and phosphorylation reactions catalyzed by 'associated' protein kinase, *FEBS Letters* **46:**285–288.

LETERRIER, J. F., RAPPAPORT, L., and NUNEZ, J., 1974, Phosphorylation and aggregation of neurotubulin and 'associated' protein-kinase, *Mol. Cell. Endocrinol.* **1:**65–76.

LEVITAN, I. B., and BARONDES, S. H., 1974, Octopamine- and serotonin-stimulated phosphorylation of specific protein in the abdominal ganglion of *Aplysia californica, Proc. Nat. Acad. Sci.* **71:**1145–1148.

MEYER, R. B. JR., SHUMAN, D. A., and ROBINS, R. K., 1974, A new purine ring closure and the synthesis of 2-substituted derivatives of adenosine cyclic 3′,5′-phosphate, *J. Am. Chem. Soc.* **96:**4962–4966.

MILLER, J. P., BOSWELL, K. H., MUNEYAMA, K., TOLMAN, R. L., SCHOLTEN, M. B., ROBINS, R. K., SIMON, L. N., and SHUMAN, D. A., 1973, Activity of tubercidin-, toyocomycin-, and sangivamycin-3′,5′-cyclic phosphates and related compounds with some enzymes of adenosine-3′,5′-cyclic phosphate metabolism, *Biochem. Biophys. Res. Commun.* **55:**843–849.

MIYAMOTO, T., 1975, Protein kinases in myelin of rat brain: Solubilization and characterization. *J. Neurochem.* **24:**503–512.

MIYAMOTO, E., and KAKIUCHI, S., 1974, *In vitro* and *in vivo* phosphorylation of myelin basic protein by exogenous and endogenous adenosine 3′,5′-monophosphate-dependent protein kinases in brain, *J. Biol. Chem.* **249:**2769–2777.

MUNEYAMA, K., SHUMAN, D. A., BOSWELL, K. H., ROBINS, R. K., SIMON, L. N., and MILLER, J. P., 1974, Synthesis and biological activity of 8-halo-adenosine 3′,5′-cyclic phosphates, *J. Carbohydrates Nucleosides Nucleotides* **1:**55–60.

NESTEROVA, M. V., SASCHENKO, L. P., VASILIEV, V. UY., and SEVERIN, E. S., 1975, Cyclic adenosine 3′,5′-monophosphate-dependent histone kinase from pig brain, Purification and some properties of the enzyme, *Biochim. Biophys. Acta* **377:** 271–281.

SCHMIDT, M. J., 1974, Effects of neonatal hyperthyroidism on activity of cyclic AMP-dependent microsomal protein kinase, *J. Neurochem.* **22:**469–471.

SEVERIN, E. S., NESTEROVA, M. V., SASHCHENKO, L. P., RASUMOVA, V. V., TUNITSKAYA, V. L., KOCHETKOV, S. N., and GULYAEV, N. N., 1975, Investigation of the adenosine 3′,5′-cyclic phosphate binding site of pig brain histone kinase with the aid of some analogues of adenosine 3′,5′-cyclic phosphate, *Biochim. Biophys. Acta* **384:**413–422.

SHIGEKAWA, B. L., and OLSEN, R. W., 1975, Resolution of cyclic AMP-stimulated protein kinase from polymerization-purified brain microtubules. *Biochem. Biophys. Res. Commun.* **63:**455–462.

SLOBODA, R. D., RUDOLPH, S. A., ROSENBAUM, J. L., and GREENGARD, P., 1975, Cyclic AMP-dependent endogeneous phosphorylation of microtubule-associated protein, *Proc. Nat. Acad. Sci.* **72:**177–181.

SOLD, G., and HOFMANN, F., 1974, Evidence for a guanosine-3′,5′-monophosphate-binding protein from rat cerebellum, *Eur. J. Biochem.* **44:**143–149.

SOIFER, D., 1975, Enzymatic activity in tubulin preparations: Cyclic-AMP dependent protein kinase activity of brain microtubule protein, *J. Neurochem.* **24:**21–33.

TAKAHASHI, T., MATSUZAKI, S., and NUNEZ, J., 1975, Modifications in soluble protein kinase and cyclic-AMP binding capacity in developing rat brain, *J. Neurochem.* **24:**303–310.

WALSH, D. A., ASHBY, C. D., GONZALEZ, C., CALKINS, D., FISCHER, E. H., and KREBS, E. G., 1971, Purification and characterization of a protein inhibitor of adenosine 3′,5′-monophosphate-dependent protein kinases, *J. Biol. Chem.* **246:**1977–1985.

WILLIAMS, M., and RODNIGHT, R., 1974, Evidence for a role for protein phosphorylation in synaptic function in the cerebral cortex mediated through a β-noradrenergic receptor, *Brain Res.* **77:**502–506.

WILLIAMS, M., and RODNIGHT, R., 1975, Stimulation of protein phosphorylation in brain slices by electrical pulses: Speed of response and evidence for net phosphorylation, *J. Neurochem.* **24:**601–603.

WILLIAMS, M., PAVLIK, A., and RODNIGHT, R., 1969, Cellular localization of phosphoproteins in guinea pig cerebral cortex slices sensitive to noradrenaline, histamine and 5-hydroxytryptamine, *Transac. Biochem. Soc.* **2:**259–261.

WILLIAMS, M., PAVLIK, A., and RODNIGHT, R., 1974, Turnover of protein phosphorus in respiring slices of guinea pig cerebral cortex: Cellular localization of phosphoprotein sensitive to electrical stimulation, *j. Neurochem.* **22:**373–376.

2.5. Phosphoprotein Phosphates

ALBIN, E. E., and NEWBURGH, R. W., 1975, Phosphoprotein phosphatase in the central nervous system of *Manduca sexta, Biochim. Biophys. Acta* **377:**381–388.

KOBAYASHI, M., KATO, K., and SATO, S., 1975, Multiple molecular forms of phosphoprotein phosphatase. III. Phosphorylase phosphatase and phosphohistone phosphatase of rabbit liver, *Biochim. Biophys. Acta* **377:**343–355.

MAENO, H., UEDA, T., and GREENGARD, P., 1975, Adenosine 3′,5′-monophosphate-dependent protein phosphatase activity in synaptic membrane fractions, *J. Cyclic Nucleotide Res.* **1**:37–48.

MIYAMOTO, E., and KAKIUCHI, S., 1975, Phosphoprotein phosphatases for myelin basic protein in myelin and cytosol fraction of brain, *Biochim. Biophys. Acta* **384**:458–465.

3.1. Cyclic AMP in Brain Slices

DE LA PAZ, R. L., DICKMAN, S. R., and GROSSER, B. I., 1975, Effects of stress on rat brain adenosine 3′,5′-monophosphate *in vivo*, *Brain Res.* **85**:171–176.

GUIDOTTI, A., CHENEY, D. L., TRABUCCHI, M., DOTEUCHI, M., WANG, C., and HAWKINS, R. A., 1974, Focussed microwave radiation: A technique to minimize postmortem changes of cyclic nucleotides, dopa and choline and to preserve brain morphology, *Neuropharmacology* **13**:1115–1122.

JONES, D. J., MEDINA, M., ROSS, D. H., and STAVINOHA, W. B., 1974, Rate of inactivation of adenyl cyclase and phosphodiesterase: Determinants of brain cyclic AMP, *Life Sci.* **14**:1577–1585.

KIMURA, H., THOMAS, E., and MURAD, F., 1974, Effects of decapitation, ether and pentobarbital on guanosine 3′,5′-phosphate and adenosine 3′,5′-phosphate levels in rat tissues, *Biochim. Biophys. Acta* **343**:519–528.

NAHORSKI, S. R., ROGERS, K. J., and SMITH, B. M., 1974, Histamine H_2-receptors and cyclic AMP in brain, *Life Sci.* **15**:1887–1894.

SATO, A., ONAYA, T., KOTANI, H., and YAMADA, T., Effects of biogenic amines on the formation of adenosine 3′,5′-monophosphate in porcine cerebral cortex, hypothalamus and anterior pituitary slices, *Endocrinology* **94**:1311–1318.

STEFANOVICH, V., and JOHN, J. P., 1974, Increase of cyclic AMP in rat brain during anoxia, *Res. Commun. Chem. Pathol. Pharmacol.* **9**:591–593.

WATANABE, H., and PASSONNEAU, J. V., 1974, The effect of trauma on cerebral glycogen and related metabolites and enzymes, *Brain. Res.* **66**:147–159.

WATANABE, H., and PASSONNEAU, J. V., 1975, Cyclic adenosine monophosphate in cerebral cortex. Alterations following trauma, *Arch. Neurol.* **32**:181–184.

3.1.2. Guinea Pig Brain Slices

BAUDRY, M., MARTRES, M. P., and SCHWARTZ, J. C., 1975, H_1- and H_2-receptors in the histamine-induced accumulation of cyclic AMP in guinea pig brain slices, *Nature* **253**:362–363.

FREE, C. A., PAIK, V. S., and SHADA, J. D., 1974, Inhibition by phenothiazines of adenylate cyclase in adrenal and brain tissue, in *The Phenothiazines and Structurally Related Drugs*, (I. S, Forrest, C. J. Carr, and E. Usin, eds.) pp. 789–748, Raven Press, New York.

ROGERS, M., DISMUKES, K., and DALY, J. W., 1975, Histamine-elicited accumulations of cyclic adenosine 3′,5′-monophosphate in guinea pig brain slices: Effect of H_1- and H_2-antagonists, *J. Neurochem.*, in press.

SATTIN, A., RALL, T. W., and ZANELLA, J., 1975, Regulation of cyclic adenosine 3′,5′-monophosphate levels in guinea-pig cerebral cortex by interaction of alpha adenergic and adenosine receptor activity, *J. Pharmacol. Exp. Ther.* **192**:22–32.

SCHULTZ, J., 1974, Inhibition of phosphodiesterase activity in brain cortical slices from guinea pig and rat, *Pharmacol. Res. Comm.* **6**:335–341.

SCHULTZ, J., 1975, Cyclic adenosine 3′,5′-monophosphate in guinea pig cerebral cortical slices: Possible regulation of phosphodiesterase activity by cyclic adenosine 3′,5′-monophosphate and calcium ions, *J. Neurochem.* **24**:495–501.

Shimizu, H., Ichishita, H., Tateishi, M., and Umeda, I., 1974, Characteristics of the amino acid receptor site mediating formation of cyclic adenosine 3′,5′-monophosphate in mammalian brains, *Mol. Pharmacol.* **11:**223–231.

Shimizu, H., Ichishita, H., and Odagiri, H., 1974, Stimulated formation of cyclic adenosine 3′,5′-monophosphate by aspartate and glutamate in cerebral cortical slices of guinea pig, *J. Biol. Chem.* **249:**5955–5962.

3.1.3. Rat Brain Slices

Blumbert, J. B., Taylor, R. E., and Sulser, F., 1975, Blockade by pimozide of a noradrenaline sensitive adenylate cyclase in the limbic forebrain: Possible role of limbic noradrenergic mechanisms in the mode of action of antipsychotics, *J. Pharm. Pharmacol.* **27:**125–128.

Forn, J., Krueger, B. K., and Greengard, P., 1974, Adenosine 3′,5′-monophosphate content in rat caudate nucleus: Demonstration of dopaminergic and adrenergic receptors, *Science* **186:**1118–1120.

Gunaga, K. P., Kawano, A., and Menon, K. M. J., 1974, *In vivo* effect of estradiol benzoate on the accumulation of adenosine 3′,5′-cyclic monophosphate in the rat hypothalamus, *Neuroendocrinology* **16:**273–281.

Munday, K. A., Poat, J. A., and Woddruff, G. N., 1974, Increase in the cyclic AMP content of rat striatum produced by a cyclic analogue of dopamine, *J. Physiol.* **241:**119–120P.

Palmer, G. C., and Manian, A. A., 1974, Effects of phenothiazines and phenothiazine metabolites on adenyl cyclase and the cyclic AMP response in the rat brain, in *The Phenothiazines and Structurally Related Drugs* (I. S. Forrest, C. J. Carr, and E. Usdin, eds.) pp. 749–767, Raven Press, New York.

Palmer, G. C., and Manian, A. A., 1974, Modification of the receptor component of adenylate cyclase in the rat brain by phenothiazine derivatives, *Neuropharmacology* **13:**851–866.

Skolnick, P., and Daly, J. W., 1975, Stimulation of adenosine 3′,5′-monophosphate formation in rat cerebral cortical slices by methoxamine: Interaction with an alpha-adrenergic receptor, *J. Pharmacol. Exp. Ther.*, **193:**549–558

Skolnick, P., Schultz, J., and Daly, J. W., 1975, Repetitive stimulation of cyclic adenosine 3′,5′-monophosphate formation by adrenergic agonists in incubated slices from rat cerebral cortex, *J. Neurochem.*, **24:**451–456.

3.1.4. Mouse Brain Slices

Barchas, J. D., Ciaranello, R. D., Dominic, J. A., Deguchi, T., Orenberg, E., Renson, J., and Kessler, S., 1974, Genetic aspects of monoamine mechanisms, *Adv. Biochem. Psychopharmacology* **12:**195–215.

Wong, P. C. L., and Henderson, J. F., 1972, Purine ribonucleotide biosynthesis intraconversion and catabolism in mouse brain *in vitro, Biochem. J.* **129:**1085–1094.

3.1.6. Conversion of Adenine and Adenosine-labeled Nucleotides to Cyclic AMP

Kuroda, J., and McIlwain, H., 1974, Uptake and release of [^{14}C]adenine derivatives at beds of mammalian cortical synaptasomes in a superfusion system, *J. Neurochem.* **22:**691–700.

Pull, I., and McLwain, H., 1974, Uptake of neurohumoral agents and cerebral metabolites on output of adenine derivatives from superfused tissues of the brain, *J. Neurochem.* **24:**695–700.

Sturgill, T. W., Schrier, M. B. K., and Gilman, A. G. 1975, Stimulation of cyclic AMP accumulation by 2-chloroadenosine: Lack of incorporation of nucleoside into cyclic nucleotides, *J. Cyclic Nucleotide Res.* **1:**21–30.

3.1.7. Effects of Drug and other Treatments of Animals on the Cyclic AMP-Generating Systems in Brain Slices

ARBUTHNOTT, G. W., ATTREE, T. J., ECCLESTON, D. LOOSE, R. W., and MARTIN, M. J., 1974, Is adenylate cyclase the dopamine receptor? *Medical Biology* **52:**350–353.

DISMUKES. K., and DALY, W., 1974, Norepinephrine-sensitive systems generating adenosine 3′,5′-monophosphate: Increased responses in cerebral cortical slices from reserpine-treated rats, *Mol. Pharmacol.* **10:**933–940.

DISMUKES, R. K. and DALY, J. W., 1975, Altered responsiveness of adenosine 3′,5′-monophosphate generating systems in brain slices from adult rats after neontal treatment with 6-hydroxydopamine, *Exp. Neurol.*, in press.

DOLBY, T. W., and KLEINSMEITH, L. J., 1974, Effects of Δ^9-tetrahydrocannabinol on the levels of cyclic adenosine 3′,5′-monophosphate in mouse brain, *Biochem. Pharmacol.* **23:**1817–1825.

FRAZER, A., PANDEY, G., MENDELS, J., NEELEY, S., KANE, M., and HESS, M. E., 1974, The effect of tri-iodothyronine in combination with imipramine on [^{3}H]-cyclic AMP production in slices of rat cerebral cortex, *Neuropharmacology* **13:**1131–1140.

FRENCH, S. W., REID, P. E., PALMER, D. S., NAROD, M. E., and RAMEY, C. W., 1974, Adrenergic subsensitivity of the rat brain during chronic ethanol ingestion, *Res. Comm. Chem. Pathol. Pharmacol.* **9:**575–578.

MISHRA, R. K., GARDNER, E. L., KATZMAN, R., and MAKMAN, M. H., 1974, Enhancement of dopamine-stimulated adenylate cyclase activity in rat caudate after lesions in substantia nigra: Evidence for denervation supersensitivity, *Proc. Nat. Acad. Sci.* **71:**3883–3887.

PALMER, G. C. and SCOTT, H. R., 1974, The cyclic AMP response to noradrenalin in young adult rat brain following post-natal injections of 6-hydroxy-dopamine, *Experientia* **30:**520–521.

PALMER, G. C., SPURGEON, H. A., and PRIOLA, D. V., 1975, Involvement of adenylate cyclase in mechanisms of denervation supersensitivity following surgical denervation of dog heart, *J. Cyclic Nucleotide Res.* **1:**89–95.

PURI, S. K., COCHIN, J., and VOLICER, L., 1975, Effect of morphine sulfate on adenylate cyclase and phosphodiesterase activities in rat corpus striatum, *Life Sci.* **16:**759–768.

SINGHAL, R. L., KACEW, S., and LAFRENIERE, R., 1973, Brain adenyl cyclase in methadone treatment of morphine dependency, *J. Pharm. Pharmacol.* **25:**1022–1024.

STRADA, S. J., and WEISS, B., 1974, Increased response to catecholamines of the cyclic AMP system of rat pineal gland induced by decreased sympathetic activity, *Arch. Biochem. Biophys.* **160:**197–204.

TANG, L. C., COTZIAS, G. C., and DUNN, M., 1974, Changing the actions of neuroactive drugs by charging brain protein synthesis, *Proc. Nat. Acad. Sci.* **71:**3350–3354.

VON VOIGTLANDER, P. F., BOUKMA, S. J., and JOHNSON G. A., 1973, Dopaminergic denervation supersensitivity and dopamine stimulated adenyl cyclase activity, *Neuropharmacology* **12:**1081–1086.

WILLIAMS, B. J., and PIRCH, J. H., 1974, Correlation between brain adenyl cyclase activity and spontaneous motor activity in rats after chronic reserpine treatment, *Brain Res.* **68:**227–234.

3.2. Cyclic GMP in Brain Slices and Neuronal Cells

FARBER, D. B., and LOLLEY, R. N., 1974, Cyclic guanosine monophosphate: Elevation in degenerating photoreceptor cells of the C3H mouse retina, *Science* **186:**449–451.

FERRENDELLI, J. A., KINSCHERF, D. A., and CHANG, M-M., 1975, Comparison of the effects of biogenic amines of cyclic GMP and cyclic AMP levels in mouse cerebellum *in vitro*, *Brain Res.* **84:**63–73.

LABORIT, H., KUNZ, E., LAMOTHE, C., and THURET, F., 1974, Sur quelques actions de la guanosine, combinée à l'acétylcholaine ou à l'insuline sur l'activité métabolique due cerveau et la glycémie. *Agressologie* **15:**239–245.

WEIGHT, F. F., PETZOLD, G., and GREENGARD, P., 1974, Guanosine 3',5'-monophosphate in sympathetic ganglia: Increase associated with synaptic transmission, *Science* **186:**942–944.

3.3. Cyclic AMP in Ganglia

BUCHER, M.-B., and SCHORDERET, M., 1974, Apomorphine-induced accumulation of cyclic AMP in isolated retinas of the rabbit, *Biochem. Pharmacol.* **23:**3079–3082.

CHATZKEL, S., ZIMMERMAN, I., and BERG, A., 1974, Modulation of cyclic-AMP synthesis in the cat superior cervical ganglion by short term presynaptic stimulation, *Brain Res.* **80:**523–526.

CRAMER, H., and LINDL, T., 1974, Release of cyclic AMP from rat superior cervical ganglia after stimulation of synthesis *in vitro, Nature* **249:**380–382.

LINDL, T., BEHRENDT, H., and HEINL-SAWAJA, M. C. B., Effects of compound 40/80 on mast cells, histamine, and cyclic AMP in isolated superior cervical ganglia, *Naunyn Schmiedebergs Arch. Pharmacol.* **286:**283–296.

LOLLEY, R. N., SCHMIDT, S. Y., and FARBER, D. B., 1974, Alterations in cyclic AMP metabolism associated with photoreceptor cell degeneration in the C3H mouse, *J. Neurochem.* **22:**701–707.

NATHANSON, J. A., and GREENGARD, P., 1974, Serotonin-sensitive adenylate cyclase in neural tissue and its similarity to the serotonin receptor: A possible site of action of lysergic acid diethylamine, *Proc. Nat. Acad. Sci.* **71:**797–801.

ROCH, P., and KALIX, P., 1975, Effects of biogenic amines on the concentration of adenosine 3',5'-monophosphate in bovine superior cervical ganglion, *Neuropharmacology* **14:**21–30.

VEDECKIS, W. V., and GILBERT, L. I., 1973, Production of cyclic AMP and adenosine by the brain and prothoracic glands of *Manduca sexta, J. Insect. Physiol.* **19:**2445–2457.

3.4. Cyclic AMP in Cells of Neuronal or Glial Origin

BENDA, P., PREMONT, J., and JARD, S., 1972, Adénylate cyclase et phosphodiestérases dans les hybrides somatiques des cellules gliales, *C. R. Acad. Sci.* **275:**1303-1306.

BROSTROM, M. A., KON, C., OLSON, D. R., and BRECKENRIDGE, B. MCL., 1974, Adenosine 3',5'-monophosphate in glial tumor cells treated with glucocorticoids, *Mol. Pharmacol.* **10:**711–720.

CLARK, R. B., YING-FU, S., GROSS, R., and PERKINS, J. P., 1974, Regulation of adenosine 3',5'-monophosphate in human astrocytoma cells by adenosine and the adenine nucleotides, *J. Biol. Chem.* **249:**5296–5303.

PENIT, J., JARD, S., and BENDA, P., 1974, Probenecide sensitive 3',5'-cyclic AMP secretion by isoproterenol stimulated glial cells in culture, *FEBS Letters* **41:**156–160.

PRASAD, K. N., and GILMER, K. N., 1974, Demonstration of dopamine-sensitive adenylate cyclase in malignant neuroblastoma cells and change in sensitivity of adenylate cyclase to catecholamines in "differentiated" cells, *Proc. Nat. Acad. Sci.* **71:**2525–2529.

PRASAD, K. N., GILMER, K. N., and SAHU, S. K., 1974, Demonstration of acetyl-choline-sensitive adenyl cyclase in malignant neuroblastoma cells in culture, *Nature* **249:**765–767.

PRASAD, K. N., GILMER, K. N., SAHU, S. K., and BECKER, G., 1975, Effect of neurotransmitters, guanosine triphosphate and divalent cations on the regulation of adenylate cyclase activity in malignant and adenosine cyclic 3',5'-monophosphate-induced "differentiated" neuroblastoma cells, *Cancer Res.* **35:**77–81.

SHARMA, S. K., NIRENBERG, M., and KLEE, W. A., 1975, Morphine receptors as regulators of adenylate cyclase activity, *Proc. Nat. Acad. Sci.* **72:**590–594.

TRABER, J., FISCHER, K., LATZIN, S., and HAMPRECHT, B., 1974, Morphine antagonizes the action of prostaglandin in neuroblastoma cells but not of prostaglandin and noradrenaline in glioma and glioma X fibroblast hybrid cells, *FEBS Letters* **49:**260–263.

TRABER, J., FISCHER, K., LATZIN, S., and HAMPRECHT, B., 1975, Morphine antagonizes action of prostaglandin in neuroblastoma and neuroblastoma X glioma hybrid cells, *Nature* **253:**120–122.

VELLIS, J-D., and BROOKER, G., 1974, Reversal of catecholamine refractoriness by inhibitors of RNA and protein synthesis, *Science* **186:**1221–1223.

4.1. Effects on Enzymatic Processes

ANAGNOSTE, B., SHIRRON, C., FRIEDMAN, E., and GOLDSTEIN, M., 1974, Effect of dibutyryl cyclic adenosine monophosphate on ^{14}C-dopamine biosynthesis in rat brain striatal slices, *J. Pharmacol. Exp. Ther.* **191:**370–376.

CUBEDDU, L., BARNES, E., and WEINER, N., 1974, Release of norepinephrine and dopamine-β-hydroxylase by nerve stimulation. II. Effects of papaverine, *J. Pharmacol. Exp. Ther.* **191:**444–457.

EBSTEIN, B., ROBERGE, C., TABACHNICK, J., AND GOLDSTEIN, M., 1974, The effect of dopamine and of apomorphine on dB-cAMP-induced stimulation of synaptasomal tyrosine hydroxylase, *J. Pharm. Pharmacol.* **26:**975–978.

EDWARDS, C., NAHORSKI, S. R., and ROGERS, K. J., 1974, *In vivo* changes in cerebral cyclic adenosine 3′,5′-monophosphate-induced by biogenic amines: association with phosphorylase activation, *J. Neurochem.* **22:**565–572.

GUIDOTTI, A., KUROSAWA, A., CHUANG, D. M., and COSTA, E., 1975, Protein kinase activation as an early event in the trans-synaptic induction of tyrosine 3-monooxygenase in adrenal medulla, *Proc. Nat. Acad. Sci.* **72:**1152–1156.

HAMPRECHT, B. and TRABER, J., 1974, Dopamine-β-hydroxylase activity in cholinergic neuroblastoma X glioma hybrid cells: Increase in activity by N^6,O^2-dibutyryl adenosine 3′,5H-cyclic monophosphate, *FEBS Letters* **42:**211–226.

HARRIS, J. E., BALDESSARINI, R. J., MORGENROTH III, V. H., and ROTH, R. H., 1975, Activation by cyclic 3′,5′-adenosine monophosphate of tyrosine hydroxylase in the rat brain, *Proc. Nat. Acad. Sci.* **72:**789–793.

HEDGE, G. A., 1971, ACTH secretion due to hypothalamo-pituitary effects of adenosine 3′,5′-monophosphate and related substances, *Endocrinology* **89:**500–506.

JAANUS, S. D., and RUBINS, R. P., 1974, Analysis of the role of cyclic adenosine 3′,5′-monophosphate in catecholamine release, *J. Physiol.* **237:**465–476.

JONES, E. R., MOSCONA, M., and MOSCONA, A. A., 1973, Does cyclic-3′,5′-AMP induce glutamine synthetase in embryonic neural retina? *Biochem. Biophys. Res. Commun.* **51:**268–274.

KEEN, P., and MCLEAN, W. G., 1974, Effect of dibutyryl-cyclic AMP and dexamethasone on noradrenaline synthesis in isolated superior cervical ganglia, *J. Neurochem.* **22:**5–10.

KUMAR, S., BECKER, G., and PRASAD, K. N., 1975, Cyclic adenosine 3′,5′-monophosphate phosphodiesterase activity in malignant and cyclic adenosine 3′,5′-monophosphate-induced "differentiated" neuroblastoma cells, *Cancer Res.* **35:**82–87.

LABORIT, L., and THURET, F., 1974, Action of inosine and of cyclic inosine monophosphate alone or in association with 5-hydroxytryptamine on three stages of energy metabolism in rat cerebral cortex, *Agressologie* **15:**377–380.

MRSULJA, B. B., 1973, The influence of antistine on glycogenolytic effect of some biogenic amines in rat brain slices, *Experientia* **29:**76–77.

MRSULJA, B. B., 1974, Cyclic nucleotides and brain glycogen, *Experientia* **30:**66–67.

MUELLER, R. A., OTTEN, U., and THOENEN, H., 1974, The role of adenosine cyclic 3',5'-monophosphate in reserpine-initiated adrenal medullary tyrosine hydroxylase induction, *Mol. Pharmacol.* **10:**855–860.

OTTEN, U., MUELLER, R. A., and THOENEN, H., 1974, Evidence against a causal relationship between increase in c-AMP and induction of tyrosine hydroxylase in the rat adrenal medulla, *Naunyn Schmiedebergs Arch. Pharmacol.* **285:**233–242.

SCHWARTZ, J. P., and PASSONNEAU, J. V., 1974, Cyclic AMP-mediated induction of the cyclic AMP phosphodiesterase of C-6 glioma cells, *Proc. Nat. Acad. Sci.* **71:**3844–3848.

SERCK-HANSSEN, G., 1974, Effects of theophylline and propranolol on acetylcholine-induced release of adrenal medullary catecholamines, *Biochem. Pharmacol.* **23:**2225–2234.

SIMANTOV, R., and SACHS, K., 1973, Regulation of acetylcholine receptors in relation to acetylcholinesterase in neuroblastoma cells, *Proc. Nat. Acad. Sci.* **70:**2902–2905.

TANEDA, M., IZUMI, F., and OKA, M., 1974, Effect of dibutyryl adenosine 3',5'-monophosphate on catecholamine synthesis in rat brain cortical slices and isolated vasa deferentia, *Jap. J. Pharmacol.* **24:**934–936.

TORDA, C., 1972, Cyclic AMP-dependent diphosphoinositide kinase, *Biochim. Biophys.. Acta* **286:**389–395.

WEISS, B., and STILLER, R. L., 1974, Dibutyryl cyclic adenosine 3',5'-monophosphate and brain lipid metabolism, *Lipids* **9:**514–519.

4.2. Cell Morphology, Differentiation, and Growth

BJERRE, J., 1974, A neuralizing influence of dibutyryl cyclic AMP on competent chick ectoderm, *Experientia* **30:**534–535.

BONDY, S. C., PRASAD, K. N., and PRUDY, J. L., 1974, Neuroblastoma: Drug-induced differentiation increase proportion of cytoplasmic RNA that contains polyadenylic acid, *Science* **186:**359–361.

CHALAZONITIS, A., and GREENE, L. A., 1974, Enhancement in excitability properties of mouse neuroblastoma cells cultured in the presence of dibutyryl cyclic AMP, *Brain Res.* **72:**340–345.

DANIELS, M. P., and HAMPRECHT, B., 1974, The ultrastructure of neuroblastoma glioma somatic cell hybrids: Expression of neuronal characteristics stimulated by dibutyryl adenosine 3',5'-cyclic monophosphate, *J. Cell Biology* **63:**691–699.

EDSTROM, A., KANJE, M., and WALUM, E., 1974, Effects of dibutyryl cyclic AMP and prostaglandin E1 on cultured human glioma cells, *Exp. Brain Res.* **85:**217–223.

LENTZ, T. L., 1972, A role of cyclic AMP in a neurotrophic process, *Nature New Biol.* **238:**154–155.

MILLER, R. A., and RUDDLE, F. H., 1974, Enucleated neuroblastoma cells form neurites when treated with dibutyryl cyclic AMP, *J. Cell Biology* **63:**295–299.

PRASAD, K. N., KUMAR, S., GILMER, K., and VERNADAKIS, A., 1973, Cyclic AMP-induced differentiated neuroblastoma cells: Changes in total nucleic acid and protein contents, *Biochem. Biophys. Res. Commun.* **50:**973–977.

SHAPIRO, D. L., 1973, Morphological and biochemical alterations in foetal rat brain cells cultured in the presence of monobutyryl cyclic AMP, *Nature* **241:**203–204.

WAHN, H. L., LIGHTBODY, L. E., TCHEN, T. T., and TAYLOR, J. D., 1975, Induction of neural differentiation in cultures of amphibian undetermined presumptive epidermis by cyclic AMP derivatives, *Science* **188:**366–369.

4.3.1. Membrane Phenomena, Central Neurons

BLOOM, F. E., 1974, To spritz or not to spritz: The doubtful value of aimless iontophoresis, *Life Sci.* **14:**1819–1834.

BLOOM, F. E., SIGGINS, G. R., and HOFFER, B. J., 1974, Interpreting the failures to confirm the depression of cerebellar Purkinje cells by cyclic AMP, *Science* **185:**627–628.

PHILLIS, J. W., 1974, The role of calcium in the central effects of biogenic amines, *Life Sci.* **14:**1189–1201.

PHILLIS, J. W., KOSTOPOULOS, G. K., and LIMACHER, J. J., 1974, Depression of corticospinal cells by various purines and pyrimidines, *Canadian J. Physiol. Pharmacol.* **52:**1226–1229.

PHILLIS, J. W., KOSTOPOULUS, G. K., and LIMACHER, J. J., 1975, A potent depressant action of adenine derivatives on cerebral cortical neurones, *Europ. J. Pharmacol* **30:**125–129.

SEGAL, M., 1974, Responses of septal nuclei neurons to microionphoretically administered putative neurotransmitters, *Life Sci.* **14:**1345–13511.

SEGAL, M., and BLOOM, F. E., 1974, The action of norepinephrine in the rat hippocampus. I. Ionotophoretic studies, *Brain Res.* **72:**79–97.

SEGAL, M., and BLOOM, F. E., 1974, The action of norepinephrine in the rat hippocampus. II. Activation of the input pathway, *Brain Res.* **72:**99–114.

SHOEMAKER, W. J., BALENTINE, L. T., SIGGINS, G. R., HOFFER, B. J., HENRICKSEN, S. J., and BLOOM, F. E., 1975, Characteristics of the release of adenosine 3′,5′-monophosphate from micropipets by microiontrophoresis, *J. Cyclic Nucleotide Res.* **1:**97–106.

SIGGINS, G. R., HOFFER, B. J., asnd UNGERSTEDT, U., 1974, Electrophysiological evidence for involvement of cyclic adenosine monophosphate in dopamine responses of caudate neurons, *Life Sci.* **15:**779–792.

STONE, T. W., TAYLOR, D. A., and BLOOM, F. E., 1974, Cyclic AMP and cyclic GMP may mediate opposite neuronal responses in the rat cerebral cortex, *Science* **187:**845–847.

YARBROUGH, G. G., LAKE, N., and PHILLIS, J. W., 1974, Calcium antagonism and its effect on the inhibitory actions of biogenic amines on cerebral cortical neurons, *Brain Res.* **67:**77–88.

4.3.2. Membrane Phenomena, Peripheral Neurons

CHADER, G. J., BENSINGER, R., JOHNSON, M., and FLETCHER, R. T., 1973, Phosphodiesterase: An important role in cyclic nucleotide regulation in the retina, *Exp. Eye Res.* **17:**483–486.

CHADER, G. J., HERZ, L. W., and FLETCHER, R. T., 1974, Light activation of phosphodiesterase activity in retinal rod outer segments, *Biochim. Biophys. Acta* **347:**491–493.

MIKI, N., KEIRNS, J. J., MARCUS, F. R., FREEMAN, J., and BITENSKY, M. W., 1973, Regulation of cyclic nucleotide concentrations in photoreceptors: An ATP-dependent stimulation of cyclic nucleotide phosphodiesterase by light, *Proc. Nat. Acad. Sci.* **70:**3820–2824.

SURIA, A., and COSTA, E., 1975, Action of diazepam, dibutyryl cGMP and GABA on presynaptic nerve terminals in bull frog sympathetic ganglia, *Brain Res.* **87:**102–106.

TORDA, C., 1974, Restorative effect of cyclic AMP on the bioelectric processes of calcium deprived ganglia, *Experientia* **30:**1154–1155.

4.3.3. Membrane Phenomena, Motor Neurons

MIYAMOTO, M. D., and BRECKENRIDGE, B. MCL., 1974, A cyclic adenosine monophosphate link in the catecholamine enhancement of transmitter release at the neuromuscular junction, *J. Gen. Physiol.* **63:**609–624.

TAKAMORI, M., ISHII, M., and MORI, M., 1973, The role of cyclic 3′,5′-adenosine monophosphate in neuromuscular transmission, *Arch. Neurol.* **29:**420–422.

VAN DE BERG, J. S., 1974, Inhibitory effects of dibutyryl and cyclic AMP on the compound action potential in the frog (*Rana pipiens*) sciatic nerve, *Experientia* **30:**1025–1026.

VAPAATALO, H., and ANTTILA, P., 1972, Effects of some inhibitors of phosphodiesterase on neuromuscular transmission, *Naunyn-Schmiedeberg's Arch. Pharmacol.* **275:**227–232.

VAPAATALO, H., 1974, Role of cyclic neucleotides in the nervous system, *Medical Biology* **52:**200–207.

WILSON, D. F., 1974, The effects of dibutyryl cyclic adenosine 3',5'-monophosphate, theophylline and aminophylline on neuromuscular transmission in the rat, *J. Pharmacol. Exp. Ther.* **188:**447–452.

YAMASAKI, Y., FUJIWARA, M., and TODA, N., 1974, Effects of intracellularly applied cyclic 3',5'-adenosine monophosphate and dibutyryl cyclic 3',5'-adenosine monophosphate on the electrical activity of sinoatrial nodal cells of the rabbit, *J. Pharmacol. Exp. Ther.* **190:**15–20.

4.4. Centrally Active Drugs and Levels of Cyclic Nucleotides in Brain.

GARELIS, E., and NEFF, N. H., 1974, Cyclic adenosine monophosphate: Selective increase in caudate nucleus after administration of *L*-dopa, *Science* **183:**532–533.

GERHARDS, H. J., CARENZI, A., and COSTA, E., 1974, Effect of Nominfensine on motor activity, dopamine turnover rate and cyclic adenosine 3',5'-monophosphate concentrations of rat striatum, *Naunyn-Schmiedeberg's Arch. Pharmacol.* **286:**49–64.

HEIKKINEN, E. R., MYLLYLA, V. V., VAPAATALO, H., and HOKKANEN, E., 1974, Urinary excretion and cerebrospinal fluid concentration of cyclic adenosine 3',5'-monophosphate in various neurological diseases, *Europ. Neurol.* **11:**270–280.

MAO, C. C., GUIDOTTO, A., and COSTA, E., 1974, Interactions between γ-aminobutyric acid and guanosine cyclic 3',5'-monophosphate in rat cerebellum, *Mol. Pharmacol.* **10:**736–746.

MAO, C. C., GUIDOTTI, A., and COSTA, E., 1975, Inhibition by diazepam of the tremor and the increase of cerebellar c-GMP content elicited by harmaline, *Brain Res.* **83:**516–519.

MYLLYLA, V. V., HEIKKINEN, E. R., SIMILA, S., HOKKANEN, E., and VAPAATALO, H., 1974, Cerebrospinal fluid concentration and urinary excretion of cyclic adenosine-3',5'-monophosphate in various diseases of children. A preliminary study, Z. Kinderheilk. **118:**259–264.

MYLLYLA, V. V., VAPAATALO, H., HOKKANEN, E., and HEIKKINEN, E. R., 1974, Cerebrospinal fluid concentration of cyclic adenosine 3',5'-monophosphate and pneumoencephalography, *Europ. Neurol.* **12:**28–32.

PALMER, G. C., and EVAN, A. P., 1974, Effect of psychotropic drugs on the urinary excretion of cyclic AMP in the rat, *Proc. West. Pharmacol. Soc.* **17:**204–209.

SEBENS, J. B., and KORF, J., 1975, Cyclic AMP in cerebrospinal fluid: Accumulation following probenecid and biogenic amines, *Exp. Neurology,* **46:**333–344.

SIEGEL, R., CONFORT, N., FELDMAN, S., and CHOWER, I., 1974, Effects of neurogenic and systemic stresses on hypothalamic and adenohypophysial cAMP content, *Neuroendocrinology* **14:**24–33.

WANG, Y.-C., PANDEY, G. N., MENDELS, J., and FRAZER, A., 1974, Platelet adenylate cyclase responses in depression: Implications for a receptor defect, *Psychopharmacologica* **36:**291–300.

4.5. Behavioral and Pharmacological Effects

BRUS, R., HERMAN, Z. S., and KOSTMAN, 1974, Behavioral effects of norepinephrine and dibutyryl cyclic 3',5'-AMP in centrally sympathectomized rats, *Pharmacol. Biochem. Behavior* **2:**719–724.

COHN, M. L., TAYLOR, F., COHN, M., and YAMAOKA, H., 1973, Dibutyryl cyclic AMP—an effective antidote against lethal amounts of amobarbital in the rat, *Res. Commun. Chem. Pathol. Pharmacol.* **6:**435–446.

COHN, M. L., COHN, M., and TAYLOR, F. H., 1974, Norepinephrine—an antagonist of dibutyryl cyclic AMP in the regulation of narcosis in the rat, *Res. Comm. Chem. Path. Pharmacol.* **7**:687–699.

DOGGETT, N. S., and SPENCER, P. S. J., 1971, Pharmacological properties of centrally administered ouabain and their modification by other drugs, *Brit. J. Pharmacol.* **42**:242–253.

DOGGETT, N. S., and SPENCER, P. S. J., 1973, Pharmacological properties of centrally-administered agents which interfere with neurotransmitter function: A comparison with the central depressant effects of ouabain, *Brit. J. Pharmacol.* **47**:26–38.

KNOPP, J., and MITRO, A., 1973, Effect of dibutyryl cyclic AMP injected into third ventricle on the thyroid ^{131}I-iodide accumulation, *Endokrinologie* **62**:237–238.

INDEX

Acetaldehyde, 10
Acetylcholine, 29, 64, 87, 102, 214, 345
Acetylsalicylate, 10
Actinomycin D, 221
Addiction, 355–356
Adenine, 79, 80
  nucleotides, 79–84, 158, 167
    involved in depressive illness, 158
Adenohypophysis, 195
Adenosine, 51, 54, 62, 65–67, 72, 75–78, 92, 94, 95, 103, 163, 167
  -amine combination, 67, 68, 75, 76
  deaminase, 133
    inhibitor, 170, 171
  diphosphate, *see* ADP
  monophosphate, *see* AMP
  triphosphate, *see* ATP
  uptake inhibitors, 170
Adenyl compounds
  drugs potentiating, 170–171
  effect on blood flow through kidney, 139
  excitatory action, 165–168
  inhibitory action, 165–168
  muscle receptors, 166
  and purinergic transmission, 164–171
Adenylate cyclase, 48–52, 90, 142
ADP, 4, 66
Adrenergic nerves, 151–152
  transmission, 28
Amine
  -adenosine combination, 67, 68, 75, 76
  biogenic, 24–32
  as inhibitors of enzymes, 24
  oxidase, 28
  and transport, 24
Amino acid, 88
  influx into brain, 23
Amino acid decarboxylase
  inhibitors, 24, 31–32
  interference, 31
γ-Aminobutyric acid, 16–17, 31
Aminooxyacetate, 15–16
  convulsion, 16
  depression, 16
Aminophylline, 101, 169
Ammonia, 12, 13, 16
  in brain, 12–13
AMP, 66, 167
  cyclic, 47–96, 101, 142, 143, 200, 230
  dibutyryl, 64, 95–97, 103
Amphetamine, 28–30, 74, 75, 105
Amygdala, 251, 261
Amyl nitrite, 163
Amytal (Amylobarbitone), 7–10
Anatomical problems, 241–242
Androgen, 273–292
  binding, 280–288
  in birds, 281–284
  chemical specificity, 288–289
  receptors, 288
  retention, 280
  saturability, 280
  stereoselectivity, 280
  trivial names, 275
  and vocal behavior, 286
3α-Androstanediol, 274, 278
Anesthetics, 5, 7, 10, 19–21
  local, 19–21
Antazoline, 133, 163, 168
Antidepressant, 28
Antiestrogens, 268–269
Apomorphine, 53
Astrocyte, 21
  and ouabain, 21

Athetosis, 158
ATP, 3, 8, 23, 26, 54, 66, 132, 133, 137, 146, 149, 151, 162–165
ATPase, 23, 133, 146
  inhibitors, 170
Atropine, 87, 105, 133
  resistance, 140
Autoradiography, 24, 245–252
Axon, unmyelinated, 143
Azide, 72

Barbiturates, 4–10
Batrachotoxin, 62, 68, 70, 76, 78
Behavior
  courtship, 286
  effects, 106–107
  sexual, 286, 292
Benzomorphan series, 330
Benzopyrimidine, 53
Binding site, 213
  high-affinity class, 213
  low-affinity class, 213
Bradykinin, 139
Brain energy metabolism
  effects of drugs on, 1–46
  energetics, 2–4
  mechanism mediating pain, 330, 340
  methods for fixing brain tissue, 104
    freeze-blowing, 104
    microwave irradiation, 104
  time of sacrifice, 249
Bufotenine, 75

Caffeine, 63, 72, 169
Calcium ion, 19, 20, 53, 199, 200
Carbachol, 75, 78, 89, 216
Carbon monoxide poisoning, 2
Catatonia, 106
Catecholamine, 29, 50, 90, 91, 216
Cation
  flux, 10
  permeability, 33
Cell body stain, 246
Cell disruption
  differentiation, 97–98
  fractionation, 256
  growth, 97–98
  morphology, 97–98
  of nervous tissue, 51
Central nervous system (CNS)
  activities, 158
  athetosis, 158
  hibernation, 158
Central nervous system (CNS) (*cont.*)
  Lesch-Nyhan syndrome, 158
  metabolism and steroid hormones, 239–328
  psychomotor retardation, 158
  self-mutilation, 158
  steroid hormones and metabolism, 239–328
Cesium, 353
Chaffinch, 283–284
Chemotransmitter theory, 195
Chicken, 284
Chlordiazepoxide, 53, 73
Chlorimipramine, 71
Chlorobutanol, 10
Chlorpromazine, 10, 26, 27, 53, 71, 74, 105
Chlorprothixene, 74
Choline acetyltransferase, 345
Cholinergic agents, 217
Cholinium ion, 70
  dependency, 70
Chromatography, thin-layer, 254
CI-*628,* 268, 270, 271
Circling movement, 106
cis-Clomiphene, 268, 270
Cocaine, 19–21
Codeine, 337
Convulsion, intermittent, 12
Cord, 143
Corticosteroid-21-*O*-acetyltransferase, 303
Corticosterone, 274, 293–305
Corticotropin releasing factor (CRF), 196, 214–215
Cortisol, 301, 302
Cortisone, 303
Courtship behavior, 286
CRF, *see* Corticotropin releasing factor
Cyanide, 72
  poisoning, 2
Cyclase
  adenylate, 48–52
  catecholamine-mediated activation of, 50
  guanylate, 52
Cycloheximide, 221
Cyproterone, 208, 289
  acetate, 266
Cytochrome oxidase, 256
Cytosol binding, 260–262, 264, 299
  fraction in high-speed supernatant, 254

2-Deoxyglucose, 15
  phosphate, 15
Depolarizing agent, 68, 76, 87, 88
  condition, 83

Depression illness, 79–84, 158, 167
  adenine nucleotides involved, 158
  manifestation, 227
  mechanism hypothesis, 158
Desimipramine, 71
Desmethylimipramine, 28
Desoxycorticosterone acetate, 311
Dexamethasone, 295, 302
Dextrorphan, 336
3,4-Dialkoxybenzyl-2-imidazolidime, 53
N,N-Dialkyltryptamine, 75
Diazepam, 53, 73
Dichloromethane, 254
Diesthylstilbestrol, 240, 242, 245, 259, 267
Dihydroergotamine, 53
[^{3}H]Dihydromorphine, 338, 349, 350
Dihydrotestosterone, 274, 277–280, 289
Dihydroxyphenylalanine, 32
3-20-Diketopregnone-21-ol, 10
2:4-Dinitrophenol, 6, 72, 169
Diphenylpropylamine, 330
Dipyridamole, 53, 73, 163, 164, 170
DNA, 256
Dopamine, 25, 29, 30, 50, 51, 64, 75, 78, 89, 90, 101, 102, 215, 345
L-Dopa pargyline test, 203
Dove, 296
Drug
  affecting cerebral transport, 1–46
  affecting energy metabolism of brain, 1–46
  uncoupling mitochondrial respiration from phosphorylation, 10

Electroconvulsive shock, 105
Energy metabolism in brain, 1–46
Energy transfer
  drugs affecting, 4–17
Enterogastric reflex, 152
Enzymes, 95–97
  proteolytic, 53
Ephedrine, 30
Epinephrine, 50, 51, 63, 67, 74, 77, 90, 91, 103
Esophagus, 134
[^{3}H]Esterone, 242
Estradiol, 240–267, 271–274, 291
  binding, 261
  retention, 265
Estrogen, 239–273
  antiestrogenic compounds, 268, 269
Ethanol, 32–33, 86
  affecting cation transport, 32
  affecting axons, 33

Ethanol (*cont.*)
  depressant action, 32
  diminished cerebral glycolysis, 32
Ethyl ether, 10
Etonitazene, 336
Etorphine, 336
  the most potent known analgesic, 336
Eye nerves, 141

Fainting, 138
Fluoracetate, 11–12
Fluoride, 49, 52
Freeze drying brain tissue, 246

GABA, see γ-Aminobutyric acid
Gastric motility, 152
  reflex inhibition of 152
Gastrointestinal tract, 134–136, 145
GH, *see* Growth hormone
Glioma cell line, 54, 91, 92, 97
Glucocorticoids, 292–305
  chemical structure of synthetic, 293
Glucogen, 223
Glucose, 4, 13
  phosphorylation, 27
Glutamate, 64, 77
  decarboxylation, 31
Glutamine, 11, 12, 16, 19
  analog, 13
  synthetase, 13
Glycine, 64, 77
Glycogen, 13
Glycolysis *in vivo*, 95
GMP, cyclic, 47, 52, 54, 56, 105
  in brain regions, 52, 87–88
Goldfish, 348
Gonadotropin, 286
GRF, *see* Growth hormone releasing factor
Growth hormone releasing factor, 196, 218, 221–223, 226
Guanylate cyclase, 52
Guinea pig, 63–73

Haloperidol, 16–17, 216
Harmaline, 30
Harmine, 30
Hexabendine, 73, 170
Hexestrol, 240, 245, 267
HHH, *see* Hormone, hypothalamic hypophysiotropic
Hibernation
  premature arousal from, 158

Hippocampus, 251
Histamine, 50, 51, 53, 61–64, 67, 75–78, 89–92, 95
Histochemical methods, 146
  autoradiography, 147
  immunofluorescence, 147
Hormones, 195–238
  see individual hormones
5-Hydroxytryptamine, 25
Hypophysiotropic hormone, 196–201
Hyperpolarization, 102, 149, 151
Hypothalamus, 250
  hormones, 195–238
Hydroxybutyrate, 15
6-Hydroxydopamine, 84, 85
3α-Hydroxy-5α-pregnan-20-one, 306, 310
17α-Hydroxy-4-pregnan-3-one, 310
20α-Hydroxy-pregnan-4-en-3-one, 310
3α-Hydroxysteroid, 278
11β-Hydroxysteroid dehydrogenase, 303
17β-Hydroxysteroid dehydrogenase, 278

Ibotenic acid, 75
ICI-*46,474*(*trans*), 268, 270
Imidazole, 53
Imidazoline, substituted, 168–169
Imidazopyrazine, 53
Imipramine, 28, 53, 74
Innervation of gastrointestinal tract
  diagram of, 153
Insulin, 223
Intestine, small, 135
Intestinointestinal reflex, 152
Iodoacetamide
  and opiate binding, 355
Iontophoresis, 304
Iproniazid, 30
Isobutylmethylxanthine, 73, 93
Isoprenone, 311
Isoproterenol, 73, 74, 84, 91, 92
  -adenosine combination, 76

Junction potential, 147–151

Ketobemidones
  correlations of anasgetic potency and opiate receptor affinity, 337
3α-Ketosteroid dehydrogenase, 276
Δ^4-3-Ketosteroid-5α-reductase, 276
Kinase, 55–56

Lactate production, 95
Lesch-Nyhan syndrome, 158
  adenine therapy, 158
Levallorphan, 337
Levorphanal, 334, 336
Lidocaine, 19–21
Lidoflazine, 170
Lithium, 75, 353
Lordosis
  behavior, 272
  response, 272
LSD, *see* Lysergic acid diethylamide
LRF, *see* Luteinizing hormone releasing factor
Lung
  and nerves, 136
Luteinizing hormone releasing factor (LRF), 196–198, 209–214
Lysergic acid diethylamide (LSD), 31, 74, 75

Medroxyprogesterone, 311
  acetate, 311
Membrane
  permeability, 9
  phenomenon, 98–103
Mepacrine, 168
Mer-*25,* 268, 270
6-Mercaptopurine, 54
Methadone, 337
Methionine sulfoximine, 12–14
α-Methyldopa, 32
α-Methylnorepinephrine, 61, 74
N-Methyltryptamine, 62
α-Methyl-p-tyrosine, 29
Methylxanthine, 53
Midbrain, 251
Microwave irradiation, 104
Mitochondrion
  calcium accumulation, 9
  and chlorpromazine, 26
  respiration inhibited by barbiturate, 7
    stimulated by ADP, 4
Monkey, 77, 78, 348
Monoamine oxidase
  and accumulation of norepinephrine, 31
  excitation, 30
  inhibitors, 24, 29–31
    administration of, 30
    reversible potent, 30
Morphine, 85, 330, 337, 345
  molecular models of structure, 330
Motor neuron, 102–103

Mouse, 76–77, 348
MRIH, 196
MSH release inhibiting factor, 196

Naloxone, 334–336
  binding, 334
  crystal applied to brain, 345
  tissue distribution, 339
Neonate, castrated, 266
Nerve
  adrenergic, 152
  cell disruption, 51
  components, diagram of, 155
  purinergic
    hyperpolarization, 151
    role, physiological, 152–158
    stimulation, 147
  reflex activity, 152
  stimulation, 161
    by ATP, 163–164
Nervous system and cyclic nucleotides, 47–107
Neuroblastoma
  cell line, 54, 93, 97
  in mouse, 93
Neuron
  and ATP, 132
  central, 98–102
  and cocaine blockage, 21
  excitation, 33
    and barbiturate, 5–7
  flux of potassium ions, 18
    of sodium ions, 18
  inactivation, 132
  intramural inhibitory substances released, 131
  membrane, 5
  model of purinergic, 132
  motor, 102–103
  peripheral, 101–102
  potassium ion flux, 18
  purinergic, 132, 134
    hypothesis, 132
    release, 132
    storage, 132
    synthesis, 132
  respiration, reduced, 26
  structures, 26
  uptake blocked by cocaine, 21
Neurosecretory cell, hypothalamic, 195
Neurotropic drugs
  and electron transfer, 4–17

Nitrous oxide, 10
  poisoning, 2
Norepinephrine, 25, 28, 30, 31, 50, 61–63, 73–78, 84, 85, 89, 91, 92, 95, 98–100, 102, 137, 345
  deamination, 28
  depletion, 28, 29
Norethynodrel, 245
Norethindrone, 311
19-Norprogesterone, 311
Nuclear binding, 252–260
  highest concentration of radioactivity in purified nuclear pellet, 252
Nucleoside, 161, 167
5′-Nucleotidase, 146
Nucleotide, cyclic, 47–129
  accumulation, 57–94
  behavioral effects, 106–107
  in brain, 103–105
  enzyme action, 48–57, 95–97
  and growth, 97–98
  intercellular, 80–83
  membrane phenomena, 98–103
  and morphology, cellular, 97–98
  role of, 94–107
Nucleus, intercollicularis
  androgen action and vocal behavior, 286
  in songbirds, 285
  vocal behavior in birds, 285

Opiate receptor
  and anasgetic potency, 337
  binding, 335, 339–345
    sodium effect on, 352–355
  in brain of monkey, 341–343
  distribution
    heterogeneity of, 345
    phylogenetic, 348–351
      absent in brain of invertebrates, 351
      present in fish, 351
    regional, 340–345
  formation, 355
    agonists favored, 355
    antagonists favored, 355
  glass filters binding stereospecifically, 336
  identification, biochemical, 334–338
  localization
  subcellular, 340–341
  at synaptic membrane, 338–340
  mechanism, 329–360
  in species, 348, 350

Opiate receptor (*cont.*)
  stereospecificity, 330
  structure, chemical, 330–331
Ouabain, 18, 21, 22, 62, 68–71, 76, 90
  and ATPase, 170
Ovulation, 272
  stimulated, 272
Oxotremorine, 105
Oxytocin, 195

Pain relief, 345
Papaverine, 53, 73, 93, 99, 101, 104, 170
Pargyline, 75, 86
Pentose phosphate pathway
  in brain, 15
Pentothal, 5, 8
Periaqueductal gray
  critical in pain relief, 345
Perphenazine, 216
Phenobarbitone, 3, 4, 6, 8
  in mice, 5, 10
Phenothiazine, 26, 49, 53, 71, 74
Phentolamine, 54, 133, 163, 168
β-Phenylethylamine, 62
Phenylpiperidine, 330
Phosphocreatine, 4
Phosphodiesterase, 52–55, 72, 93, 142
  inhibitor, 53, 93
Phosphatase, 56
Phosphorylation, 8, 10, 55
PIF, *see* Prolactin release inhibitory factor
Pituitary secretion, 199
Poisoning
  carbon monoxide, 2
  cyanide, 2
  nitrous oxide, 2
Polypeptide hormones, 64
Potassium ion, 68–71, 76–78, 90, 95, 353
Pregnanedione, 306, 310
Prenylamine, 71
Primate, 77–79
Procaine, 19–21
Progesterone
  action, specific, 309–311
  distribution in brain, 307
  localization, 307
  mating behavior, 308–309
  retention, 305
    saturability of, 307
  specificity, 309–311
  structure, chemical, 310
Progestin, 305–311
Prolactin, 223
  secretion, 215
Prolactin release inhibiting factor (PIF), 196, 215–218
  bioassay, 215
Prostaglandin, 64, 75, 78, 93, 94
Protein factor
  in brain homogenate, 53
Protein kinase, 55–56
Proteolytic enzymes, 53
Protoveratrine, 9, 12, 18, 23–24
Protriptyline, 74
Psilocybin, 75
Pulsation, electrical, 70
Purine, 161
Purinergic
  hypothesis, 163
  nerves
    development, 171–175
    distribution, 133–143
    evolution, 171–175
    fine structure, 143–147
    localization, 146–147
    response in single cell, 151–152
    role, physiological, 152–158
    structure, fine, 143–147
    transmitter, 147, 158–164
  transmission, 131–194
Purkinje cell, 100
  hyperpolarization, 100
Puromycin, 54, 221
2-2′-Pyridylisatogen, 133, 163, 169

Quinidine, 133, 163, 168
Quinine, 168

Rabbit, 61–63
Rat, 73–76, 93, 97, 339, 348
Reproduction
  organs, 140–141
Reserpine, 25–26, 53, 85, 105
Respiration, mitochondrial, 10
Rhesus monkey, 77
RO *20-1724*, 53
Rubidium, 353

Saxitonin, 19
Scintillation counting of dissected brain areas, 241
Scintillometry, liquid, 133

Self-mutilation
  as a disorder of purine metabolism, 158
Serine, 55
Serotonin, 31, 62, 64, 74, 75, 78, 90, 95
Sexual behavior in rat, 308
Sexual differentiation, 291
Slime hag, 348
Sodium ion, 20–23, 353–354
  conductance, 19–21
Somatotropin release inhibiting factor (SRIF), 196
Somatostatin, 196, 223
Somatostatin–somatotropin release inhibiting factor, 218–227
Spiny dogfish, 348
Spore receptor concept, 204
Squirrel monkey, 78
Stereoselectivity, evidence for, 244–245
Steroids facilitating lordosis, 310
5α-Steroid reductase, 278, 279
Stimulation, electrical, 95, 99
Stimulus-secretion coupling, 200
Stomach, 134
Stress response, 215
Synaptosome, 339

Tachyphylaxis, 163
Testosterone, 245, 273–278, 285–289, 291
  localization, cellular, 273
  metabolism in brain, 278–280
Tetrodotoxin, 12, 17–19, 133, 136
Thaw-mount method for brain tissue, 246
Theophylline, 53, 62, 63, 65, 69, 72, 75, 78, 88–91, 94, 102–104
Thiobarbiturate, 10
Thiopental, 5
Thyroid hormone, 201, 225
Thyrotropin, 223
Thyrotropin releasing factor (TRF), 196–199, 201–209
Tolazoline, 163, 168
Tolbutamide, 53
Trachea, 136–137
Transfer, electron
  affecting neurotropic drugs, 4–17
Translocation artifacts, 246
Transmitter, postsynaptic, 151
Transport, cerebral, 1–46
TRF, *see* Thyrotropin releasing factor
Triamcinolone, 302
Tribromethanol, 10
Tryptamine, 31
TSH releasing factor, 196, 197, 201, 205
d-Tubocurarine, 103
Tyramine, 75
Tyrosine hydroxylase, 273, 346
  regional differences, 346

U-11, 100A, 268
Urinogenital system, 140–161

Varicosity, terminal
  in autonomic nerves, 144
Vascular system, 137–139
Vasoconstriction, 137
Vasodilatation, 137–139
Ventricles, 344
Veratridine, 62, 68–71, 76–78
Vesicles, 133
Viadril, 10

Yohimbine, 168